Insurance Handbook
for the Medical Office

STUDENT WORKBOOK

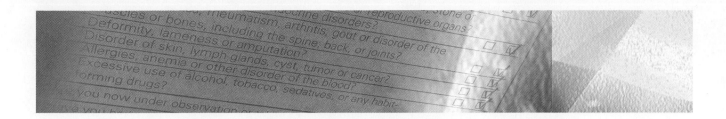

Insurance Handbook
for the Medical Office

STUDENT WORKBOOK

NINTH EDITION

Marilyn Takahashi Fordney, CMA-AC, CMT
Formerly Instructor of Medical Insurance, Medical Terminology,
Medical Machine Transcription, and Medical Office Procedures
Ventura College
Ventura, California

TECHNICAL COLLABORATOR AND CONTRIBUTING AUTHOR:

Brenda K. Burton, CCP
Director, MEDEXTEND
Fayetteville, Georgia

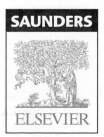

SAUNDERS

ELSEVIER

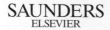

SAUNDERS
ELSEVIER

11830 Westline Industrial Drive
St. Louis, Missouri 63146

Notice

Neither the Publisher nor the Author assumes any responsibility for any loss or injury and/or damage to persons or property arising out of or related to any use of the material contained in this book. It is the responsibility of the treating practitioner, relying on independent expertise and knowledge of the patient, to determine the best treatment and method of application for the patient.

The Publisher

Acquisitions Editor: Susan Cole
Associate Developmental Editor: Colin Odell
Publishing Services Manager: Patricia Tannian
Senior Project Manager: Anne Altepeter
Design Coordinator: Teresa McBryan

Printed in the United States of America

Last digit is the print number: 9 8 7 6 5 4 3 2 1

Working together to grow
libraries in developing countries

www.elsevier.com | www.bookaid.org | www.sabre.org

ELSEVIER   BOOK AID International   Sabre Foundation

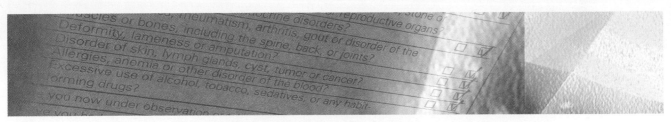

Acknowledgments

This edition of the *Workbook for Insurance Handbook for the Medical Office* has had considerable input from many medical professionals. Expert consultation has been necessary because of the complexities of the managed care environment, intricacies of procedural and diagnostic coding, impact of technology on insurance claims processing, and the more sophisticated role the insurance billing specialist has in today's work force.

I owe an immense debt of gratitude to Brenda K. Burton, CCP, director of MEDEXTEND, Fayetteville, Georgia; and David Smith, vice president of sales and marketing, and Lathe Bigler, vice president of marketing, of AltaPoint Data Systems, LLC. These individuals helped in inputting data into the AltaPoint practice management software for the *Workbook* software assignments.

Also a debt of gratitude is extended to Linda French, CMA-C, NCICS, CPC, and Karen Hawkins, RN, who acted as technical collaborators and helped me update the clinical and coding information of the patient records in the *Workbook* exercises and tests for the previous edition.

Thank you to my assistants, Barbara Evans and Gemma Hiranuma, who enthusiastically and competently did the typing, filing, mailing, and many other tasks necessary to meet the target dates.

Most importantly, I express overwhelming gratitude to the professional consultants who provided vital information to make this *Workbook* better than previous editions, and they are:

Deborah Emmons, CMA
President
S.T.A.T. Transcription Service
Port Hueneme, California

Sandy Gutt
Instructor
Southern California Regional Occupational Center
Torrance, California

Ronna Jurow, MD
Active Staff and Attending Physician in Obstetrics, Gynecology, and Infertility
Community Memorial Hospital
Ventura, California

Karen Levein
Instructor
Monrovia Adult School
Monrovia, California

Lucille M. Loignon, MD, FACS
Diplomate, American Board of Ophthalmology
Oxnard, California

Maria Reyes
Ventura Anesthesia Medical Group
Ventura, California

Walter A. Shaff
President
CPR
Lake Oswego, Oregon

Lita Starr
Office Manager
Oxnard, California

Paul Wertlake, MD
Medical Director and Chief Pathologist
Unilab Corporation
Tarzana, California

Shirley Wertlake, CLS
Technical Specialist
Clinical Laboratories
University of California—Los Angeles Medical Center
Los Angeles, California

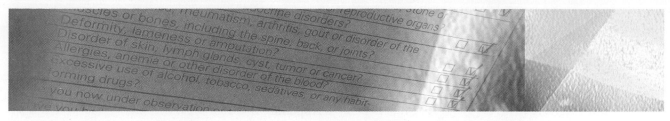

Contents

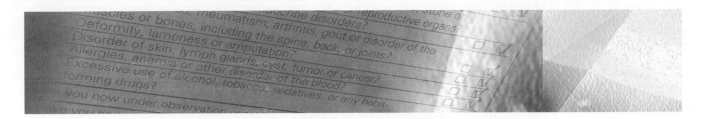

Instruction Guide to the Workbook

LEARNING OBJECTIVES

The student will be able to:

- Define and spell key terms for each chapter.
- Answer self-study review questions for each chapter of the *Handbook*.
- Complete assignments to enhance and develop better critical thinking skills.
- Define abbreviations as they appear on a patient record.
- Abstract subjective and objective data from patient records.
- Review documentation on patient records.
- Prepare legally correct medicolegal forms and letters.
- Code professional services properly, using the *Current Procedural Terminology* (CPT) Code Book or Appendixes A and B.
- Select diagnostic code numbers, using the *International Classification of Diseases, Ninth Revision, Clinical Modification* (ICD-9-CM).
- Locate errors on insurance claims before submission to insurance companies.
- Locate errors on returned insurance claims.
- Complete an insurance claim tracer form.
- Carry out collection procedures on delinquent accounts.
- Execute financial management procedures for tracing managed care plans.
- Abstract information necessary to complete insurance claim forms from patient records and billing statement/ledger cards.
- Complete and electronically transmit insurance claim forms commonly used in medical offices.
- Post payments, adjustments, and balances to patients' statement/ledger cards when submitting insurance claims.
- Compute mathematical calculations for Medicare and TRICARE cases.
- Analyze insurance claims in both hospital inpatient and outpatient settings.
- Prepare a cover letter, resume, job application, and follow-up letter when searching for employment.
- Access the Internet and visit Web sites to research and/or obtain data.

Instructions to the Student

The ninth edition of *Workbook for Insurance Handbook for the Medical Office* has been prepared for those who use the textbook, *Insurance Handbook for the Medical Office* (hereafter referred to as the *Handbook*). It is designed to assist the learner in a practical approach to doing insurance billing and coding. It will also develop a better understanding of the differences among the insurance programs when completing and electronically transmitting the CMS-1500 health insurance claim form.

The key terms are repeated for quick reference when studying. Each chapter's outline will serve as a lecture guide to use for note taking. Self-study review questions in the form of short answer, true/false, multiple choice, and matching are presented to reinforce learning of key concepts for each topic. Answers are found in Appendix D.

Some assignments give students hands-on experience in typing claim forms for optical character recognition (OCR) scanning equipment, which is used in many states for insurance claims processing and payment. Insurance claim forms and other sample documents that are easily removable are included for typing practice.

Current procedural and diagnostic code exercises are used throughout to facilitate and enhance coding skills for submitting a claim or making up an itemized billing statement.

Icons appearing throughout the *Workbook* are used to indicate assignment types. An illustration of each icon, along with its description, is outlined below.

Self-study assignments encompass important points from each chapter and allow you to study at your own pace.

Critical thinking assignments require skills that help prepare you for real-world scenarios encountered in insurance billing.

The **Practice Management and Billing Software CD-ROM** found at the back of the *Handbook* is required for completing selected assignments in Chapters 8 through 14.

Internet assignments point you to the World Wide Web for resources.

Key Terms

Key terms are presented for each chapter, and definitions may be located in the glossary at the end of the *Handbook*. It is suggested that you make up 3- by 5-inch index cards for each term and write in the definitions as you encounter them while reading each chapter in the *Handbook*. This will reinforce your knowledge and help you learn the words. Your instructor may wish to select certain words to study for "pop" quizzes.

Note Taking

Taking notes is an important key to success in studying and learning. Note taking helps an individual pay attention during class and retain information. Each chapter has a study outline for organizational purposes, and the outline may be used as a guide for writing down key points during lectures or when studying or reviewing from the *Handbook* for tests. Use file cards, note pads, or a notebook for taking notes. Underline or highlight important words or phrases. To improve the usefulness of notes, try the following format:

1. On a notepad sheet or file card, draw a margin 3 inches from the left.
2. Use the left side for topic headings and the right side for notes.
3. Skip a few lines when the topic changes.
4. Write numbers or letters to indicate sub-ideas under a heading.
5. Be brief; do not write down every word except when emphasizing a quotation, rule, or law. Write notes in your own words, since that is what you will understand.
6. Use abbreviations that you know how to translate.
7. Listen carefully to the lecture.
8. After the lecture, reread your notes. Highlight the word(s) on the left side of the page to identify the topic of the notes on the right.
9. For study purposes, cover the right side and see if you can explain to yourself or someone else the topic or word.
10. Remember—learning is by doing, and doing is up to you. So take notes for better understanding.

Self-Study Assignments

Review questions have been designed to encompass important points for each chapter to assist you in studying insurance billing and coding theory. Answers are located in Appendix D. With this edition, the review questions are presented as self-study assignments so that students and instructors will have more time in class to cover other important issues related to billing and coding.

Simulation Assignments

Assume that you have been hired as an insurance billing specialist and that you are working in a clinic setting for an incorporated group of medical doctors, other allied health specialists, and a podiatrist. You will be asked to complete various assignments. These doctors will be on the staff of a nearby hospital. Appendix A details this clinic's policies and procedures, which you must read completely before beginning the competency-based assignments. Within each chapter, the simulation assignments progress from easy to more complex. Some assignments are given with critical thinking problems, which the instructor may use for class discussion.

Always read the assignment entirely before beginning it. There are *Workbook* assignments. Table I-1 is a reference guide that lists chapter numbers and titles, along with the corresponding assignment numbers.

Medical Terminology and Abbreviations

A list of abbreviations is provided in Appendix A to help you learn how to abstract and read physicians' notes. Decode any abbreviations that you do not understand or that are unfamiliar to you. To reinforce learning these abbreviations, write their meanings on the assignment pages. If you do not have a background in medical terminology, it may be wise to use a good medical dictionary as a reference or, better yet, enroll in a terminology course to master that skill.

Patient Records

Patient records, financial accounting records (ledgers), and encounter forms are presented as they might appear in a physician's office, so the learner may have the tools needed to extract information to complete claim forms. Patient records have been abbreviated because of space and page constraints. The records contain pertinent data for each type of case, but it was necessary to omit a lengthy physical examination. Because detailed documentation is encouraged in medical practices, the records all appear typewritten rather than in handwritten notes. The physician's signature will appear after each dated entry on the record.

All the materials included in the assignments have been altered to prevent identification of the cases or parties involved. The names and addresses are fictitious, and no reference to any person living or dead is intended. No evaluation of medical practice or medical advice is to be inferred from the patient records, nor is any recommendation made toward alternative treatment methods or prescribed medications.

Financial Records

Financial accounting record (ledger) assignments will provide you with experience in posting, totaling the fees, and properly recording appropriate information on the ledger when the insurance claim is submitted. Financial accounting record statement/ledger cards are

TABLE I-1		
***Workbook* Assignments**		
Handbook **Chapter**	**Corresponding *Workbook* Chapter**	**Assignments**
1	Role of an Insurance Billing Specialist	1–1 through 1–4
2	Compliance and the E-Health Initiative	2–1 through 2–5
3	Basics of Health Insurance	3–1 through 3–7
4	Medical Documentation	4–1 through 4–7
5	Diagnostic Coding	5–1 through 5–13
6	Procedural Coding	6–1 through 6–10
7	The Health Insurance Claim Form	7–1 through 7–6
8	Electronic Data Interchange (EDI)	8–1 through 8–9
9	Receiving Payments and Insurance Problem Solving	9–1 through 9–9
10	Office and Insurance Collection Strategies	10–1 through 10–7
11	The Blue Plans, Private Insurance, and Managed Care Plans	11–1 through 11–6
12	Medicare	12–1 through 12–10
13	Medicaid and Other State Programs	13–1 through 13–5
14	TRICARE and CHAMPVA	14–1 through 14–6
15	Workers' Compensation	15–1 through 15–6
16	Disability Income Insurance and Disability Benefit Program	16–1 through 16–6
17	Hospital Billing	17–1 through 17–9
18	Seeking a Job and Attaining Professional Advancement	18–1 through 18–8

also included for typing practice. Refer to Appendix A to obtain information about the Mock Fee Schedule and the physicians' fees for posting to the statements.

CMS-1500 Claim Form

If you have access to a computer, use the practice management software that accompanies the *Handbook* to complete each assignment and print it out for evaluation. To complete the CMS-1500 claim form properly for each type of program, refer to the section in Chapter 7 of the *Handbook* that describes in detail the correct information to be put in each block. Also view the templates found at the end of Chapter 7 for each insurance type.

Complete all insurance forms in OCR style, since this is the format in which insurance carriers process claims most expediently. Chapter 7 gives instructions on OCR do's and don'ts. If you do not have access to a computer, type or neatly write in the information on the insurance form as you abstract it from the patient record.

Performance Evaluation Checklist

This ninth edition features a competency-based format for each assignment indicating performance objectives to let you know what is to be accomplished. The task (job assignment), conditions (elements needed to perform and complete the task), and standards (time management), as well as directions for the specific task, are included. Use of a checklist with points projected and points earned assists in scoring the assignments and helps you develop the skill of speed in completing tasks.

A two-part performance evaluation checklist used when completing a CMS-1500 claim form is depicted in Figures I-1 and I-2. Reproduce these sheets only for

the assignments that involve completing the CMS-1500 claim form. Your instructor will give you the number of points to be assigned for each step.

Appendices

Refer to Table I-2, which shows what is included in each of the appendices.

Student Reference Notebook

A *student reference notebook* is recommended so that you can access information quickly to help you complete the *Workbook* assignments. Before beginning the assignments, tear out Appendix A and place it in a three-ring binder with chapter indexes. Appendix A includes the clinic policies and guidelines, data about the clinic staff, medical and laboratory abbreviations, and mock fee schedule used while working as an insurance billing specialist for the College Clinic.

Besides these suggestions, you may wish either to tear out or make photocopies of other sections of the *Handbook* for your personal use. In addition, your instructor may give you handouts from time to time, pertaining to regional insurance program policies and procedures, to place in your notebook.

Content Suggestions from *Workbook*

✓ Appendix A: College Clinic policies, data about staff physicians, medical and laboratory abbreviations, and mock fee schedule
✓ Appendix B: HCPCS codes
✓ CMS-1500 claim form (photocopy if extra copies are needed for making rough drafts or retyping an assignment)

TABLE I-2	
Appendix	**Contents**
A	College Clinic Staff (Provider) Information
	College Clinic and Contract Facilities Information
	Medical Abbreviations and Symbols
	Laboratory Abbreviations
	College Clinic Mock Fee Schedule
B	Medicare Level II Healthcare Common Procedure Code System (HCPCS) Codes
C	Medi-Cal Abbreviations
	Medi-Cal Self-Study Review Questions
D	Answers to Self-Study Review Questions for Chapters

PERFORMANCE EVALUATION CHECKLIST

Assignment No. _____

Name:_____ Date:_____

Performance Objective

Task: Given access to all necessary equipment and information, the student will complete a CMS-1500 health insurance claim form.

Standards: Claim Productivity Management
Time _____ minutes
Note: Time element may be given by instructor.

Directions: See assignment.

NOTE TIME BEGAN_____ **NOTE TIME COMPLETED**_____

PROCEDURE STEPS	ASSIGNED POINTS	STEP PERFORMED SATISFACTORY	COMMENTS
1. Assembled CMS-1500 claim form, patient record, E/M code slip, ledger card, typewriter or computer, pen or pencil, and code books.	_____	_____	_____
2. Posed ledger card correctly.	_____	_____	_____
3. Proofread form for spelling and typographical errors while form remained in typewriter or on computer screen.	_____	_____	_____
4. Points earned for correct completion of CMS-1500 block-by-block data.	_____	_____	_____

Figure I–1

Content Suggestions from *Handbook*

✓ Evaluation and Management CPT codes: Tables 6–1 and 6–2

✓ Insurance form templates from Chapter 7: Figures 7–6 through 7–15

✓ Medical terminology (lay and medical terms): Table 4–1

✓ Terminology used in coding procedures: Table 4–2 CMS-1500 block-by-block claim form instructions from Chapter 7

✓ Glossary

PERFORMANCE EVALUATION CHECKLIST

BLOCK	INCORRECT	MISSING	NOT NEEDED	REMARKS	BLOCK	INCORRECT	MISSING	NOT NEEDED	REMARKS
					18				
1A					19				
2					20				
3					21				
4									
5					22				
6					23				
7					24A				
8					24B				
					24C				
9					24D				
9A									
9B									
9C					24E				
9D									
					24F				
10A					24G				
10B					24H, 24I				
10C					24J				
10D					24K				
11					25, 26				
11A					27				
11B					28				
11C					29				
11D									
12					30				
13									
14					31				
15									
16					32				
17									
17A					33				
					Reference Initials				

TOTAL POINTS EARNED: _____   TOTAL POINTS POSSIBLE: _____

Evaluator's signature _____   NEED TO REPEAT: _____

Figure I–2

Tests

Tests are provided at the end of the *Workbook* to provide a complete, competency-based educational program.

Reference Material

To do the assignments in this *Workbook* and gain expertise in coding and insurance claims completion, an individual must have access to the books listed here. Addresses for obtaining these materials are given in parentheses. Additional books and booklets on these topics, as well as Medicaid, Medicare, TRICARE, and more, are listed in the Resources at the end of each chapter of the *Handbook*.

Dictionary

Dorland's Illustrated Medical Dictionary, 29th edition, Elsevier Science, WB Saunders Company, 2000 (6277 Sea Harbor Drive, Orlando, FL 32821-9989; 1-800-545-2522).

Code Books

Current Procedural Terminology, American Medical Association, published annually (515 North State Street, Chicago, IL 60610; 1-800-621-8335).

International Classification of Diseases, Ninth Revision, Clinical Modification (An inexpensive soft-cover generic physician version of Volumes 1 through 3 is available from Channel Publishing Limited, 4750 Longley Lane, Suite 100, Reno, NV 89502; 1-800-248-2882.)

Word Book

Medical Abbreviations and Eponyms by Sheila Sloane, Elsevier Science, WB Saunders Company, 1997 (6277 Sea Harbor Drive, Orlando, FL 32821-9989; 1-800-545-2522).

Pharmaceutical Book

Optional publications for drug names and descriptions might be either drug books used by nurses (e.g., Mosby's Gen RX, Elsevier, published annually [11830 Westline Industrial Drive, St. Louis, MO 63146; 1-800-325-4177; *www.elsevier.com*]) or ones used by physicians (e.g., *Physician's Disk Reference [PDR]*, Medical Economics Company, published annually [5 Paragon Drive, Montvale, NJ, 07645; 1-800-432-4570]).

Employee Insurance Procedural Manual

If you currently work in a medical office, you may custom design an insurance manual for your physician's practice as you complete insurance claims in this *Workbook*. Obtain a three-ring binder with indexes and label them "Group Plans," "Private Plans," "Medicaid," "Medicare," "Managed Care Plans," "State Disability," "TRICARE," and "Workers' Compensation." If many of your patients have group plans, complete an insurance data or fact sheet (Figure I-3) for each plan and organize them alphabetically by group plan. For managed care plans, type a form as shown in Figure 11-5 of the *Handbook*.

An insurance manual with fact sheets listing benefits can keep you up-to-date on policy changes and ensure maximum reimbursement. Fact sheets can be prepared from information obtained when patients bring in their benefit booklets. Obtain and insert a list of the procedures that must be performed as an outpatient and those that must have second opinions for each of the insurance plans.

As you complete the assignments in this *Workbook*, place them in the insurance manual as examples of completed claims for each particular program.

PRACTICE MANAGEMENT AND BILLING SOFTWARE

Because more and more medical practices use computer technology to perform financial operations, Elsevier has teamed up with the software company AltaPoint to provide students with a real-life practice management and billing software experience. The CD that accompanies the *Handbook* contains the program off which exercises in this *Workbook* are based. By following the instructions starting on page 175 of the *Workbook*, you can install the practice management software on your computer to complete the corresponding exercises.

INSURANCE DATA

1. Employer's name _____

2. Address _____ Telephone Number _____

3. Insurance Company Contact Person _____

4. Insurance Carrier _____

5. Address _____ Telephone Number to Call for Benefits _____

6. Group Policy Number _____

7. Group Account Manager _____ Telephone Number _____

8. **Insurance Coverage:**

   Annual Deductible _____ Patient Copayment Percentage _____

   Noncovered Procedures _____

   Maximum Benefits _____

9. **Diagnostic Coverage:**

   Limited Benefits _____

   Maximum Benefits _____

   Noncovered Procedures _____

10. **Major Medical:**

    Annual Deductible _____ Patient Copayment Percentage _____

    Limited Benefits _____

    Maximum Benefits _____

    Noncovered Procedures _____

Mandatory Outpatient Surgeries _____

Second Surgical Opinions _____

Preadmission Certification   Yes _____ No _____   Authorized Labs _____

Payment Plan:

UCR _____ Schedule of Benefits _____ CPT _____ RVS _____

Send claims to: _____

_____

Date Entered _____ Date Updated _____

Figure I–3

SPECIAL FEATURES

AltaPoint Practice Management Software

AltaPoint Data Systems, LLC, is a private software company that has developed practice management systems for professionals in fields such as medical, dental, legal, optometric/ophthalmologic, chiropractic, and veterinary. Through a special partnership, Elsevier has customized AltaPoint's innovative practice management system into the CD-ROM that accompanies the *Handbook*. More information regarding AltaPoint can be found at *www.altapoint.com*

Source Documents

Authentic source documents such as encounter forms (p. 284), explanation of benefits, insurance checks, patient records, and more are provided to give students the opportunity to enter pertinent information into the software as they would in an actual practice environment.

Practice Management Functions

In addition to source document–based exercises, assignments also offer the student practice in everyday functions such as View an Insurance Aging Report, Print a Remaining Authorization Report, and Electronically Print a Collection letter (p. 265).

Fee Schedule/Billing Codes

Based on the College Clinic fee schedule printed in the back of this and past *Workbooks*, fees automatically appear when the CPT and diagnostic codes are entered. Additionally, students can choose a Place of Service depending on the exercise.

Claims Transmission

Using the software and specialized assignments in the *Workbook*, students can transmit an insurance claim electronically or on hard copy to individual insurance companies.

Patient Database

To provide an authentic practice management setting, Elsevier has customized the practice management software program to include a database of patients including names, telephone numbers, birthdates, addresses, photographs, and outstanding balances.

Detailed Instructions

Beginning with the first software assignment and throughout, detailed instructions are provided to explain simple procedures or more complex functions of the software. For each set of instructions, screen shots are provided. Examples of the screen shots are depicted here.

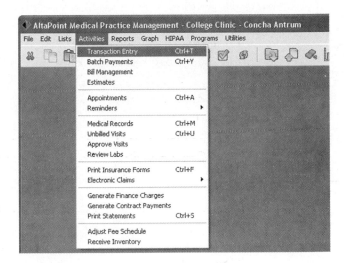

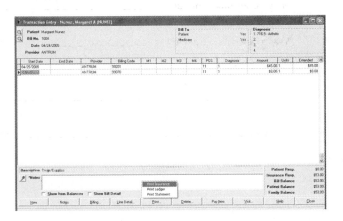

Software installation instructions begin on p. 175 of the *Workbook*.

keyboarding knowledge of insurance carriers + medicare policies

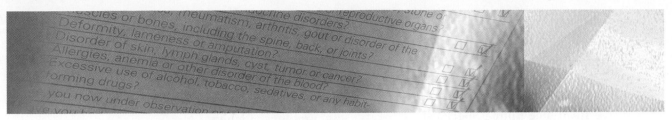

Role of an Insurance Billing Specialist

KEY TERMS

Your instructor may wish to select some specific words pertinent to this chapter for a test. For definitions of the terms, further study, and/or reference, the words, phrases, and abbreviations may be found in the glossary at the end of the Handbook. *Key terms for this chapter follow.*

American Health Information Management
  Association (AHIMA)

American Medical Association (AMA)

cash flow

claims assistant professional (CAP)

ethics

etiquette

insurance billing specialist

list service (listserv)

multiskilled health practitioner (MSHP)

reimbursement specialist

respondeat superior

PERFORMANCE OBJECTIVES

The student will be able to:

■ Define and spell the key terms for this chapter, given the information from the *Handbook* glossary, within a reasonable time period and with enough accuracy to obtain a satisfactory evaluation.

■ Answer the self-study review questions, after reading the chapter, with enough accuracy to obtain a satisfactory evaluation.

■ Use critical thinking to write one or two grammatically correct paragraphs with sufficient information to obtain a satisfactory evaluation.

STUDY OUTLINE

Background of Insurance Claims, Coding, and Billing
Role of the Insurance Billing Specialist
    Job Responsibilities
    Educational and Training Requirements
    Career Advantages
    Qualifications
Medical Etiquette

Medical Ethics
Confidentiality
Employer Liability
Employee Liability
Scope of Practice
Future Challenges

SELF-STUDY **1-1** ▸ **REVIEW QUESTIONS**

Review the objectives, key terms, and chapter information before completing the following review questions.

1. Read the job descriptions in Chapter 1 in the *Handbook*. Abilities to read handwritten and transcribed documents in the medical record, interpret information, and enter accurate code data into the computer system are technical skills required in the job of a/an ___hospital coder & specialist for an acute/or ambulatory care setting, Health Info./medical Record technician___

2. Name some of the facilities where hospital billing is used.
    a. ___acute care hospital___
    b. ___skilled nursing facility___
    c. ___long-term care facility___
    d. ___rehab or ambulatory surgical center___

3. Name examples of nonphysician practitioners (NPPs).
    a. ___Nurse practitioner___
    b. ___physical therapist___
    c. ___speech therapist___
    d. ___licensed clinical social worker___
    e. ___Certified (RN) practioner___

4. Identify three career opportunities (job titles) available after training in diagnostic and procedural coding and insurance claims completion.
    a. ___medical biller, electronic claims professional___
    b. ___claims assistance professional___
    c. ___insurance billing specialist___

5. List some of the responsibilities and duties an insurance billing specialist might perform generally as well as when acting as a collection manager.

Review diagnostic & procedural codes for correction & completness

b. Submit insurance claims promptly

c. collect data from hospitals, labs, + other physicians.

d. Discuss practices financial policies + insurance coverage + payment dates.

e. Answer inquiries related to account balances + insur. submissions

f. Assist patients in budgeting

g. Check up on delinquent accounts by tracing denied, adjusted, or unpaid claims.

6. List the duties of a claims assistance professional.

a. Help patents organize, file, + negotiate health insurance claims / aging

b. Assist consumer in obtaining max benefits from insur. companies.

c. tell patent what checks to write to providers in order to eliminate over paying.

7. Insurance claims must be promptly submitted within __1-5__ business days to ensure continuous cash flow.

8. Define cash flow.

Amount of actual money available to the medical practice

9. Reasons for a medical practice's large accounts receivable are:

a. failure to verify insur. plan benefits

b. failure to obtain authorization or precertification

c. failure to collect co-pays or deductibles

d. inadequat claims filing

10. Skills required for an insurance billing specialist are

a. Knowledge of compliance issues

b. precise reading shills

c. knowledge of medical terminology

d. knowledge of insurance terminology

e. proficiency in completing insur. claims

f. <u>computer skills, basic typing   or keyboarding</u>

g. <u>medicale   knowledge</u>

<u>knowledge of insurance carriers + medicare polices</u>

i. <u>basic math + use of calculators</u>

j. <u>billing + collection techniques</u>

11. Standards of conduct by which an insurance billing specialist determines the propriety

    of his or her behavior in a relationship are known as <u>medical ethics</u>.

12. Complete these statements with either the word *illegal* or *unethical*.

    a. To report incorrect information to the Aetna Casualty Company
       is <u>unethical</u>.

    b. To report incorrect information to a Medicare fiscal intermediary
       is <u>illegal</u>.

    c. It is <u>unethical</u> for two physicians to treat the same patient for
       the same condition.

13. When a physician is legally responsible for an employee's conduct performed during

    employment, this is known as <u>vicarious liability</u> <u>respondeat superior</u>

14. A claims assistance professional neglects to submit an insurance claim to a Medicare
    supplemental insurance carrier within the proper time limit. What type of insurance
    is needed for protection against this loss for the client?

    <u>Errors + Omissions insurance</u>

To check your answers to this self-study assignment, see Appendix D.

CRITICAL THINKING

To enhance your critical thinking skills, problems will be interspersed throughout the *Workbook*. Thinking is the goal of instruction and a student's responsibility. When trying to solve a problem by critical thinking, it is desirable to have more than one solution and to take time to think out answers. Remember that an answer may be changed when additional information is provided in a classroom setting.

A S S I G N M E N T **1 – 2** ▸ **CRITICAL THINKING**

Performance Objective

Task: Describe why you are training to become an insurance billing specialist.

Conditions: Use one or two sheets of white typing paper and pen or pencil.

Standards: Time:_____ minutes

                 Accuracy: _____

                 (Note: The time element and accuracy criteria may be given by your instructor.)

Directions: Write one or two paragraphs describing why you are training to become an insurance billing specialist. Or, if enrolled in a class that is part of a medical assisting course, explain why you are motivated to seek a career as a medical assistant. Make sure grammar, punctuation, and spelling are correct.

ASSIGNMENT **1–3** ▸ **VISIT WEB SITES**

Performance Objective

Task: Access the Internet and visit several Web sites of the World Wide Web.

Conditions: Use a computer with printer and/or pen or pencil to make notes.

Standards: Time: _____ minutes

                 Accuracy: _____

                 (Note: The time element and accuracy criteria may be given by your
                 instructor.)

Directions: If you have access to the Internet, visit the World Wide Web and do the
following three site searches.

1. Access an Internet server and find one of the Web search engines (Yahoo, Excite,
   Google, Alta Vista). Begin a Web search (e.g., key in "insurance billers") to search for
   information about insurance billers or go to Web site: http://www.careerpath.com.
   List three to five Web sites found. Go to one or more of those resources and list the
   benefits that those sites might have for a student in locating job opportunities or
   networking with others for professional growth and knowledge. Bring the Web site
   addresses to share with the class.

2. Site-search information on standards of ethical coding by visiting the Web site of
   the American Health Information Management Association (http://www.ahima.org).
   At the search site box insert "ethics" and click "Go." Review the topics on the list and
   click on "HIMSS Code of Ethics." Print a hard copy of this code developed by
   AHIMA.
   Next, obtain information on eHealth code of ethics by visiting the Web site of the
   Internet Healthcare Coalition organization at: http://www.ihealthcoalition.org. Click
   on "eHealth Code of Ethics," download the file, print a hard copy, read the document,
   and respond to the following:

   A. Write a brief definition for each of the following terms: health information, health
      products, and health services.
   B. State the eight guiding principles of organizations and individuals who provide
      health information over the Internet.

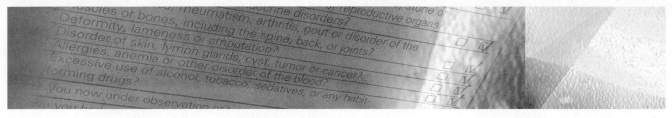

Compliance and the E-Health Initiative

KEY TERMS

Your instructor may wish to select some specific words pertinent to this chapter for a test. For definitions of the terms, further study, and/or reference, the words, phrases, and abbreviations may be found in the glossary at the end of the Handbook. *Key terms for this chapter follow.*

abuse

authorization form

breach of confidential communication

business associate

clearinghouse

code set

compliance

compliance plan

confidential communication

confidentiality

consent form

covered entity

disclosure

e-health information management (eHIM)

electronic media

embezzlement

fraud

health care provider

individually identifiable health information (IIHI)

nonprivileged information

phantom billing

privacy

privacy officer, privacy official

privileged information

protected health information (PHI)

standard

state preemption

transaction

use

PERFORMANCE OBJECTIVES

The student will be able to:

- Define and spell the key terms for this chapter, given the information from the *Handbook* glossary, within a reasonable time period and with enough accuracy to obtain a satisfactory evaluation.
- Answer the self-study review questions, after reading the chapter, with enough accuracy to obtain a satisfactory evaluation.

- Make decisions after reading scenarios whether the situations are considered fraud, abuse, or neither.
- Decide when a situation is an incidental disclosure, HIPAA violation, or neither.
- Make a choice after reading scenarios whether to ask for consent or authorization, or perform other office procedures.
- Visit Web sites and site-search information.

STUDY OUTLINE

Compliance Defined

Health Information Using Electronic Technologies
E-Health Information Management
National Health Information Infrastructure
Health Level Seven

Systemized Nomenclature of Human and Veterinary Medicine (SNOMED) International

Health Insurance Portability and Accountability Act (HIPAA)
Title I: Health Insurance Reform
Title II: Administrative Simplification
Defining Roles and Relationships: Key Terms
HIPAA in the Practice Setting

The Privacy Rule: Confidentiality and Protected Health Information
Confidential Information
Patients' Rights
Privacy Rules: Patient Rights Under HIPAA
Right to Notice of Privacy Practices
Right to Request Restrictions on Certain Uses and Disclosures of PHI
Right to Request Confidential Communications
Right to Access, Inspect, and Obtain PHI
Right to Request Amendment of PHI
Right to Receive an Accounting of Disclosures of PHI

Organization and Staff Responsibilities in Protecting Patient Rights
Verification of Identity and Authority
Validating Patient Permission
Training
Safeguards: Ensuring that Confidential Information is Secure
Complaints to Health Care Practice and Workforce Sanctions
Mitigation
Refraining from Intimidating or Retaliatory Acts

Transaction and Code Set Regulations: Streamlining Electronic Data Interchange
Standard Unique Identifiers

The Security Rule: Administrative, Physical, and Technical Safeguards

Application to Practice Setting
Guidelines for HIPAA Privacy Compliance

Consequences of Noncompliance with HIPAA

Office of the Inspector General
Fraud and Abuse Laws
Federal False Claims Act
Qui Tam "Whistleblower"
Civil Monetary Penalties Law
Criminal False Claims Act
Stark Laws
Anti-Kickback Statute
Safe Harbors
Additional Laws and Compliance
Operation Restore Trust
Medicare Integrity Program
Correct Coding Initiative
Increased Staffing and Expanded Penalties for Violations
Special Alerts, Bulletins, and Guidance Documents
Exclusion Program

Compliance Program Guidance for Individual and Small Group Physician Practices
Increased Productivity and Decreased Penalties with Plan

Seven Basic Components of a Compliance Plan
Conducting Internal Monitoring and Auditing
Implementing Compliance and Practice Standards
Designating a Compliance Officer or Contact
Conducting Appropriate Training and Education
Responding Appropriately to Detected Offenses and Developing Corrective Action
Developing Open Lines of Communication
Enforcing Disciplinary Standards Through Well-Publicized Guidelines

What to Expect From Your Health Care Practice

Compliance Lessons Learned

Internet Resources

SELF-STUDY 2-1 ▸ REVIEW QUESTIONS

Review the objectives, key terms, and chapter information before completing the following review questions.

1. Compliance is the process of meeting regulations, recommendations & expectations of federal/state agencies that pay for health care services & regulate the industry.

2. Transactions in which health care information is accessed, processed, stored, and transferred using electronic technologies is known as e-Health information management and its acronym is e HIM.

3. Baby Nelson was born on January 20, 2005, at 7:15 AM. When using the required Health Level 7 (HL7) format for transmission, how would this appear?

   200501200715

4. A code system used for managing patient electronic health records, informatics, indexing, and billing laboratory procedures is called Systematized Nomenclature of Human & Veterinary Medicine and its acronym is SNOMED.

5. What is the primary purpose of HIPAA Title I: Insurance Reform? Provide continuos insurance coverage for workers & their insured dependents when they change or lose jobs.

6. The focus on the health care practice setting and reduction of administrative costs and burdens are the goals of which part of HIPAA?
   Title II, Administrative Simplification

7. A third-party administrator that receives insurance claims from the physician's office, performs edits, and transmits claims to insurance carriers is known as
   a/an Clearinghouse

8. Under HIPAA guidelines, a health care coverage carrier, such as Blue Cross/Blue Shield that transmits health information in electronic form in connection with a transaction is called a/an Covered entity.

9. Dr. John Doe contracts with an outside billing company to manage claims and accounts receivable. Under HIPAA guidelines, the billing company is considered

a/an ___business associate___ of the provider.

10. An individual designated to assist the provider by putting compliance policies and procedures in place and training office staff is known as a/an _privacy officer or privacy official_ under HIPAA guidelines.

11. If you give, release, or transfer information to another entity, this is known as _disclosure_.

12. Define protected health information (PHI). _Data that identifies an individual & describes his/her health status, age, sex, ethnicity, or other demographic characteristics whether or not that information is stored or transmitted electronically._

13. Unauthorized release of a patient's health information is called _breach of confidential communication._

14. A confidential communication related to the patient's treatment and progress that may be disclosed only with the patient's permission is known as _privileged communication._

15. Exceptions to the right of privacy are those records involving

    a. _____

    b. _____

    c. _____

    d. _____

    e. _____

    f. _____

16. At a patient's first visit under HIPAA guidelines, the document that must be given so the patient acknowledges the provider's confidentiality of their protected health

information is the _____.

17. Under HIPAA Privacy Regulation, state the types of information that patients do not have the right to access.

    a. _____

    b. _____

    c. _____

18. Name the three main sections of the HIPAA Security Rule for protecting electronic health information.

    a. _____

    b. _____

    c. _____

19. Indicate whether the situation is one of *fraud* or *abuse* in the following situations.

    a. Billing a claim for services not medically necessary.   _____

    b. Changing a figure on an insurance claim form to get increased payment.   _____

    c. Dismissing the copayment owed by a Medicare patient.   _____

    d. Neglecting to refund an overpayment to the patient.   _____

    e. Billing for a complex fracture when the patient suffered a simple break. _____

ASSIGNMENT 2-2 ▶ **CRITICAL THINKING: INCIDENTAL DISCLOSURE VERSUS HIPAA VIOLATION**

Performance Objective

Task: Make a decision using your best judgment after reading each case study, whether it should be considered an incidental disclosure, an HIPAA violation, or neither.

Conditions: Use pen or pencil.

Standards: Time: _____ minutes

                Accuracy: _____

                Note: The time element and accuracy criteria may be given by your instructor.)

Directions: Read through each case study. Use your best judgment and circle whether you think it is an incidental disclosure issue (ID), an HIPAA violation (V), or neither (N).

Scenarios

1. Dr. Practon's office sign-in sheets ask patients to fill in their names, appointment times, and physicians' names.

   ID   V   N

2. It is Monday morning and you are inundated with work that needs to be done. You receive a telephone call and give patient information without confirming who is on the line.

   ID   V   N

3. You send a fax but accidentally you switch the last two digits of the fax number by mistake and the patient's billing information is received in the wrong location.

   ID   V   N

4. You are in a high-traffic area where patients might overhear protected health information and you are careful to keep your voice down.

   ID   V   N

5. It is 10:30 AM and you go on a coffee break leaving two patients' charts on the checkout counter.

   ID   V   N

6. In the reception room, a patient, Martha Havasi, overhears your telephone conversation even though you spoke quietly and shut the glass window.

   ID   V   N

7. You telephone a patient, Alex Massey, to remind him of tomorrow's appointment and leave a voice mail on his answering machine.

   ID   V   N

8. Three patients near the reception area of the office overhear you telling another staff member that Daisy Dotson is scheduled for a Pap smear tomorrow at 4:00 PM.

   ID   V   N

9. You telephone a patient, Janet Hudson. She is not home so you leave a message on her answering machine that her breast cancer biopsy results came back negative.

   ID   V   N

10. You call out Fran O'Donnell's name in the waiting room where other patients are sitting.

    ID   V   N

11. You do not close the glass window to the reception room when talking on the telephone with your sister.

    ID   V   N

12. The office nurse tells a patient, Hugo Wells, his test results in front of his relatives.

    ID   V   N

13. You leave Katy Zontag's medical chart open at the receptionist's counter.

    ID   V   N

14. You telephone a patient, Jose Ramirez, and leave your name, the physician's name, and telephone number on his answering machine.

    ID   V   N

15. A patient, Kim Lee, is in the examination room and overhears a conversation concerning blood test results of another patient in an adjoining room.

    ID   V   N

16. While waiting in the reception room, a patient, Xavier Gomez, overhears a receptionist talking with another patient about a colonoscopy appointment.

    ID   V   N

17. Betty Burton, a patient who is being weighed on the office scale by the medical assistant, overhears a conversation between an insurance billing specialist and an insurance company representative in which she is trying to obtain preauthorization for another patient's medical procedure.

    ID   V   N

18. In a restaurant, a waitress overhears an insurance biller talking to a friend and telling her about a famous actress that visited her physician's office yesterday.

    ID   V   N

ASSIGNMENT **2-3** ▶ **CRITICAL THINKING: FRAUD VERSUS ABUSE**

Performance Objective

Task: Make a decision after reading each case study, whether it is considered fraud, abuse, or neither.

Conditions: Use pen or pencil.

Standards: Time: _____ minutes

                        Accuracy: _____

                        (Note: the time element and accuracy criteria may be given by your instructor.)

Directions: Read through each scenario and circle whether it is a fraud (F) issue, practice of abuse (A), or neither (N).

Scenarios

1. Dr. Pedro Atrics has a friend and his child needs elective surgery. He agrees to perform the surgery and bill as an "insurance only" case.

   F   A   N

2. A patient, Carl Skinner, calls the office repeatedly about his prescriptions. When seen in the office the next time, Dr. Input bills a higher level of evaluation and management service to allow for the additional time.

   F   A   N

3. Dr. Skeleton sets a simple fracture and puts a cast on Mr. Davis. He bills for a complex fracture.

   F   A   N

4. A patient, Maria Gomez, asks a friendly staff member to change the dates on the insurance claim form. The medical assistant complies with the request.

   F   A   N

5. A patient, Roberto Loren, asks the physician to restate a diagnosis so the insurance company will pay because payment would be denied based on the present statement. The physician complies with the request.

   F   A   N

6. Dr. Rumsey sees a patient twice on the same day but bills as though the patient was seen on two different dates.

   F   A   N

7. A Medicare patient, Joan O'Connor, is seen by Dr. Practon, and the insurance claim shows a charge to the Medicare fiscal intermediary at a fee schedule rate higher than and different from that of non-Medicare patients.

   F   A   N

8. A patient, Hazel Plunkett, receives a service that is not medically necessary to the extent rendered and an insurance claim is submitted.

   F   A   N

9. A patient, Sun Cho, paid for services that were subsequently declared not medically necessary, and Dr. Cardi failed to refund the payment to the patient.

   F   A   N

10. Dr. Ulibarri tells the insurance biller not to collect the deductible and copayments from Mrs. Gerry Coleman.

    F   A   N

ASSIGNMENT 2–4 ▸ CRITICAL THINKING: CONSENT VERSUS AUTHORIZATION

Performance Objective

Task: Make a decision using your best judgment after reading each scenario, and determine whether you should ask for consent or authorization or do other procedures.

Conditions: Use pen or pencil.

Standards: Time: _____ minutes

                Accuracy: _____

                (Note: The time element and accuracy criteria may be given by your instructor. Class discussion may offer other possible ways of handling the given situations.)

Directions: Read through each case study and determine whether you should ask for consent or authorization, or perform other office procedures.

Scenarios

1. Dr. Practon's patient, Mary Ann Bailey, goes to the College Hospital's emergency department complaining of severe stomach cramps. Subsequently she is admitted to the hospital for pancreatitis. The floor nurse at the hospital telephones Dr. Practon's office asking for the patient's medical records to be brought over immediately. What should you do?

   Response _____

   _____

   _____

2. Robert Fellow, a patient, telephones the College Clinic and states that he has hired a lawyer and is filing a lawsuit against another driver for an automobile accident that happened about a month ago. The attorney for the other driver needs your patient's medical records to find out what injuries your patient suffered as a result of the accident. The attorney also wants to know if there are any preexisting injuries. Mr. Fellow requests that you send a copy of his medical records to the other attorney. What should you do?

   Response _____

   _____

   _____

3. Consuelo Lopez, the mother of a minor patient, Johnnie Lopez, telephones your office stating that Johnnie is having difficulty staying focused and loses his concentration during classroom activities at school. Mrs. Lopez has made an appointment for him to be seen by a psychologist and has requested that you

send his medical records to the psychologist before the date of the appointment.
What should you do?

Response _____

_____

_____

4. Eric Jacobs, a patient, receives psychiatric counseling as well as treatment for diabetes at the College Clinic. The patient requests a copy of his medical record. (A) Is it necessary to remove the documentation pertaining to the psychiatric counseling sessions before giving the patient a copy of his medical record? (B) Can you disclose to the patient his medical records?

Response (A) _____

_____

(B) _____

_____

ASSIGNMENT **2–5** ▸ **VISIT WEB SITES**

Performance Objective

Task: Access the Internet and visit several Web sites of the World Wide Web.

Conditions: Use a computer with printer and/or pen or pencil to make notes.

Standards: Time: _____ minutes

                 Accuracy: _____

                 (Note: The time element and accuracy criteria may be given by your
                 instructor.)

Directions: If you have access to the Internet, visit the World Wide Web and do the
following three site searches.

1. Site-search information on patient confidentiality by visiting the Web site of the
   American Medical Association (http://www.ama-assn.org/). Under "ethics, education,
   science, public health, quality, and accreditation," Click on "legal issues of physicians."
   Then click on "patient-physician relationship issues." Then click on "patient
   confidentiality." Make notes or print a hard copy of the pages while remaining online.

2. Site-search information on patient confidentiality by visiting the Web site of the
   American Health Information Management Association (http://www.ahima.org). Click
   on site search at that Web site. Key in "patient confidentiality." Then click on "search
   for matching documents." List a recent question asked about this topic and record the
   answer or print a hard copy of all the questions and answers while remaining online.

3. Site search for information on fraud and abuse by visiting one or more of the federal
   Web sites. See what you can discover and either print out or take notes and bring back
   information to share with the class for discussion. Try one or more of the following
   Web sites:
   http://www.cms.gov/medicare/fraud/defini2.htm
   http://www.cms.gov/medicaid/mbfrud.htm
   http://www.govmedicaid/medicaid.htm

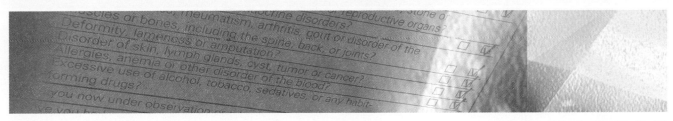

Basics of Health Insurance

KEY TERMS

Your instructor may wish to select some words pertinent to this chapter for a test. For definitions of the terms, further study, and/or reference, the words, phrases, and abbreviations may be found in the glossary at the end of the Handbook. *Key terms for this chapter follow.*

accounts receivable management

applicant

assignment

blanket contract

capitation

Civilian Health and Medical Program of the Department of Veterans Affairs (CHAMPVA)

claim

coinsurance

competitive medical plan (CMP)

conditionally renewable

contract

daysheet

deductible

disability income insurance

electronic signature

eligibility

emancipated minor

encounter form

exclusions

exclusive provider organization (EPO)

expressed contract

extended

financial accounting record

foundation for medical care (FMC)

guaranteed renewable

guarantor

health insurance

health maintenance organization (HMO)

high risk

implied contract

indemnity

independent or individual practice association (IPA)

insured

major medical

Maternal and Child Health Program (MCHP)

Medicaid (MCD)

Medicare (M)

Medicare/Medicaid (Medi-Medi)

member

noncancelable policy

nonparticipating provider (nonpar)

optionally renewable

participating provider (par)

patient registration form

personal insurance

point-of-service (POS) plan

posted

preauthorization

precertification

predetermination

preferred provider organization (PPO)

premium

running balance

State Disability Insurance (SDI)

subscriber

TRICARE

Unemployment Compensation Disability (UCD)

Veterans Affairs (VA) outpatient clinic

workers' compensation (WC) insurance

PERFORMANCE OBJECTIVES

The student will be able to:

■ Define and spell the key terms for this chapter, given the information from the textbook glossary, within a reasonable time period and with enough accuracy to obtain a satisfactory evaluation.

■ Answer the self-study review questions after reading the chapter with enough accuracy to obtain a satisfactory evaluation.

■ Arrange 12 administrative processing steps of an insurance claim in proper sequence, given data from the textbook, within a reasonable time period and with enough accuracy to obtain a satisfactory evaluation.

■ Use critical thinking to explain some of the differences in insurance key terms, given data from the textbook, within a reasonable time period and with enough accuracy to obtain a satisfactory evaluation.

■ Prepare a financial accounting record, given data from the textbook, within a reasonable time period and with enough accuracy to obtain a satisfactory evaluation.

■ Abstract data from some insurance identification cards, given data from the textbook, within a reasonable time period and with enough accuracy to obtain a satisfactory evaluation.

STUDY OUTLINE

History

Insurance in the United States

Legal Principles of Insurance
  Insurance Contracts

Physician–Patient Contracts and Financial Obligation
  Implied or Expressed Contracts

The Insurance Policy
  Policy Application
  Policy Renewal Provisions
  Policy Terms
  Coordination of Benefits
  General Policy Limitations

Choice of Health Insurance
  Group Contract
  Individual Contract
  Prepaid Health Plan

Types of Health Insurance Coverage
  CHAMPVA
  Competitive Medical Plan
  Disability Income Insurance

  Exclusive Provider Organization
  Foundation for Medical Care
  Health Maintenance Organization
  Independent or Individual Practice Association
  Maternal and Child Health Program
  Medicaid
  Medicare
  Medicare/Medicaid
  Point-of-Service Plan
  Preferred Provider Organization
  TRICARE
  Unemployment Compensation Disability
  Veterans Affairs Outpatient Clinic
  Workers' Compensation Insurance

Examples of Insurance Billing

Keeping Up to Date

Procedure: Handling and Processing Insurance Claims

Procedure: Prepare and Post to a Patient's Financial Accounting Record

SELF-STUDY 3-1 ▶ REVIEW QUESTIONS

Review the objectives, key terms, glossary definitions to key terms, chapter information, and figures before completing the following review questions.

1. A/an _____ is a legally enforceable agreement or contract.

2. An individual promising to pay for medical services rendered is known as a/an _____

_____.

3. List five health insurance policy renewal provisions.

   a. _____

   b. _____

   c. _____

   d. _____

   e. _____

4. Insurance reimbursement or payment is also called _____.

5. Name two general health insurance policy limitations.

   a. _____

   b. _____

6. The act of finding out whether treatment is covered under an individual's health

   insurance policy is called _____.

7. The procedures to obtain permission for a procedure before it is done, to see whether

   the insurance program agrees it is medically necessary, is termed _____.

8. Determining the maximum dollar amount the insurance company will pay for a

   procedure before it is done is known as _____.

9. Name three ways an individual may obtain health insurance.

   a. _____

   b. _____

   c. _____

10. List four methods a physician's practice may use to submit insurance claims to insurance companies.

    a. _____

    b. _____

    c. _____

    d. _____

11. A document signed by the insured directing the insurance company to pay benefits

    directly to the physician is known as a/an _____.

12. A patient service slip personalized to the practice of the physician and used as a communications/billing tool during routing of the patient is also known as a/an

    a. _____

    b. _____

    c. _____

    d. _____

13. Electronic access to computer data may consist of the following verification or access methods.

    a. _____   d. _____

    b. _____   e. _____

    c. _____   f. _____

14. Guidelines for avoiding unauthorized use and preventing problems when a medical practice uses a facsimile signature stamp are:

    a. _____

    b. _____

    c. _____

    d. _____

15. Match the following insurance terms in the right column with their descriptions and fill in the blank with the appropriate letter.

_____ An insurance company takes into account benefits payable by another carrier in determining its own liability.	a. adjuster
_____ Benefits paid by an insurance company to an insured person.	b. assignment
_____ Transfer of one's right to collect an amount payable under an insurance contract.	c. carrier
_____ Time that must elapse before an indemnity is paid.	d. coordination of benefits
_____ Acts for insurance company or insured in settlement of claims.	e. deductible
_____ Periodic payment to keep insurance policy in force.	f. exclusions
_____ Amount insured person must pay before policy will pay.	g. indemnity
_____ Time period in which a claim must be filed.	h. premium
_____ Certain illnesses or injuries listed in a policy that the insurance company will not cover.	i. subscriber
_____ Insurance company that carries the insurance.	j. time limit
_____ One who belongs to an insurance plan.	k. waiting period

To check your answers to this self-study assignment, see Appendix D.

ASSIGNMENT 3-2 ▸ CRITICAL THINKING: ADMINISTRATIVE
SEQUENCE OF PROCESSING AN INSURANCE
CLAIM

Performance Objective

Task: Number from 1 to 12 the proper sequence of processing an insurance
                   claim.

Conditions: Use given data and pen or pencil.

Standards: Time: _____minutes

                   Accuracy: _____

                   (Note: The time element and accuracy criteria may be given by your
                   instructor.)

Directions: Arrange the listed steps 1-12 in proper sequence by placing the correct
number to the left of the statement.

_____ Bank deposit made and unpaid claims followed up

_____ Patient account established in practice management software

_____ Insurance information obtained and verified

_____ Claim processed by insurance payer and payment posted

_____ Patient's financial data posted

_____ Appointment made and patient registration obtained

_____ CMS-1500 paper claim forms submitted or electronic (HIPAA X12 837)
                 claims transmitted

_____ Insurance claims generated

_____ HIPAA Notice of Privacy Practices presented

_____ Claim transaction completed and patient's financial account is zero

_____ Patient's signature obtained on release of information document

_____ Services performed and encounter form completed

ASSIGNMENT **3-3** ▸ **CRITICAL THINKING: DIFFERENCES IN INSURANCE KEY TERMS**

Performance Objective

Task: Describe and/or explain your response to five questions.

Conditions: Use one or two sheets of white typing paper and pen or pencil.

Standards: Time: _____ minutes

              Accuracy: _____

              (Note: The time element and accuracy criteria may be given by your instructor.)

Directions: Respond verbally or in writing to these questions or statements.

1. Explain the difference between the following:

   Blanket contract _____

   Individual contract _____

2. Explain the difference between a participating provider and a nonparticipating provider for the following:

   Commercial insurance company or managed care plan participating provider:

   _____

   Commercial insurance company or managed care plan nonparticipating provider:

   _____

   Medicare participating provider:

   _____

   Medicare nonparticipating provider:

   _____

3. State the difference between the following:

   Implied contract _____

   Expressed contract _____

4. Explain the birthday law (rule) and when it is used. _____

   _____

ASSIGNMENT 3–4 ► **PREPARE A FINANCIAL ACCOUNTING RECORD**

Performance Objective

Task: Prepare, insert descriptions, and post fees, payments, credit adjustments, and balances due to a patient's ledger card. If you have access to copy equipment, make a photocopy.

Conditions: Use one patient accounts or ledger form (Figure 3–1), pen or pencil, and calculator.

Standards: Time: _____ minutes

               Accuracy: _____

               (Note: The time element and accuracy criteria may be given by your instructor.)

Directions:

1. Locate a financial accounting record (ledger) (Figure 3–1) form. Refer to the step-by-step procedures at the end of Chapter 3 in the *Handbook*. In addition, see Figures 3–18, 10–2, and 12–15 in the *Handbook* for graphic examples of financial accounting records (ledgers).

2. Insert the patient's name and address, including ZIP code in the box.

3. Enter the patient's personal data.

4. Ledger lines: Insert date of service (DOS), reference (CPT code number, check number or dates of service for posting adjustments or when insurance was billed), description of the transaction, charge amounts, payments, adjustments, and running current balance. The posting date is the actual date the transaction is recorded. If the DOS differs from the posting date, list the DOS in the reference or description column.

    Line 2: _____

    Line 3: _____

    Line 4: _____

    Line 5: _____

    Line 6: _____

    Line 7: _____

Note: A good bookkeeping practice is to use a red pen to draw a line across the financial accounting record (ledger) from left to right to indicate the last entry billed to the insurance company.

Account No. ____3-3____

FINANCIAL STATEMENT
PRACTION MEDICAL GROUP, INC.
4567 Broad Avenue
Woodland Hills, XY 12345-0001
Tel. 555-486-9002
Fax No. 555-487-8976

Phone No. (H) _____   (W) _____   Birthdate _____

Primary Insurance Co. _____   Policy/Group No. _____

| | REFERENCE | DESCRIPTION | CHARGES | CREDITS | | BALANCE |
				PYMNTS.	ADJ	
			BALANCE FORWARD ⟶			

PLEASE PAY LAST AMOUNT IN BALANCE COLUMN ⇧

THIS IS A COPY OF YOUR FINANCIAL ACCOUNT AS IT APPEARS ON OUR RECORDS

Figure 3–1

Scenario: A new patient, Miss Carolyn Wachsman, of 4590 Ashton Street, Woodland Hills, XY 12345, was seen by Dr. Practon; her account number is 2-3. Her home telephone number is (555) 340-8876 and her work telephone number is (555) 509-7091. She was born on 5-8-75. She is insured by Blue Cross, and her subscriber number is 540-xx-3209.

Miss Wachsman was seen on March 24 of the current year for a level III evaluation and management office visit ($). She also received an ECG ($). Locate these fees in the Mock Fee Schedule in Appendix A of this *Workbook*.

An insurance claim form was sent to Blue Cross on March 25. On May 15, Blue Cross sent an explanation of benefits stating the patient had previously met her deductible. Check number 433 for $76 was attached to the EOB and $19 was indicated as the adjustment to be made by the provider. On May 25, the patient was billed for the balance.

After the instructor has returned your work to you, either make the necessary corrections and place it in a three-ring notebook for future reference, or, if you received a high score, place it in your portfolio for reference when applying for a job.

ASSIGNMENT 3-5 ▸ ABSTRACT DATA FROM AN INSURANCE IDENTIFICATION CARD

Performance Objective

Task: Answer questions in reference to an insurance identification card for Case A.

Conditions: Use an insurance identification card (Figure 3-2), the questions presented, and pen or pencil.

Standards: Time: _____ minutes

Accuracy: _____

(Note: The time element and accuracy criteria may be given by your instructor.)

Directions: An identification card provides much of the information needed to establish a patient's insurance coverage. You have photocopied the front and back sides of three patients' cards and placed copies in their patient records, returning the originals to the patients. Answer the questions by abstracting or obtaining the data from the cards.

CASE A

1. Name of patient covered by the policy _____

2. Provide the insurance policy's effective date. _____

3. List the telephone number for preauthorization. _____

4. State name and address of insurance company. _____

5. List the telephone number to call for provider access. _____

6. Name the type of insurance plan. _____

7. List the insurance identification number (a.k.a. subscriber, certificate, or member numbers). _____

8. Furnish the group number. Plan or coverage code. _____

9. State the copay requirements _____

10. Does the card indicate the patient has hospital coverage? _____

Figure 3-2

ASSIGNMENT **3-6** ▸ **ABSTRACT DATA FROM AN INSURANCE IDENTIFICATION CARD**

Performance Objective

Task: Answer questions in reference to the insurance identification card for Case B.

Conditions: Use an insurance identification card (Figure 3–3), the questions presented, and pen or pencil.

Standards: Time: _____ minutes

Accuracy: _____

(Note: The time element and accuracy criteria may be given by your instructor.)

1. Patient's name covered by the policy. _____

2. Provide the insurance policy's effective date. _____

3. List the telephone number for preauthorization. _____

4. State name of insurance company. _____

5. List the telephone number to call for patient benefits and eligibility. _____

6. Name the type of insurance plan. _____

7. List the insurance identification number (a.k.a. subscriber,

   certificate, or member numbers). _____

8. Furnish the group number. Plan or coverage code. _____

9. State the copay requirements, if any. _____

10. List the Bluc Shield Web site. _____

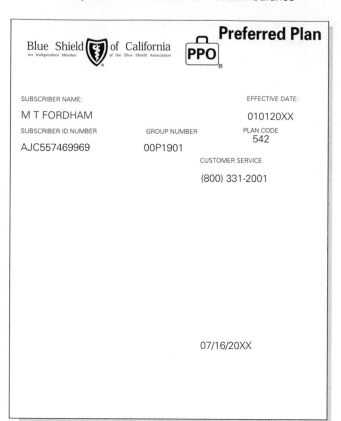

Use Blue Shield of California Preferred Physicians and Hospitals to receive maximum benefits.

Carry the Blue Shield Identification Card with you at all times and present it whenever you or one of your covered dependents receives medical services. Read your employee booklet/Health Services Agreement which summarizes the benefits, provisions, limitations and exclusions of your plan. Your health plan may require prior notification of any hospitalization and notification, within one business day, of an emergency admission. Review of selected procedures may be required before some services are performed. To receive hospital pre-admission and pre-service reviews, call 1-800-343-1691. Your failure to call may result in a reduction of benefits.

For questions, including those related to benefits, and eligibility, call the customer service number listed on the front of this card.

The PPO logo on the front of this ID Card identifies you to preferred providers outside the state of California as a member of the Blue Card PPO Program.

When you are outside of California call 1-800-810-2583 to locate the nearest PPO Provider. Remember, any services you receive are subject to the policies and provisions of your group plan.

ID-23200-PPO REVERSE   www.blueshieldca.com

Figure 3–3

ASSIGNMENT **3-7** ▸ **ABSTRACT DATA FROM AN INSURANCE IDENTIFICATION CARD**

Performance Objective

Task: Answer questions in reference to the insurance identification card for Case C.

Conditions: Use an insurance identification card (Figure 3–4), the questions presented, and pen or pencil.

Standards: Time: _____ minutes

                 Accuracy: _____

                 (Note: The time element and accuracy criteria may be given by your instructor.)

1. Patient's name covered by the policy. _____

2. Provide the insurance policy's effective date, if there is one. _____

3. List the number to call for out-of-network preauthorization. _____

4. State name and address of insurance company. _____

5. List the telephone number to call for member inquiries. _____

6. Name the type of insurance plan. _____

7. List the insurance identification number (a.k.a. subscriber, certificate,

   or member numbers). _____

8. Furnish the group number. _____

9. State the copay requirements, if any. _____

10. Who is the patient's primary care physician? _____

UNITEDhealthcare

LINDA L. FLORES
Member # 52170-5172

CALMAT

Group # 176422
COPAY: Office Visit $10 ER $50
  Urgent $35

Electronic Claims Payor ID 87726

Call 800-842-5751 for Member Inquiries

POS PCP Plan
WITH RX D - UHC
and MH/CD
PCP: G. LOMAN
805-643-9973

MTH

This identification card is not proof of membership nor does it guarantee coverage. Persons with coverage that remains in force are entitled to benefits under the terms and conditions of this group health benefit plan as detailed in your benefit description.

IMPORTANT MEMBER INFORMATION
In non-emergencies, call your Primary Care Physician to receive the highest level of benefits. If you have an emergency and are admitted to a hospital, you are required to call your Primary Care Physician within two working days.
For out of network services that require authorization, call the Member Inquiries 800 number on the front of this card.

Claim Address: P.O. Box 30990, Salt Lake City, UT 84130-0990

Figure 3–4

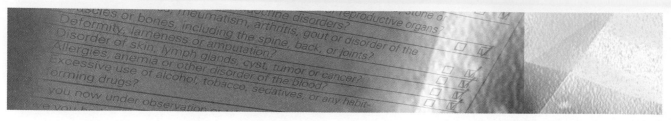

Medical Documentation

KEY TERMS

Your instructor may wish to select some words pertinent to this chapter for a test. For definitions of the terms, further study, and/or reference, the words, phrases, and abbreviations may be found in the glossary at the end of the Handbook. *Key terms for this chapter follow.*

acute

attending physician

chief complaint (CC)

chronic

comorbidity

comprehensive (C)

concurrent care

consultation

consulting physician

continuity of care

counseling

critical care

detailed (D)

documentation

electronic health record (EHR)

emergency care

eponym

established patient

expanded problem focused (EPF)

external audit

facsimile (fax)

family history (FH)

health record/medical record

high complexity (HC)

history of present illness (HPI)

internal review

low complexity (LC)

medical necessity

medical report

moderate complexity (MC)

new patient (NP)

ordering physician

past history (PH)

physical examination (PE or PX)

primary care physician (PCP)

problem focused (PF)

prospective review

referral

referring physician

resident physician

retrospective review

review of systems (ROS)

social history (SH)

straightforward (SF)

subpoena

subpoena duces tecum

teaching physician

treating or performing physician

treating practitioner

PERFORMANCE OBJECTIVES

The student will be able to:

▨ Define and spell the key terms for this chapter, given the information from the *Handbook* glossary, within a reasonable time period and with enough accuracy to obtain a satisfactory evaluation.

▨ Answer the self-study review questions after reading the chapter with enough accuracy to obtain a satisfactory evaluation.

▨ Use critical thinking to solve an office problem about patients' medical records.

▨ Abstract subjective and objective data from patient records, within a reasonable time period and with enough accuracy to obtain a satisfactory evaluation.

▨ Review a patient record and obtain answers to questions about the documentation presented, within a reasonable time period and with enough accuracy to obtain a satisfactory evaluation.

▨ Select the correct medicolegal form, create a letter with appropriate content, prepare an envelope, and properly complete U.S. Postal Service documents for the physician's signature, given the patients' chart notes and ledger cards, within a reasonable time period and with enough accuracy to obtain a satisfactory evaluation.

STUDY OUTLINE

S E L F - S T U D Y **4-1** ▸ **R E V I E W   Q U E S T I O N S**

Review the objectives, key terms, glossary definitions to key terms, chapter information, and figures before completing the following review questions.

1. Written or graphic information about patient care is termed a/an _____.

2. _____ is written or dictated to record chronologic facts and observations about a patient's health.

3. Match the following terms in the right column with their descriptions and fill in the blank with the appropriate letter.

_____	Renders a service to a patient	a. Attending physician
_____	Directs selection, preparation, and administration of tests, medication, or treatment	b. Consulting physician
_____	Legally responsible for the care and treatment given to a patient	c. Ordering physician
_____	Gives an opinion regarding a specific problem that is requested by another doctor	d. Primary care physician
_____	Sends the patient for tests or treatment or to another doctor for consultation	e. Referring physician
_____	Oversees care of patients in managed care plans and refers patients to see specialists when needed	f. Teaching physician
_____	Responsible for training and supervising medical students	g. Treating or performing physician
_____	Clinical nurse specialist or physician assistant treating a patient for a medical problem	h. Treating practitioner

4. Performance of services or procedures consistent with the diagnosis, done with standards of good medical practice and a proper level of care given in the appropriate setting is known as

_____

_____

5. If a medical practice is audited by Medicare officials and intentional miscoding is discovered, _____

_____ may be levied and providers may be _____.

6. A list of all staff members' names, job titles, signatures, and their initials is known as a/an

_____

_____

7. How should an insurance billing specialist correct an error on a patient's record?

_____

_____

8. Name the five documentation components of a patient's history.

   a. _____

   b. _____

   c. _____

   d. _____

   e. _____

9. An inventory of body systems by documenting responses to questions about symptoms that a patient

   has experienced is called a/an _____.

10. Define the following terms in relationship to billing.

    a. New patient _____

    _____

    b. Established patient_____

    _____

11. Explain the difference between a consultation and the referral of a patient.

    a. Consultation _____.

    b. Referral _____.

12. Medical care for a patient who has received treatment for an illness and is referred to a second physician for treatment of the same condition is a situation called

    _____.

13. If two physicians see the same patient on the same day, one for the patient's heart condition and the other for a diabetic situation, this medical care situation is called

    _____.

14. When faxing a patient's medical records, a signed document for _____ must be obtained from the patient.

15. Action to take when a faxed medical document is misdirected is _____

    _____.

16. What must the former physician have from the patient before a record can be given to a new physician?

    _____.

17. What must an insurance billing specialist do if he or she receives a request from another physician for certain

records? _____

_____.

18. What must a physician have from the patient before he or she can give information to an attorney?

_____.

19. Indicate either indefinite retention or number of years for keeping records in the following situations:

   a. Computerized payroll records   _____

   b. Insurance claim for Medicare patient   _____

   c. Medical record of a deceased patient   _____

   d. Active patient medical records   _____

   e. Letter to a patient about balance due after insurance paid   _____

20. Is it proper for an insurance billing specialist to receive a subpoena for his or her

physician? _____

21. Can a physician terminate a contract with a patient?_____ If so, how?

_____.

To check your answers to this self-study assignment, see Appendix D.

S E L F - S T U D Y **4 – 2** ▸ **R E V I E W   Q U E S T I O N S**

Diagnostic Terminology and Abbreviations

In the *Handbook*, review Table 4–1 and anatomic figures, as well as Appendix A in the *Workbook*, which has a list of abbreviations and symbols.

1. Match the following terms in the right column with the descriptions and fill in the blank with the appropriate letter.

_____	Pertaining to both sides	a. acute
_____	Decubitus ulcer	b. chronic
_____	Condition that runs a short but severe course	c. menopause
_____	Change of life	d. bilateral
_____	Tinnitus	e. bed sore
_____	Condition persisting over a long period of time	f. ringing sensation in ears

2. Write in the meaning for these abbreviations and/or symbols commonly encountered in a patient's medical record.

RLQ _____

DC _____

WNL _____

R/O _____

URI _____

c̄ _____

+ _____

3. When documenting incisions, the unit of measure length should be listed in _____

_____.

Multiple Choice: Circle the letter that gives the best answer to each question.

4. If a physician called and asked for a patient's medical record STAT, what would he or she mean?

a. The physician wants a statistic from a patient's record.

b. The physician wants the record delivered on Tuesday.

c. The physician wants the record delivered immediately.

5. If a physician asks you to locate the results of the last UA, what would you be searching for?

     a. a urinalysis report

     b. an x-ray report of the ulna

     c. uric acid test results

6. If a physician telephoned and asked for a copy of the last H&P to be faxed, what is being requested?

     a. heart and pulmonary findings

     b. H_2 antagonist test results

     c. a history and physical

7. If a hospital nurse telephoned and asked you to read the results of the patient's last CBC, what would you be searching for?

     a. carcinoma basal cell report

     b. complete blood count

     c. congenital blindness, complete report

8. If you were asked to make a photocopy of the patient's last CT, what would you be searching for?

     a. chemotherapy record

     b. connective tissue report

     c. computed tomography scan

To check your answers to this self-study assignment, see Appendix D.

ASSIGNMENT **4-3** ► **CRITICAL THINKING: SOLVE AN OFFICE PROBLEM**

Performance Objective

Task: Answer questions after reviewing the case study using critical thinking skills.

Conditions: Use a case study and a pen or pencil.

Standards: Time: _____ minutes

                         Accuracy: _____

Directions: Answer questions after reviewing the case study using your critical thinking skills. Record your answer on the blank lines.

1. A patient comes into the office for treatment. He does not return, because he is dissatisfied with Dr. Practon's treatment. Is it necessary to keep his records when

   he obviously will not return? _____ Why? _____

   _____

ASSIGNMENT 4–4 ► ABSTRACT SUBJECTIVE OBSERVATIONS AND OBJECTIVE FINDINGS FROM PATIENT RECORDS

Performance Objective

Task: List subjective observations and objective findings after reading each of the case studies.

Conditions: Use a pencil and four case studies.

Standards: Time: _____ minutes

              Accuracy: _____

              (Note: The time element and accuracy criteria may be given by your instructor.)

Case Study 1: Mrs. Smith is 25 years old and was brought into the emergency department of College Hospital with complaints of difficulty in breathing and chest pain. Her vital signs show an elevated temperature of 101° F and pulse of 90. Respirations are labored and 30/min. BP is 140/80. Her skin is warm and diaphoretic (perspiring). She states, "This condition has been going on for the past 3 days."

Subjective observations: _____

Objective findings: _____

Case Study 2: Mr. Jones is 56 years old and was admitted to the hospital with chest pains and elevated pulse and blood pressure. His skin is cold and clammy.

Subjective observations: _____

Objective findings: _____

Case Study 3: You are assisting the radiology technician with Sally Salazar, a 6-year-old Hispanic girl, who was brought into the pediatrician's office with a suspected fracture of the right arm. Sally states she was "running at school, tripped on my shoelace, and fell." She tells you her "arm hurts," points out how "funny my arm looks," and starts to cry. You notice her arm looks disfigured and is covered with dirt. Sally is cradling her arm against her body and is unwilling to let go because "it's going to fall off."

Subjective observations: _____

Objective findings: _____

Case Study 4: You are working in the business office of College Hospital. A former patient in your hospital comes in complaining of his billing. He states he was never catheterized, never had any of the medications listed on his itemized bill, and has "never been in this hospital for that length of time." His face is red, his voice is gradually getting louder, and you notice he is standing with the aid of crutches because his left leg is in a full cast.

Subjective observations: _____

Objective findings: _____

ASSIGNMENT **4–5** ▸ **REVIEW OF A PATIENT RECORD**

Performance Objective

Task: Answer questions after reviewing a patient's record.

Conditions: Use a pencil, internal record review sheet, medical dictionary, abbreviation reference list, drug reference book (i.e., *Mosby's MD Consult*, and laboratory reference book.

Standards: Time: _____ minutes

                   Accuracy: _____

                   (Note: The time element and accuracy criteria may be given by your instructor.)

Directions: In many instances, when developing the skill of reviewing a patient record, you may need critical thinking in addition to efficient use of reference books. Answer only those questions you think can be justified by the documentation presented in the patient's record. Because each record content is variable, you may or may not have answers to all eight questions.

   Answer the questions by recording on the blank the documentation found identifying the components from the patient's record.

   If your answers vary, perhaps you have a reason for them that may or may not be valid. List your reasons in the response section. Differences may be reviewed with your instructor privately or via class discussion.

Patient Record

10-21-20xx   HPI This new pt is an 80-year-old white male who has had problems with voiding since 9-5-20xx.

   During the night the pt had only 50 cc output and was catheterized this morning because of his poor urinary output (200 cc). He was thought to have a distended bladder; he complains of pressure in the suprapubic region. He has not had any gross hematuria. He has voiding difficulty especially lying down and voiding in the supine position. His voiding pattern is improved while standing and sitting.

Gene Ulibarri, MD

mtf

Check off:

_____ 1. Location: In what body system is the sign or symptom occurring?

   _____

_____ 2. Quality: Is the symptom or pain burning, gnawing, stabbing, pressure-like, squeezing, fullness?

   _____

_____ 3. Severity: How would you rank the symptom or pain (slight, mild, severe, persistent)?

   _____

_____   4. Duration: How long has symptom been present or how long does it last?

_____

_____   5. Timing: When do (does) sign(s) or symptom(s) occur (AM, PM, after or before meals)?

_____

_____   6. Context: Is the pain/symptom associated with big meals, dairy products, etc.?

_____

_____   7. Modifying factors: What actions make symptoms worse or better?

_____

_____   8. Associated signs and symptoms: What other system or body area produces complaints when the presenting problem occurs? (Example: chest pain leads to shortness of breath.)

_____

ASSIGNMENT 4-6 ▸ KEY A LETTER OF WITHDRAWAL

Performance Objective

Task: Key letter for physician's signature with envelope, prepare U.S. Postal Service forms, and complete an authorization form.

Conditions: Use one sheet of letterhead (Figure 4–1), U.S. Postal Service forms for certified mail with return receipt requested (Figure 4–2), Authorization for Release of Information form (Figure 4–3), a number 10 envelope, thesaurus, English dictionary, medical dictionary, computer, printer, and pen or pencil.

Standards: Time: _____ minutes

               Accuracy: _____

               (Note: The time element and accuracy criteria may be given by your instructor.)

Directions: Mrs. Mclean is negligent about following Dr. Ulibarri's advice after she received surgery. Refer to *Workbook* Assignment 7–2 for information from the patient record of Mrs. Merry M. Mclean. Use a letterhead and type in modified block style an appropriate letter to Mrs. Mclean advising her of the doctor's withdrawal from the case (see *Handbook* Figure 4–20). Date the letter June 30 of the current year. Dr. Ulibarri will be available to this patient for 30 days after receipt of this letter.

This letter must be prepared for Dr. Ulibarri's signature because it is a legal document. Type Mrs. Mclean's address on a number 10 envelope, referring to *Workbook* Figure 4–4. Send the letter by certified mail with return receipt requested, referring to *Handbook* Figure 4–21, *A–C* and enclose a completed Authorization for Release of Information form *Workbook* Figure 4–3.

After the instructor has returned your work to you, either make the necessary corrections and place it in a three-ring notebook for future reference, or, if you receive a high score, place it in your portfolio for reference when applying for a job.

1. Assemble materials, determine the recipient's address, and decide on modified or full block letter style or format.
2. Turn on the computer and select the word processing program. Open a blank document.
3. Key the dateline beginning at least three lines below the letterhead and make certain it is in the proper location for the chosen style.
4. Double-space down and insert the inside address and make certain it is in the proper location for the chosen style. Select a style to insert an attention line, if necessary.
5. Double-space and key the salutation. Use either open or mixed punctuation.
6. Double-space and enter the reference line ("Re:" or "Subject:") in the location for the chosen letter style.
7. Double-space and key the body (content) of the letter in single-space and make certain the paragraph style is proper for the format chosen. Double-space between paragraphs. Save the letter to the computer hard drive every 15 minutes.
8. Proofread the letter on the computer screen for composition.
9. Proofread the letter on the computer screen for typographical, spelling, grammatical, and mechanical errors. Use the spell-check feature of the word processing program and reference books to check for correct spelling, meaning, or usage.
10. Key the second page heading (name, page number, and date) in vertical or horizontal format if a second page is needed.
11. Key a complimentary close and make certain it is in the proper location for the chosen style.
12. Drop down four spaces and key the sender's name and title or credentials as printed on the letterhead.
13. Double-space and insert the sender's and typist's reference initials.
14. Single- or double-space to insert copy ("CC") or enclosure ("Enclosure" or "Enc"), or attachment notations.
15. Double-space to insert a postscript ("P.S."), if necessary.

Text continued on p. 51

College Clinic
4567 Broad Avenue
Woodland Hills, XY 12345-0001
Telephone: 555-486-9002   Fax: 555-487-8976

Figure 4–1

UNITED STATES POSTAL SERVICE

First-Class Mail
Postage & Fees Paid
USPS
Permit No. G-10

• Sender: Please print your name, address, and ZIP+4 in this box •

SENDER: *COMPLETE THIS SECTION*

■ Complete items 1, 2, and 3. Also complete item 4 if Restricted Delivery is desired.
■ Print your name and address on the reverse so that we can return the card to you.
■ Attach this card to the back of the mailpiece, or on the front if space permits.

1. Article Addressed to:

COMPLETE THIS SECTION ON DELIVERY

A. Received by (*Please Print Clearly*) | B. Date of Delivery

C. Signature
X
☐ Agent
☐ Addressee

D. Is delivery address different from item 1? ☐ Yes
If YES, enter delivery address below: ☐ No

3. Service Type
☐ Certified Mail ☐ Express Mail
☐ Registered ☐ Return Receipt for Merchandise
☐ Insured Mail ☐ C.O.D.

4. Restricted Delivery? (*Extra Fee*) ☐ Yes

2. Article Number (*Copy from service label*)

PS Form 3811, July 1999   Domestic Return Receipt   102595-00-M-0952

U.S. Postal Service
CERTIFIED MAIL RECEIPT
(*Domestic Mail Only; No Insurance Coverage Provided*)

CERTIFIED MAIL

PLACE STICKER AT TOP OF ENVELOPE TO THE RIGHT OF RETURN ADDRESS. FOLD AT DOTTED LINE

7000 0520 0020 3886 3112
7000 0520 0020 3886 3112

Postage | $
Certified Fee
Return Receipt Fee (Endorsement Required)
Restricted Delivery Fee (Endorsement Required)
Total Postage & Fees | $

Postmark Here

Recipient's Name (*Please Print Clearly*) (*To be completed by mailer*)
Street, Apt. No.; or PO Box No.
City, State, ZIP+4

PS Form 3800, February 2000   See Reverse for Instructions

Figure 4–2

AUTHORIZATION FOR RELEASE OF INFORMATION

Section A: Must be completed for all authorizations.

I hereby authorize the use or disclosure of my individually identifiable health information as described below.
I understand that this authorization is voluntary. I understand that if the organization to receive the information is not a health plan or health care provider, the released information may no longer be protected by federal privacy regulations.

Patient name: _____   ID Number: _____

Persons/organizations providing information: Persons/organizations receiving information:

Specific description of information [including date(s)]: _____

Section B: Must be completed only if a health plan or a health care provider has requested the authorization.

1. The health plan or health care provider must complete the following:
   a. What is the purpose of the use or disclosure? _____
   b. Will the health plan or health care provider requesting the authorization receive financial or in-kind compensation in exchange for using or disclosing the health information described above? Yes____ No____

2. The patient or the patient's representative must read and initial the following statements:
   a. I understand that my health care and the payment of my health care will not be affected if I do not sign this form.
   Initials:_____
   b. I understand that I may see and copy the information described on this form if I ask for it, and that I get a copy of this form after I sign it.
   Initials:_____

Section C: Must be completed for all authorizations.

The patient or the patient's representative must read and initial the following statements:

1. I understand that this authorization will expire on ____/____/____ (DD/MM/YR).
   Initials:_____
2. I understand that I may revoke this authorization at any time by notifying the providing organization in writing, but if I do not it will not have any effect on actions they took before they received the revocation.
   Initials:_____

_____   _____
Signature of patient or patient's representative   **Date**
(Form MUST be completed before signing)

Printed name of patient's representative: _____

Relationship to patient: _____

YOU MAY REFUSE TO SIGN THIS AUTHORIZATION
You may not use this form to release information for treatment or payment except
when the information to be released is psychotherapy notes or certain research information.

Figure 4–3

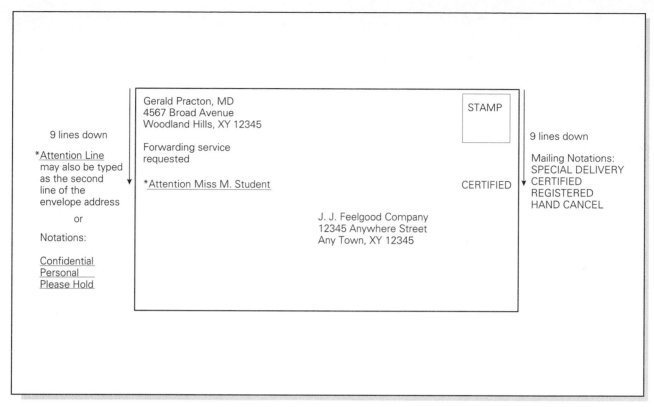

Figure 4–4

16. Save the file before printing a hard copy and proofread the letter once more. Make corrections, if needed.
17. Print the final copy to be sent and proofread. Make a copy to be retained in the files in case it is needed for future reference.
18. Save the file to a CD-ROM to be stored for future reference.
19. Prepare an envelope and use the format for optical scanning recommended by the U.S. Postal Service. Insert special mailing instructions in the correct location on the envelope if sending by certified mail.
20. Prepare Authorization for Release of Information form.
21 Prepare U.S. Postal Service certified mail documents.
22. Clip attachments to the letter and give it to the physician for review and signature.

ASSIGNMENT **4–7** ▸ **KEY A LETTER TO CONFIRM DISCHARGE BY THE PATIENT**

Performance Objective

Task: Key letter for the physician's signature.

Conditions: Use one sheet of letterhead (Figure 4–5), number 10 envelope, and U.S. Postal Service forms for certified mail with return receipt requested (Figure 4–6).

Standards: Time: _____ minutes

                   Accuracy: _____

                   (Note: The time element and accuracy criteria may be given by your instructor.)

Directions: Mr. Walter J. Stone telephones on June 3, sounding extremely upset and irrational. He says that he is unable to return to work on June 22 and that he does not want to be seen by Dr. Input again. Type a letter to confirm this discharge by the patient (see *Handbook* Figure 4–22). Suggest that he contact the local medical society for the names of three internists for further care. This letter must be prepared for Dr. Input's signature because it is a legal document. Refer to Assignment 7–4 for information from the patient record. Use a letterhead and key in modified block style as shown in *Handbook* Figure 4–22. Use current date. Key Mr. Stone's address on a number 10 envelope, referring to *Workbook* Figure 4–4. Send the letter by certified mail with return receipt requested, referring to *Handbook* Figure 4–21, *A–C*.

After the instructor has returned your work to you, either make the necessary corrections and place it in a three-ring notebook for future reference, or, if you receive a high score, place it in your portfolio for reference when applying for a job.

1. Assemble materials, determine the recipient's address, and decide on modified or full block letter style or format.
2. Turn on the computer and select the word processing program. Open a blank document.
3. Key the dateline beginning at least three lines below the letterhead and make certain it is in the proper location for the chosen style.
4. Double-space down and insert the inside address. Make certain it is in the proper location for the chosen style. Select a style to insert an attention line, if necessary.
5. Double-space and key the salutation. Use either open or mixed punctuation.
6. Double-space and enter the reference line ("Re:" or "Subject:") in the location for the chosen letter style.
7. Double-space and key the body (content) of the letter in single-space and make certain the paragraph style is proper for the format chosen. Double-space between paragraphs. Save the letter to the computer hard drive every 15 minutes.
8. Proofread the letter on the computer screen for composition.
9. Proofread the letter on the computer screen for typographical, spelling, grammatical, and mechanical errors. Use the spell-check feature of the word processing program and reference books to check for correct spelling, meaning, or usage.
10. Key the second page heading (name, page number, and date) in vertical or horizontal format if a second page is needed.
11. Key a complimentary close and make certain it is in the proper location for the chosen style.
12. Drop down four spaces and key the sender's name and title or credentials as printed on the letterhead.
13. Double-space and insert the sender's and typist's reference initials.
14. Single- or double-space to insert copy ("CC") or enclosure ("Enclosure" or "Enc"), or attachment notations.
15. Double-space to insert a postscript ("P.S."), if necessary.
16. Save the file before printing a hard copy and proofread the letter once more. Make corrections, if needed.

Text continued on p. 57

COLLEGE CLINIC
4567 Broad Avenue
Woodland Hills, XY 12345-0001
Telephone: 555-486-9002   Fax: 555-487-8976

Figure 4–5

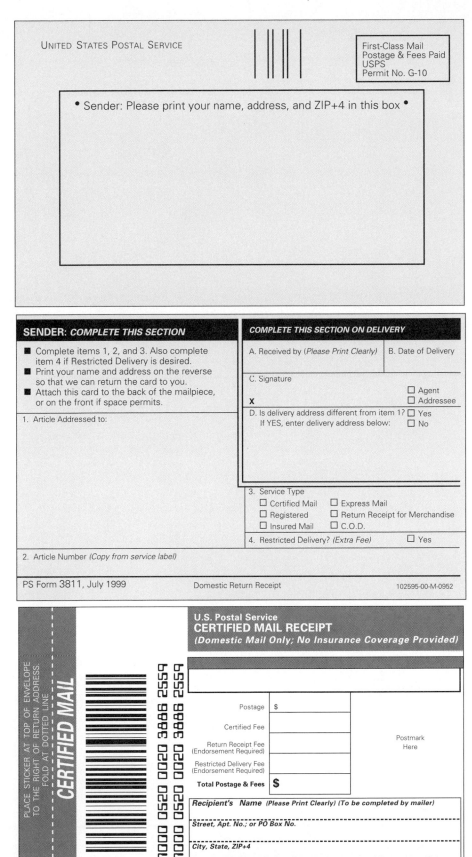

Figure 4–6

17. Print the final copy to be sent and proofread. Make a copy to be retained in the files in case it is needed for future reference.
18. Save the file to a CD-ROM to be stored for future reference.
19. Prepare an envelope and use the format for optical scanning recommended by the U.S. Postal Service. Insert special mailing instructions in the correct location on the envelope if sending by certified mail.
20. Prepare U.S. Postal Service certified mail documents.
21. Clip attachments to the letter and give it to the physician for review and signature.

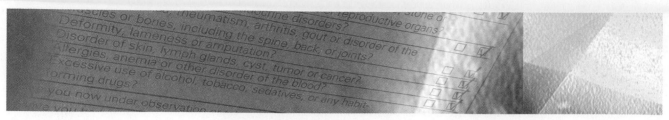

Diagnostic Coding

KEY TERMS

Your instructor may wish to select some words pertinent to this chapter for a test. For definitions of the terms, further study, and/or reference, the words, phrases, and abbreviations may be found in the glossary at the end of the Handbook. *Key terms for this chapter follow.*

adverse effect

benign tumor

chief complaint (CC)

combination code

complication

E codes

etiology

in situ

International Classification of Diseases, Ninth Revision, Clinical Modification (ICD-9-CM)

intoxication

italicized code

late effect

malignant tumor

not elsewhere classifiable (NEC)

not otherwise specified (NOS)

physician's fee profile

poisoning

primary diagnosis

principal diagnosis

secondary diagnosis

slanted brackets

syndrome

V codes

PERFORMANCE OBJECTIVES

The student will be able to:

■ Define and spell the key terms for this chapter, given the information from the *Handbook* glossary, within a reasonable time period and with enough accuracy to obtain a satisfactory evaluation.

■ Answer the self-study review questions after reading the chapter with enough accuracy to obtain a satisfactory evaluation.

■ Assignment 5–3: Indicate main terms, subterms, subterms to subterms, and carryover lines, given a section of a page from the ICD-9-CM code book, with enough accuracy to obtain a satisfactory evaluation.

■ Assignment 5–4: Answer questions given a section of a page from the ICD-9-CM code book with enough accuracy to obtain a satisfactory evaluation.

■ Assignment 5–5: Select the correct diagnostic code numbers, given a series of diagnoses using Volumes 1 and 2 of the ICD-9-CM code book, with enough accuracy to obtain a satisfactory evaluation.

■ Assignments 5–6 through 5–13: Select the correct diagnostic code numbers, given a series of scenarios and diagnoses using Volumes 1 and 2 of the ICD-9-CM code book, with enough accuracy to obtain a satisfactory evaluation.

STUDY OUTLINE

The Diagnostic Coding System
  Types of Diagnostic Codes
  Reasons for the Development and Use
    of Diagnostic Codes
  Physician's Fee Profile
History of Coding Diseases
International Classification of Diseases
  History
  Organization and Format
  Contents
How to Use the Diagnostic Code Books
  Properly
  Coding Instructions

Rules for Coding
  Signs, Symptoms, and Ill-Defined Conditions
  Sterilization
  Neoplasms
  Circulatory System Conditions
  Diabetes Mellitus
  Pregnancy, Delivery, or Abortion
  Admitting Diagnoses
  Burns
  Injuries and Late Effects
ICD-10-CM Diagnosis and Procedure Codes
Procedure: Basic Steps in Selecting Diagnostic
  Codes

SELF-STUDY **5-1** ▸ **ICD-9-CM REVIEW QUESTIONS**

Review the objectives, key terms, and chapter information before completing the following review questions.

1. Why is it important that diagnostic ICD-9-CM coding become routinely used in the physician's office?

ensure accuracy of reporting a patients' diagnosis & so that the physician's future profiles reflect more realistic payments

2. For retrieving types of diagnoses related to pathology by an institution within an institution, the coding system is found in a book entitled *Systematized Nomenclature of Human & veterinary medicine*

3. The system for coding and billing diagnoses is found in a book entitled *International Classification of diseases, ninth revision.*

4. The abbreviation ICD-9-CM means *International Classification of Disease, 9th revision*

5. Volume 1, Diseases, is a/an *tabular or numerical* listing of code numbers.

6. Volume 2, Diseases, is a/an _____ index or listing of code numbers.

7. The coding in ICD-9-CM varies from _____ to _____ characters.

8. The abbreviation NEC appearing in the ICD-9-CM code book means

  _____.

9. To code using Volume 2, the Alphabetic Index, the main term, the _____ is looked up rather than the anatomic part.

10. E codes are a supplementary classification of coding for _____ rather than disease and of coding

  for _____.

To check your answers to this self-study assignment, see Appendix D.

SELF-STUDY 5-2 ▸ ICD-10 REVIEW QUESTIONS

Directions: Multiple Choice. Circle the letter that gives the best answer to each statement.

1. ICD-10 was published by:

   a. National Center for Health Statistics

   b. World Health Organization

   c. Centers for Disease Control

   d. Centers for Medicare and Medicaid Services

2. ICD-10-CM is being clinically modified by:

   a. National Center for Health Statistics

   b. World Health Organization

   c. Centers for Disease Control

   d. Centers for Medicare and Medicaid Services

3. ICD-10-PCS (Procedure Coding System) was developed by 3M Health Information systems under contract with the:

   a. National Center for Health Statistics

   b. World Health Organization

   c. Centers for Disease Control

   d. Centers for Medicare and Medicaid Services

4. The disease codes in ICD-10-CM have a maximum of:

   a. 3 digits

   b. 4 digits

   c. 5 digits

   d. 6 digits

   e. 7 digits

5. Reason(s) the Clinical Modification was developed is/are:

   a. Removal of procedural codes

   b. Removal of unique mortality codes

   c. Removal of multiple codes

d. Only a and c

e. Only b

f. All of the above

6. One of the reasons for ICD-10-PCS is that:

a. ICD-9-CM was not capable of necessary expansion.

b. ICD-9-CM was not as comprehensive as it should be.

c. ICD-9-CM included diagnostic information.

d. All of the above.

7. The letters "I" and "O" are (were) used in:

a. ICD-9-CM

b. ICD-10-CM Diseases

c. ICD-10-PCS

d. None of the above

To check your answers to this self-study assignment, see Appendix D.

ASSIGNMENT 5-3 ▸ IDENTIFY FORMAT COMPONENTS OF ICD-9-CM, VOLUME 2

Performance Objective

Task: Identify seven format components of ICD-9-CM, Volume 2.

Conditions: Use the abstracted section from ICD-9-CM, Volume 2, and pen or pencil.

Standards: Time: _____ minutes

                   Accuracy: _____

                   (Note: The time element and accuracy criteria may be given by your instructor.)

Directions: Label the line indicated as either main term, subterm, subterm of subterm, or carryover line. Refer to Chapter 5 in the *Handbook*, section on "Diabetes Mellitus," and locate Figure 5–2, which graphically illustrates the format components.

1. ——————————————▸ **Saccharomyces** infection (*see also*
2. ————————————————▸ Candidiasis) 112.9
    Sacroiliitis NEC 720.2
    Sacrum—*see* condition
    Saddle
3. ————————————————▸ back 737.8
    embolus, aorta 444.0
    nose 738.0
4. ————————————————▸ congenital 754.0
    due to syphilis 090.5
5. ——————————▸ **Salicylism**
    correct substance properly administered
    535.4
    Salmonella choleraesuis (enteritidis)
6. ————————————————▸ (gallinarum) (suipestifer)
    (typhimurium) (see also Infection Salmonella) 003.9
7. ————————————————▸ arthritis 003.23
    carrier (suspected) of V02.3

ASSIGNMENT **5 – 4** ▶ **I C D - 9 - C M , V O L U M E 2**

Performance Objective

Task: Answer questions pertaining to categories **320** and **321** of ICD-9-CM, Volume 2.

Conditions: Use abstracted section from ICD-9-CM, Volume 2 (Figure 5–1) and pen or pencil.

Standards: Time: _____ minutes

                     Accuracy: _____

                     (Note: The time element and accuracy criteria may be given by your instructor.)

Directions: Refer to a section from a page of ICD-9-CM, Volume 2 (see Figure 5–1) and answer questions pertaining to categories 320 and 321.

1. Locate the section title _____

2. Refer to the INCLUSION TERMS listed under category code 320, entitled "Bacterial meningitis." Place an "X" in front of each of the following diagnostic statements that are included in category 320.

       _____ purulent meningitis

       _____ bacterial meningomyelitis

       _____ meningitis

       _____ meningoencephalitis

       _____ pyogenic meningitis

       _____ meningococcal

3. Refer to the EXCLUSION TERMS located under code 320.7, entitled "Meningitis in other bacterial diseases classified elsewhere." Place an "X" in front of the following code number(s) which are excluded.

       _____ secondary syphilis 091.81

       _____ acquired syphilis 097.9

       _____ gonococcal meningitis 098.82

       _____ congenital syphilis 090.42

       _____ primary syphilis 091.2

       _____ gram-negative anaerobes 320.81

6. NERVOUS SYSTEM AND SENSE ORGANS (320-389)

INFLAMMATORY DISEASES OF THE CENTRAL NERVOUS SYSTEM (320-326)

320 Bacterial meningitis

Includes: arachnoiditis
leptomeningitis
meningitis
meningoencephalitis } bacterial
meningomyelitis
pachymeningitis

320.0 *Haemophilus* meningitis
Meningitis due to *Haemophilus influenzae* [*H. Influenzae*]

320.1 Pneumococcal meningitis

320.2 Streptococcal meningitis

320.3 Staphylococcal meningitis

320.7 Meningitis in other bacterial diseases classified elsewhere

Code first underlying diseases as:
actinomycosis (039.8)
listeriosis (027.0)
typhoid fever (002.0)
whooping cough (033.0-033.9)
Excludes: *meningitis (in):*
epidemic (036.0)
gonococcal (098.82)
meningococcal (036.0)
salmonellosis (003.21)
syphilis:
NOS (094.2)
congenital (090.42)
meningovascular (094.2)
secondary (091.81)
tuberculous (013.0)

320.8 Meningitis due to other specified bacteria

320.81 Anaerobic meningitis
Bacteroides (fragilis)
Gram-negative anaerobes

320.82 Meningitis due to gram-negative bacteria, not elsewhere classified

Aerobacter aerogenes	*Klebsiella pneumoniae*
Escherichia coli [E. coli]	*Proteus morganii*
Friedländer bacillus	*Pseudomonas*

Excludes: *gram-negative anaerobes (320.81)*

320.89 Meningitis due to other specified bacteria
Bacillus pyocyaneus

320.9 Meningitis due to unspecified bacterium
Meningitis:
bacterial NOS
purulent NOS
pyogenic NOS
suppurative NOS

321   Meningitis due to other organisms

Includes: arachnoiditis
leptomeningitis } due to organisms
meningitis   other than bacteria
pachymeningitis

321.0   Cryptococcal meningitis
Code first underlying disease (117.5)

Figure 5–1

4. Place an "X" in front of each of the following diagnostic statements included in category code 320 and its subcategories.

_____ leptomeningitis

_____ meningitis resulting from *E. coli*

_____ pyogenic meningitis

_____ epidemic meningitis

_____ tuberculous meningitis

5. Write the code numbers for category 320 that require fifth digits.

_____

DIAGNOSTIC CODING ASSIGNMENTS

In this chapter, the points awarded for assignments that require diagnostic codes are one point for each correct digit.

ASSIGNMENT 5-5 ▸ OBTAIN GENERAL DIAGNOSTIC CODES FOR CONDITIONS

Performance Objective

Task: Locate the correct diagnostic code for each diagnosis listed.

Conditions: Use pen or pencil and ICD-9-CM diagnostic code book.

Standards: Time: _____ minutes

                    Accuracy: _____

                    (Note: The time element and accuracy criteria may be given by your instructor.)

Directions: Using the *International Classification of Diseases, Ninth Revision, Clinical Modification* (ICD-9-CM) code book, read each diagnosis and locate the condition in Volume 2, the alphabetical index. Match the definition to the written description as close as possible and assign the correct code, entering it on the blank line.

Problems:

1. Breast mass   _____

2. *Klebsiella* pneumonia   _____

3. Acute lateral wall myocardial infarction; initial episode   _____

4. Acute cerebrovascular accident   _____

5. Arteriosclerotic cardiovascular disease   _____

6. Dyspnea, R/O cystic fibrosis   _____

7. Ileitis   _____

8. Arthritis of elbow   _____

9. Ringing in the ears   _____

10. Acute exacerbation of chronic asthmatic bronchitis   _____

Scoring Grid

	Problem 1	Problem 2	Problem 3	Problem 4	Problem 5	Problem 6	Problem 7	Problem 8	Problem 9	Problem 10
Locate the main term or condition in the Alphabetic Index, Volume 2 (1 pt)										
Refer to any notes under the main term. (1 pt)										
Read any notes or terms enclosed in parentheses after the main term. (1 pt)										
Look for appropriate subterm. (1 pt)										
Look for appropriate sub-subterm and follow any cross-reference instructions. (1 pt)										
Write down the code. (1 pt)										
Verify the code number in the Tabular List, Volume 1. (1 pt)										
Read and be guided by any instructional terms in the Tabular List. (1 pt)										
Read complete description and then code to the highest specificity. (1 pt)										
Assign the code (3 to 5 pts)										
(Total Points Preferred)	(12 to 14)	(12 to 14)	(12 to 14)	(12 to 14)	(12 to 14)	(12 to 14)	(12 to 14)	(12 to 14)	(12 to 14)	(12 to 14)
Total Points Earned										

ASSIGNMENT 5–6 ▸ CODE DIAGNOSES FROM MEDICAL RECORDS

Performance Objective

Task: Locate the correct diagnostic code for each case scenario.

Conditions: Use pen or pencil and ICD-9-CM diagnostic code book.

Standards: Time: _____ minutes

                       Accuracy: _____

                       (Note: The time element and accuracy criteria may be given by your instructor.)

Directions: This exercise will give you experience in basic diagnostic coding for physicians' insurance claims. First list the ICD-9-CM code for the diagnosis, condition, problem, or other reason for the admission and/or encounter (visit) shown in the medical record to be chiefly responsible for the services provided. Then list additional diagnostic codes that describe any coexisting conditions that affect patient care. Always assign codes to their highest level of specificity—the more digits, the more specific. Do not code probable, rule out, suspected, or questionable conditions. Assign the correct code(s), entering it (them) on the blank line.

Problems:

Problem 1. A patient, Mrs. Jennifer Hanson, calls Dr. Input's office stating she has blood in her stool. Dr. Input suspects a GI bleed and tells Mrs. Hanson to come in immediately. It is discovered that the reason for the blood in the stool is a bleeding duodenal ulcer. Code the diagnosis to be listed on the insurance claim for the office visit.   _____

Problem 2. a. Jason Belmen comes in with a fractured humerus. He also has chronic obstructive pulmonary disease (COPD), which is not treated. Code the diagnosis.   a. _____

b. Assume Mr. Belmen needs general anesthesia for open reduction of the fractured humerus. The COPD could now be considered a risk factor. List the diagnostic code in the second part of this scenario.   b. _____

Problem 3. Margarita Sanchez came into the office for removal of sutures. Code the diagnosis.   _____

Problem 4. A patient, George Martin, has benign prostatic hypertrophy (BPH). He is seen for catheterization because of urinary retention. Code the primary and secondary diagnoses for the office visit. (Note: BPH is an enlargement of   a. _____
the prostate gland, due to overgrowth of androgen-sensitive glandular elements, which occurs naturally with aging.)   b. _____

Problem 5. Mia Bartholomew is seen in the office complaining of a sore throat. A throat culture is done and the specimen is sent to an outside laboratory for a culture and sensitivity study to determine the presence of *Streptococcus*. List the diagnostic code the physician would use if the insurance claim is submitted before the results are known.   a. _____
List the diagnostic code if the physician submits the insurance claim after the laboratory report is received indicating *Streptococcus* is present.   b. _____

Scoring Grid

	Problem 1	Problem 2a	Problem 2b	Problem 3	Problem 4a	Problem 4b	Problem 5a	Problem 5b
Locate the main term or condition in the Alphabetic Index, Volume 2 **(1 pt)**								
Refer to any notes under the main term. **(1 pt)**								
Read any notes or terms enclosed in parentheses after the main term. **(1 pt)**								
Look for appropriate subterm. **(1 pt)**								
Look for appropriate subterm and follow any cross-reference instructions. **(1 pt)**								
Write down the code. **(1 pt)**								
Verify the code number in the Tabular List, Volume 1. **(1 pt)**								
Read and be guided by any instructional terms in the Tabular List. **(1 pt)**								
Read complete description and then code to the highest specificity. **(1 pt)**								
Assign the code **(3 to 5 pts)**								
(Total Points Preferred)	(12 to 14)	(12 to 14)	(12 to 14)	(12 to 14)	(12 to 14)	(12 to 14)	(12 to 14)	(12 to 14)
Total Points Earned								

ASSIGNMENT 5–7 ▸ CODE DIAGNOSES USING V CODES

Performance Objective

Task: Locate the correct diagnostic code for each case scenario.

Conditions: Use pen or pencil and ICD-9-CM diagnostic code book.

Standards: Time: _____ minutes

               Accuracy: _____

               (Note: The time element and accuracy criteria may be given by your instructor.)

Directions: In this exercise you will be reviewing V codes in the ICD-9-CM code book. Assign the correct code, entering it on the blank line. These are some key words under which V codes may be located in Volume 2:

admission	checking/checkup	donor	insertion of	status post
aftercare	conflict	evaluation	maintenance	vaccination
attention to	contact	examination	observation	
border	contraception	fitting of	person with	
care of	counseling	follow-up	problem with	
carrier	dialysis	history of	screening	

Problems:

1. Kathy Osborn, a patient, is seen in the office for an annual checkup.   _____.

2. Daniel Matsui is seen in the office for adjustment of a lumbosacral corset.   _____.

3. Philip O'Brien comes into the office to receive a prophylactic flu shot.   _____.

4. Bernadette Murphy is seen in the office for a pregnancy test.   _____.

5. Michiko Fujita is seen in the office for a fractured rib.
   No x-rays are taken because Mrs. Fujita thinks she
   is pregnant.
   a. _____
   b. _____

6. Dr. Perry Cardi sees Kenneth Pickford in the office for cardiac
   pacemaker adjustment. The pacemaker was implanted because of
   sick sinus syndrome.
   _____

7. Frank Meadows returns for follow-up, postoperative transurethral
   prostatic resection (TURP) for prostate cancer after treatment has
   been completed.
   a. _____
   b. _____

Scoring Grid

	Problem 1	Problem 2	Problem 3	Problem 4	Problem 5a	Problem 5b	Problem 6	Problem 7a	Problem 7b
Locate the main term or condition in the Alphabetic Index, Volume 2 **(1 pt)**									
Refer to any notes under the main term. **(1 pt)**									
Read any notes or terms enclosed in parentheses after the main term. **(1 pt)**									
Look for appropriate subterm. **(1 pt)**									
Look for appropriate sub-subterm and follow any cross-reference instructions. **(1 pt)**									
Write down the code. **(1 pt)**									
Verify the code number in the Tabular List, Volume 1. **(1 pt)**									
Read and be guided by any instructional terms in the Tabular List. **(1 pt)**									
Read complete description and then code to the highest specificity. **(1 pt)**									
Assign the code **(3 to 5 pts)**									
(Total Points Preferred)	(12 to 14)	(12 to 14)	(12 to 14)	(12 to 14)	(12 to 14)	(12 to 14)	(12 to 14)	(12 to 14)	(12 to 14)
Total Points Earned									

ASSIGNMENT 5-8 ▸ CODE NEOPLASTIC DIAGNOSES

Performance Objective

Task: Locate the correct diagnostic code for each diagnosis listed.

Conditions: Use pen or pencil and ICD-9-CM diagnostic code book.

Standards: Time: _____ minutes

                   Accuracy: _____

                   (Note: The time element and accuracy criteria may be given by your instructor.)

Directions: In this exercise, you will be reviewing diagnostic codes in the ICD-9-CM code book involving neoplasms. The morphology of neoplasm is found in Appendix A of Volume 1. Neoplasms are classified according to their histology. Morphology (M) codes are sometimes used to supplement a diagnostic code. M codes are not used on insurance forms when submitting claims by physicians; therefore, they will not be used in this assignment. M codes are never used as a primary diagnostic code. Assign the correct code, entering it on the blank line.

1. Leiomyoma, uterus   _____

2. Ewing's sarcoma, forearm   _____

3. Adenocarcinoma, right breast, central portion   _____

4. Dyspnea resulting from carcinoma of the breast with metastasis   a. _____
   to the lung

                                                         b. _____

5. Patient is seen for a yearly examination 1 year after a mastectomy   a. _____
   for breast cancer; she is disease-free at this time.

                                                         b. _____

6. Patient comes in for chemotherapy because of lymphosarcoma   a. _____
   of the intrathoracic lymph nodes.

                                                         b. _____

Scoring Grid

	Problem 1	Problem 2	Problem 3	Problem 4a	Problem 4b	Problem 5a	Problem 5b	Problem 6a	Problem 6b
Locate the main term or condition in the Alphabetic Index, Volume 2 **(1 pt)**									
Refer to any notes under the main term. **(1 pt)**									
Read any notes or terms enclosed in parentheses after the main term. **(1 pt)**									
Look for appropriate subterm. **(1 pt)**									
Look for appropriate sub-subterm and follow any cross-reference instructions. **(1 pt)**									
Write down the code. **(1 pt)**									
Verify the code number in the Tabular List, Volume 1. **(1 pt)**									
Read and be guided by any instructional terms in the Tabular List. **(1 pt)**									
Read complete description and then code to the highest specificity. **(1 pt)**									
Assign the code **(3 to 5 pts)**									
(Total Points Preferred)	(12 to 14)	(12 to 14)	(12 to 14)	(12 to 14)	(12 to 14)	(12 to 14)	(12 to 14)	(12 to 14)	(12 to 14)
Total Points Earned									

ASSIGNMENT 5-9 ▸ CODE DIAGNOSES FOR PATIENTS WITH DIABETES

Performance Objective

Task: Locate the correct diagnostic code for each diagnosis listed.

Conditions: Use pen or pencil and ICD-9-CM diagnostic code book.

Standards: Time: _____ minutes

               Accuracy: _____

               (Note: The time element and accuracy criteria may be given by your instructor.)

Directions: In this exercise, you will review diagnostic codes in the ICD-9-CM code book involving cases of patients with diabetes. When coding diabetes, first find out the type of diabetes being treated, type I or type II. Then look to see whether the diabetes is under control. These two answers determine the assignment of the fifth digit.

For diabetic complications, determine whether the complication is due to the diabetes and whether the diabetes is out of control. These points need to be regarded as two distinctly different issues. A patient can have controlled diabetes but still have a complication caused by diabetes. Complications arising from diabetes must be coded. The code for the complication is listed after the subterm in brackets.

Example: If a patient with type II uncontrolled diabetes is treated for a skin ulcer on the lower extremity, look up "diabetes" in Volume 2 and find the subterm "ulcer." The diabetes code listed is 250.8 and under the subterm "ulcer" is a sub-subterm of "lower extremity" with the code 707.1 in brackets. Go to Volume 1 and verify the diabetes code and assign a fifth digit. The correct code is 250.82 (2 for type II, uncontrolled). Now verify the ulcer code in Volume 1. You will see that code 707.1 does not mention diabetes. If diabetes is the cause of the ulcer, code the diabetes first and the ulcer second. If the patient's diabetes is under control and is not being treated at the visit, code the ulcer first and diabetes second as an underlying disease. Other complications, such as bone changes (731.8) may tell you to code the underlying disease first. Therefore, always verify all codes in Volume 1 before assigning them.

Assign the correct code(s) for each case involving diabetes, entering it (them) on the blank line.

1. Diabetes mellitus   _____

2. Uncontrolled noninsulin-dependent diabetes mellitus   _____
    with ketoacidosis

3. Diabetic gangrene (type I diabetes, out of control)   a. _____

                                                b. _____

4. Controlled type II diabetes with cataract.   a. _____

                                                b. _____

5. Type I diabetes with diabetic polyneuropathy and   a. _____
    retinopathy

                                                b. _____

                                                c. _____

                                                d. _____

Scoring Grid

	Problem 1	Problem 2	Problem 3a	Problem 3b	Problem 4a	Problem 4b	Problem 5a	Problem 5b	Problem 5c	Problem 5d
Locate the main term or condition in the Alphabetic Index, Volume 2 **(1 pt)**										
Refer to any notes under the main term. **(1 pt)**										
Read any notes or terms enclosed in parentheses after the main term. **(1 pt)**										
Look for appropriate subterm. **(1 pt)**										
Look for appropriate subsubterm and follow any cross-reference instructions. **(1 pt)**										
Write down the code. **(1 pt)**										
Verify the code number in the Tabular List, Volume 1. **(1 pt)**										
Read and be guided by any instructional terms in the Tabular List. **(1 pt)**										
Read complete description and then code to the highest specificity. **(1 pt)**										
Assign the code **(3 to 5 pts)**										
(Total Points Preferred)	(12 to 14)	(12 to 14)	(12 to 14)	(12 to 14)	(12 to 14)	(12 to 14)	(12 to 14)	(12 to 14)	(12 to 14)	(12 to 14)
Total Points Earned										

ASSIGNMENT 5–10 ▸ CODE DIAGNOSES FOR PATIENTS WITH HYPERTENSION

Performance Objective

Task: Locate the correct diagnostic code for each diagnosis listed.

Conditions: Use pen or pencil and ICD-9-CM diagnostic code book.

Standards: Time: _____ minutes

Accuracy: _____

(Note: The time element and accuracy criteria may be given by your instructor.)

Directions: In this exercise, you will review diagnostic codes in the ICD-9-CM code book involving patients who have hypertension. To begin coding, look in Volume 2 under "hypertension" and find the Hypertension Table. This is designed to simplify coding conditions caused by, or associated with, hypertension or hypertensive disease. At the beginning of the table, many terms are listed in parentheses. These terms are nonessential modifiers, which means that the absence or presence of one of these terms does not change the meaning of the code. From the table, the codes relating to hypertension begin with 401. Go to this number in Volume 1 and look through this section to become familiar with it.

Assign the correct code(s) for each case, entering it (them) on the blank line.

1. High blood pressure   _____

2. Malignant hypertension   _____

3. Antepartum hypertension complicating pregnancy   _____

4. Hypertension with kidney disease   _____

5. Hypertension due to arteriosclerotic cardiovascular disease   _____
   (ASCVD) and congestive heart failure (CHF)

6. Myocarditis and CHF due to malignant hypertension   a. _____

                                                            b. _____

Scoring Grid

	Problem 1	Problem 2	Problem 3	Problem 4	Problem 5	Problem 6a	Problem 6b
Locate the main term or condition in the Alphabetic Index, Volume 2 (1 pt)							
Refer to any notes under the main term. (1 pt)							
Read any notes or terms enclosed in parentheses after the main term. (1 pt)							
Look for appropriate subterm. (1 pt)							
Look for appropriate subterm and follow any cross-reference instructions. (1 pt)							
Write down the code. (1 pt)							
Verify the code number in the Tabular List, Volume 1. (1 pt)							
Read and be guided by any instructional terms in the Tabular List. (1 pt)							
Read complete description and then code to the highest specificity. (1 pt)							
Assign the code (3 to 5 pts)							
(Total Points Preferred)	(12 to 14)	(12 to 14)	(12 to 14)	(12 to 14)	(12 to 14)	(12 to 14)	(12 to 14)
Total Points Earned							

ASSIGNMENT 5–11 ▸ CODE DIAGNOSES FOR INJURIES, FRACTURES, BURNS, LATE EFFECTS, AND COMPLICATIONS

Performance Objective

Task: Locate the correct diagnostic code for each diagnosis listed.

Conditions: Use pen or pencil and ICD-9-CM diagnostic code book.

Standards: Time: _____ minutes

                 Accuracy: _____

(Note: The time element and accuracy criteria may be given by your instructor.)

Directions: In this exercise, you will review diagnostic codes from the ICD-9-CM code book involving patients who have suffered injuries, burns, fractures, and late effects. Some guidelines for coding injuries, fractures, burns, late effects, and complications are:

Injuries
✔ Code injuries separately according to their general type and then by anatomic site. Fifth digits are commonly used in the injury section to specify anatomic sites and severity.
✔ Code injuries separately if they are classifiable to more than one subcategory unless the diagnosis does not support separate injuries or the Alphabetic Index provides instructions to use combination code.

Fractures
✔ Fractures are presumed to be closed unless otherwise specified.
✔ Fracture/dislocations are coded as fractures.
✔ Pathologic fractures are coded first and the cause (disease process) coded second.

Burns
✔ Multiple burns at the same site, but of different degrees, are coded to the most severe degree.

✔ Code the extent of body surface involved (percentage of body surface), when specified, as an additional code.

Late Effects
✔ A residual, late effect is defined as the current condition resulting from a previous acute illness or injury that is no longer the current problem. Late effects are coded using the residual or late effect as the primary diagnosis. The cause of the residual or late effect is coded second.

Complications
✔ For conditions resulting from the malfunction of internal devices, use the subterm "mechanical" found under the main term "complication."
✔ Postoperative complications are sometimes found under the subterm "postoperative," which appears under the main term identifying the condition. If not found there, look for a subterm identifying the type of procedure, type of complication, or surgical procedure under the main term "complication."

Assign the correct code(s) for each case, entering it (them) on the blank line.

1. Supracondylar fracture of right femur   _____

2. Fracture of left humerus and left foot   a. _____

                                                 b. _____

3. Comminuted fracture of left radius and ulna

4. Pathologic fracture of right hip due to drug-induced osteoporosis   a. _____

                                                 b. _____

5. Lacerations of arm, with embedded glass   _____

6. Burns on the face and neck   .   _____

7. Second- and third-degree burns on chest wall; 20% of body
   involved, 10% third-degree

   a. _____

   b. _____

8. Bursitis of the knee resulting from crushing injury to the
   knee 1 year ago

   a. _____

   b. _____

Scoring Grid

	Problem 1	Problem 2a	Problem 2b	Problem 3	Problem 4a	Problem 4b	Problem 5	Problem 6	Problem 7a	Problem 7b	Problem 8a	Problem 8b
Locate the main term or condition in the Alphabetic Index, Volume 2 (1 pt)												
Refer to any notes under the main term. (1 pt)												
Read any notes or terms enclosed in parentheses after the main term. (1 pt)												
Look for appropriate subterm. (1 pt)												
Look for appropriate sub-subterm and follow any cross-reference instructions. (1 pt)												
Write down the code. (1 pt)												
Verify the code number in the Tabular List, Volume 1. (1 pt)												
Read and be guided by any instructional terms in the Tabular List. (1 pt)												
Read complete description and then code to the highest specificity. (1 pt)												
Assign the code (3 to 5 pts)												
(Total Points Preferred)	(12 to 14)	(12 to 14)	(12 to 14)	(12 to 14)	(12 to 14)	(12 to 14)	(12 to 14)	(12 to 14)	(12 to 14)	(12 to 14)	(12 to 14)	(12 to 14)
Total Points Earned												

ASSIGNMENT 5-12 ▸ CODE DIAGNOSES FOR PREGNANCY, DELIVERY, AND NEWBORN CARE

Performance Objective

Task: Locate the correct diagnostic code for each case scenario.

Conditions: Use pen or pencil and ICD-9-CM diagnostic code book.

Standards: Time: _____ minutes

                 Accuracy: _____

                 (Note: The time element and accuracy criteria may be given by your instructor.)

Directions: In this exercise, you will review diagnostic codes from the ICD-9-CM code book involving patients who have conditions involving pregnancy and delivery, and newborn infants.

For the supervision of a normal pregnancy, turn to Volume 2 and look up "pregnancy." This is a long category. Look up the subterm "supervision" and find the sub-subterm "normal" (NEC V22.1) and "first" (V22.0). Check Volume 1 to verify these codes. Also see code V22.2 "pregnancy state, incidental." This code is used in the second position to tell the insurance carrier that the patient is pregnant in addition to any other diagnosis.

If a patient develops complications, turn to Volume 2 and look under the main term "pregnancy." Find the subterm "complicated by," and find the sub-subterm stating the complication. These are codes from ICD-9-CM Chapter 11: "Complications of Pregnancy, Childbirth, and Puerperium" (630-677).

Delivery in a completely normal case is coded 650 and is listed under the main term "delivery, uncomplicated." Normal is described as "delivery without abnormality or complication and with spontaneous cephalic delivery, without mention of fetal manipulation or instrumentation." A different code must be used to describe any complication or deviation from this description of normal.

When coding deliveries, always include a code for the status of the infant. Look up "outcome of delivery" in Volume 2 and you will find various V27 codes listing possible outcomes. These codes would be listed as secondary codes on the insurance claim form for the delivery.

On the insurance claim form for the newborn, turn to "newborn" in Volume 2. You will find V codes from V30.X to V39.X describing the birth of the newborn. Use these codes in the first position when billing for services for the newborn infant.

Assign the correct code(s) for each case entering it (them) on the blank line.

1. A pregnant patient who is due to deliver in 6 weeks presents in the office with preeclampsia.   _____ _____

2. A patient presents with a chief complaint of severe episodes of pain and vaginal hemorrhage. The physician determines that the patient has an incomplete spontaneous abortion complicated by excessive hemorrhage; she was 6 weeks' pregnant.   _____

3. A patient comes in who is diagnosed with a kidney stone; the patient is also pregnant.

a. _____

b. _____

4. A patient delivers twins by cesarean section because of cephalopelvic disproportion, which caused an obstruction.

a. _____

b. _____

c. _____

Scoring Grid

	Problem 1	Problem 2	Problem 3a	Problem 3b	Problem 4a	Problem 4b	Problem 4c
Locate the main term or condition in the Alphabetic Index, Volume 2 **(1 pt)**							
Refer to any notes under the main term. **(1 pt)**							
Read any notes or terms enclosed in parentheses after the main term. **(1 pt)**							
Look for appropriate subterm. **(1 pt)**							
Look for appropriate subterm and follow any cross-reference instructions. **(1 pt)**							
Write down the code. **(1 pt)**							
Verify the code number in the Tabular List, Volume 1. **(1 pt)**							
Read and be guided by any instructional terms in the Tabular List. **(1 pt)**							
Read complete description and then code to the highest specificity. **(1 pt)**							
Assign the code **(3 to 5 pts)**							
(Total Points Preferred)	(12 to 14)	(12 to 14)	(12 to 14)	(12 to 14)	(12 to 14)	(12 to 14)	(12 to 14)
Total Points Earned							

ASSIGNMENT **5–13** ▸ **CODE DIAGNOSES USING E CODES**

Performance Objective

Task:	Locate the correct diagnostic code for each diagnosis listed.
Conditions:	Use pen or pencil and the ICD-9-CM diagnostic code book.
Standards:	Time: _____ minutes
	Accuracy: _____

(Note: The time element and accuracy criteria may be given by your instructor.)

Directions: In this exercise you will be reviewing diagnostic codes from the ICD-9-CM code book involving patients who may have been in an accident, had an adverse effect from ingesting a toxic substance, or suffered an injury. Read the definitions for poisoning and drug intoxication in the *Handbook*.

✔ E codes are not used to describe the primary reason for a patient's visit but identify external environmental events, circumstances, and conditions as the cause of injury, poisoning, and other adverse effects (unfavorable results).

✔ E codes that identify external environmental events, such as an injury, are used only as supplemental codes to describe how an injury occurred. These codes are listed in the back of Volume 2 and provide a more descriptive clinical picture for the insurance carrier.

They may or may not be required and in some cases may speed up the payment of the claim.

✔ E codes are used for coding adverse effects of drugs and chemicals but are not required when coding a poisoning. Use the Table of Drugs and Chemicals at the back of Volume 2 and go to the column titled "Therapeutic Use." In addition, it is necessary to use a code to describe the adverse effect of using a particular drug or medicine. Find this in Volume 2 and verify it in Volume 1.

Assign the correct code(s) for each case and enter it (them) on the blank line.

1. Light-headedness caused by digitalis intoxication

  a._____

  b. _____

2. Treatment of a rash after an initial dose of penicillin is given

  a. _____

  b. _____

3. Accidental overdose of meperidine (Demerol)

  a. _____

  b. _____

4. A 20-month-old baby accidentally ingests approximately 15 aspirin and is severely nauseated

  a. _____

  b._____

  c. _____

5. A patient presents in the physician's office with a vague complaint of not
feeling well. The physician notices that the patient has ataxia (a staggering
gait). After reviewing the patient's history, the physician determines
the ataxia is due to the meprobamate the patient is taking.

a. _____

b. _____

6. Internal bleeding: abnormal reaction to a combination
chloramphenicol and warfarin (Coumadin)

a. _____

b. _____

c. _____

Scoring Grid

	Problem 1a	Problem 1b	Problem 2a	Problem 2b	Problem 3a	Problem 3b	Problem 4a	Problem 4b	Problem 4c	Problem 5a	Problem 5b	Problem 6a	Problem 6b	Problem 6c
Locate the main term or condition in the Alphabetic Index, Volume 2 (1 pt)														
Refer to any notes under the main term. (1 pt)														
Read any notes or terms enclosed in parentheses after the main term. (1 pt)														
Look for appropriate subterm. (1 pt)														
Look for appropriate sub-subterm and follow any cross-reference instructions. (1 pt)														
Write down the code. (1 pt)														
Verify the code number in the Tabular List, Volume 1. (1 pt)														
Read and be guided by any instructional terms in the Tabular List. (1 pt)														
Read complete description and then code to the highest specificity. (1 pt)														
Assign the code (3 to 5 pts)														
(Total Points Preferred)	(12 to 14)	(12 to 14)	(12 to 14)	(12 to 14)	(12 to 14)	(12 to 14)	(12 to 14)	(12 to 14)	(12 to 14)	(12 to 14)	(12 to 14)	(12 to 14)	(12 to 14)	
Total Points Earned														

Procedural Coding

KEY TERMS

Your instructor may wish to select some words pertinent to this chapter for a test. For definitions of the terms, further study, and/or reference, the words, phrases, and abbreviations may be found in the glossary at the end of the Handbook. *Key terms for this chapter follow.*

alternative billing codes (ABCs)

bilateral

bundled codes

comprehensive code

conversion factor

Current Procedural Terminology (CPT)

customary fee

downcoding

fee schedule

global surgery policy

Healthcare Common Procedure Coding System (HCPCS)

modifier

procedure code numbers

professional component (PC)

reasonable fee

relative value studies (RVS)

relative value unit (RVU)

resource-based relative value scale (RBRVS)

surgical package

technical component (TC)

unbundling

upcoding

usual, customary, and reasonable (UCR)

PERFORMANCE OBJECTIVES

The student will be able to:

■ Define and spell the key terms for this chapter, given the information from the *Handbook* glossary, within a reasonable time period and with enough accuracy to obtain satisfactory evaluation.

■ Answer the self-study review questions after reading the chapter with enough accuracy to obtain a satisfactory evaluation.

■ Select the five-digit procedure code numbers, modifiers, and/or descriptors of each service, given

a series of problems relating to various medical procedures and services and using the *Current Procedural Terminology* (CPT) code book or the Mock Fee Schedule in Appendix A of the *Workbook* with enough accuracy to obtain a satisfactory evaluation.

■ Fill in the correct meaning of each abbreviation given in a list of common medical abbreviations and symbols that appear in chart notes, and with enough accuracy to obtain a satisfactory evaluation.

STUDY OUTLINE

Understanding the Importance of Procedural Coding Skills

Coding Compliance Plan
Current Procedural Terminology

Methods of Payment
Fee Schedule
Usual, Customary, and Reasonable
Developing a Fee Schedule Using Relative Value Studies Conversion Factors

How to Use the CPT Code Book
Category I, II, and III Codes
Code Book Symbols
Evaluation and Management Section
Surgery Section

Unlisted Procedures
Coding Guidelines for Code Edits
Code Monitoring

Helpful Hints in Coding
Office Visits
Drugs and Injections
Adjunct Codes
Basic Life or Disability Evaluation Services

Code Modifiers
Correct Use of Common CPT Modifiers
Comprehensive List of Modifier Codes

Procedure: Determine Conversion Factors

Procedure: Choose Correct Procedural Codes for Professional Services

 SELF-STUDY **6–1** ▸ **REVIEW QUESTIONS**

Review the objectives, key terms, and chapter information before completing the following review questions.

1. The coding system used for billing professional medical services and procedures is

   found in a book titled _____.

2. The Medicare program uses a system of coding composed of three levels, and this is

   called _____.

3. Complications or special circumstances about a medical service or procedure may be

   shown by using a CPT code with a/an _____.

4. A relative value scale or schedule is a listing of procedure codes indicating the relative

   value of services performed, which is shown by_____.

5. Name three methods for basing payments adopted by insurance companies and state and federal programs.

   a. _____

   b. _____

   c. _____

6. List four situations that can occur in a medical practice when referring to charges and payments from a fee schedule.

   a. _____

b. _____

c. _____

d. _____

7. Name the eight main sections of CPT.

a. _____

b. _____

c. _____

d. _____

e. _____

f. _____

g. _____

h. _____

8. Match the symbol in the first column with the definitions in the second column.
   Write the correct letters on the blanks.

   _____   ►◄   a. New code

   _____   ●   b. Modifier -51 exempt

   _____   ⊃   c. Add-on code

   _____   ⊘   d. New or revised text

   _____   +   e. Revised code

   _____   ▲   f. Reference material

   _____   ⊙   g. Conscious sedation

9. Name five hospital departments where critical care of a patient may take place.

a. _____

b. _____

c. _____

d. _____

e. _____

10. A surgical package includes

    a. _____

    b. _____

    c. _____

    d. _____

    e. _____

    f. _____

    g. _____

11. Medicare global surgery policy includes

    a. _____

    b. _____

    c. _____

    d. _____

    e. _____

    f. _____

    g. _____

    h. _____

12. A function of computer software that performs online checking of codes on an insurance claim to detect improper code submission is called a/an _____.

13. A single code that describes two or more component codes bundled together as one unit is known as a/an _____ _____.

14. Two group-related codes together is commonly referred to as _____.

15. Use of many procedural codes to identify procedures that may be described by one code is termed _____.

16. A code used on a claim that does not match the code system used by the insurance carrier and is converted to the closest code rendering less payment is termed _____.

17. Intentional manipulation of procedural codes to generate increased reimbursement is called _____.

18. Give eight reasons for using modifiers on insurance claims.

    a. _____

    b. _____

    c. _____

    d. _____

    e. _____

    f. _____

    g. _____

    h. _____

19. Match the symbol in the first column with the definitions in the second column.
    Write the correct letters on the blanks.

    _____   -21   a. Unusual procedural services

    _____   -22   b. Multiple procedures

    _____   -25   c. Staged or related procedure

    _____   -26   d. Decision for surgery

    _____   -51   e. Significant, separately identifiable E/M service by the same physician
                        on the same day of the procedure or other service

    _____   -52   f. Prolonged evaluation and management services

    _____   -57   g. Reduced services

    _____   -58   h. Professional component

20. What modifier is usually used when billing for an assistant surgeon? _____

21. Explain when to use the -99 modifier code. _____

    _____

    _____

To check your answers to this self-study assignment, see Appendix D.

SELF-STUDY ASSIGNMENT 6-2 ▸ DEFINE MEDICAL ABBREVIATIONS

To reinforce abbreviations you have learned, let's review some of those encountered during the *Workbook* assignments presented in this chapter. You should be able to decode these abbreviations without a reference. However, if you have difficulty with one or two, simply refer to Appendix A of this *Workbook*.

I & D _____

IM _____

Pap _____

ER _____

EEG _____

DPT _____

ECG _____

IUD _____

OB _____

D & C _____

OV _____

KUB _____

GI _____

Hgb _____

new pt _____

rt _____

UA _____

est pt _____

ASHD _____

tet. tox. _____

CBC _____

E/M _____

CPT _____

Ob-Gyn _____

TURP _____

cm _____

T & A _____

mL _____

inj _____

hx _____

NC _____

To check your answers to this self-study assignment, see Appendix D.

PROCEDURE CODING ASSIGNMENTS

In this chapter, the points awarded for assignments that require procedure codes are one point for each correct digit.

ASSIGNMENT 6-3 ▸ **INTRODUCTION TO CPT AND CODING EVALUATION AND MANAGEMENT SERVICES**

Performance Objective

Task: Locate the correct information and/or procedure code for each question and/or case scenario.

Conditions: Use pen or pencil and the *Current Procedural Terminology* code book.

Standards: Time: _____ minutes

            Accuracy: _____

            (Note: The time element and accuracy criteria may be given by your instructor.)

1. To become acquainted with the sections of the *Current Procedure Terminology* code book, match the code number in the left column with the appropriate description in the right column by writing the letters in the blanks. Locate each code number in the *Current Procedural Terminology* code book. As you progress though the assignment, the problems get more difficult and complex.

   99231   _____   a. Chest x-ray

   59400   _____   b. Anesthesia for procedures on cervical spine and cord

   71010   _____   c. Subsequent hospital care

   00600   _____   d. Supplies and materials

   85031   _____   e. Routine OB care, ante- and postpartum

   99070   _____   f. CBC

2. Name the section of the CPT where each of the following codes is located.

   a. 65091 _____

   b. 86038 _____

   c. 92596 _____

   d. 75982 _____

   e. 0010T _____

   f. 00600 _____

   g. 99321 _____

   h. 0503F _____

3. Evaluation and Management (E/M) codes are used by physicians to report a significant portion of their services. Remember, it is the physician's responsibility to assign E/M codes, and the exercises presented are only for familiarization. The problems will acquaint you with terminology for this section of the CPT code book. Select the appropriate **new patient** office visit codes using the key components:

a. This is a Level 3 case: Detailed history

   Detailed examination

   Low-complexity decision making   _____

b. This is a Level 1 case: Problem-focused history

   Problem-focused examination

   Straightforward decision making   _____

c. This is a Level 5 case: Comprehensive history

   Comprehensive examination

   High-complexity decision making   _____

	Problem 3a	Problem 3b	Problem 3c
Use the code book index. **(1 pt)**			
Read the introduction to the section. **(1 pt)**			
Locate code number in code section or subsection. **(1 pt)**			
Select the code. **(5 pts)**			
Determine if modifier(s) is needed. **(1 pt)**			
(Total Points Preferred)	(9)	(9)	(9)
Total Points Earned			

4. Select the appropriate **established patient** office visit codes using the key components. Coding these cases illustrates consideration of two of three components.

   a. This is a Level 4 case: Detailed history

      Detailed examination

      Low-complexity decision making.   _____

   b. This is a Level 5 case: Comprehensive history

      Comprehensive examination

      Moderate-complexity decision making   _____

   c. This is a Level 5 case: Detailed history

      Comprehensive examination

      High-complexity decision making   _____

	Problem 4a	Problem 4b	Problem 4c
Use the code book index. **(1 pt)**			
Read the introduction to the section. **(1 pt)**			
Locate code number in code section or subsection. **(1 pt)**			
Select the code. **(2 pts)**			
Determine if modifier(s) is needed. **(2 pts)**			
(Total Points Preferred)	(7)	(7)	(7)
Total Points Earned			

5. Evaluation and Management (E/M) codes **99201** to **99239** are used for services provided in the physician's office or in an outpatient or hospital facility. Read the brief statement and then locate the code number in the *Current Procedural Terminology* code book.

   a. Office visit of a 20-year-old patient seen within the past 3 years for instruction in diabetes injection sites by RN (minimal problem). Patient not seen by physician at this brief visit.   _____

   b. Office visit of a 30-year-old new patient with allergic rhinitis. This case had an expanded problem-focused hx & exam and straightforward decision making.   _____

   c. Discussion of medication with the son of an 80-year-old patient with dementia on discharge from the observation unit.   _____

   d. Admission to hospital of 60-year-old established patient in acute respiratory distress with bronchitis. Comprehensive hx & exam and medical decision making of moderate complexity.   _____

   e. Hospital visit of a 4-year-old boy, now stable, who will be discharged the next day. This is a problem-focused interval hx & exam and medical decision making of low complexity.   _____

   f. New patient seen in the office for chest pain, congestive heart failure, and hypertension. Comprehensive hx & exam and highly complex decision making.   _____

	Problem 5a	Problem 5b	Problem 5c	Problem 5d	Problem 5e	Problem 5f
Use the code book index. **(1 pt)**						
Read the introduction to the section. **(1 pt)**						
Locate code number in code section or subsection. **(1 pt)**						
Select the code. **(5 pts)**						
Determine if modifier(s) is needed. **(1 pt)**						
(Total Points Preferred)	(9)	(9)	(9)	(9)	(9)	(9)
Total Points Earned						

6. Evaluation and Management codes **99241** to **99275** are used for consultations provided in the physician's office or in an outpatient or inpatient hospital facility. A consultation is a service provided by a physician whose opinion about a case is requested by another physician. Read the brief statement and then locate the code number in the *Current Procedural Terminology* code book.

a. Office consultation for a 30-year-old woman complaining of palpitations and chest pains. Her family physician described a mild systolic click. This is an expanded problem-focused hx & exam and straightforward decision making. _____

b. Follow-up inpatient consultation for a 64-year-old woman, who is now stable, admitted 2 days ago for a bleeding ulcer. This case is a problem-focused hx & exam and low-complexity decision making. _____

c. Office consultation for a 14-year-old boy with poor grades in school and suspected alcohol abuse. This is a comprehensive hx & exam and medical decision making of moderate complexity. _____

d. Follow-up inpatient consultation for a 70-year-old man who is diabetic and is suffering with fever, chills, gangrenous heel ulcer, rhonchi, and dyspnea (difficulty breathing), an unstable condition. The patient appears lethargic and tachypneic (rapid breathing). This case is detailed hx & exam with highly complex medical decision making. _____

e. Initial emergency department consultation for a senior who presents with thyrotoxicosis, exophthalmos, cardiac arrhythmia, and congestive heart failure. This case is a comprehensive hx & exam with highly complex medical decision making. _____

f. Initial hospital consultation for a 30-year-old woman, postabdominal surgery, who is exhibiting a fever. This case is an expanded problem-focused hx & exam and straightforward medical decision. _____

	Problem 6a	Problem 6b	Problem 6c	Problem 6d	Problem 6e	Problem 6f
Use the code book index. **(1 pt)**						
Read the introduction to the section. **(1 pt)**						
Locate code number in code section or subsection. **(1 pt)**						
Select the code. **(5 pts)**						
Determine if modifier(s) is needed. **(1 pt)**						
(Total Points Preferred)	(9)	(9)	(9)	(9)	(9)	(9)
Total Points Earned						

7. Evaluation and Management codes **99281** to **99499** are used for emergency department, critical care, nursing facility, rest home, custodial care, home, prolonged, physician standby, and preventive medicine services. Read the brief statement and then locate the code number in the *Current Procedural Terminology* code book.

   a. First hour of critical care of a senior who, following major surgery, suffers a cardiac arrest from a pulmonary embolus. _____

   b. A 40-year-old woman is admitted to the OB unit, and the primary care physician has requested the neonatologist to stand by for possible cesarean section and neonatal resuscitation. Code for a 1-hour standby. _____

   c. A child is seen in the emergency department with a fever, diarrhea, abdominal cramps, and vomiting. This case had an expanded problem-focused hx & exam and a moderately complex medical decision was made. _____

   d. A patient is seen for an annual visit at a nursing facility for detailed hx & comprehensive exam and straightforward medical decision making. _____

   e. An initial visit is made to a domiciliary care facility for a developmentally disabled individual with a mild rash on hands and face. This case had a problem-focused hx & exam and low-complexity medical decision making. _____

   f. A 50-year-old man with a history of asthma comes into the office with acute bronchospasm and moderate respiratory distress. Office treatment is initiated. The case requires intermittent physician face-to-face time with the patient for 2 hours and prolonged services. Assume the appropriate E & M code has been assigned for this case. _____

	Problem 7a	Problem 7b	Problem 7c	Problem 7d	Problem 7e	Problem 7f
Use the code book index. (1 pt)						
Read the introduction to the section. (1 pt)						
Locate code number in code section or subsection. (1 pt)						
Select the code. (5 pts)						
Determine if modifier(s) is needed. (1 pt)						
(Total Points Preferred)	(9)	(9)	(9)	(9)	(9)	(9)
Total Points Earned						

ASSIGNMENT **6-4** ▸ **CODE ANESTHESIA PROBLEMS**

Performance Objective

Task: Locate the correct procedure and modifier, if necessary, for each
                    question and/or case scenario.

Conditions: Use pen or pencil and *Current Procedural Terminology* code book.

Standards: Time: _____ minutes

                    Accuracy: _____

                    (Note: The time element and accuracy criteria may be given by your instructor.)

Directions: Anesthesia codes **00100** to **01999** may be used by anesthesiologists as well as physicians. Some plastic surgeons, other medical specialists, and large clinics may have a room set aside to perform surgical procedures that might be performed in a hospital outpatient surgical department. For Medicare claims, some regions do not use the Anesthesia Section of CPT for billing but use a surgical code with an HCPCS modifier appended. Read the brief statement and then locate the code number in the *Current Procedural Terminology* code book. Special modifiers **P1** through **P6** may be needed when coding for this section, as well as code numbers for cases that have difficult circumstances. Definitions for abbreviations may be found in Appendix A.

a. Cesarean delivery following neuraxial labor anesthesia, normal healthy patient   _____

b. Reduction mammoplasty of a woman with mild systemic disease   _____

c. Total right hip replacement, 71-year-old patient, normal healthy patient   _____

d. Repair of cleft palate, newborn infant, normal healthy patient   _____

e. TURP, normal healthy male   _____

	Problem a	Problem b	Problem c	Problem d	Problem e
Use the code book index. **(1 pt)**					
Read the introduction to the section. **(1 pt)**					
Locate code number in code section or subsection. **(1 pt)**					
Select the code. **(5 pts)**					
Determine if modifier(s) is needed. **(2 pts)**					
(Total Points Preferred)	(10)	(10)	(12)	(12)	(10)
Total Points Earned					

ASSIGNMENT 6-5 ► CODE SURGICAL PROBLEMS

Performance Objective

Task: Locate the correct procedure code and modifier, if necessary, for each
                     question and/or case scenario.

Conditions: Use pen or pencil and *Current Procedural Terminology* code book.

Standards: Time: _____ minutes

                     Accuracy: _____

                     (Note: The time element and accuracy criteria may be given by your instructor.)

Directions: Surgery codes **10040** to **69979** are used for each anatomic part of the body. Read over each case carefully. It is preferable to use the *Current Procedural Terminology* code book, but if you do not have one then refer to the Mock Fee Schedule found in Appendix A of this *Workbook* to obtain the correct code number for each descriptor given. Full descriptors for services rendered have been omitted in some instances to give you practice in abstracting the correct descriptor from the available information. Indicate the correct two-digit modifier if necessary. The skill of critical thinking enters this section of the assignment, in that you may have to use your own judgment to code because the cases do not contain full details. Definitions for abbreviations may be found in Appendix A. Remember to use the index at the back of the CPT code book.

a. Suppose you work in an office that has an encounter form listing code 36530.
    Check your edition of CPT and see whether you can locate this code number.
    If the code does not appear, what code number are you directed to use?   _____

Integumentary System 10040–19499

b. Removal of benign lesion from the back (1.0 cm) and left foot (0.5 cm)   _____

c. Drainage of deep breast abscess   _____

d. Laser destruction of two benign facial lesions   _____

	Problem a	Problem b	Problem c	Problem d
Use the code book index. **(1 pt)**				
Read the introduction to the section. **(1 pt)**				
Locate code number in code section or subsection. **(1 pt)**				
Select the code. **(5 pts)**				
Determine if modifier(s) is needed. **(2 pts)**				
(Total Points Preferred)	(10)	(15)	(10)	(15)
Total Points Earned				

Musculoskeletal System 20000–29909

e. Aspiration of fluid (arthrocentesis) from right knee joint; not infectious   _____

f. Deep tissue biopsy of left upper arm   _____

g. Fracture of the left tibia, closed treatment   _____

   Does the procedural code include the application and removal of the first cast?   _____

   If done as an office procedure, may supplies be coded?   _____

   If so, what is the code number from the Medicine section?   _____

   Does the procedural code include subsequent replacement of a cast for follow-up care?   _____

   If not, list the code number for application of a walking short leg cast.   _____

Respiratory System 30000–32999

h. Parietal pleurectomy   _____

i. Removal of two nasal polyps, simple   _____

j. Diagnostic bronchoscopy with biopsy   _____

	Problem e	Problem f	Problem g	Problem h	Problem i	Problem j
Use the code book index. (1 pt)						
Read the introduction to the section. (1 pt)						
Locate code number in code section or subsection. (1 pt)						
Select the code. (5 pts)						
Determine if modifier(s) is needed. (2 pts)						
(Total Points Preferred)	(10)	(10)	(15)	(10)	(10)	(10)
Total Points Earned						

Cardiovascular System 33010–37799

k. Pacemaker insertion with transvenous electrode, atrial   _____

l. Thromboendarterectomy with patch graft   _____

m. Introduction of intracatheter and injection procedure for contrast venography   _____

Hemic/Lymphatic/Diaphragm 38100–39599

n. Repair, esophageal/diaphragmatic hernia   _____

o. Partial splenectomy   _____

p. Excision, two deep cervical nodes   _____

	Problem k	Problem l	Problem m	Problem n	Problem o	Problem p
Use the code book index. (1 pt)						
Read the introduction to the section. (1 pt)						
Locate code number in code section or subsection. (1 pt)						
Select the code. (5 pts)						
Determine if modifier(s) is needed. (2 pts)						
(Total Points Preferred)	(10)	(10)	(10)	(10)	(10)	(10)
Total Points Earned						

Digestive System 40490–49999

q. T & A, 12-year-old boy   _____

r. Balloon dilation of esophagus   _____

Urinary System/Male and Female Genital 50010–55980

s. Removal of urethral diverticulum from female patient   _____

t. Anastomosis of single ureter to bladder   _____

Laparoscopy/Peritoneoscopy/Hysteroscopy/Female Genital/Maternity 56300–59899

u. Routine OB care, ante- and postpartum care   _____

v. Therapeutic D & C, nonobstetric   _____

	Problem q	Problem r	Problem s	Problem t	Problem u	Problem v
Use the code book index. **(1 pt)**						
Read the introduction to the section. **(1 pt)**						
Locate code number in code section or subsection. **(1 pt)**						
Select the code. **(5 pts)**						
Determine if modifier(s) is needed. **(2 pts)**						
(Total Points Preferred)	(10)	(10)	(10)	(10)	(10)	(10)
Total Points Earned						

ASSIGNMENT 6-6 ▸ CODE PROBLEMS FOR RADIOLOGY AND PATHOLOGY

Performance Objective

Task: Locate the correct procedure code and modifier, if necessary, for each question and/or case scenario.

Conditions: Use pen or pencil and *Current Procedural Terminology* code book.

Standards: Time: _____ minutes

                        Accuracy: _____

                        (Note: The time element and accuracy criteria may be given by your instructor.)

Radiologists as well as other physicians in many specialties perform these studies. A physician who interprets, dictates, and signs a report may not bill for the report separately because it is considered part of the radiology procedure.

   Some medical practices perform basic laboratory tests under a waived test certificate that complies with the rules of the Clinical Laboratory Improvement Amendments (CLIA) of 1988, implemented in September 1992.

a. Upper GI x-ray study with films and KUB   _____

b. Ultrasound, pregnant uterus after first trimester, multiple gestation   _____

c. Routine urinalysis with microscopy, nonautomated   _____

d. Hemoglobin (Hgb), electrophoretic method.   _____

	Problem a	Problem b	Problem c	Problem d
Use the code book index. **(1 pt)**				
Read the introduction to the section. **(1 pt)**				
Locate code number in code section or subsection. **(1 pt)**				
Select the code. **(5 pts)**				
Determine if modifier(s) is needed. **(2 pts)**				
(Total Points Preferred)	(10)	(10)	(10)	(10)
Total Points Earned				

ASSIGNMENT 6-7 ▸ PROCEDURE CODE AND MODIFIER PROBLEMS

Performance Objective

Task: Locate the correct procedure code and modifiers, if necessary, for each case scenario.

Conditions: Use pen or pencil and *Current Procedural Terminology* code book.

Standards: Time: _____ minutes

               Accuracy: _____

               (Note: The time element and accuracy criteria may be given by your instructor.)

Directions: Find the correct procedure codes and modifiers, if necessary. This assignment will reinforce what you have already learned about procedural coding, because code numbers for the case scenarios presented are located in all the sections of the CPT code book. Also search for codes in the Medicine Section, if necessary. The CPT list of modifiers may be found in the *Handbook*.

1. A new patient had five benign skin lesions on the right arm destroyed with surgical curettement. Complete the coding for the surgery.

   Code Number   *Description*

   a. _____   Level 3, detailed history and exam with low-complexity decision
                         making, initial new pt office visit

   b. _____   Destruction of benign skin lesion rt arm

   c. _____   Destruction of second, third, fourth, and fifth lesions

	Problem 1a	Problem 1b	Problem 1c
Use the code book index. **(1 pt)**			
Read the introduction to the section. **(1 pt)**			
Locate code number in code section or subsection. **(1 pt)**			
Select the code. **(5 pts)**			
Determine if modifier(s) is needed. **(2 pts)**			
(Total Points Preferred)	(10)	(10)	(10)
Total Points Earned			

2. Mrs. Stayman had four moles on her back. Dr. Davis excised the multiple nevi in one office visit. The information on the pathology report stated nonmalignant lesions measuring 2.2 cm, 1.5 cm, 1 cm, and 0.75 cm.

Code Number		*Description*
a. _____	_____	Initial OV
b. _____	_____	Excision, benign lesion 2.2 cm
c. _____	_____	Excision, benign lesion 1.5 cm
d. _____	_____	Excision, benign lesion 1 cm
e. _____	_____	Excision, benign lesion 0.75 cm

	Problem 2a	Problem 2b	Problem 2c	Problem 2d	Problem 2e
Use the code book index. **(1 pt)**					
Read the introduction to the section. **(1 pt)**					
Locate code number in code section or subsection. **(1 pt)**					
Select the code. **(5 pts)**					
Determine if modifier(s) is needed. **(2 pts)**					
(Total Points Preferred)	(10)	(10)	(10)	(10)	(10)
Total Points Earned					

In another case, if a patient required removal of a 1-cm lesion on the back and a 0.5-cm

lesion on the neck, the procedural codes would be _____ for the

back lesion and _____ for the neck lesion.

3. Dr. Davis stated on his operative report that Mr. Allen was suffering from a complex, complicated nasal fracture. Dr. Davis debrided the wound, because it was contaminated, and performed an open reduction with internal fixation in a complex and complicated procedure.

Code Number   *Description*

_____ _____   Initial OV, complex hx & exam, moderate-complexity decision making

_____   Open tx nasal fracture complicated

_____ _____   Debridement, skin, subcutaneous tissue, muscle, and bone

4. An RN, an established patient (est pt), age 40 years, sees the doctor for an annual physical. A Pap (Papanicolaou) smear is obtained and sent to an outside laboratory. The patient also has a furuncle on the right axilla at the time of the visit, which the doctor incises and drains (I & D).

Code Number   *Description*

_____   Periodic physical examination

_____   Handling of specimen

_____   I & D, furuncle, right axilla

_____   5-mL penicillin inj IM

5. While making his rounds in the hospital during the noon hour, Dr. James sees a new patient in the ED (emergency department) for a laceration of the forehead, 5 cm long. The doctor does a workup for a possible concussion.

Code Number   *Description*

_____   ED care, expanded problem-focused history, expanded problem-focused examination, low-complexity decision making

_____   Repair of laceration, simple, face

6. The physician sees a new patient in the office with the same condition as the patient in Problem 5; however, an infection has developed and the patient is seen for daily dressing changes. On day 11, the sutures are removed, and on day 12 a final dressing change is made, and the patient is discharged.

Code Number   *Description*

_____   Level 3, detailed history and exam with low-complexity decision making, initial new patient office visit

_____   Repair of laceration

_____   Tet tox (tetanus toxoid) 0.5 cc

_____ Minimal service, OV, dressing change (2 days)

_____ OV, suture removal (4 days)

Note: Some fee schedules allow no follow-up days; Medicare fee schedule allows
10 follow-up days for the procedural code number for repair of laceration.

7. The physician sees 13-year-old Bobby Jones (est pt) for a Boy Scout physical. Bobby
is in good health and well groomed. His troop is going for a 1-week camping trip in
12 days. The physician reviewed safety issues with Bobby, talked to him about school,
and counseled him about not getting into drugs or alcohol. Bobby denied any
problems with that or of being sexually active. He said that he plays baseball.
He has no allergies. The physician performed a detailed examination. The physician
completed information for scouting papers and cleared him for camping activity.

Code Number   *Description*

_____ _____ Periodic preventive evaluation and management

8. A new patient, David Ramsey, age 15 years, was seen by Dr. Menter for lapses
of memory and frequent headaches. The doctor performed an EEG
(electroencephalogram) and some psychological tests (including psychodiagnostic
assessment of personality and psychopathology tests [Rorschach and MMPI]).
Dr. Astro Parkinson was called in as a consultant. All the tests were negative, and the
patient was advised to come in for weekly psychotherapy.

Code Number   *Description*

Dr. Menter's bill:

_____ OV, comp hx & exam, moderate-complexity decision making

_____ EEG, extended monitoring (1 hr)

_____ Psychological tests (Rorschach and MMPI)

_____ Psychotherapy (50 min)

Dr. Parkinson's bill:

_____ Consultation, expanded problem-focused hx and exam
straightforward decision making

9. An est pt, age 70 years, requires repair of a bilateral initial inguinal hernia. The code

for this initial procedure is _____ _____.

	Problem 3	Problem 4	Problem 5	Problem 6	Problem 7	Problem 8	Problem 9
Use the code book index. **(1 pt)**							
Read the introduction to the section. **(1 pt)**							
Locate code number in code section or subsection. **(1 pt)**							
Select the code. **(5 pts)**							
Determine if modifier(s) is needed. **(2 pts)**							
(Total Points Preferred)	(30)	(40)	(20)	(50)	(10)	(50)	(10)
Total Points Earned							

ASSIGNMENT 6–8 ▸ HCPCS/MODIFIER CODE MATCH

Performance Objective

Task: Locate the correct HCPCS code and modifier, if necessary, for each medical drug, supply item, or service presented.

Conditions: Use pen or pencil and HCPCS code reference list in Appendix B of this *Workbook*.

Standards: Time: _____ minutes

               Accuracy: _____

               (Note: The time element and accuracy criteria may be given by your instructor.)

Directions: Match the HCPCS code in the first or second column with the description of the drug, supply item, or service presented in the third or fourth column. Write the correct letters on the blanks.

E0962 _____	J0760 _____	a. Vitamin B$_{12}$, 1000 µg	k. Blood (whole) for to transfusion/unit
E0141 _____	A9150 _____	b. injection, insulin	l. One-inch cushion, for wheelchair
J0290 _____	J2000 _____	c. Rigid walker, wheeled, without seat	m. Ampicillin inj, up to 500 mg
J3420 _____	L0160 _____	d. Waiver of liability statement on file	n. Dimethyl sulfoxide, DMSO inj
J1815 _____	L3100-RT _____	e. Nonemergency transportation, taxi	o. Urine strips
P9010 _____	A4250 _____	f. Inj of colchicine	p. Vancomycin (Vancocin) inj
J1212 _____	J2590 _____	g. Cervical occipital/ mandibular support	q. Oxytocin (Pitocin) inj
J3370 _____	A4930 _____	h. Inj of lidocaine (Xylocaine)	r. Standard youth wheelchair, new equipment
E1091-NU _____	A0100 _____	i. gloves, sterile	s. Rt hallux valgus night
A4211 _____	-GA _____	j. supplies for self-administered drug	t. Aspirin, nonprescription injections

ASSIGNMENT 6-9 ▸ **PROCEDURAL CODING CASE SCENARIOS**

Performance Objective

Task: Locate the correct procedure code and modifier, if necessary, for each case scenario.

Conditions: Use pen or pencil and *Current Procedural Terminology* code book.

Standards: Time: _____ minutes

                   Accuracy: _____

                   (Note: The time element and accuracy criteria may be given by your instructor.)

Directions: Find the correct procedure codes and modifiers, if necessary, for each case scenario.

1. The physician sees Horace Hart, a 60-year-old new patient, in the office for bronchial asthma, ASHD (arteriosclerotic heart disease), and hypertension. He performs an ECG (electrocardiogram) and UA (urinalysis) without microscopy, and obtains x-rays. Comprehensive metabolic and lipid panels and a CBC (complete blood count) are done by an outside laboratory.

   Code Number   *Description*

   Physician's bill:

   _____   Initial OV, comp hx & exam, high-complexity decision
                          making

   _____   ECG with interpret and report

   _____   UA, routine, nonautomated

   _____   Chest x-ray, 2 views

   _____   Routine venipuncture for handling of specimen

   Laboratory's bill:

   _____   Comprehensive metabolic panel: albumin, bilirubin, calcium,
                          carbon dioxide, chloride, creatinine, glucose, phosphatase
                          (alkaline), potassium, protein, sodium, ALT, AST, and urea nitrogen

   _____   Lipid panel

   _____   CBC, completely automated with complete differential

   If the doctor decides to have the chest x-rays interpreted by a radiologist, the procedural

   code billed by the radiologist would be _____   _____.

2. Mr. Hart is seen again in the office on May 12. On May 25 he is seen at home at 2 AM with asthma exacerbation, possible myocardial infarct, and congestive heart failure. The doctor consulted with a thoracic cardiovascular surgeon by telephone. He also called to make arrangements for hospitalization. These services required 2 hours and 40 minutes to complete the patient care.

Code Number   *Description*

_____   OV, problem-focused hx & exam, straightforward decision making

_____   Home visit, detailed interval hx & exam, high-complexity decision making

_____   Detention time, prolonged (list time required)

3. On June 9, Horace Hart is seen again in the hospital. The thoracic cardiovascular surgeon who was telephoned the previous day was called in for consultation to formally examine him and says that surgery is necessary, which is scheduled the following day. The patient's physician sees the patient for his asthmatic condition and acts as assistant surgeon. The surgeon does the follow-up care and assumes care in the case.

Code Number   *Description*

Primary care physician/assistant surgeon's bill:

_____   Hospital visit, problem-focused hx & exam, low-complexity decision making

_____ _____   Pericardiotomy

Thoracic cardiovascular surgeon's bill:

_____ _____   Consultation, comp hx & exam, moderate-complexity decision making

_____   Pericardiotomy

	Problem 1	Problem 2	Problem 3
Use the code book index. (1 pt)			
Read the introduction to the section. (1 pt)			
Locate code number in code section or subsection. (1 pt)			
Select the code. (5 pts)			
Determine if modifier(s) is needed. (2 pts)			
(Total Points Preferred)	(80)	(40)	(40)
Total Points Earned			

ASSIGNMENT **6–10** ▸ **CASE SCENARIO FOR CRITICAL THINKING**

Performance Objective

Task: Locate the correct procedure codes and modifiers, if necessary, for a case scenario.

Conditions: Use pen or pencil and *Current Procedural Terminology* code book.

Standards: Time: _____ minutes

                    Accuracy: _____

                    (Note: The time element and accuracy criteria may be given by your instructor.)

Directions: Read through this progress note on Roy A. Takashima. Abstract information from the note about the subjective symptoms, objective findings, and diagnoses. List the diagnostic and procedure codes you think this case would warrant.

```
Takashima, Roy A.
October 5, 20xx

   Pt. has many things going on. First, he's had no difficulties following the feral
cat bite, and the cat was normal on quarantine.
   He seemed to be recovering from the flu but is plagued with a very persisting
cough and pain down the center of his chest without fever or grossly discolored
phlegm.
   Physical exam shows expiratory rhonchi and gross exacerbation of his cough on
forced expiration. Spirometry before and after bronchodilator was remarkably good;
nonetheless, it is improved and he is symptomatically improved with a Proventil
inhaler, which he is given as a sample. I don't think other antibiotics would help.
   His reflux is under good control with proprietary antacids with a clear exam.
   He has several areas of seborrheic keratoses on his face and head that need
attention.
   Finally, in follow-up of all the above, he needs a complete physical exam.

                                                              Ting Cho, MD
```

Diagnosis: Influenza and acute bronchitis.

Subjective symptoms   _____

                       _____

                       _____

Objective findings   _____

                       _____

                       _____

Diagnosis and Dx code _____

_____

_____

_____

E/M code _____

Spirometry code _____

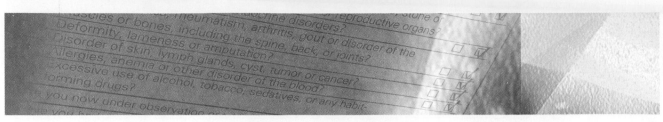

The Paper Claim: CMS-1500

KEY TERMS

Your instructor may wish to select some specific words pertinent to this chapter for a test. For definitions of the terms, further study, and/or reference, words, phrases, and abbreviations may be found in the glossary at the end of the Handbook. *Key terms for this chapter follow.*

clean claim
dirty claim
durable medical equipment (DME) number
electronic claim
employer identification number (EIN)
facility provider number
group provider number
Health Insurance Claim Form (CMS-1500)
incomplete claim

intelligent character recognition (ICR)
invalid claim
National Provider Identifier (NPI)
optical character recognition (OCR)
"other" claims
paper claim
pending claim
physically clean claim
provider identification number (PIN)
rejected claim
Social Security number (SSN)
state license number
unique provider identification number (UPIN)

PERFORMANCE OBJECTIVES

The student will be able to:

- Define and spell the key terms for this chapter, given the information from the *Handbook* glossary, within a reasonable time period and with enough accuracy to obtain a satisfactory evaluation.

- After reading the chapter, answer the self-study review questions with enough accuracy to obtain a satisfactory evaluation.
- Given a handwritten CMS-1500 form, type a CMS-1500 Health Insurance Claim Form and list

the reasons why the claim was either rejected or delayed within a reasonable time period and with enough accuracy to obtain a satisfactory evaluation.

▪ Given the patients' medical chart notes, ledger cards, encounter forms, and blank insurance claim forms, complete each CMS-1500 Health Insurance Claim Form for billing within a reasonable time period and with enough accuracy to obtain a satisfactory evaluation.

▪ Using the Mock Fee Schedule in Appendix A in this *Workbook*, correctly post payments, adjustments, and balances to the patients' ledger cards within a reasonable time period and with enough accuracy to obtain a satisfactory evaluation.

▪ Given a list of common medical abbreviations and symbols that appear in chart notes, fill in the correct meaning of each abbreviation within a reasonable time period and with enough accuracy to obtain a satisfactory evaluation.

STUDY OUTLINE

History

Compliance Issues Related to Insurance Claim Forms

Types of Claims
Claim Status

Abstracting from Medical Records
Cover Letter Accompanying Insurance Claims
Life or Health Insurance Applications

Health Insurance Claim Form (CMS-1500)
Basic Guidelines for Submitting a Claim
Completion of Insurance Claim Forms

Common Reasons Why Claim Forms Are Delayed or Rejected
Additional Reasons Why Claim Forms Are Delayed

Optical Scanning Format Guidelines
Optical Character Recognition
Do's and Don'ts for Optical Character Recognition

Procedure: Instructions for the Health Insurance Claim Form (CMS-1500)
Insurance Program Templates

SELF-STUDY **7–1** ▸ REVIEW QUESTIONS

Review the objectives, key terms, chapter information, glossary definitions of key terms, and figures before completing the following review questions.

1. Who developed the Standard Form? _____

2. State the name of the insurance form approved by the American Medical Association.

   _____

3. Does Medicare accept the CMS-1500 claim form? _____

4. What important document must you have before an insurance company can

   photocopy a patient's chart? _____

5. What is dual coverage? _____

6. The insurance company with the first responsibility for payment of a bill for medical

   services is known as _____.

7. Match the types of claims listed in the right column with their descriptions, and fill in the blanks with the appropriate letters.

_____ Claim missing required information

_____ Phrase used when a claim is held back from payment

_____ Claim that is submitted and then optically scanned by the insurance carrier and converted to electronic form

_____ Claim that needs manual processing because of errors or to solve a problem

_____ Claim that needs clarification and answers to some questions

_____ Claim that is submitted via telephone, fax, or claim computer modem

_____ Claim that is submitted within the time limit and claim correctly completed

_____ Medicare claim that contains information that is complete and necessary but is illogical or incorrect

a. clean claim

b. paper claim

c. invalid claim

d. dirty claim

e. electronic

f. suspense

g. rejected

h. incomplete claim

8. If the patient brings in a private insurance form that is not group insurance, where do

you send the form after completion? _____

9. Match the types of numbers listed in the right column with their descriptions, and fill in the blanks with the appropriate letters.

_____ A number issued by the federal government to each individual for personal use

_____ A Medicare lifetime provider number

_____ A number listed on a claim when submitting insurance claims to insurance companies under a group name

_____ A number issued by the Medicare program to each physician who treats patients and submits claims to this program

_____ A number that a physician must obtain to practice in a state

_____ A number used when billing for supplies and equipment

a. state license number

b. employer identification number

c. Social Security number

d. provider identification number

e. unique provider identification number

f. group provider number

_____ A number issued to a hospital

g. National Provider Identifier

_____ An individual physician's federal tax identification number issued by the Internal Revenue Service

h. durable medical equipment

_____ A number issued by the insurance carrier to every physician who renders services to patients

i. facility provider number

10. An insurance claim is returned for the reason "diagnosis incomplete." State one or more solutions to this problem on how you would try to obtain reimbursement.

_____

_____

_____

11. Indicate whether the following statements are true (T) or false (F).

   a. A photocopy of a claim form may be optically scanned.   _____

   b. Handwriting is permitted on optically scanned insurance claims.   _____

   c. Do not fold or crease an insurance form that will be optically scanned. _____

   d. Never strike over errors when making a correction on a claim form
      that is to be optically scanned.   _____

12. When preparing a claim that is to be optically scanned, birth dates are keyed

   in with how many digits? _____

13. Define this abbreviation: MG/MCD. _____

14. A CMS-assigned National Provider Identifier (NPI) number consists

   of _____ characters.

To check your answers to this self-study assignment, see Appendix D in this *Workbook*.

ASSIGNMENT 7-2 ▸ **COMPLETE A HEALTH INSURANCE CLAIM
FORM FOR A PRIVATE CASE**

Performance Objective

Task: Complete a health insurance claim form and post the information to the patient's financial
               account record/statement.

Conditions: Use Merry M. McLean's E/M code slip (Figure 7–1), patient record (Figure 7–2), and
               financial account record/statement (Figure 7–3); one health insurance claim form (Figure 7–4);
               a typewriter, computer, or pen; procedural and diagnostic code books; and Appendices A and B
               in the *Workbook*.

Standards: Claim Productivity Measurement

               Time: _____ minutes

               Accuracy: _____

               (Note: The time element and accuracy criteria may be given by your instructor.)

E/M Code Slip

Patient _McLean, Merry M._   Date _5-6-XX_
     CPT Code _____
     Dx Code _____

HISTORY

☐ Problem Focused
  Chief complaint; Brief history of present illness

☐ Expanded Problem Focused
  Chief complaint; Brief history of present illness;
  Problem pertinent system review

☑ Detailed
  Chief complaint: Extended history of present illness;
  Extended system review; Pertinent past family, social history

☐ Comprehensive
  Chief complaint; Extended history of present illness;
  Complete system review; Complete past family, social history

EXAMINATION

☐ Problem Focused
  Exam limited to affected body area or organ system

☐ Expanded Problem Focused
  Exam extended to other symptomatic or related organ
  systems

☑ Detailed
  Extended exam of affected area(s) and other
  symptomatic or related systems

☐ Comprehensive
  Complete single system specialty exam or complete
  multi-system exam

MEDICAL DECISION MAKING

Medical Decision	Number of Dx Options	Amount of Data	Risk M and M
☐ Straightforward	minimal 1 dx	minimal	minimal
☑ Low Complexity	limited 1-2 dx	limited	low
☐ Moderate Complexity	multiple 1-2 dx	moderate	moderate
☐ High Complexity	extensive 2-3 dx	extensive	high

☐ Counseling ☐ Time _____
☐ Consult ☐ Referring Dr. _Emdee Fine_
Diagnosis _See Pt record_

NP ☑   Est pt _____

Figure 7–1

Directions: Complete the Health Insurance Claim* Form, using OCR or ICR guidelines, and send the form to the Prudential Insurance Company for Mrs. Merry M. McLean by referring to her E/M code slip, patient record, and financial account record/statement. Date the claim June 15. Refer to Appendix A in this Workbook to fill in the fees on the financial account record/statement.

1. Use your CPT code book or Appendix A in this *Workbook* to determine the correct five-digit code number and modifiers for each professional service rendered.
2. Record on the financial account record/statement when you have billed the insurance company.
3. A Performance Evaluation Checklist may be reproduced from the "Instruction Guide to the Workbook" chapter if your instructor wishes you to submit it to assist with scoring and comments.
4. After the instructor has returned your work to you, either make the necessary corrections and place your work in a three-ring notebook for future reference or, if you received a high score, place it in your portfolio for reference when applying for a job.

Abbreviations pertinent to this record:

NP	_____	LC	_____
UA	_____	MDM	_____
Dx	_____	HV	_____
ptr	_____	PF	_____
Cysto	_____	SF	_____
Pt	_____	RTO	_____
Cont	_____	postop	_____
adm	_____	OV	_____
hosp	_____	lb	_____
C	_____	adv	_____
Hx	_____	retn	_____
exam	_____	est	_____

---

*See Chapter 7 in the *Handbook* for help in completing this form.

PATIENT RECORD NO. 7-2

McLean	Merry	M.	02-02-48	F	555-486-1859
LAST NAME	FIRST NAME	MIDDLE NAME	BIRTH DATE	SEX	HOME PHONE

4919 Dolphin Way	Woodland Hills,	XY	12345
ADDRESS	CITY	STATE	ZIP CODE

555-430-7709	555-098-3456	555-486-1859	McLean@WB.net
CELL PHONE	PAGER NO.	FAX NO.	E-MAIL ADDRESS

459-XX-9989	M0039857
PATIENT'S SOC. SEC. NO.	DRIVER'S LICENSE

Secretary	Porter Company
PATIENT'S OCCUPATION	NAME OF COMPANY

5490 Wilshire Blvd., Merck, XY 12346	555-446-7781
ADDRESS OF EMPLOYER	PHONE

Harry L. McLean	Computer programmer
SPOUSE OR PARENT	OCCUPATION

IBM Corporation	5616 Wilshire Blvd., Merck, XY 12346	555-664-9023
EMPLOYER	ADDRESS	PHONE

Prudential Insurance Co., 5621 Wilshire Blvd., Merck, XY 12346	Harry L. McLean
NAME OF INSURANCE	INSURED OR SUB SCRIBER

459-XX-9989	8832
POLICY/CERTIFICATE NO.	GROUP NO.

REFERRED BY:Emdee Fine, MD, 5000 Wilshire Blvd., Merck, XY 12346   NPI # 73027175XX

DATE	PROGRESS NOTES	No. 7-2
5-6-xx	NP presents in office with constant dribbling and wetting at night; uses 15 pads/day.	
	Began March 10, 20xx. Pelvic exam done—normal findings. No bladder or uterine	
	prolapse noted. UA dipstick performed (nonautomated with microscopy); few bacteria,	
	few urates. Dx: urinary incontinence. ptr 4 days for cystourethroscopy.	
	GU/llf	*Gene Ulibarri, MD*
5-10-xx	Cysto performed—revealed fistula of bladder with an opening into urinary bladder	
	and copious leakage into vagina. Schedule surgery to repair fistula. Pt cont to work.	
	GU/llf	*Gene Ulibarri, MD*
5-16-xx	Adm to College hosp. C hx/exam LC MDM. Dx: vesicovaginal fistula.	
	GU/llf	*Gene Ulibarri, MD*
5-17-xx	Closure of vesicovaginal fistula; abdominal approach.	
	GU/llf	*Gene Ulibarri, MD*
5-18-xx thru	Saw patient in hospital (HV) PF hx/exam SF MDM.	
5-21-xx	GU/llf	*Gene Ulibarri, MD*
5-22-xx	Discharge from hospital. RTO 2 weeks.	
	GU/llf	*Gene Ulibarri, MD*
6-5-xx	Post-op OV. Patient presents complaining of pain near operative site. Pt reports she has	
	been walking daily and lifting more than 5 lb objects. Pt adv no excessive walking,	
	no lifting, stooping, or bending until surgical site is completely healed. Retn to clinic in	
	1 wk. Est return to work 7-1-xx. PF hx/exam SF MDM.	
	GU/llf	*Gene Ulibarri, MD*

Figure 7–2

Acct No. 7-2

STATEMENT
Financial Account
COLLEGE CLINIC
4567 Broad Avenue
Woodland Hills, XY 12345-0001
Tel. 555-486-9002
Fax No. 555-487-8976

Merry McLean
4919 Dolphin Way
Woodland Hills, XY 12345

Phone No. (H) (555) 486-1859   (W) (555) 446-7781   Birthdate   02-02-48

Primary Insurance Co.   Prudential Insurance Co.   Policy/Group No.   459-XX-9989/8832

	REFERENCE	DESCRIPTION	CHARGES	CREDITS PYMNTS.	ADJ.	BALANCE	
20XX			BALANCE FORWARD				
05-06-xx		OV NP					
05-06-xx		UA					
05-10-xx		Cystourethroscopy					
5-16-xx		Initial hosp care					
05-17-xx		Repair vesicovaginal fistula					
05-18 to 05-22-xx		HV					
05-22-xx		Discharge					
06-05-xx		PO-OV					

PLEASE PAY LAST AMOUNT IN BALANCE COLUMN

THIS IS A COPY OF YOUR FINANCIAL ACCOUNT AS IT APPEARS ON OUR RECORDS

Figure 7–3

PLEASE
DO NOT
STAPLE
IN THIS
AREA

HEALTH INSURANCE CLAIM FORM

PICA		PICA

1. MEDICARE MEDICAID CHAMPUS CHAMPVA GROUP HEALTH PLAN FECA BLK LUNG OTHER

(Medicare #) (Medicaid #) (Sponsor's SSN) (VA File #) (SSN or ID) (S SN) (ID)

1a. INSURED'S I.D. NUMBER (FOR PROGRAM IN ITEM 1)

2. PATIENT'S NAME (Last Name, First Name, Middle Initial)

3. PATIENT'S BIRTH DATE MM DD YY SEX M F

4. INSURED'S NAME (Last Name, First Name, Middle Initial)

5. PATIENT'S ADDRESS (No., Street)

6. PATIENT RELATIONSHIP TO INSURED Self Spouse Child Other

7. INSURED'S ADDRESS (No., Street)

CITY STATE

8. PATIENT STATUS Single Married Other

Employed Full-Time Student Part-Time Student

CITY STATE

ZIP CODE TELEPHONE (Include Area Code)

ZIP CODE TELEPHONE (INCLUDE AREA CODE)

9. OTHER INSURED'S NAME (Last Name, First Name, Middle Initial)

10. IS PATIENT'S CONDITION RELATED TO:

11. INSURED'S POLICY GROUP OR FECA NUMBER

a. OTHER INSURED'S POLICY OR GROUP NUMBER

a. EMPLOYMENT? (CURRENT OR PREVIOUS) YES NO

a. INSURED'S DATE OF BIRTH MM DD YY SEX M F

b. OTHER INSURED'S DATE OF BIRTH MM DD YY SEX M F

b. AUTO ACCIDENT? PLACE (State) YES NO

b. EMPLOYER'S NAME OR SCHOOL NAME

c. EMPLOYER'S NAME OR SCHOOL NAME

c. OTHER ACCIDENT? YES NO

c. INSURANCE PLAN NAME OR PROGRAM NAME

d. INSURANCE PLAN NAME OR PROGRAM NAME

10d. RESERVED FOR LOCAL USE

d. IS THERE ANOTHER HEALTH BENEFIT PLAN? YES NO *If yes*, return to and complete item 9 a-d.

READ BACK OF FORM BEFORE COMPLETING & SIGNING THIS FORM.

12. PATIENT'S OR AUTHORIZED PERSON'S SIGNATURE I authorize the release of any medical or other information necessary to process this claim. I also request payment of government benefits either to myself or to the party who accepts assignment below.

SIGNED _____ DATE _____

13. INSURED'S OR AUTHORIZED PERSON'S SIGNATURE I authorize payment of medical benefits to the undersigned physician or supplier for services described below.

SIGNED _____

14. DATE OF CURRENT: MM DD YY ILLNESS (First symptom) OR INJURY (Accident) OR PREGNANCY(LMP)

15. IF PATIENT HAS HAD SAME OR SIMILAR ILLNESS. GIVE FIRST DATE MM DD YY

16. DATES PATIENT UNABLE TO WORK IN CURRENT OCCUPATION MM DD YY FROM TO MM DD YY

17. NAME OF REFERRING PHYSICIAN OR OTHER SOURCE

17a. I.D. NUMBER OF REFERRING PHYSICIAN

18. HOSPITALIZATION DATES RELATED TO CURRENT SERVICES MM DD YY FROM TO MM DD YY

19. RESERVED FOR LOCAL USE

20. OUTSIDE LAB? $ CHARGES YES NO

21. DIAGNOSIS OR NATURE OF ILLNESS OR INJURY. (RELATE ITEMS 1,2,3 OR 4 TO ITEM 24E BY LINE)

1. ___ 3. ___
2. ___ 4. ___

22. MEDICAID RESUBMISSION CODE ORIGINAL REF. NO.

23. PRIOR AUTHORIZATION NUMBER

24. A						B	C	D		E	F	G	H	I	J	K
DATE(S) OF SERVICE From — To						Place of Service	Type of Service	PROCEDURES, SERVICES, OR SUPPLIES (Explain Unusual Circumstances) CPT/HCPCS | MODIFIER		DIAGNOSIS CODE	$ CHARGES	DAYS OR UNITS	EPSDT Family Plan	EMG	COB	RESERVED FOR LOCAL USE
MM	DD	YY	MM	DD	YY											

25. FEDERAL TAX I.D. NUMBER SSN EIN

26. PATIENT'S ACCOUNT NO.

27. ACCEPT ASSIGNMENT? (For govt. claims, see back) YES NO

28. TOTAL CHARGE $

29. AMOUNT PAID $

30. BALANCE DUE $

31. SIGNATURE OF PHYSICIAN OR SUPPLIER INCLUDING DEGREES OR CREDENTIALS (I certify that the statements on the reverse apply to this bill and are made a part thereof.)

SIGNED _____ DATE _____

32. NAME AND ADDRESS OF FACILITY WHERE SERVICES WERE RENDERED (If other than home or office)

33. PHYSICIAN'S, SUPPLIER'S BILLING NAME, ADDRESS, ZIP CODE & PHONE #

PIN# GRP#

(APPROVED BY AMA COUNCIL ON MEDICAL SERVICE 8/88) *PLEASE PRINT OR TYPE*

APPROVED OMB-0938-0008 FORM CMS-1500 (12-90), FORM RRB-1500, APPROVED OMB-1215-0055 FORM OWCP-1500, APPROVED OMB-0720-0001 (CHAMPUS)

CARRIER PATIENT AND INSURED INFORMATION PHYSICIAN OR SUPPLIER INFORMATION

EXAMPLE ONLY

Figure 7–4

ASSIGNMENT **7-3** ▸ **COMPLETE A HEALTH INSURANCE CLAIM FORM**
FOR A PRIVATE CASE

Performance Objective

Task: Complete a health insurance claim form and post the information to the patient's financial
                 account record/statement.

Conditions: Use Billy S. Rubin's E/M code slip (Figure 7–5), patient record (Figure 7–6), and financial account
                 record/statement (Figure 7–7); one health insurance claim form (Figure 7–8); a typewriter,
                 computer, or pen; procedural and diagnostic code books; and Appendices A and B in this *Workbook*.

Standards: Claim Productivity Measurement

                 Time: _____ minutes

                 Accuracy: _____

                 (Note: The time element and accuracy criteria may be given by your instructor.)

Directions: Complete the Health Insurance Claim Form* on Mr. Billy S. Rubin for processing and send it to
Aetna Life and Casualty Company by referring to Mr. Rubin's E/M code slip, patient record, and financial account
record/statement. Date the claim August 30. Refer to Appendix A in this *Workbook* to fill in the fees on the financial
statement. Use OCR guidelines.

_____

*See Chapter 7 in the *Handbook* for help in completing this form.

E/M Code Slip

Patient _Rubin, Billy S._   Date *_____
                                                                             CPT Code_____
                                                                             Dx code_____

HISTORY   EXAMINATION

☑ Problem Focused   ☑ Problem Focused
  Chief complaint; Brief history of present illness   Exam limited to affected body area or organ system

☐ Expanded Problem Focused   ☐ Expanded Problem Focused
  Chief complaint; Brief history of present illness;   Exam extended to other symptomatic or related organ
  Problem pertinent system review   systems

☐ Detailed   ☐ Detailed
  Chief complaint: Extended history of present illness;   Extended exam of affected area(s) and other
  Extended system review; Pertinent past family, social history symptomatic or related symptoms

☐ Comprehensive   ☐ Comprehensive
  Chief complaint; Extended history of present illness;   Complete single system specialty exam or complete
  Complete system review; Complete past family, social history multi-system exam

MEDICAL DECISION MAKING

	Medical Decision	Number of Dx Options	Amount of Data	Risk M and M
☐	Straightforward	minimal 1 dx	minimal	minimal
☑	Low Complexity	limited 1-2 dx	limited	low
☐	Moderate Complexity	multiple 1-2 dx	moderate	moderate
☐	High Complexity	extensive 2-3 dx	extensive	high

☐ Counseling ☐ Time _____
☐ Consult ☑ Referring Dr. _U.R. Wright_
Diagnosis _see pt. record_

NP_____   Est pt ☑

* For space constraints, this E/M code slip is being used for 8-7-00, 8-14-00, and 8-16-00

Figure 7–5

1. Use your CPT code book or Appendix A in this *Workbook* to determine the correct five-digit code number and modifiers for each professional service rendered. Do not include no charge entries on the claim form.
2. Record when you have billed the insurance company on the financial account record/statement.
3. On September 1, Mr. Rubin sends you check No. 421 in the amount of $200 to apply to his account. Post this entry and calculate the balance due.
4. A Performance Evaluation Checklist may be reproduced from the "Instruction Guide to the Workbook" chapter if your instructor wishes you to submit it to assist with scoring and comments.
5. After the instructor has returned your work to you, either make the necessary corrections and place your work in a three-ring notebook for future reference, or, if you received a high score, place it in your portfolio for reference when applying for a job.

Abbreviations pertinent to this record:

est	_____	TURP	_____
pt	_____	wks	_____
CC	_____	HV	_____
BC	_____	PF	_____
diff	_____	hx	_____
PSA	_____	exam	_____
bx	_____	SF	_____
STAT	_____	MDM	_____
PTR	_____	Disch	_____
CA	_____	hosp	_____
adm	_____	postop	_____
surg	_____		

Additional Coding

1. Determine CPT codes that you would use to bill for College Hospital from the following services mentioned in the patient's progress notes.

A. Blood draw (venipuncture)

_____

B. Complete blood cell count (CBC) (automated) with differential

_____

C. Prostate-specific antigen (PSA) (total)

_____

D. Ultrasonography with guided fine-needle biopsy

_____

PATIENT RECORD NO. 7-3

Rubin	Billy	S.	11-09-53	M	555-893-5770
LAST NAME	FIRST NAME	MIDDLE NAME	BIRTH DATE	SEX	HOME PHONE

547 North Oliver Rd.	Woodland Hills	XY	12345	
ADDRESS	CITY	STATE	ZIP CODE	

555-430-9080	555-987-7790	555-893-5770	Rubin@WB.net
CELL PHONE	PAGER NO.	FAX NO.	E-MAIL ADDRESS

505-XX-1159	R0398056
PATIENT'S SOC. SEC. NO.	DRIVER'S LICENSE

salesman	Nate's Clothier's
PATIENT'S OCCUPATION	NAME OF COMPANY

7786 East Chabner Blvd., Dorland, XY 12347	555-449-6605
ADDRESS OF EMPLOYER	PHONE

Lydia B. Rubin (wife)
SPOUSE OR PARENT

EMPLOYER	ADDRESS	PHONE

Aetna Life and Casualty Co., 3055 Wilshire Blvd., Merck, XY 12345	Billy S. Rubin
NAME OF INSURANCE	INSURED OR SUB SCRIBER

42107	2641
POLICY/CERTIFICATE NO.	GROUP NO.

REFERRED BY: U. R. Wright, MD, 5010 Wrong Road, Torres, XY 12349   555-907-5440   NPI # 271385554XX

DATE	PROGRESS NOTES	No. 7-3
8-7-xx	Office exam est pt. CC: urinary hesitancy, frequency and posturinary dribbling since	
	July 15 of this year. Exam revealed hard nodule in prostate. Sent pt to College Hospital for	
	laboratory work; CBC (automated with diff) and PSA (total). PTR in 1 wk.	
	GU/llf	*Gene Ulibarri, MD*
8-14-xx	Office exam. PSA elevated (5.6), CBC normal. Explained to pt that biopsy is needed at this	
	point; may be done as outpatient at College Hospital. Pt elected to have immediate	
	bx;arrangements made for stat. ultrasound with guided fine needle bx. PTR in 2 days for	
	results.	
	GU/llf	*Gene Ulibarri, MD*
8-16-xx	Pt returns for bx report; positive for CA in situ of prostate. Advised patient that an	
	operation is necessary and explained surgical procedure, risks, and complications.	
	Arranged for adm to College Hospital on 8/22/xx.	
	GU/llf	*Gene Ulibarri, MD*
8-22-xx	Admit to College Hospital. Surg: TURP. Pt tolerated surg well and is comfortable in the	
	recovery room. Pt last worked 8/21/xx; est disability 6 to 8 wks. Est return to work on	
	10/22/xx.	
	GU/llf	*Gene Ulibarri, MD*
8-23-xx thru	HV (PF hx/exam SF MDM)	
8-26-xx	GU/llf	*Gene Ulibarri, MD*
8-27-xx	Disch from hosp. Pt confined at home for 1 week at which time patient will return to	
	office for postop check.	
	GU/llf	*Gene Ulibarri, MD*

Figure 7–6

Acct No. _7-3_

STATEMENT
Financial Account
COLLEGE CLINIC
4567 Broad Avenue
Woodland Hills, XY 12345-0001
Tel. 555-486-9002
Fax No. 555-487-8976

Billy S. Rubin
547 North Oliver Road
Woodland Hills, XY 12345

Phone No. (H)_ (555) 893-5770 _   (W)_ (555) 449-6605 _   Birthdate_ 11-09-53 _

Primary Insurance Co._ Aetna Life and Casualty Co. _   Policy/Group No. _ 421074/2641 _

	REFERENCE	DESCRIPTION	CHARGES	CREDITS PYMNTS.	ADJ.	BALANCE	
20XX			BALANCE FORWARD ➡				
08-07-xx		OV Est Pt					
08-14-xx		OV Est Pt					
08-16-xx		OV Est Pt					
08-22-xx		TURP					
08-23 to 08-26-xx		HV					
08-27-xx		Discharge					

PLEASE PAY LAST AMOUNT IN BALANCE COLUMN ⬆

THIS IS A COPY OF YOUR FINANCIAL ACCOUNT AS IT APPEARS ON OUR RECORDS

Figure 7–7

PLEASE
DO NOT
STAPLE
IN THIS
AREA

CARRIER

HEALTH INSURANCE CLAIM FORM

PICA | | | PICA | |

1. MEDICARE ☐ (Medicare #)   MEDICAID ☐ (Medicaid #)   CHAMPUS ☐ (Sponsor's SSN)   CHAMPVA ☐ (VA File #)   GROUP HEALTH PLAN ☐ (SSN or ID)   FECA BLK LUNG ☐ (S SN)   OTHER ☐ (ID)
1a. INSURED'S I.D. NUMBER   (FOR PROGRAM IN ITEM 1)

2. PATIENT'S NAME (Last Name, First Name, Middle Initial)
3. PATIENT'S BIRTH DATE MM DD YY   SEX M ☐ F ☐
4. INSURED'S NAME (Last Name, First Name, Middle Initial)

5. PATIENT'S ADDRESS (No., Street)
6. PATIENT RELATIONSHIP TO INSURED   Self ☐ Spouse ☐ Child ☐ Other ☐
7. INSURED'S ADDRESS (No., Street)

CITY   STATE
8. PATIENT STATUS   Single ☐ Married ☐ Other ☐
CITY   STATE

ZIP CODE   TELEPHONE (Include Area Code))
Employed ☐ Full-Time Student ☐ Part-Time Student ☐
ZIP CODE   TELEPHONE (INCLUDE AREA CODE)

9. OTHER INSURED'S NAME (Last Name, First Name, Middle Initial)
10. IS PATIENT'S CONDITION RELATED TO:
11. INSURED'S POLICY GROUP OR FECA NUMBER

a. OTHER INSURED'S POLICY OR GROUP NUMBER
a. EMPLOYMENT? (CURRENT OR PREVIOUS) YES ☐ NO ☐
a. INSURED'S DATE OF BIRTH MM DD YY   SEX M ☐ F ☐

b. OTHER INSURED'S DATE OF BIRTH MM DD YY SEX M ☐ F ☐
b. AUTO ACCIDENT?   PLACE (State) YES ☐ NO ☐
b. EMPLOYER'S NAME OR SCHOOL NAME

c. EMPLOYER'S NAME OR SCHOOL NAME
c. OTHER ACCIDENT? YES ☐ NO ☐
c. INSURANCE PLAN NAME OR PROGRAM NAME

d. INSURANCE PLAN NAME OR PROGRAM NAME
10d. RESERVED FOR LOCAL USE
d. IS THERE ANOTHER HEALTH BENEFIT PLAN? YES ☐ NO ☐ *If yes*, return to and complete item 9 a-d.

READ BACK OF FORM BEFORE COMPLETING & SIGNING THIS FORM.
12. PATIENT'S OR AUTHORIZED PERSON'S SIGNATURE I authorize the release of any medical or other information necessary to process this claim. I also request payment of government benefits either to myself or to the party who accepts assignment below.
SIGNED _____ DATE _____
13. INSURED'S OR AUTHORIZED PERSON'S SIGNATURE I authorize payment of medical benefits to the undersigned physician or supplier for services described below.
SIGNED _____

14. DATE OF CURRENT: ILLNESS (First symptom) OR INJURY (Accident) OR PREGNANCY(LMP) MM DD YY
15. IF PATIENT HAS HAD SAME OR SIMILAR ILLNESS. GIVE FIRST DATE MM DD YY
16. DATES PATIENT UNABLE TO WORK IN CURRENT OCCUPATION FROM MM DD YY TO MM DD YY

17. NAME OF REFERRING PHYSICIAN OR OTHER SOURCE
17a. I.D. NUMBER OF REFERRING PHYSICIAN
18. HOSPITALIZATION DATES RELATED TO CURRENT SERVICES FROM MM DD YY TO MM DD YY

19. RESERVED FOR LOCAL USE
20. OUTSIDE LAB? YES ☐ NO ☐ $ CHARGES

21. DIAGNOSIS OR NATURE OF ILLNESS OR INJURY. (RELATE ITEMS 1,2,3 OR 4 TO ITEM 24E BY LINE)
1. _____ 3. _____
2. _____ 4. _____
22. MEDICAID RESUBMISSION CODE   ORIGINAL REF. NO.
23. PRIOR AUTHORIZATION NUMBER

24. A DATE(S) OF SERVICE From MM DD YY To MM DD YY	B Place of Service	C Type of Service	D PROCEDURES, SERVICES, OR SUPPLIES (Explain Unusual Circumstances) CPT/HCPCS MODIFIER	E DIAGNOSIS CODE	F $ CHARGES	G DAYS OR UNITS	H EPSDT Family Plan	I EMG	J COB	K RESERVED FOR LOCAL USE
1										
2										
3										
4										
5										
6										

25. FEDERAL TAX I.D. NUMBER SSN ☐ EIN ☐
26. PATIENT'S ACCOUNT NO.
27. ACCEPT ASSIGNMENT? (For govt. claims, see back) YES ☐ NO ☐
28. TOTAL CHARGE $
29. AMOUNT PAID $
30. BALANCE DUE $

31. SIGNATURE OF PHYSICIAN OR SUPPLIER INCLUDING DEGREES OR CREDENTIALS (I certify that the statements on the reverse apply to this bill and are made a part thereof.)
SIGNED _____ DATE _____
32. NAME AND ADDRESS OF FACILITY WHERE SERVICES WERE RENDERED (If other than home or office)
33. PHYSICIAN'S, SUPPLIER'S BILLING NAME, ADDRESS, ZIP CODE & PHONE #
PIN# _____ GRP# _____

(APPROVED BY AMA COUNCIL ON MEDICAL SERVICE 8/88)   **PLEASE PRINT OR TYPE**
APPROVED OMB-0938-0008 FORM CMS-1500 (12-90), FORM RRB-1500,
APPROVED OMB-1215-0055 FORM OWCP-1500,   APPROVED OMB-0720-0001 (CHAMPUS)

Figure 7–8

ASSIGNMENT 7-4 ▸ COMPLETE TWO HEALTH INSURANCE CLAIM FORMS FOR A PRIVATE CASE

Performance Objective

Task: Complete two health insurance claim forms and post the information to the patient's financial account record/statement.

Conditions: Use Walter J. Stone's E/M code slip (Figure 7–9), patient record (Figure 7–10), and financial account record/statement (Figure 7–11); one health insurance claim form (Figure 7–12) and a photocopy of this form to use for the second claim; a typewriter, computer, or pen; procedural and diagnostic code books; and Appendices A and B in this *Workbook.*

Standards: Claim Productivity Measurement

Time: _____ minutes

Accuracy: _____

(Note: The time element and accuracy criteria may be given by your instructor.)

Directions: You will be billing for all services listed on the patient's progress notes for Dr. Gaston Input. Note that the patient was hospitalized twice, which necessitates two claim forms.

Figure 7–9

Complete two Health Insurance Claim Forms,* addressing them to Travelers Insurance Company for Mr. Walter J. Stone by referring to his E/M code slip, patient record, and financial account record/statement. Date the claims June 1. Refer to Appendix A in this *Workbook* to fill in the fees on the financial account record/statement. Use OCR guidelines.

1. Use your CPT code book or Appendix A in this *Workbook* to determine the correct five-digit code number and modifiers for each professional service rendered. The surgeon, Dr. Cutler, is charging $714.99 for the cholecystectomy. You are submitting a claim for the assistant surgeon, Dr. Input, and calculating a standard 20% of the surgeon's fee.
2. On May 14, the insurance company sends the physician a check, number 48572, for $25. Post this entry.
3. Record on the financial account record/statement when you have billed the insurance company.
4. A Performance Evaluation Checklist may be reproduced from the "Instruction Guide to the Workbook" chapter if your instructor wishes you to submit it to assist with scoring and comments.
5. After the instructor has returned your work to you, either make the necessary corrections and place your work in a three-ring notebook for future reference or, if you received a high score, place it in your portfolio for reference when applying for a job.

Abbreviations pertinent to this record:

est	_____	exam	_____
pt	_____	LC	_____
ER	_____	MDM	_____
BP	_____	EGD	_____
Dx	_____	bx	_____
GI	_____	ofc	_____
HV	_____	wk	_____
PF	_____	OV	_____
hx	_____	adv	_____

Additional Coding

1. Refer to Mr. Stone's patient record, abstract information, and code the procedures for services that would be billed by the hospital.

Description of Service   *Code*

a. _____   _____

b. _____   _____

c. _____   _____

---

*See Chapter 7 in the *Handbook* for help in completing this form.

PATIENT RECORD NO. 7-4

Stone	Walter	J.	03-14-49	M	555-345-0776
LAST NAME	FIRST NAME	MIDDLE NAME	BIRTH DATE	SEX	HOME PHONE

2008 Converse Street	Woodland Hills	XY	12345
ADDRESS	CITY	STATE	ZIP CODE

555-980-7750	555-930-5674	555-345-0776	Stone@WB.net
CELL PHONE	PAGER NO.	FAX NO.	E-MAIL ADDRESS

456-XX-9989	H9834706
PATIENT'S SOC. SEC. NO.	DRIVER'S LICENSE

advertising agent	R. V. Black and Associates
PATIENT'S OCCUPATION	NAME OF COMPANY

1267 Broad Street, Woodland Hills, XY 12345	555-345-6012
ADDRESS OF EMPLOYER	PHONE

widower
SPOUSE OR PARENT

EMPLOYER	ADDRESS	PHONE

Travelers Insurance Co. 5460 Olympic Blvd., Woodland Hills, XY 12345	Walter J. Stone
NAME OF INSURANCE	INSURED OR SUB SCRIBER

456-XX-9989	6754
POLICY/CERTIFICATE NO.	GROUP NO.

REFERRED BY: John B. Stone (brother), former patient of Dr. Input

DATE	PROGRESS NOTES	No. 7-4
5-3-xx	Est pt presented in ER after experiencing sudden onset of profuse rectal bleeding with	
	nausea and severe abdominal pains. Elevated BP 180/100. Dr. Input called to ER by	
	Dr. Cutler who recommended pt be admitted for further evaluation and diagnostic workup.	
	Dr. Input performed a comprehensive history and examination with moderate complexity	
	decision making and admitted the pt to College Hospital. Dx: Unspecified GI hemorrhage.	
	Pt disabled from work.	
	GI/llf	*Gaston Input, MD*
5-4-xx	HV (PF hx/exam LC MDM). Pt symptoms have subsided somewhat. Cholecystography	
	with oral contrast and complete abdominal ultrasound confirmed inflammatory gallbladder	
	with stones. EGD with bx confirmed prepyloric gastric ulcer.	
	GI/llf	*Gaston Input, MD*
5-5-xx	Discharged to home. Pt to be seen in ofc in 1 wk.	
	GI/llf	*Gaston Input, MD*
5-12-xx	Pt returns for an OV. Pt complains of ongoing GI distress. Continued elevated	
	BP of 186/98 shows a concern for hypertension. Adv to see Dr. Cutler for further	
	evaluation and possible surgery. DX: Acute prepyloric gastric ulcer with hemorrhage,	
	cholecystitis with cholelithiasis, benign hypertension.	
	GI/llf	*Gaston Input, MD*
5-16-xx	Pt admitted to College Hospital by surgeon, Dr. Cutler. He performed a laparoscopic	
	cholecystectomy in which I assisted. Pt will resume work on 6/22/xx.	
	GI/llf	*Gaston Input, MD*

Figure 7–10

Acct No. _7-4_

STATEMENT
Financial Account
COLLEGE CLINIC
4567 Broad Avenue
Woodland Hills, XY 12345-001
Tel. 555-486-9002
Fax No. 555-487-8976

Walter J. Stone
2008 Converse Street
Woodland Hills, XY 12345

Phone No. (H) _(555) 345-0776_   (W) _(555) 345-6012_   Birthdate _03-14-49_

Primary Insurance Co. _Travelers Insurance Co,_   Policy/Group No. _456-XX9989/6754_

20XX	REFERENCE	DESCRIPTION	CHARGES		CREDITS PYMNTS.	ADJ.		BALANCE	
20XX				BALANCE FORWARD ➡					
01-03-xx	99214	OV	61	51				61	51
01-15-xx	01-03-xx	Billed Travelers Ins.						61	51
03-02-xx	Ck 95268	ROA Travlers Ins.			49	21		12	30
03-03-xx	99213	OV	40	20				52	50
04-03-xx	3-3-xx	Billed Travelers Ins.						52	50
05-03-xx		Initial hosp care							
05-04-xx		HV							
05-05-xx		Discharge							
05-12-xx		OV							
05-16-xx		Cholecystectomy Asst.							

PLEASE PAY LAST AMOUNT IN BALANCE COLUMN ⬆

THIS IS A COPY OF YOUR FINANCIAL ACCOUNT AS IT APPEARS ON OUR RECORDS

Figure 7–11

PLEASE
DO NOT
STAPLE
IN THIS
AREA

CARRIER

HEALTH INSURANCE CLAIM FORM

| | PICA | | | | | | | | PICA | | |

1. MEDICARE ☐ (Medicare #) MEDICAID ☐ (Medicaid #) CHAMPUS ☐ (Sponsor's SSN) CHAMPVA ☐ (VA File #) GROUP HEALTH PLAN ☐ (SSN or ID) FECA BLK LUNG ☐ (S SN) OTHER ☐ (ID)   **1a.** INSURED'S I.D. NUMBER   (FOR PROGRAM IN ITEM 1)

2. PATIENT'S NAME (Last Name, First Name, Middle Initial)

3. PATIENT'S BIRTH DATE MM | DD | YY   SEX M ☐ F ☐

4. INSURED'S NAME (Last Name, First Name, Middle Initial)

5. PATIENT'S ADDRESS (No., Street)

6. PATIENT RELATIONSHIP TO INSURED   Self ☐ Spouse ☐ Child ☐ Other ☐

7. INSURED'S ADDRESS (No., Street)

CITY   STATE

8. PATIENT STATUS   Single ☐ Married ☐ Other ☐

CITY   STATE

ZIP CODE   TELEPHONE (Include Area Code) ( )

Employed ☐ Full-Time Student ☐ Part-Time Student ☐

ZIP CODE   TELEPHONE (INCLUDE AREA CODE)

9. OTHER INSURED'S NAME (Last Name, First Name, Middle Initial)

10. IS PATIENT'S CONDITION RELATED TO:

11. INSURED'S POLICY GROUP OR FECA NUMBER

a. OTHER INSURED'S POLICY OR GROUP NUMBER

a. EMPLOYMENT? (CURRENT OR PREVIOUS) YES ☐ NO ☐

a. INSURED'S DATE OF BIRTH MM | DD | YY   SEX M ☐ F ☐

b. OTHER INSURED'S DATE OF BIRTH MM | DD | YY   SEX M ☐ F ☐

b. AUTO ACCIDENT?   PLACE (State) YES ☐ NO ☐

b. EMPLOYER'S NAME OR SCHOOL NAME

c. EMPLOYER'S NAME OR SCHOOL NAME

c. OTHER ACCIDENT? YES ☐ NO ☐

c. INSURANCE PLAN NAME OR PROGRAM NAME

d. INSURANCE PLAN NAME OR PROGRAM NAME

10d. RESERVED FOR LOCAL USE

d. IS THERE ANOTHER HEALTH BENEFIT PLAN? YES ☐ NO ☐ *If yes*, return to and complete item 9 a-d.

READ BACK OF FORM BEFORE COMPLETING & SIGNING THIS FORM.
12. PATIENT'S OR AUTHORIZED PERSON'S SIGNATURE I authorize the release of any medical or other information necessary to process this claim. I also request payment of government benefits either to myself or to the party who accepts assignment below.

SIGNED _____   DATE _____

13. INSURED'S OR AUTHORIZED PERSON'S SIGNATURE I authorize payment of medical benefits to the undersigned physician or supplier for services described below.

SIGNED _____

PATIENT AND INSURED INFORMATION

EXAMPLE ONLY

14. DATE OF CURRENT: MM | DD | YY ◄ ILLNESS (First symptom) OR INJURY (Accident) OR PREGNANCY(LMP)

15. IF PATIENT HAS HAD SAME OR SIMILAR ILLNESS. GIVE FIRST DATE MM | DD | YY

16. DATES PATIENT UNABLE TO WORK IN CURRENT OCCUPATION FROM MM | DD | YY TO MM | DD | YY

17. NAME OF REFERRING PHYSICIAN OR OTHER SOURCE

17a. I.D. NUMBER OF REFERRING PHYSICIAN

18. HOSPITALIZATION DATES RELATED TO CURRENT SERVICES FROM MM | DD | YY TO MM | DD | YY

19. RESERVED FOR LOCAL USE

20. OUTSIDE LAB? $ CHARGES YES ☐ NO ☐

21. DIAGNOSIS OR NATURE OF ILLNESS OR INJURY. (RELATE ITEMS 1,2,3 OR 4 TO ITEM 24E BY LINE)

1. L___   3. L___
2. L___   4. L___

22. MEDICAID RESUBMISSION CODE   ORIGINAL REF. NO.

23. PRIOR AUTHORIZATION NUMBER

24. A DATE(S) OF SERVICE						B	C	D PROCEDURES, SERVICES, OR SUPPLIES		E	F	G	H	I	J	K
From			To			Place of Service	Type of Service	(Explain Unusual Circumstances)		DIAGNOSIS CODE	$ CHARGES	DAYS OR UNITS	EPSDT Family Plan	EMG	COB	RESERVED FOR LOCAL USE
MM	DD	YY	MM	DD	YY			CPT/HCPCS	MODIFIER							
1																
2																
3																
4																
5																
6																

25. FEDERAL TAX I.D. NUMBER SSN ☐ EIN ☐

26. PATIENT'S ACCOUNT NO.

27. ACCEPT ASSIGNMENT? (For govt. claims, see back) YES ☐ NO ☐

28. TOTAL CHARGE $

29. AMOUNT PAID $

30. BALANCE DUE $

31. SIGNATURE OF PHYSICIAN OR SUPPLIER INCLUDING DEGREES OR CREDENTIALS (I certify that the statements on the reverse apply to this bill and are made a part thereof.)

SIGNED _____   DATE _____

32. NAME AND ADDRESS OF FACILITY WHERE SERVICES WERE RENDERED (If other than home or office)

33. PHYSICIAN'S, SUPPLIER'S BILLING NAME, ADDRESS, ZIP CODE & PHONE #

PIN#   GRP#

PHYSICIAN OR SUPPLIER INFORMATION

(APPROVED BY AMA COUNCIL ON MEDICAL SERVICE 8/88)   ***PLEASE PRINT OR TYPE***   APPROVED OMB-0938-0008 FORM CMS-1500 (12-90), FORM RRB-1500,
APPROVED OMB-1215-0055 FORM OWCP-1500,   APPROVED OMB-0720-0001 (CHAMPUS)

Figure 7–12

ASSIGNMENT 7–5 ▶ LOCATE ERRORS ON A COMPLETED HEALTH INSURANCE CLAIM FORM

Performance Objective

Task: Complete a health insurance claim form and post the information to the patient's ledger card.

Conditions: Use Tom N. Parkinson's completed insurance claim (Figure 7–13), one health insurance claim form (Figure 7–14), and either a typewriter and/or computer or a pen.

Standards: Time: _____ minutes

                Accuracy: _____

                (Note: The time element and accuracy criteria may be given by your instructor.)

Guidance: To alleviate frustration and ease the process of completing a claim form for the first time, you will be editing a claim and then taking the correct information and inserting it on a blank CMS-1500 form (see Figure 7–14). Refer to Chapter 7 in the Handbook for block-by-block private payer instructions for completing the CMS-1500 insurance claim form. Refer to Figure 7–6 in the Handbook for visual placement of data. Refer to Appendix A in this Workbook for the physician/clinic information and the clinic's mock fee schedule. The billing physician is Gerald Practon. The name of the insurance carrier is ABC Insurance Company at 111 Main Street in Denver, CO, 80210.

Directions: Study the completed claim form (see Figure 7–13) and search for missing or incorrect information. If possible, verify all information. Highlight or circle in red all incorrect or missing information. Insert the correct information on the claim form. Now transfer all the data to a blank CMS-1500 claim form (see Figure 7–14). If mandatory information is missing, insert the word "NEED" in the corresponding block of the claim form.

   A Performance Evaluation Checklist may be reproduced from the "Instruction Guide to the Workbook" chapter if your instructor wishes you to submit it to assist with scoring and comments.

Optional: List, in block-by-block order, the reasons why the claim may be either rejected or delayed according to the errors found.

General Directions for Claim Form Completion

Assume that the Health Insurance Claim Form* CMS-1500 is printed in red ink for processing by OCR or ICR. Complete the form using OCR/ICR guidelines pertinent to the type of carrier that you are billing (e.g., private, Medicare, TRICARE) and send it to the proper insurance carrier. Refer to Chapter 7 in the *Handbook* for block instructions for each major type of insurance carrier. All blocks are clearly labeled, and each major carrier has an icon that is color coded for easy reference. Claim form templates have been completed to use as visual examples for placement of data; they may be found at the end of Chapter 7 in the *Handbook*. Screened areas on each form do not apply to the insurance program example shown and should be left blank.

   Many physicians complete an evaluation and management (E/M) code slip for each patient encounter. Chapter 7 assignments feature this form as a reference for part of each exercise and are used to assist you with E/M *Current Procedural Terminology* (CPT) code selection. In future assignments, you identify key components for E/M services in the medical record. All physicians in College Clinic accept assignment of benefits for all types of insurance that you will be billing for; indicate this by checking "yes" in Block 27. For each claim completed, be sure to insert your initials at the lower left corner of the claim form. When coding services from the Surgery Section of CPT, be sure to check the Mock Fee Schedule in Appendix A in this *Workbook* to determine how many follow-up days are included in the surgical or global package. Services provided during the surgical/global package time frame should not be included on the claim form; however, such services should be documented on the financial accounting record,

---

*See Chapter 7 in the *Handbook* for help in completing this form.

referenced with code 99024 (postoperative follow-up visit; included in global service), and listed as no charge (N/C). Refer to the *Handbook* for detailed information about surgical/global package and follow-up days.

A list of abbreviations pertinent to the medical record have been provided as an exercise to reinforce learning. Not all medical offices use abbreviations in medical record documentation. In the College Clinic scenario, abbreviations are used in patient progress notes to give you an opportunity to practice reading and interpreting them.

7/9/07

PLEASE DO NOT STAPLE IN THIS AREA

[redacted]

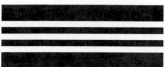

ABC INSURANCE COMPANY
111 MAIN STREET
DENVER CO 80210

okay

CARRIER

PICA

HEALTH INSURANCE CLAIM FORM

PICA

needs to be checked →

1. MEDICARE (Medicare #) ☐ MEDICAID (Medicaid #) ☐ CHAMPUS (Sponsor's SSN) ☐ CHAMPVA (VA File #) ☐ GROUP HEALTH PLAN (SSN or ID) ☐ FECA BLK LUNG (SSN) ☐ OTHER (ID) ☐

1a. INSURED'S I.D. NUMBER (FOR PROGRAM IN ITEM 1): PX4278A — Social #

2. PATIENT'S NAME (Last Name, First Name, Middle Initial): PARKINSON TOM N

3. PATIENT'S BIRTH DATE MM DD YY: 04 06 1993 — SEX M ☒ F ☐

4. INSURED'S NAME (Last Name, First Name, Middle Initial): PARKINSON, JAMIE B — no punctuation

5. PATIENT'S ADDRESS (No., Street): 4510 SOUTH A STREET

6. PATIENT RELATIONSHIP TO INSURED: Self ☐ Spouse ☐ Child ☒ Other ☐

7. INSURED'S ADDRESS (No., Street): ~~4510 SOUTH A STREET~~ same

CITY: WOODLAND HILLS — STATE: XY

8. PATIENT STATUS: Single ☒ Married ☐ Other ☐

CITY: ~~WOODLAND HILLS~~ same — STATE: ~~XY~~

ZIP CODE: 12345 — TELEPHONE (Include Area Code): (555) 742-1560 — no dash

Employed ☐ Full-Time Student ☒ Part-Time Student ☐

ZIP CODE: ~~12345~~ same — TELEPHONE (INCLUDE AREA CODE): (555) 742 1560 — same

9. OTHER INSURED'S NAME (Last Name, First Name, Middle Initial)

10. IS PATIENT'S CONDITION RELATED TO:

11. INSURED'S POLICY GROUP OR FECA NUMBER

a. OTHER INSURED'S POLICY OR GROUP NUMBER

a. EMPLOYMENT? (CURRENT OR PREVIOUS) ☐ YES ☒ NO

a. INSURED'S DATE OF BIRTH MM DD YY — SEX M ☐ F ☐

leave blank if no one insurance

b. OTHER INSURED'S DATE OF BIRTH MM DD YY — SEX M ☐ F ☐

b. AUTO ACCIDENT? ☐ YES ☒ NO — PLACE (State)

b. EMPLOYER'S NAME OR SCHOOL NAME

c. EMPLOYER'S NAME OR SCHOOL NAME

c. OTHER ACCIDENT? ☐ YES ☒ NO

c. INSURANCE PLAN NAME OR PROGRAM NAME

d. INSURANCE PLAN NAME OR PROGRAM NAME

10d. RESERVED FOR LOCAL USE

d. IS THERE ANOTHER HEALTH BENEFIT PLAN? ☐ YES ☒ NO — *If yes*, return to and complete item 9 a-d.

READ BACK OF FORM BEFORE COMPLETING & SIGNING THIS FORM.

12. PATIENT'S OR AUTHORIZED PERSON'S SIGNATURE I authorize the release of any medical or other information necessary to process this claim. I also request payment of government benefits either to myself or to the party who accepts assignment below.

SIGNED (SOF) missing signature DATE

13. INSURED'S OR AUTHORIZED PERSON'S SIGNATURE I authorize payment of medical benefits to the undersigned physician or supplier for services described below.

SIGNED needs Signature → SOF

EXAMPLE ONLY

14. DATE OF CURRENT: MM DD YY ◀ ILLNESS (First symptom) OR INJURY (Accident) OR PREGNANCY(LMP)

15. IF PATIENT HAS HAD SAME OR SIMILAR ILLNESS. GIVE FIRST DATE MM DD YY

16. DATES PATIENT UNABLE TO WORK IN CURRENT OCCUPATION FROM MM DD YY TO MM DD YY

17. NAME OF REFERRING PHYSICIAN OR OTHER SOURCE — only for referals

17a. I.D. NUMBER OF REFERRING PHYSICIAN

18. HOSPITALIZATION DATES RELATED TO CURRENT SERVICES FROM MM DD YY TO MM DD YY

19. RESERVED FOR LOCAL USE — ok to leave blank

20. OUTSIDE LAB? ☐ YES ☒ NO — $ CHARGES

21. DIAGNOSIS OR NATURE OF ILLNESS OR INJURY. (RELATE ITEMS 1,2,3 OR 4 TO ITEM 24E BY LINE)

1. ____ 3. ____
2. ____ 4. ____

needs diagnosis — ICD-9

22. MEDICAID RESUBMISSION CODE — ORIGINAL REF. NO.

23. PRIOR AUTHORIZATION NUMBER

24. A DATE(S) OF SERVICE From MM DD YY	To MM DD YY	B Place of Service	C Type of Service	D PROCEDURES, SERVICES, OR SUPPLIES (Explain Unusual Circumstances) CPT/HCPCS MODIFIER	E DIAGNOSIS CODE	F $ CHARGES	G DAYS OR UNITS	H EPSDT Family Plan	I EMG	J COB	K RESERVED FOR LOCAL USE
1 07 1420 XX				99242	✓	80 24	1			✓	needs
2 07 1420 XX				71020	1	38 96	1			46	278897XX
3											
4											
5											
6											

needs pos — DRS NPI #

PHYSICIAN OR SUPPLIER INFORMATION

PATIENT AND INSURED INFORMATION

25. FEDERAL TAX I.D. NUMBER: 70 34597XX — SSN ☐ EIN ☐

26. PATIENT'S ACCOUNT NO. — Assignment #7-5

27. ACCEPT ASSIGNMENT? (For govt. claims, see back) ☒ YES ☐ NO

28. TOTAL CHARGE $ 119 20

29. AMOUNT PAID $

30. BALANCE DUE $ — same as #28

pg 202 wkbk

31. SIGNATURE OF PHYSICIAN OR SUPPLIER INCLUDING DEGREES OR CREDENTIALS (I certify that the statements on the reverse apply to this bill and are made a part thereof.)
GERALD PRACTON MD
07 14 20XX
SIGNED Signature missing DATE

32. NAME AND ADDRESS OF FACILITY WHERE SERVICES WERE RENDERED (If other than home or office)
SAME → entered

33. PHYSICIAN'S, SUPPLIER'S BILLING NAME, ADDRESS, ZIP CODE & PHONE #
COLLEGE CLINIC 555 486 9002
4567 BROAD AVENUE
WOODLAND HILLS XY 12345
PIN# — GRP# 3664021XX

(APPROVED BY AMA COUNCIL ON MEDICAL SERVICE 8/88)

PLEASE PRINT OR TYPE

APPROVED OMB-0938-0008 FORM CMS-1500 (12-90), FORM RRB-1500, APPROVED OMB-1215-0055 FORM OWCP-1500, APPROVED OMB-0720-0001 (CHAMPUS)

Figure 7–13

MES

PLEASE
DO NOT
STAPLE
IN THIS
AREA

CARRIER

HEALTH INSURANCE CLAIM FORM

PICA | | PICA

1. MEDICARE (Medicare #) **MEDICAID** (Medicaid #) **CHAMPUS** (Sponsor's SSN) **CHAMPVA** (VA File #) **GROUP HEALTH PLAN** (SSN or ID) **FECA BLK LUNG** (SSN) **OTHER** (ID)

1a. INSURED'S I.D. NUMBER (FOR PROGRAM IN ITEM 1)

2. PATIENT'S NAME (Last Name, First Name, Middle Initial)

3. PATIENT'S BIRTH DATE MM DD YY **SEX** M F

4. INSURED'S NAME (Last Name, First Name, Middle Initial)

5. PATIENT'S ADDRESS (No., Street)

6. PATIENT RELATIONSHIP TO INSURED Self Spouse Child Other

7. INSURED'S ADDRESS (No., Street)

CITY STATE

8. PATIENT STATUS Single Married Other / Employed Full-Time Student Part-Time Student

CITY STATE

ZIP CODE TELEPHONE (Include Area Code))

ZIP CODE TELEPHONE (INCLUDE AREA CODE)

9. OTHER INSURED'S NAME (Last Name, First Name, Middle Initial)

10. IS PATIENT'S CONDITION RELATED TO:

11. INSURED'S POLICY GROUP OR FECA NUMBER

a. OTHER INSURED'S POLICY OR GROUP NUMBER

a. EMPLOYMENT? (CURRENT OR PREVIOUS) YES NO

a. INSURED'S DATE OF BIRTH MM DD YY **SEX** M F

b. OTHER INSURED'S DATE OF BIRTH MM DD YY **SEX** M F

b. AUTO ACCIDENT? PLACE (State) YES NO

b. EMPLOYER'S NAME OR SCHOOL NAME

c. EMPLOYER'S NAME OR SCHOOL NAME

c. OTHER ACCIDENT? YES NO

c. INSURANCE PLAN NAME OR PROGRAM NAME

d. INSURANCE PLAN NAME OR PROGRAM NAME

10d. RESERVED FOR LOCAL USE

d. IS THERE ANOTHER HEALTH BENEFIT PLAN? YES NO *If yes*, return to and complete item 9 a-d.

READ BACK OF FORM BEFORE COMPLETING & SIGNING THIS FORM.
12. PATIENT'S OR AUTHORIZED PERSON'S SIGNATURE I authorize the release of any medical or other information necessary to process this claim. I also request payment of government benefits either to myself or to the party who accepts assignment below.

SIGNED _____ DATE _____

13. INSURED'S OR AUTHORIZED PERSON'S SIGNATURE I authorize payment of medical benefits to the undersigned physician or supplier for services described below.

SIGNED _____

PATIENT AND INSURED INFORMATION

14. DATE OF CURRENT: MM DD YY ILLNESS (First symptom) OR INJURY (Accident) OR PREGNANCY(LMP)

15. IF PATIENT HAS HAD SAME OR SIMILAR ILLNESS. GIVE FIRST DATE MM DD YY

16. DATES PATIENT UNABLE TO WORK IN CURRENT OCCUPATION FROM MM DD YY TO MM DD YY

17. NAME OF REFERRING PHYSICIAN OR OTHER SOURCE

17a. I.D. NUMBER OF REFERRING PHYSICIAN

18. HOSPITALIZATION DATES RELATED TO CURRENT SERVICES FROM MM DD YY TO MM DD YY

19. RESERVED FOR LOCAL USE

20. OUTSIDE LAB? YES NO **$ CHARGES**

21. DIAGNOSIS OR NATURE OF ILLNESS OR INJURY. (RELATE ITEMS 1,2,3 OR 4 TO ITEM 24E BY LINE)
1. _____ 3. _____
2. _____ 4. _____

22. MEDICAID RESUBMISSION CODE ORIGINAL REF. NO.

23. PRIOR AUTHORIZATION NUMBER

24.

A. DATE(S) OF SERVICE From MM DD YY To MM DD YY	B. Place of Service	C. Type of Service	D. PROCEDURES, SERVICES, OR SUPPLIES (Explain Unusual Circumstances) CPT/HCPCS MODIFIER	E. DIAGNOSIS CODE	F. $ CHARGES	G. DAYS OR UNITS	H. EPSDT Family Plan	I. EMG	J. COB	K. RESERVED FOR LOCAL USE
1										
2										
3										
4										
5										
6										

25. FEDERAL TAX I.D. NUMBER SSN EIN

26. PATIENT'S ACCOUNT NO.

27. ACCEPT ASSIGNMENT? (For govt. claims, see back) YES NO

28. TOTAL CHARGE $

29. AMOUNT PAID $

30. BALANCE DUE $

31. SIGNATURE OF PHYSICIAN OR SUPPLIER INCLUDING DEGREES OR CREDENTIALS (I certify that the statements on the reverse apply to this bill and are made a part thereof.)

SIGNED _____ DATE _____

32. NAME AND ADDRESS OF FACILITY WHERE SERVICES WERE RENDERED (If other than home or office)

33. PHYSICIAN'S, SUPPLIER'S BILLING NAME, ADDRESS, ZIP CODE & PHONE #

PIN# GRP#

PHYSICIAN OR SUPPLIER INFORMATION

(APPROVED BY AMA COUNCIL ON MEDICAL SERVICE 8/88)   ***PLEASE PRINT OR TYPE***   APPROVED OMB-0938-0008 FORM CMS-1500 (12-90),   FORM RRB-1500, APPROVED OMB-1215-0055 FORM OWCP-1500,   APPROVED OMB-0720-0001 (CHAMPUS)

Figure 7–14

SELF-STUDY **7-6** ▸ **REVIEW PATIENT RECORD ABBREVIATIONS**

Performance Objective

Task: Insert meanings of abbreviations.

Conditions: Use a pencil or pen.

Standards: Time: _____ minutes

                   Accuracy: _____

                   (Note: The time element and accuracy criteria may be given by your instructor.)

Directions: After completing all the patient records in the *Workbook* that are pertinent to this chapter, you will be able to answer the next two questions.

1. What do these abbreviations mean?

    a. PTR   _____   f. Dx   _____

    b. TURP   _____   g. BP   _____

    c. HX   _____   h. CC   _____

    d. IVP   _____   i. UA   _____

    e. c̄   _____   j. PE   _____

2. Give the abbreviations for the following terms.

    A. return _____

    B. cancer, carcinoma _____

    C. patient _____

    D. established _____

    E. discharged _____

    F. gallbladder _____

    G. initial _____

To check your answers to this self-study assignment, see Appendix D in this *Workbook*.

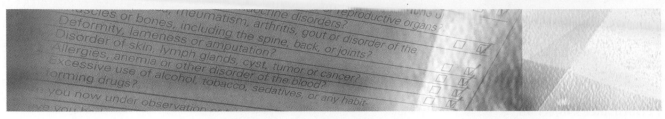

Electronic Data Interchange: Transactions and Security

KEY TERMS

Your instructor may wish to select some specific words pertinent to this chapter for a test. For definitions of the terms, further study, and/or reference, the words, phrases, and abbreviations may be found in the glossary at the end of the Handbook. *Key terms for this chapter follow.*

Accredited Standards Committee ×12 (ASC ×12)

application service provider (ASP)

back up

batch

business associate agreement

cable modem

clearinghouse

code sets

covered entity

data elements

direct data entry (DDE)

digital subscriber line (DSL)

electronic data interchange (EDI)

electronic funds transfer (EFT)

electronic remittance advice (ERA)

encoder

encryption

HIPAA Transaction and Code Set (TCS) rule

National Standard Format (NSF)

password

real time

standard transactions

T-1

taxonomy codes

trading partner agreement

PERFORMANCE OBJECTIVES

The student will be able to:

- Define and spell the key terms for this chapter, given the information from the *Handbook* glossary, within a reasonable time period and with enough accuracy to obtain a satisfactory evaluation.
- After reading the chapter, answer the self-study review questions with enough accuracy to obtain a satisfactory evaluation.
- Decide whether keyed medical and nonmedical data elements are required, situational, or not used when electronically submitting the 837P health care claim.
- Decide which medical and nonmedical code sets for 837P electronic claims are required, situational, or not used.
- Input data into the element for place of service codes for 837P electronic claims submission.
- Indicate the patient's relationship to the insured by using the individual relationship code numbers for 837P electronic claims submission.
- Select the correct individual relationship code number for 837P electronic claims submission.

- Select the correct taxonomy codes for the specialists for submission of 837P electronic claims submission.
- Locate errors, given computer-generated insurance forms, within a reasonable time period and with enough accuracy to obtain a satisfactory evaluation.
- Transmit electronic insurance claims for private cases using practice management software, within a reasonable time period and with enough accuracy to obtain a satisfactory evaluation.
- Print a batch claim report using practice management software, within a reasonable time period and with enough accuracy to obtain a satisfactory evaluation.
- Fill in the correct meaning of each abbreviation, given a list of common medical abbreviations and symbols that appear in chart notes, with enough accuracy to obtain a satisfactory evaluation.

STUDY OUTLINE

Electronic Data Interchange
Electronic Claims
Advantages of Electronic Claim Submission
Clearinghouses
Transaction and Code Set Regulations: Streamlining Electronic Data Interchange
 Transaction and Code Set Standards
Transition from Paper CMS-1500 to Electronic Standard HIPAA 837
 Levels of Information for 837P Standard Transaction Format
Claims Attachments Standards
 Standard Unique Identifiers
Practice Management System
Building the Claim
 Encounter or Multipurpose Billing Forms
 Scannable Encounter Form
 Keying Insurance Data for Claim Transmission
 Encoder
 Clean Electronic Claims Submission
Putting HIPAA Standard Transactions to Work
 Interactive Transactions

Electronic Remittance Advice
Driving the Data
Methods for Sending Claims
Computer Claims Systems
 Payer or Carrier-Direct
 Clearinghouse
Transmission Reports
 Electronic Processing Problems
 Billing and Account Management Schedule
 Administrative Simplification Enforcement Tool (ASET)
 The Security Rule: Administrative, Physical, and Technical Safeguards
HIPAA: Application to the Practice Setting
Computer Confidentiality
 Confidentiality Statement
 Prevention Measures
Records Management
 Data Storage
 Electronic Power Protection

SELF-STUDY 8-1 ▶ REVIEW QUESTIONS

Review the objectives, key terms, glossary definitions of key terms, chapter information, and figures before completing the following review questions.

1. Exchange of data in a standardized format through computer systems is a technology

   known as _____.

2. The act of converting computerized data into a code so that unauthorized users are

   unable to read it is a security system known as _____.

3. Payment to the provider of service of an electronically submitted insurance claim

   may be received in approximately _____.

4. List benefits of using HIPAA standard transactions and code sets.

   a. _____

   b. _____

   c. _____

   d. _____

   e. _____

   f. _____

5. Dr. Morgan has 10 or more full-time employees and submits insurance claims for

   his Medicare patients. Is his medical practice subject to the HIPAA transaction rules? _____

6. Dr. Maria Montez does not submit insurance claims electronically and has five

   full-time employees. Is she required to abide by HIPAA transaction rules? _____

7. Name the standard code sets used for the following:

   a. physician services _____

   b. diseases and injuries _____

   c. pharmaceuticals and biologics _____

8. Refer to Table 8-3 in the *Handbook* to complete these statements.

   a. The staff at College Clinic submits professional health care claims for each of their

      providers and must use the industry standard electronic format called _____

      _____ to transmit them electronically.

b. The billing department at College Hospital must use the industry standard

electronic format called _____

to transmit health care claims electronically.

c. The Medicare fiscal intermediary (insurance carrier) uses the industry standard

electronic format called _____

to transmit payment information to the College Clinic and College Hospital.

d. It has been 3 weeks since Gordon Marshall's health care claim was transmitted
to the XYZ insurance company and you wish to inquire about the status of the
claim. The industry standard electronic format that must be used to transmit

this inquiry is called _____

e. Dr. Practon's insurance billing specialist must use the industry standard electronic

format called _____ to obtain information

about Beatrice Garcia's health policy benefits and coverage from the insurance plan.

9. The family practice taxonomy code is _____.

10. A Medicare patient, Charles Gorman, signed a signature authorization form, which is

on file. The patient's signature source code for data element #1351 is _____.

11. Name the levels for data collected to construct and submit an electronic claim.

a. _____

b. _____

c. _____

d. _____

e. _____

f. _____

12. The most important function of a practice management system is

_____.

13. To look for and correct all errors before the health claim is transmitted to the

insurance carrier, you may _____ or _____

_____.

14. Add-on software to a practice management system that can reduce the time it takes

to build or review a claim before batching is known as a/an _____

_____.

15. Software that is used in a network that serves a group of users working on a related

project allowing access to the same data is called a/an _____

_____.

To check your answers to this self-study assignment, see Appendix D.

ASSIGNMENT 8-2 ▸ **CRITICAL THINKING FOR MEDICAL AND NONMEDICAL CODE SETS FOR 837P ELECTRONIC CLAIMS SUBMISSION**

Performance Objective

Task: Decide whether keyed medical and nonmedical data elements are required, situational, or not used when electronically submitting the 837P health care claim.

Conditions: List of keyed data elements (Table 8-6 in Handbook) and pen or pencil.

Standards: Time: _____ minutes

Accuracy: _____

(Note: The time element and accuracy criteria may be given by your instructor.)

Directions: When submitting the 837P health care claim, supporting code sets of medical and nonmedical data are composed of "Required" and "Situational" data elements. Read each keyed data element and answer whether you think it is **R** for required, **S** for situational, or **N** for not used.

a. Patient's last menstrual period   _____

b. Patient's telephone number   _____

c. Insured's name   _____

d. Diagnosis code   _____

e. Provider's PIN   _____

f. Procedure code   _____

g. Provider's signature   _____

h. Employer's name   _____

i. Type of service   _____

j. Procedure modifier   _____

ASSIGNMENT 8-3 ▸ **INPUT DATA INTO ELEMENT FOR PLACE OF SERVICE CODES FOR 837P ELECTRONIC CLAIMS SUBMISSIONS**

Performance Objective

Task: Insert the correct place of service code for each location description where medical professional service was rendered.

Conditions: Place of service codes reference (Figure 8–1), list of places where medical care was rendered, and pen or pencil.

Standards: Time: _____ minutes

Accuracy: _____

(Note: The time element and accuracy criteria may be given by your instructor.)

Directions: When submitting the 837P electronic claim, place of service codes must be entered in data element 1331. Refer to the place of service codes reference list and insert the correct code for each place of service for the following locations.

a. Inpatient psychiatric facility _____

b. Doctor's office _____

c. Outpatient hospital _____

d. Intermediate nursing facility _____

e. Independent clinic _____

f. Independent laboratory _____

g. Birthing center _____

h. End-stage renal disease treatment facility _____

i. Inpatient hospital _____

j. Hospice _____

PLACE OF SERVICE CODES	
Codes	**Place of Service**
00-02	Unassigned
03	School
04	Homeless shelter
05	Indian health service free-standing facility
06	Indian health service provider-based facility
07	Tribal 638 free-standing facility
08	Tribal 638 provider-based facility
09-10	Unassigned
11	Doctor's office
12	Patient's home
13	Assisted living facility
14	Group home
15	Mobile unit
16-19	Unassigned
20	Urgent care facility
21	Inpatient hospital
22	Outpatient hospital
23	Emergency department—hospital
24	Ambulatory surgical center
25	Birthing center
26	Military treatment facility/uniformed service treatment facility
27-30	Unassigned
31	Skilled nursing facility (swing bed visits)
32	Nursing facility (intermediate/long-term care facilities)
33	Custodial care facility (domiciliary or rest home services)
34	Hospice (domiciliary or rest home services)
35-40	Unassigned
41	Ambulance—land
42	Ambulance—air or water
43-48	Unassigned
49	Independent clinic
50	Federally qualified health center
51	Inpatient psychiatric facility
52	Psychiatric facility—partial hospitalization
53	Community mental health care (outpatient, 24-hours-a-day services, admission screening, consultation, and educational services)
54	Intermediate care facility/mentally retarded
55	Residential substance abuse treatment facility
56	Psychiatric residential treatment center
58-59	Unassigned
60	Mass immunization center
61	Comprehensive inpatient rehabilitation facility
62	Comprehensive outpatient rehabilitation facility
63-64	Unassigned
65	End-stage renal disease treatment facility
66-70	Unassigned
71	State or local public health clinic
72	Rural health clinic
73-80	Unassigned
81	Independent laboratory
82-98	Unassigned
99	Other place of service

Figure 8–1

ASSIGNMENT 8-4 ▸ **SELECT THE CORRECT INDIVIDUAL RELATIONSHIP CODE NUMBER FOR 837P ELECTRONIC CLAIMS SUBMISSION**

Performance Objective

Task: Insert the correct individual relationship code for the patient's relationship to the insured.

Conditions: Individual relationship code number reference (Figure 8–2), list of individuals or entities, and pen or pencil.

Standards: Time: _____ minutes

                 Accuracy: _____

                 (Note: The time element and accuracy criteria may be given by your instructor.)

Directions: Refer to the individual relationship code number list, choose the correct code for the patient's relationship to the insured for the following persons, and insert it on the lines.

a. Mother   _____

b. Spouse   _____

c. Child   _____

d. Father   _____

e. Stepdaughter   _____

f. Emancipated minor   _____

g. Adopted child   _____

h. Handicapped dependent   _____

i. Stepson   _____

j. Sponsored dependent   _____

Individual Relationship Code	
Code	**Relationship**
01	Spouse
04	Grandfather or grandmother
05	Grandson or granddaughter
07	Nephew or niece
09	Adopted child
10	Foster child
15	Ward
17	Stepson or stepdaughter
19	Child
20	Employee
21	Unknown
22	Handicapped dependent
23	Sponsored dependent
24	Dependent of a minor dependent
29	Significant other
32	Mother
33	Father
34	Other adult
36	Emancipated minor
39	Organ donor
40	Cadaver donor
41	Injured plaintiff
43	Child where insured has no financial responsibility
53	Life partner
G8	Other relationship

Figure 8–2

ASSIGNMENT 8–5 ▸ **SELECT THE CORRECT TAXONOMY CODES
FOR MEDICAL SPECIALIST FOR 837P
ELECTRONIC CLAIMS SUBMISSION**

Performance Objective

Task: Choose the correct taxonomy code for each specialist for submission of 837P electronic claims by referring to the Healthcare Provider Taxonomy code list.

Conditions: Healthcare Provider Taxonomy code list (Figure 8–3), list of providers of service, and pen or pencil.

Standards: Time: _____ minutes

             Accuracy: _____

             (Note: The time element and accuracy criteria may be given by your instructor.)

Directions: Refer to the Healthcare Provider Taxonomy code list, choose the correct code for each of the following specialists, and insert the code numbers on the lines.

a. Raymond Skeleton, MD, orthopedist   _____

b. Gaston Input, MD, gastroenterologist   _____

c. Vera Cutis, MD, dermatologist   _____

d. Gene Ulibarri, MD, urologist   _____

e. Bertha Caesar, MD, obtetrician/gynecologist _____

f. Gerald Practon, MD, general practitioner   _____

g. Pedro Atrics, MD, pediatrician   _____

h. Astro Parkinson, MD, neurosurgeon   _____

i. Brady Coccidioides, MD, pulmonary disease _____

j. Max Glutens, RPT, physical therapist   _____

College Clinic Staff		
Health Care Provider Taxonomy Codes		
Name	**Speciality**	**Taxonomy Code**
Concha Antrum, MD	Otolaryngologist	207Y00000X
Pedro Atrics, MD	Pediatrician	208000000X
Bertha Caesar, MD	Obstetrician/Gynecologist	207V00000X
Perry Cardi, MD	Cardiologist	207RC0000X
Brady Coccidioides, MD	Pulmonary disease	207RP1001X
Vera Cutis, MD	Dermatologist	207N00000X
Clarence Cutler, MD	General surgeon	208600000X
Dennis Drill, DDS	Dentist	122300000X
Max Glutens, RPT	Physical therapist	208100000X
Cosmo Graff, MD	Plastic surgeon	208200000X
Malvern Grumose, MD	Pathologist	207ZP0105X
Gaston Input, MD	Gastroenterologist	207RG0100X
Adam Langerhans, MD	Endocrinologist	207RE0101X
Cornell Lenser, MD	Ophthalmologist	207W00000X
Michael Menter, MD	Psychiatrist	2084P0800X
Arthur O. Dont, DDS	Orthodontist	1223X0400X
Astro Parkinson, MD	Neurosurgeon	207T00000X
Nick Pedro, MD	Podiatrist	213E00000X
Gerald Practon, MD	General practitioner	208D00000X
Walter Radon, MD	Radiologst	2085R0202X
Rex Rumsey, MD	Proctologist	208C00000X
Sensitive E. Scott, MD	Anesthesiologist	207L00000X
Raymond Skeleton, MD	Orthopedist	207X00000X
Gene Ulibarri, MD	Urologist	208800000X

Figure 8–3

ASSIGNMENT 8–6 ▸ COMPOSE ELECTRONIC MAIL MESSAGES

Performance Objective

Task: Compose brief messages for electronic mail transmission after reading each scenario.

Conditions: List of scenarios, one sheet of 8½- × 11-inch plain typing paper, and either a typewriter and/or computer or a pen.

Standards: Time: _____ minutes

Accuracy: _____

(Note: The time element and accuracy criteria may be given by your instructor.)

Directions: Read each scenario. Compose polite, effective, and brief messages that, on the job, would be transmitted via electronic mail (e-mail). Use the guidelines presented in the *Handbook*. Be sure to list a descriptive subject line as the first item in each composition. Single-space the message. Insert a short signature at the end of the message to include your name and affiliation, and create an e-mail address for yourself if you do not have one.

Scenario 1:

Ask an insurance biller, Mary Davis, in a satellite office to locate and fax you a copy of the billing done on account number 43500 for services rendered to Margarita Sylva on March 2, 20xx. Explain that you must telephone the patient about her account. Mary Davis' e-mail address is mdavis@aal.com.

Checklist

1. Used Times New Roman font, or other recommended font, in 12 or 14 point. _____

2. Inserted the recipient's e-mail address. _____

3. Inserted a subject line. _____

4. Inserted a salutation. _____

5. Composed a single-spaced, left-justified message in the body of the letter. _____

6. Appended closing signature line(s) at the end of the message. _____

7. Printed a hard copy of the e-mail message. _____

Scenario 2:

Patient Ellen Worth was recently hospitalized; her hospital number is 20-9870-11. Compose an e-mail message to the medical record department at College Hospital (collegehospmedrecords@rrv.net) for her final diagnosis and the assigned diagnostic code needed to complete the insurance claim form.

Checklist

1. Used Times New Roman font, or other recommended font, in 12 or 14 point. _____

2. Inserted the recipient's e-mail address. _____

3. Inserted a subject line. _____

4. Inserted a salutation. _____

5. Composed a single-spaced, left-justified message in the body of the letter.   _____

6. Appended closing signature line(s) at the end of the message.   _____

7. Printed a hard copy of the e-mail message.   _____

Scenario 3:

You are working for a billing service and receive an encounter form that is missing the information about the patient's professional service received on August 2, 20xx. The patient's account number is 45098. You have the diagnosis data. Compose an e-mail message to Dr. Mason (pmason@email.mc.com) explaining what you must obtain to complete the billing portion of the insurance claim form.   *Checklist*

1. Used Times New Roman font, or other recommended font, in 12 or 14 point.   _____

2. Inserted the recipient's e-mail address.   _____

3. Inserted a subject line.   _____

4. Inserted a salutation.   _____

5. Composed a single-spaced, left-justified message in the body of the letter.   _____

6. Appended closing signature line(s) at the end of the message.   _____

7. Printed a hard copy of the e-mail message.   _____

Scenario 4:

A new patient, John Phillips, has e-mailed your office to ask what the outstanding balance is on his account. The account number is 42990. You look up the financial record and note the service was for an office visit on June 14, 20xx. The charge was $106.11. Compose an e-mail response to Mr. Phillips, whose e-mail address is: bphillips@hotmail.com.   *Checklist*

1. Used Times New Roman font, or other recommended font, in 12 or 14 point.   _____

2. Inserted the recipient's e-mail address.   _____

3. Inserted a subject line.   _____

4. Inserted a salutation.   _____

5. Composed a single-spaced, left-justified message in the body of the letter.   _____

6. Appended closing signature line(s) at the end of the message.   _____

7. Printed a hard copy of the e-mail message.   _____

Scenario 5:

You are having difficulty deciding whether the codes 13101, 13102, and 13132 with modifier -51 selected for a case are appropriate. Compose an e-mail message that will be posted on the Part B News Internet listserv (PartB-L@usa.net) asking for comments.

The case involves a 12-year-old boy who fell against a bicycle, lacerating the left side of his chest to the pectoralis muscle through a 12-cm gaping wound. He also sustained a 5-cm laceration to his left cheek. Complex repairs were required for these two wounds and totaled 17 cm. Find out whether modifier -15 should be appended to the second code or to the third code.

Checklist

1. Used Times New Roman font, or other recommended font, in 12 or 14 point.   _____

2. Inserted the recipient's e-mail address.   _____

3. Inserted a subject line.   _____

4. Inserted a salutation.   _____

5. Composed a single-spaced, left-justified message in the body of the letter.   _____

6. Appended closing signature line(s) at the end of the message.   _____

7. Printed a hard copy of the e-mail message.   _____

After the instructor has returned your work to you, either make the necessary corrections and place your work in a three-ring notebook for future reference or, if you received a high score, place it in your portfolio for use when applying for a job.

ASSIGNMENT 8-7 ▶ **PROOFREAD A COMPUTER-GENERATED HEALTH INSURANCE CLAIM FORM AND LOCATE INCORRECT AND MISSING DATA**

Performance Objective

Task: Locate and designate blocks on the computer-generated insurance claim form that have incorrect information or need completion; correct or add data before submission to the insurance company.

Conditions: Use Brad E. Diehl's patient record (Figure 8–4), completed insurance claim (Figure 8–5), and a highlighter and a red ink pen.

Standards: Time: _____ minutes

                Accuracy: _____

                (Note: The time element and accuracy criteria may be given by your instructor.)

Directions: Proofread the insurance claim form (Figure 8–5) and locate blocks that need correction or completion before submission to the insurance company. Highlight all errors you discover. Refer to the patient's record (Figure 8–4) to verify pertinent demographic and insurance information. Refer to the progress notes to verify procedures and determine diagnoses. Verify all entries on the claim form, including dates, codes, rounded out fees, and physician identification numbers. Insert all corrections and missing information in red. If you cannot locate the necessary information but know it is mandatory, write "NEED" in the corresponding block.

Optional: Retype a blank CMS-1500 claim form with all corrections and changes. Or if you have access to a computer, use the AltaPoint CD that accompanies the *Handbook* and go to the Handouts folder and print a blank CMS-1500 claim form for manual completion.

Additional Coding

1. Assume that Mr. Diehl followed Dr. Input's treatment plan. Refer to his record, abstract information, and locate procedure codes that would be billed by providers outside of the office.

Site	*Description of Service*	*Code*
a. ABC Radiology	_____	_____
b. College Hospital	_____	_____
c. College Hospital	_____	_____

2. Code the symptoms Mr. Diehl was complaining about when he presented for the January 5, 20xx, office visit.

Symptom	*Code*
a. _____	_____
b. _____	_____
c. _____	_____
d. _____	_____

PATIENT RECORD NO. 8-7

Diehl	Brad	E.	09-21-46	M	555-222-0123
LAST NAME	FIRST NAME	MIDDLE NAME	BIRTH DATE	SEX	HOME PHONE

3975 Hills Road	Woodland Hills	XY	12345
ADDRESS	CITY	STATE	ZIP CODE

555-703-6600	555-321-0988	555-222-0123	Diehl@WB.net
CELL PHONE	PAGER NO.	FAX NO.	E-MAIL ADDRESS

561-XX-1501	M0983457
PATIENT'S SOC. SEC. NO.	DRIVER'S LICENSE

radio advertising salesman	KACY Radio
PATIENT'S OCCUPATION	NAME OF COMPANY

4071 Mills Road, Woodland Hills, XY 12335	555-201-6666
ADDRESS OF EMPLOYER	PHONE

Tak E. Diehl (birthdate 4-7-45)	legal secretary
SPOUSE OR PARENT	OCCUPATION

Attys. Dilman, Forewise & Gilson,	12 West Dix Street, Woodland Hills, XY 12345	555-222-6432
EMPLOYER	ADDRESS	PHONE

Aetna Insurance Co., 2412 Main Street, Woodland Hills, XY 12345	Brad E. Diehl
NAME OF INSURANCE	INSURED OR SUB SCRIBER

403119	
POLICY/CERTIFICATE NO.	GROUP NO.

REFERRED BY: Raymond Skeleton, MD

DATE	PROGRESS NOTES	No. 8-7
1-5-20xx	NP pt comes in complaining of coughing and sneezing; some difficulty breathing.	
	Occasional dizziness and epigastric abdominal pain with cramping. Symptoms started in	
	July of last year. Performed a detailed history and physical examination with low	
	complexity medical decision making. AP & lat chest x-rays taken; neg findings. BP 178/98.	
	Pt to have cholecystography with oral contrast at ABC Radiology. Diagnostic colonoscopy	
	(flexible) to be scheduled at College Hospital. Dx: hypertension and respiratory distress;	
	R/O irritable colon. No disability at this time.	
	GI/llf *Gaston Input, MD*	
1-20-xx	Pt retns for a EPF hx/exam LC MDM. Oral cholecystography reveals a single 1.5 cm	
	radiolucent calculus within the cholecyst. Colonoscopy confirmed irritable bowel	
	syndrome. Blood drawn and CBC (auto with diff) performed in office indicates	
	WBC 10,000. DX: cholecistitis with cholelithiasis. Adv. cholecystectomy	
	(abdominal approach) as soon as possible; to be scheduled at College Hospital.	
	GI/llf *Gaston Input, MD*	

Figure 8–4

PLEASE
DO NOT
STAPLE
IN THIS
AREA

CARRIER

HEALTH INSURANCE CLAIM FORM

PICA		PICA

1. MEDICARE MEDICAID CHAMPUS CHAMPVA GROUP HEALTH PLAN FECA BLK LUNG OTHER	1a. INSURED'S I.D. NUMBER (FOR PROGRAM IN ITEM 1)
☐ (Medicare #) ☐ (Medicaid #) ☐ (Sponsor's SSN) ☐ (VA File #) ☒ (SSN or ID) ☐ (S SN) ☐ (ID)	403119

2. PATIENT'S NAME (Last Name, First Name, Middle Initial)	3. PATIENT'S BIRTH DATE SEX	4. INSURED'S NAME (Last Name, First Name, Middle Initial)
DIEHL BRAD E	MM 09 DD 21 YY 1946 M ☐ F ☐	SAME

5. PATIENT'S ADDRESS (No., Street)	6. PATIENT RELATIONSHIP TO INSURED	7. INSURED'S ADDRESS (No., Street)
3975 HILLS ROAD	Self ☐ Spouse ☐ Child ☐ Other ☐	

CITY	STATE	8. PATIENT STATUS	CITY	STATE
WOODLAND HILLS	XY	Single ☐ Married ☒ Other ☐		

ZIP CODE	TELEPHONE (Include Area Code)		ZIP CODE	TELEPHONE (INCLUDE AREA CODE)
12345	(555) 222 0123	Employed ☒ Full-Time Student ☐ Part-Time Student ☐		( )

9. OTHER INSURED'S NAME (Last Name, First Name, Middle Initial)	10. IS PATIENT'S CONDITION RELATED TO:	11. INSURED'S POLICY GROUP OR FECA NUMBER
a. OTHER INSURED'S POLICY OR GROUP NUMBER	a. EMPLOYMENT? (CURRENT OR PREVIOUS) ☐ YES ☒ NO	a. INSURED'S DATE OF BIRTH MM DD YY M ☐ F ☐
b. OTHER INSURED'S DATE OF BIRTH MM DD YY SEX M ☐ F ☐	b. AUTO ACCIDENT? PLACE (State) ☐ YES ☒ NO	b. EMPLOYER'S NAME OR SCHOOL NAME
c. EMPLOYER'S NAME OR SCHOOL NAME	c. OTHER ACCIDENT? ☐ YES ☒ NO	c. INSURANCE PLAN NAME OR PROGRAM NAME
d. INSURANCE PLAN NAME OR PROGRAM NAME	10d. RESERVED FOR LOCAL USE	d. IS THERE ANOTHER HEALTH BENEFIT PLAN? ☐ YES ☒ NO *If yes,* return to and complete item 9 a-d.

READ BACK OF FORM BEFORE COMPLETING & SIGNING THIS FORM.

12. PATIENT'S OR AUTHORIZED PERSON'S SIGNATURE I authorize the release of any medical or other information necessary to process this claim. I also request payment of government benefits either to myself or to the party who accepts assignment below.

SIGNED _____   DATE _____

13. INSURED'S OR AUTHORIZED PERSON'S SIGNATURE I authorize payment of medical benefits to the undersigned physician or supplier for services described below.

SIGNED _____

14. DATE OF CURRENT: ILLNESS (First symptom) OR INJURY (Accident) OR PREGNANCY(LMP) MM DD YY	15. IF PATIENT HAS HAD SAME OR SIMILAR ILLNESS. GIVE FIRST DATE MM DD YY	16. DATES PATIENT UNABLE TO WORK IN CURRENT OCCUPATION FROM MM DD YY TO MM DD YY
17. NAME OF REFERRING PHYSICIAN OR OTHER SOURCE RAYMOND SKELETON MD	17a. I.D. NUMBER OF REFERRING PHYSICIAN	18. HOSPITALIZATION DATES RELATED TO CURRENT SERVICES FROM MM DD YY TO MM DD YY
19. RESERVED FOR LOCAL USE		20. OUTSIDE LAB? ☐ YES ☐ NO $ CHARGES

21. DIAGNOSIS OR NATURE OF ILLNESS OR INJURY. (RELATE ITEMS 1,2,3 OR 4 TO ITEM 24E BY LINE)	22. MEDICAID RESUBMISSION CODE ORIGINAL REF. NO.
1. 564 1 3. ⌐	
2. ⌐ 4. ⌐	23. PRIOR AUTHORIZATION NUMBER

24. A DATE(S) OF SERVICE		B Place of Service	C Type of Service	D PROCEDURES, SERVICES, OR SUPPLIES (Explain Unusual Circumstances)		E DIAGNOSIS CODE	F $ CHARGES	G DAYS OR UNITS	H EPSDT Family Plan	I EMG	J COB	K RESERVED FOR LOCAL USE
From MM DD YY	To MM DD YY			CPT/HCPCS	MODIFIER							
01 0520 XX		11		99203			70 92	1			32	783127XX
01 0520 XX		11		71020		1	80 00	1			32	783127XX
01 2020 XX		11		99213		1	40 20	1			32	783127XX
01 2020 XX		11		85025		1	25 00	1			32	783127XX
01 2020 XX		11				1		1			32	783127XX

25. FEDERAL TAX I.D. NUMBER SSN EIN ☐ ☐	26. PATIENT'S ACCOUNT NO. 8-7	27. ACCEPT ASSIGNMENT? (For govt. claims, see back) ☒ YES ☐ NO	28. TOTAL CHARGE $	29. AMOUNT PAID $	30. BALANCE DUE $

31. SIGNATURE OF PHYSICIAN OR SUPPLIER INCLUDING DEGREES OR CREDENTIALS (I certify that the statements on the reverse apply to this bill and are made a part thereof.) 01 25 20XX SIGNED DATE	32. NAME AND ADDRESS OF FACILITY WHERE SERVICES WERE RENDERED (If other than home or office) SAME	33. PHYSICIAN'S, SUPPLIER'S BILLING NAME, ADDRESS, ZIP CODE & PHONE # COLLEGE CLINIC 4567 BROAD AVENUE WOODLAND HILLS XY 12345 555 486 9002 PIN# GRP# 3664021XX

reference initials
(APPROVED BY AMA COUNCIL ON MEDICAL SERVICE 8/88)

PLEASE PRINT OR TYPE

APPROVED OMB-0938-0008 FORM CMS-1500 (12-90),   FORM RRB-1500,
APPROVED OMB-1215-0055 FORM OWCP-1500,   APPROVED OMB-0720-0001 (CHAMPUS)

Figure 8–5

ASSIGNMENT **8 – 8** ► **PROOFREAD A COMPUTER-GENERATED HEALTH INSURANCE CLAIM FORM AND LOCATE INCORRECT AND MISSING DATA**

Performance Objective

Task: Locate and designate blocks on the computer-generated insurance claim form that have incorrect information or need completion; correct or add data before submission to the insurance company.

Conditions: Use Evert I. Strain's patient record (Figure 8–6), completed insurance claim (Figure 8–7), and a highlighter and a red ink pen.

Standards: Time: _____ minutes

Accuracy: _____

(Note: The time element and accuracy criteria may be given by your instructor.)

Directions: Proofread the insurance claim form (Figure 8–7) and locate blocks that need correction or completion before submission to the insurance company. Highlight all errors you discover. Refer to the patient's record (Figure 8–6) to verify pertinent demographic and insurance information. Refer to the progress notes to verify procedures and determine diagnoses. Verify all entries on the claim form, including dates, codes, rounded out fees, and physician identification numbers. Insert all corrections and missing information in red. If you cannot locate the necessary information but know it is mandatory, write "NEED" in the corresponding block.

Optional: Retype a blank CMS-1500 claim form with all corrections and changes. Or if you have access to a computer, use the AltaPoint CD that accompanies the *Handbook* and go to the Handouts Folder and print a blank CMS-1500 claim form for manual completion.

Additional Coding

1. Refer to Mr. Strain's medical record, abstract information, and code procedures that would be billed by outside providers.

Site	*Description of Service*	*Code*
a. ABC Laboratory	_____	_____
b. ABC Radiology	_____	_____

PATIENT RECORD NO. 8-8

Strain,	Evert	I		09-11-46	M	555-678-0211
LAST NAME	FIRST NAME	MIDDLE NAME		BIRTH DATE	SEX	HOME PHONE

7650 None Such Road	Woodland Hills	XY	12345
ADDRESS	CITY	STATE	ZIP CODE

555-430-2101	555-320-9980	555-678-0211		Strain@WB.net
CELL PHONE	PAGER NO.	FAX NO.		E-MAIL ADDRESS

453-XX-4739	Y0923658
PATIENT'S SOC. SEC. NO.	DRIVER'S LICENSE

mechanical engineer	R & R Company
PATIENT'S OCCUPATION	NAME OF COMPANY

2400 Davon Road, Woodland Hills, XY 12345	555-520-8977
ADDRESS OF EMPLOYER	PHONE

Ester I. Strain (wife)	administrative assistant
SPOUSE OR PARENT	OCCUPATION

University College, 4021 Book Road, Woodland Hills, XY 12345		555-450-9908
EMPLOYER	ADDRESS	PHONE

ABC Insurance Co., P.O.Box 130, Woodland Hills, XY 12345	Evert I. Strain
NAME OF INSURANCE	INSURED OR SUBSCRIBER

453-XX-4739	96476A
POLICY/CERTIFICATE NO.	GROUP NO.

REFERRED BY: Gerald C. Jones, MD, 1403 Haven Street, Woodland Hills, XY 12345   NPI # 54754966XX

DATE	PROGRESS NOTES	No. 8-8
1-8-20xx	Est pt comes in complaining of frequent urination, headaches, polyphagia; unable to	
	remember current events. These problems have been present for almost a year.	
	A comprehensive history is taken and compared to his last H & P 2 years ago.	
	A com PX is performed. BP 160/110; pt was prescribed antihypertensive medication but	
	discontinued it when the prescription ran out. Lab report, hand carried by pt from an	
	urgent care center indicates SGOT in normal range and cholesterol elevated. Fasting blood	
	sugar extremely high. Dx: diabetes mellitus, malignant hypertensive, and ASCVD.	
	Pt to have 3 hour GTT tomorrow a.m. at ABC laboratory. STAT CT scan of head s̄ contrast	
	ordered at ABC radiology to follow lab work. Arrangement will be made for pt to be	
	admitted to College Hospital. Disability 1/9 through 1/31.	
	GI/llf *Gerald Practon, MD*	
1-9-xx	Admit to College Hospital (C hx/exam MC MDM).	
	GI/llf *Gerald Practon, MD*	
1-10-xx	Hosp visit (PF hx/exam SF MDM). CT scan of head reviewed, neg. findings. Pt alert and	
	comfortable. If blood sugar and BP remain stable, discharge planned for tomorrow.	
	BP 130/85.	
	GI/llf *Gerald Practon, MD*	
1-11-xx	DC from hosp. Pt to be seen in one week in ofc.	
	GI/llf *Gerald Practon, MD*	

Figure 8–6

PLEASE
DO NOT
STAPLE
IN THIS
AREA

HEALTH INSURANCE CLAIM FORM

| | PICA | | | | | | | | | PICA | |

1. MEDICARE	MEDICAID	CHAMPUS	CHAMPVA	GROUP HEALTH PLAN	FECA BLK LUNG	OTHER	1a. INSURED'S I.D. NUMBER	(FOR PROGRAM IN ITEM 1)
☐ (Medicare #)	☐ (Medicaid #)	☐ (Sponsor's SSN)	☐ (VA File #)	☒ (SSN or ID)	☐ (S SN)	☐ (ID)	453 XX 4739	96476A

2. PATIENT'S NAME (Last Name, First Name, Middle Initial)
STRAIN EVERT I

3. PATIENT'S BIRTH DATE MM DD YY   SEX   M ☒   F ☐

4. INSURED'S NAME (Last Name, First Name, Middle Initial)
SAME

5. PATIENT'S ADDRESS (No., Street)
7650 NONE SUCH ROAD

6. PATIENT RELATIONSHIP TO INSURED
Self ☐   Spouse ☒   Child ☐   Other ☐

7. INSURED'S ADDRESS (No., Street)

CITY
WOODLAND HILLS   STATE **XY**

8. PATIENT STATUS
Single ☐   Married ☒   Other ☐

CITY   STATE

ZIP CODE   TELEPHONE (Include Area Code) ( )

Employed ☒   Full-Time Student ☐   Part-Time Student ☐

ZIP CODE   TELEPHONE (INCLUDE AREA CODE) ( )

9. OTHER INSURED'S NAME (Last Name, First Name, Middle Initial)

10. IS PATIENT'S CONDITION RELATED TO:

11. INSURED'S POLICY GROUP OR FECA NUMBER

a. OTHER INSURED'S POLICY OR GROUP NUMBER

a. EMPLOYMENT? (CURRENT OR PREVIOUS)   ☐ YES   ☒ NO

a. INSURED'S DATE OF BIRTH MM DD YY   SEX   M ☐   F ☐

b. OTHER INSURED'S DATE OF BIRTH MM DD YY   SEX M ☐   F ☐

b. AUTO ACCIDENT?   PLACE (State)   ☐ YES   ☒ NO

b. EMPLOYER'S NAME OR SCHOOL NAME

c. EMPLOYER'S NAME OR SCHOOL NAME

c. OTHER ACCIDENT?   ☐ YES   ☒ NO

c. INSURANCE PLAN NAME OR PROGRAM NAME

d. INSURANCE PLAN NAME OR PROGRAM NAME

10d. RESERVED FOR LOCAL USE

d. IS THERE ANOTHER HEALTH BENEFIT PLAN?
☐ YES   ☐ NO   *If yes*, return to and complete item 9 a-d.

READ BACK OF FORM BEFORE COMPLETING & SIGNING THIS FORM.
12. PATIENT'S OR AUTHORIZED PERSON'S SIGNATURE I authorize the release of any medical or other information necessary to process this claim. I also request payment of government benefits either to myself or to the party who accepts assignment below.

SIGNED **SOF**   DATE _____

13. INSURED'S OR AUTHORIZED PERSON'S SIGNATURE I authorize payment of medical benefits to the undersigned physician or supplier for services described below.

SIGNED **SOF**

14. DATE OF CURRENT: MM DD YY ◀ ILLNESS (First symptom) OR INJURY (Accident) OR PREGNANCY(LMP)

15. IF PATIENT HAS HAD SAME OR SIMILAR ILLNESS. GIVE FIRST DATE MM DD YY

16. DATES PATIENT UNABLE TO WORK IN CURRENT OCCUPATION
FROM MM DD YY   TO MM DD YY

17. NAME OF REFERRING PHYSICIAN OR OTHER SOURCE
GERALD C JONES MD

17a. I.D. NUMBER OF REFERRING PHYSICIAN
690235

18. HOSPITALIZATION DATES RELATED TO CURRENT SERVICES
FROM **01 09 20XX**   TO **01 11 20XX**

19. RESERVED FOR LOCAL USE

20. OUTSIDE LAB?   ☐ YES   ☒ NO $ CHARGES

21. DIAGNOSIS OR NATURE OF ILLNESS OR INJURY. (RELATE ITEMS 1,2,3 OR 4 TO ITEM 24E BY LINE)
1. **25000**   3. **414.0**
2. **401.1**   4. _____

22. MEDICAID RESUBMISSION CODE   ORIGINAL REF. NO.

23. PRIOR AUTHORIZATION NUMBER

24. A. DATE(S) OF SERVICE From MM DD YY	To MM DD YY	B. Place of Service	C. Type of Service	D. PROCEDURES, SERVICES, OR SUPPLIES (Explain Unusual Circumstances) CPT/HCPCS	MODIFIER	E. DIAGNOSIS CODE	F. $ CHARGES	G. DAYS OR UNITS	H. EPSDT Family Plan	I. EMG	J. COB	K. RESERVED FOR LOCAL USE
1	01 0820 XX		11		99215			75 00	1			46	278897XX
2	01 0920 XX		21		99222			120 80	1			46	278897XX
3	01 1020 XX		21		99231			37 74	1			46	278897XX
4	01 1120 XX		21		99231			37 74	1			46	278897XX
5													
6													

25. FEDERAL TAX I.D. NUMBER   SSN EIN
70 34597XX   ☐ ☒

26. PATIENT'S ACCOUNT NO.
8-8

27. ACCEPT ASSIGNMENT? (For govt. claims, see back)
☒ YES   ☐ NO

28. TOTAL CHARGE $ **71 28**

29. AMOUNT PAID $

30. BALANCE DUE $ **71 28**

31. SIGNATURE OF PHYSICIAN OR SUPPLIER INCLUDING DEGREES OR CREDENTIALS (I certify that the statements on the reverse apply to this bill and are made a part thereof.)
01 25 20XX
SIGNED   DATE

32. NAME AND ADDRESS OF FACILITY WHERE SERVICES WERE RENDERED (If other than home or office)

33. PHYSICIAN'S, SUPPLIER'S BILLING NAME, ADDRESS, ZIP CODE & PHONE #
COLLEGE CLINIC
4567 BROAD AVENUE
WOODLAND HILLS XY 12345
555 486 9002
PIN#   GRP# **3664021XX**

(APPROVED BY AMA COUNCIL ON MEDICAL SERVICE 8/88)   **PLEASE PRINT OR TYPE**   APPROVED OMB-0938-0008 FORM CMS-1500 (12-90),   FORM RRB-1500,
APPROVED OMB-1215-0055 FORM OWCP-1500,   APPROVED OMB-0720-0001 (CHAMPUS)

EXAMPLE ONLY

Figure 8–7

SELF-STUDY 8–9 ▸ DEFINE PATIENT RECORD ABBREVIATIONS

Performance Objective

Task: Insert definitions of abbreviations.

Conditions: Use pencil or pen.

Standards: Time: _____ minutes

             Accuracy: _____

             (Note: The time element and accuracy criteria may be given by your instructor.)

Directions: After completing the assignments in this chapter, you will be able to define the abbreviations shown here.

Abbreviations pertinent to the record of Brad E. Diehl:

NP _____	R/O _____
LC _____	auto _____
pt _____	retn _____
MDM _____	diff _____
AP _____	EPF _____
cm _____	WBC _____
lat _____	hx _____
neg _____	DX _____
BP _____	exam _____
CBC _____	adv _____

Abbreviations pertinent to the record of Evert I. Strain:

est _____	PX _____
CT _____	MC _____
pt _____	BP _____
C _____	MDM _____
H & P _____	lab _____
hx _____	hosp _____
comp _____	SGOT _____
exam _____	PF _____

Dx _____   GTT _____

SF _____   DC _____

ASCVD_____   STAT _____

neg _____   ofc _____

To check your answers to this self-study assignment, see Appendix D.

FINDING YOUR WAY AROUND THE PRACTICE MANAGEMENT AND BILLING SOFTWARE

(Portions of these general program tips and instruction reprinted with permission from AltaPoint Data Systems, LLC, Midvale, Utah.)

Important Message to New Users

If you are no stranger to using the computer, then you know how important it is to protect your data files. It cannot be said enough, "Back up your data!" It is strongly recommended that you back up data files *every* time you use this program.

Cycle the media you use for your backups. In other words, use more than one CD/disk and rotate them throughout the week. For example, if you use the program three times in a week, each day you access it and back up the files, there should be a separate CD/disk. In this case, there should be three separate CDs/disks, perhaps labeled "Monday," "Wednesday," and "Friday." This way, you will be assured that a damaged data set can be replaced with a current good backup and if one backup CD/disk becomes lost or damaged, there will be a complete set of data files available to recover. Instructions for Backup Data Files appear near the end of this section.

Initial Access and Log On to the AltaPoint Software

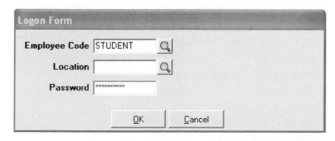

After inserting the CD and installing the software onto your computer, double click on the AltaPoint program icon on the desktop.

Initially, you will be asked to enter an "Employee Code," "Location," and "Password." Until you set yourself up as a user, the Employee Code "STUDENT" will be the only usable choice, so select this in order to set up your own user name. Disregard the "Location" at this time. The initial access password is "STUDENT." NOTE: The asterisks in the Password field ****** are inserted by the program and do not indicate the presence of a password.

Next, set up an Employee Code that identifies you as a system user. Click on "File" and select "Providers and Employees."

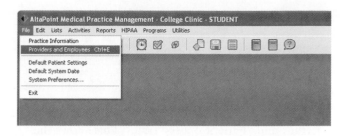

The list of employees appears. Click on "New" to create a new Employee Code (user).

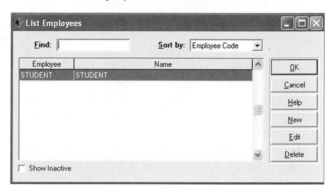

The Employee Code can be up to 10 alphanumeric characters. For example, SMITH123 would be an acceptable Employee Code. Ideally, the Employee Code should be your last name. Follow your instructor's direction on what to enter for your Employee Code. Click "OK."

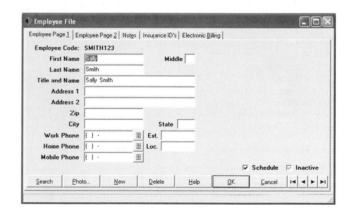

Setting User Password and Security

As a safety precaution, at least one employee (student) must have access to the Password Maintenance feature under the File option. This way, users do not accidentally lock themselves out of the program indefinitely. For multi-user or client servers, the instructor should have access to this feature.

NOTE: *Important! Check with your instructor for information before setting the user password and security levels.*

1. For single-user desktops, after logging in, select the employee (student) for whom you wish to set up password clearance. This should be you. Go to HIPAA on the menu and select passwords and security.

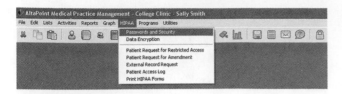

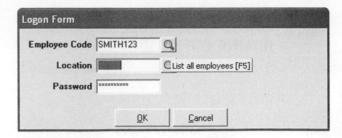

2. Click to place a checkmark in "Employee Audit Trail" and "Patient Access Trail." This allows the system to track the user's access to files and link activity to the *Workbook* assignments. An audit trail will be kept for this employee (student), tracking any record deletions or edits made by this employee (student).
3. Click "Check All" at the bottom of the dialog box *or* check the checkboxes for each item that you would like the employee (student) to have access to when working in the program.
4. Type in the password for this employee (student).
5. Verify the password by retyping the password to ensure that the password was typed correctly. Click "OK."

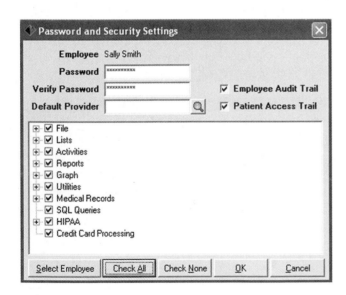

HELPFUL FEATURES AND NOTES

Program Start Up

Pressing the magnifying glass (look up) icon or the F5 key on the keyboard allows the user to select from a list of possible employee/student codes. The employee/student code assigned to each student makes it easier for more than one individual to work in the same system and maintain separate user activity logs that correspond with each *Workbook* assignment. Enter your employee/student code and password in the appropriate fields to gain access to the system for completing the electronic exercises in the *Workbook* assignments.

Toolbar Icons

Like most software programs, you can pass your mouse over any icon to see a description of functionality for that particular icon. Each of the functions associated with an icon can be accessed through the menu options as well (Figure 8–8).

Getting Help

The "Help" feature in AltaPoint answers a wide range of questions. To access assistance, just click on the "?" icon on the main toolbar.

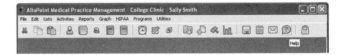

Using Shortcut and Alt Keys

There are several shortcut keys in the program for the user's convenience. These shortcut keys take you directly to certain functions in the software without having to work through any menus. The shortcuts are generally a series of keystrokes. (They are also listed throughout the program next to their respective menu items.)

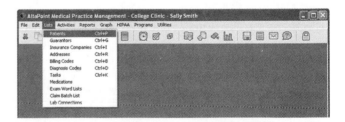

Here, you can access a patient file in one of two ways:

1. Click on "Lists" and then click on "Patients"
   or
2. Press the "Ctrl" key and then the letter "P" on the keyboard. The Patient List pops open. (**NOTE:** If you press this sequence without being in the program, likely your Print window will open!)

The following are examples of shortcut keys. The entire list can be found in the AltaPoint Help file.

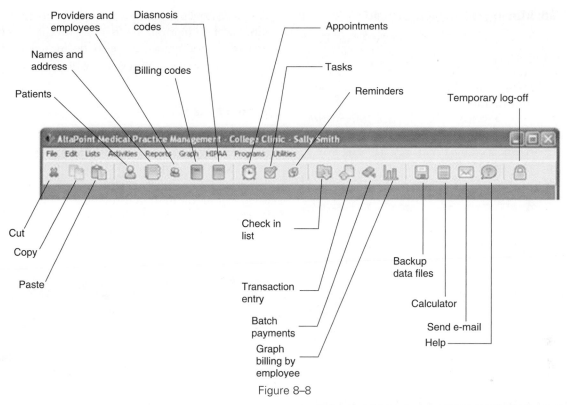

Figure 8–8

Keystrokes	Feature
Ctrl + A	Appointments
Ctrl + B	Billing Code File
Ctrl + C	Copy
Ctrl + D	Diagnosis Code File

Temporary Log Off

A user has the ability to log off of the program without exiting the program. This feature is helpful in controlling who has access to the data in your program. Additionally, HIPAA guidelines mandate that a health care provider control who sees the patient information in the practice. This feature helps an organization be compliant with this HIPAA requirement.

There are two ways to temporarily log off from the program:

1. Click on "File" and then "Log off." This means that another user can log on without having to launch the program again.
2. Press the security lock icon on the toolbar.

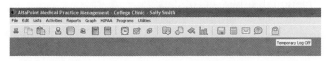

Exiting the Program

To exit AltaPoint, click on "File" and then "Exit."

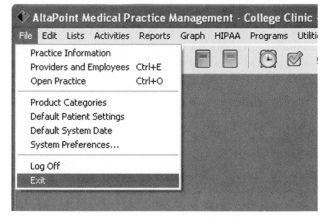

A screen prompts the user to "Backup Data Files," "Cancel," or "Exit AltaPoint." Click the desired action. Selecting "Exit AltaPoint" shuts down the program completely without a backup.

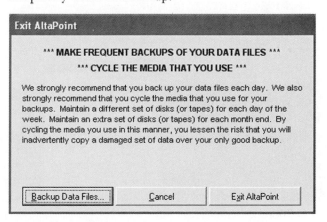

Enter or Tab: Moving from Field to Field

Using the "Tab" key is the Windows standard. However, you can use the "Enter" key to move from field to field. It is simply a matter of user preference. To choose between the "Enter" and "Tab" keys, select "File" and then "Practice Information."

In the "Options" tab from the Practice Information screen, place a checkmark in the "Use Enter Key for Next Field" box to use the Enter key. (If this box is checked, you may use both keys.)

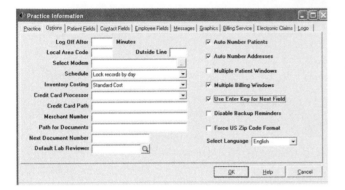

System Date and Date Spin

When performing exercises, you will key in dates. In most date fields throughout the program you have the ability to advance the date forward or backward by pressing the "+" or "−" keys on the number pad on the right side of your keyboard. By default, the current system date will be displayed. Also, if a date field is blank, pressing the "+" or "-" key will input the current system date. Remember to hold down the "Shift" key while depressing the "+"; otherwise, you are pressing the "=" symbol!

Utilities–Data File Backup and Restore Options

Use the "Backup Data Files" and "Restore Data Files" options from the Utilities menu to perform routine backups (as an alternative to running a backup from the Exit AltaPoint option) and restore data when necessary.

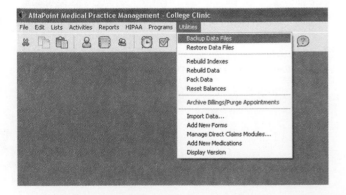

Before backing up or restoring, read through this entire section to avoid any issues with the system. This area of the program may also be locked from other user's access to avoid unnecessary problems.

Backup Data Files

Select "Backup Data Files" from the Utilities menu to access this option. This feature allows the user to specify a location for the data file backup and proceed to back up the data. A backup reminder pops up or appears when exiting the system if this option is selected in the Practice Information feature under the Options tab. Once this option is selected from the Utilities menu, the following screen appears.

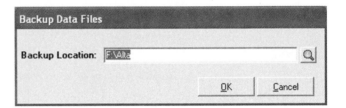

Enter the path for the backup in the "Backup Location" field. The user may also browse to a specific drive, folder, or access point by pressing the lookup button (magnifying glass button to the right of the field). Press the OK button and the system compresses and backs up the files to the specified location.

Restore Data Files

Contact your instructor if you have issues with damaged data and only perform "Restore Data" when absolutely necessary. This option allows flexibility in deciding which files to restore to your current data set or system. It may have several purposes, including the following:

Simple examples:
- Restoring over existing data that may have problems

Advanced examples:
- Restoring specific insurance, procedure, or diagnosis files when duplicating a data set for another doctor or for billing services that have a need to duplicate information in other sets of data
- Restoring an old set of data from an old backup to a separately created set of data if archived or deleted data need to be recalled and evaluated.

1. From the main menu, click on "Utilities" and then select "Restore Data Files." The following will appear.

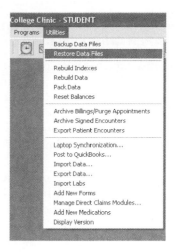

2. As a default, all available options are selected. If resolving an issue wherein a full restoration is necessary, leave all boxes selected. If a specific file is in question, select only that option when restoring the data.

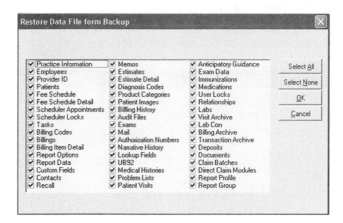

3. Press "Select All" or "Select None" to expedite the selection process. Press the OK button to proceed to the next option; the following will appear (**NOTE:** AltaPoint pulls the data to be restored from the most current backup— remember how important it was to back up data daily!)

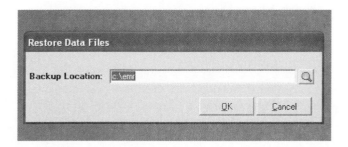

If the location of the backup file to be used as the source of data does not automatically appear, press the Lookup button to browse to the desired directory that contains the backup file if necessary. Press OK and all selected (checked) files will be restored to the currently open data set.

Hands-On Exercises

The student will use the practice management software for "electronic exercises" throughout Chapters 8 through 14. The directions for these assignments are in the *Workbook* and allow for both paper and electronic-based exercises.

MORE TECHNICAL HELP AND INFORMATION

Access the Help functionality in AltaPoint for more detailed information and troubleshooting. Or, via email contact technical.support@elsevier.com.

PRACTICE MANAGEMENT AND BILLING SOFTWARE ASSIGNMENTS

NOTE: For assignment purposes, the Social Security, state license, federal tax ID, UPIN, PIN, and NPI numbers associated with the patients and providers have been entered with a mix of zeros and x's so that they are not realistic.

e hint   **General Instructions for Entering a TRANSACTION**

1. Click on "Activities."
2. Select "Transaction Entry."

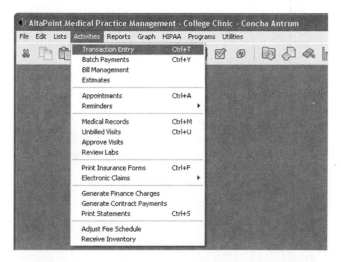

3. [Patient field:] Click the magnifying glass (lookup) and find the patient (example: Margaret A. Nunez).
4. Double-click on the desired patient's name. This opens the patient's account and allows a "Transaction Entry" to be posted.

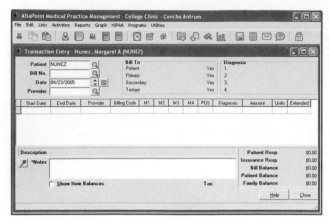

5. [Bill No. field:] A bill number is automatically assigned by the system, so Enter/Tab through this field.

6. [Date field:] This date is the date the transaction was posted. As a result, the current computer system date will be filled in when you Enter/Tab through this field. **However, when completing the *Workbook* exercises, use the last service date as identified on the encounter form.**

7. [Provider field:] Click the magnifying glass (lookup) and find the provider of services (example: Gene Ulibarri, MD).

8. [Start Date field:] Enter/Tab or click on the "Start Date" field and enter the date of service. Key in the desired date. Remember, the current system date is the default and you can use the "Date Spin" hotkey to toggle the date up or down.

9. [End Date field:] This is generally the same date of service for office visits, so Enter or Tab through.

10. [Billing Code field:] Click on the "..." button and scroll to find the CPT code. You can select by double clicking *or* highlighting and pressing "OK."

11. [POS field:] In the "Place of Service" code, click on the "..." button and select the correct option, depending on the *Workbook* assignment.

12. [Diagnosis field:] Click on the "..." and select the proper diagnosis code by clicking on the magnifying glass under "Diagnosis for this bill." Then click "OK."

13. When finished posting transactions, click on "Close" at the bottom of the screen to close the billing screen.

HELPFUL HINTS when Entering a TRANSACTION

▪ For the system to record and save the entry, there must be a valid SERVICE DATE, PROVIDER, and BILLING CODES!

▪ If there is more than one transaction to post while the "Transaction Entry" screen is open for the same patient, Enter/Tab at the end of the first line entry. This saves the information and compiles it with subsequent lines of entry.

(e hint) General Instructions for Printing a PAPER CMS 1500 CLAIM

1. After a date of service has been posted, a paper CMS 1500 claim form can be printed. For *Workbook* exercises, unless otherwise indicated, one claim form will be generated per individual patient. A batch made up of several claims produces several patients' billings at a time.

2. After posting an entry in the "Transaction Entry" window, click on "Print" at the bottom of the screen and select "Print Insurance."

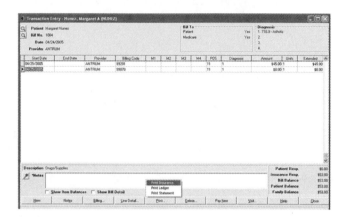

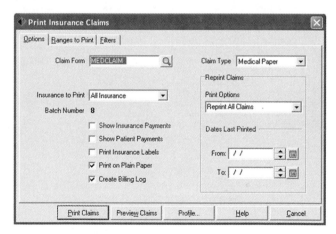

3. In the [Claim Form] field, choose "MEDCLAIM" (the CMS 1500 form).

4. Be sure the [Claim Type] field is "Medical Paper."

5. Click on "Print Claims" button. Hand the completed form in to your instructor as directed.

HELPFUL HINTS when Printing a PAPER CMS 1500 CLAIM

▪ You can reprint claims once they have been generated.

▪ In the "Print Insurance Claims" screen, go to [Print Options] and click on the down arrow. From there, choose "Reprint All Claims."

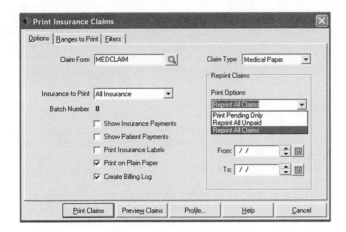

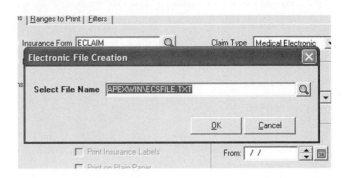

find the folder or CD/floppy drive that the file is to be saved to.

(e hint) General Instructions for TRANSMISSION OF AN ELECTRONIC CLAIM (A SINGLE CLAIM)

An electronic claim is essentially a text file (filename.txt) that is sent to the clearinghouse. So, when an electronic claim is generated, the file must be saved in a directory that will subsequently be sent to the clearinghouse. Think of writing a document in Microsoft Word. The document is then saved to a specific directory in order to be easily accessed later.

1. Follow your instructor's direction and either set up a dedicated folder on your desktop to send the file to or use a CD/floppy.
2. To create an electronic claim after a transaction has been entered, follow the steps for printing a paper claim *except* under [Claim Type] field, the drop down box should be changed to "Medical Electronic" and the [Insurance Form] should be "ECLAIM" unless otherwise specified by your instructor.

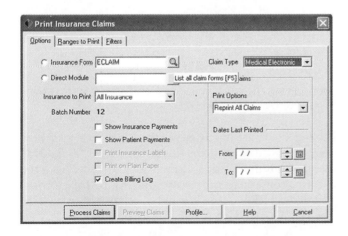

3. Click on "Process Claims" at the bottom of the screen. A screen will open asking what directory to send the file to. Click on the magnifying glass to

4. After clicking on the magnifying glass, you can browse and select the proper directory where the electronic claim is to be saved. Again, this can be a folder on the desktop or a CD/floppy designated for your *Workbook* assignments.

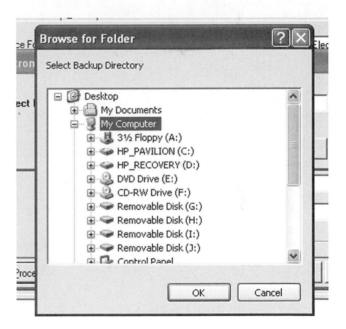

(e hint) General Instructions for TRANSMISSION OF A BATCH OF ELECTRONIC CLAIMS (SEVERAL CLAIMS AT ONCE)

1. To create a batch of electronic claims after several transactions have been entered, click on "Activities" menu, then "Electronic Claims," and, finally, the "Create Electronic Claims" option.
   The familiar "Print Insurance Claims" screen will appear.
2. In the [Insurance to Print] field, select "All Insurance."
3. Follow the previous instructions for saving the .txt to file to the given directory.

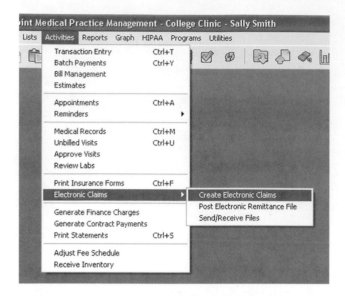

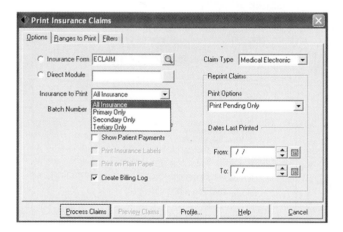

HELPFUL HINTS when performing TRANSMISSION OF ELECTRONIC CLAIMS

- An HIPAA-compliant ANSI format looks something like this when opened as a text (.txt) file:

ISA*00* *01*51333 *ZZ*0007 *ZZ*REC ID *040806*1206*U*00401*000000121*1*T*:~GS*HC*0007*REC ID*20040806*1206*121*X*004010X098A1~ST*837*0121~BHT*0019*00*000000121*20040806*1206*CH~REF*87*004010X098~NM1*41*2*COLLEGE CLINIC*****46*0007~PER*IC*STACEY*TE*8015699360~NM1*40*2*REC NAME*****46*REC ID~HL*1**20*1~NM1*85*2*CREEKSIDE CLINIC*****24*95-8888555~N3*5252 BIG BEAVER RD.~N4*MIDVALE*UT*84047~REF*1C*444444~HL*2*1*22*0~SBR*P*18*******~NM1*IL*1*NUNEZ*MARGARET*A***MI*SPEE-00000~N3*3851 W. COBBLE RIDGE #6-107~N4*WEST JORDAN*UT*84088~DMG*D8**~NM1*PR*2*UNITED WEST-ERN BENEFIT*****PI*ECPID~N3*151 SOUTH MARKET STREET~N4*SALT LAKE CITY*UT*84111~CLM*SPEE-00000B14*100***::1*Y*C*N*N*~DTP*454*D8*20040203~DTP*304*D8*20040409~NM1*DN*1*SPEER*JUSTIN~REF*1G*222222~NM1*82*1*LYNDON*JEFFERY****24*123456~REF*G2*585858~NM1*DQ*1*ANTRUM*CONCHA****34*~LX*1~SV1*HC:99214*100*UN*1*****N~DTP*472*D8*20040409~SE*32*0121~GE*1*121~IEA*1*000000121~

- An electronic claim output that is not in HIPAA format (one of the old NSF versions) looks something like this when opened as a text file:

```
                    MEDICARE
               X
NUNEZ, MARGARET A  08 04 1947  X NUNEZ, MARGARET A
1912 BROOK LANE        X      1912 BROOK LANE
SPRING OAK        XY   X  SPRING OAK          XY
12345                       12345
               X    08 04 1947   X
               X
               X
                    X
                    X
  716.9
04252005   11    99201   1    45 00  1
04252005   11    99070   1    8 00  1
74-10640XX    X  NUNEZ    X    53 00    53 00
               COLLEGE CLINIC
               4567 BROAD AVENUE
SIGNATURE ON FILE,   WOODLAND HILLS, XY 12345-0001
               12458977XX
```

For ease in grading *Workbook* exercises, your instructor may choose to only use the [Insurance Form] "ECLAIM" because it is more readable than an ANSI file. Also, the clearinghouse may still accept the "ECLAIM" format, but under HIPAA, the clearinghouse must translate it to the HIPAA-standard ANSI.

ASSIGNMENT 8-10 ▸ TRANSMIT AN ELECTRONIC INSURANCE CLAIM
FOR A PRIVATE CASE

Performance Objective

Task: Transmit an electronic insurance claim form and post the information to the patient's financial account record.

Conditions: Use Margaret A. Nunez's encounter form (Figure 8–9), patient's electronic data, and computer.

Standards: Productivity Measurement

Time: _____ minutes

Accuracy: _____

(Note: The time element and accuracy criteria may be given by your instructor.)

Directions:

1. Electronically prepare an insurance claim form by referring to Margaret A. Nunez's encounter form in the *Workbook* and her electronic personal and medical data. Follow the step-by-step general directions for transmission of an insurance claim.

2. Enter the patient's data into the software to obtain the procedural and diagnostic codes and College Clinic fee amounts.

3. Transmit the insurance claim to Aetna Health Plan.

4. Print a hard copy of the insurance claim to hand in to your instructor to receive a score.

5. A Performance Evaluation Checklist may be reproduced from the "Instruction Guide to the Workbook" chapter if your instructor wishes you to submit it to assist with scoring and comments.

After the instructor has returned your work to you, either make the necessary corrections and place your work in a three-ring notebook for future reference or, if you received a high score, place it in your portfolio for reference when applying for a job.

TAX ID #3664021CC
Medicaid #HSC12345F

College Clinic

4567 Broad Avenue
Woodlands Hills, XY
12345-0001
Tel (555) 486-9002
Fax (555) 487-8976

Doctors No. _____

☒ PRIVATE   ☐ MANAGED CARE   ☐ MEDICAID   ☐ MEDICARE   ☐ TRICARE   ☐ W/C

ACCOUNT #	PATIENT'S LAST NAME	FIRST	INITIAL	TODAY'S DATE
001	*Nunez*	*Margaret*	*A.*	*1/19/2007*

ASSIGNMENT: I hereby assign payment directly to College Clinic of the surgical and/or medical benefits, if any, otherwise payable to me for his/her services as described below.
SIGNED (Patient, or Parent, if Minor) *Margaret A. Nunez*   DATE: *1/19/2007*

✓	DESCRIPTION	CPT-4/MD	FEE	✓	DESCRIPTION	CPT-4/MD	FEE	✓	DESCRIPTION	CPT-4/MD	FEE
	OFFICE VISIT-NEW PATIENT				**WELL BABY EXAM**				**LABORATORY**		
	Level 1	99201			Intial	99381			Glucose Blood	82962	
	Level 2	99202			Periodic	99391			Heamatocrit	85013	
	Level 3	99203			**OFFICE PROCEDURES**				Occult Blood	82270	
	Level 4	99204			Anscopy	46600		✓	Urine Dip	81000	*8.00*
	Level 5	99205			ECG 24-hr	93224			**X-RAY**		
	OFFICE VISIT-ESTAB, PATIENT				Fracture Rpr Foot	28470			Foot - 2 View	73620	
✓	Level 1	99211	*16 07*		I & D	10060			Forearm - 2 View	73090	
	Level 2	99212			Suture Repair				Nasal Bone - 3	70160	
	Level 3	99213							Spine LS - 2 view	72100	
	Level 4	99214			**INJECTIONS/VACCINATIONS**						
	Level 5	99215			DPT	90701			**MISCELLANEOUS**		
	OFFICE CONSULT-NP/EST				IM-Antibiotic	90788			Handling of Spec	99000	
	Level 3	99243			OPU-Poliovirus	90712			Supply	99070	
	Level 4	99244			Tetanus	90703			Venipuncture	36415	
	Level 5	99245									

COMMENTS:

Physician: *Gene Ulibarri, M.D.*

RETURN APPOINTMENT

___/___ Week(s)   _____ Month(s)

DIAGNOSIS: DESCRIPTION   CODE
Primary: *Urinary tract infection*   *599.0*
Secondary: _____ _____
_____ _____

REC'D BY:
☐ BANK CARD
☐ CASH
☐ CHECK
_____

PREVIOUS BALANCE   *-0-*
TODAY'S FEE   *24.07*
AMOUNT REC'D/CO-PAY *-0-*
BALANCE   *24.07*

Figure 8–9

ASSIGNMENT 8–11 ▸ **TRANSMIT AN ELECTRONIC INSURANCE CLAIM FOR A PRIVATE CASE**

Performance Objective

Task: Transmit an electronic insurance claim form and post the information to the patient's financial account record.

Conditions: Use Samantha L. Walker's encounter form (Figure 8–10), patient's electronic data, and computer.

Standards: Productivity Measurement

Time: _____ minutes

Accuracy: _____

(Note: The time element and accuracy criteria may be given by your instructor.)

Directions:

1. Electronically prepare an insurance claim form by referring to Samantha L. Walker's encounter form in the *Workbook* and her electronic personal and medical data. Follow the step-by-step general directions for transmission of an insurance claim.

2. Enter the patient's data into the software to obtain the procedural and diagnostic codes and College Clinic fee amounts.

3. Transmit the insurance claim to Monarch Medical Insurance.

4. Print a hard copy of the insurance claim to hand in to your instructor to receive a score.

5. A Performance Evaluation Checklist may be reproduced from the "Instruction Guide to the Workbook" chapter if your instructor wishes you to submit it to assist with scoring and comments.

    After the instructor has returned your work to you, either make the necessary corrections and place your work in a three-ring notebook for future reference or, if you received a high score, place it in your portfolio for reference when applying for a job.

TAX ID #3664021CC
Medicaid #HSC12345F

College Clinic

4567 Broad Avenue
Woodlands Hills, XY
12345-0001
Tel (555) 486-9002
Fax (555) 487-8976

Doctors No. _____

☒ PRIVATE   ☐ MANAGED CARE   ☐ MEDICAID   ☐ MEDICARE   ☐ TRICARE   ☐ W/C

ACCOUNT #	PATIENT'S LAST NAME	FIRST	INITIAL	TODAY'S DATE
002	Walker	Samantha	L.	7/16/2007

ASSIGNMENT: I hereby assign payment directly to College Clinic of the surgical and/or medical benefits, if any, otherwise payable to me for his/her services as described below.
SIGNED (Patient, or Parent, if Minor)   Samantha L. Walker   DATE: 7/16/2007

✓	DESCRIPTION	CPT-4/MD	FEE	✓	DESCRIPTION	CPT-4/MD	FEE	✓	DESCRIPTION	CPT-4/MD	FEE
	OFFICE VISIT-NEW PATIENT				**WELL BABY EXAM**				**LABORATORY**		
	Level 1	99201			Intial	99381		✓	Culture screen	87081	25.00
	Level 2	99202			Periodic	99391			Heamatocrit	85013	
	Level 3	99203			**OFFICE PROCEDURES**				Occult Blood	82270	
	Level 4	99204			Anscopy	46600			Urine Dip	81000	
	Level 5	99205			ECG 24-hr	93224			**X-RAY**		
	OFFICE VISIT-ESTAB, PATIENT				Fracture Rpr Foot	28470			Foot - 2 View	73620	
	Level 1	99211			I & D	10060			Forearm - 2 View	73090	
✓	Level 2	99212	28.55		Suture Repair				Nasal Bone - 3	70160	
	Level 3	99213							Spine LS - 2 view	72100	
	Level 4	99214			**INJECTIONS/VACCINATIONS**						
	Level 5	99215			DPT	90701			**MISCELLANEOUS**		
	OFFICE CONSULT-NP/EST				IM-Antibiotic	90788			Handling of Spec	99000	
	Level 3	99243			OPU-Poliovirus	90712			Supply	99070	
	Level 4	99244			Tetanus	90703			Venipuncture	36415	
	Level 5	99245									

COMMENTS:

Physician: Concha Antrum, M.D.

RETURN APPOINTMENT

____/____ Week(s)   _____ Month(s)

DIAGNOSIS: DESCRIPTION   CODE
Primary: Influenza w/pharyngitis   487.1
Secondary: _____ _____
_____ _____

REC'D BY:
☐ BANK CARD
☐ CASH
☐ CHECK
_____

PREVIOUS BALANCE	-0-
TODAY'S FEE	53.55
AMOUNT REC'D/CO-PAY	-0-
BALANCE	53.55

Figure 8–10

ASSIGNMENT 8-12 ► **TRANSMIT AN ELECTRONIC INSURANCE CLAIM FOR A PRIVATE CASE**

Performance Objective

Task: Transmit an electronic insurance claim form and post the information to the patient's financial account record.

Conditions: Use Richard D. Jameson's encounter form (Figure 8–11), patient's electronic data, and computer.

Standards: Productivity Measurement

Time: _____ minutes

Accuracy: _____

(Note: The time element and accuracy criteria may be given by your instructor.)

Directions:

1. Electronically prepare an insurance claim form by referring to Richard D. Jameson's encounter form in the *Workbook* and his electronic personal and medical data. Follow the step-by-step general directions for transmission of an insurance claim.

2. Enter the patient's data into the software to obtain the procedural and diagnostic codes and College Clinic fee amounts.

3. Transmit the insurance claim to Royal Pacific Insurance Company.

4. Print a hard copy of the insurance claim to hand in to your instructor to receive a score.

5. A Performance Evaluation Checklist may be reproduced from the "Instruction Guide to the Workbook" chapter if your instructor wishes you to submit it to assist with scoring and comments.

After the instructor has returned your work to you, either make the necessary corrections and place your work in a three-ring notebook for future reference or, if you received a high score, place it in your portfolio for reference when applying for a job.

TAX ID #3664021CC
Medicaid #HSC12345F

College Clinic

4567 Broad Avenue
Woodlands Hills, XY
12345-0001
Tel (555) 486-9002
Fax (555) 487-8976

Doctors No. _____

☒ PRIVATE ☐ MANAGED CARE ☐ MEDICAID ☐ MEDICARE ☐ TRICARE ☐ W/C

ACCOUNT #	PATIENT'S LAST NAME	FIRST	INITIAL	TODAY'S DATE
003	Jameson	Richard	D.	9/29/2007

ASSIGNMENT: I hereby assign payment directly to College Clinic of the surgical and/or medical benefits, if any, otherwise payable to me for his/her services as described below.
SIGNED (Patient, or Parent, if Minor)   Richard D. Jameson   DATE: 9/29/2007

✓	DESCRIPTION	CPT-4/MD	FEE	✓	DESCRIPTION	CPT-4/MD	FEE	✓	DESCRIPTION	CPT-4/MD	FEE
	OFFICE VISIT-NEW PATIENT				**WELL BABY EXAM**				**LABORATORY**		
	Level 1	99201			Intial	99381			Glucose Blood	82962	
	Level 2	99202			Periodic	99391			Heamatocrit	85013	
	Level 3	99203			**OFFICE PROCEDURES**				Occult Blood	82270	
	Level 4	99204			Anscopy	46600			Urine Dip	81000	
	Level 5	99205			ECG 24-hr	93224			**X-RAY**		
	OFFICE VISIT-ESTAB. PATIENT				Fracture Rpr Foot	28470			Foot - 2 View	73620	
	Level 1	99211			I & D	10060			Forearm - 2 View	73090	
	Level 2	99212			Suture Repair				Nasal Bone - 3	70160	
✓	Level 3	99213	40.20						Spine LS - 2 view	72100	
	Level 4	99214			**INJECTIONS/VACCINATIONS**			✓	Chest-2 view	71020	40.97
	Level 5	99215			DPT	90701			**MISCELLANEOUS**		
	OFFICE CONSULT-NP/EST				IM-Antibiotic	90788		✓	Handling of Spec	99000	5.00
	Level 3	99243			OPU-Poliovirus	90712			Supply	99070	
	Level 4	99244			Tetanus	90703		✓	Venipuncture	36415	10.00
	Level 5	99245									

COMMENTS:

Physician: Brady Coccidioides, M.D.

RETURN APPOINTMENT

__2__ Week(s) _____ Month(s)

DIAGNOSIS:	DESCRIPTION	CODE
Primary:	Influenza w/pneumonia	487.0
Secondary:		

REC'D BY:
☐ BANK CARD
☐ CASH
☐ CHECK
  # _____

PREVIOUS BALANCE   127.49
TODAY'S FEE   96.17
AMOUNT REC'D/CO-PAY
BALANCE   223.66

Figure 8–11

ASSIGNMENT 8-13 ▸ **TRANSMIT AN ELECTRONIC INSURANCE CLAIM FOR A PRIVATE CASE**

Performance Objective

Task: Transmit an electronic insurance claim form and post the information to the patient's financial account record.

Conditions: Use Cameron R. Tushla's encounter form (Figure 8–12), patient's electronic data, and computer.

Standards: Productivity Measurement

                 Time:_____ minutes

                 Accuracy:_____

                 (Note: The time element and accuracy criteria may be given by your instructor.)

Directions:

1. Electronically prepare an insurance claim form by referring to Cameron R. Tushla's encounter form in the *Workbook* and his electronic personal and medical data. Follow the step-by-step general directions for transmission of an insurance claim.

2. Enter the patient's data into the software to obtain the procedural and diagnostic codes and College Clinic fee amounts.

3. Transmit the insurance claim to Prudential Insurance Company.

4. Print a hard copy of the insurance claim to hand in to your instructor to receive a score.

5. A Performance Evaluation Checklist may be reproduced from the "Instruction Guide to the Workbook" chapter if your instructor wishes you to submit it to assist with scoring and comments.

   After the instructor has returned your work to you, either make the necessary corrections and place your work in a three-ring notebook for future reference or, if you received a high score, place it in your portfolio for reference when applying for a job.

TAX ID #3664021CC
Medicaid #HSC12345F

College Clinic

4567 Broad Avenue
Woodlands Hills, XY
12345-0001
Tel (555) 486-9002
Fax (555) 487-8976

Doctors No. _____

☒ PRIVATE   ☐ MANAGED CARE   ☐ MEDICAID   ☐ MEDICARE   ☐ TRICARE   ☐ W/C

ACCOUNT #	PATIENT'S LAST NAME	FIRST	INITIAL	TODAY'S DATE
004	Tushla	Cameron	R.	8/31/2007

ASSIGNMENT: I hereby assign payment directly to College Clinic of the surgical and/or medical benefits, if any, otherwise payable to me for his/her services as described below.
SIGNED (Patient, or Parent, if Minor)   *Cameron R. Tushla*   DATE: *8/31/2007*

✓	DESCRIPTION	CPT-4/MD	FEE	✓	DESCRIPTION	CPT-4/MD	FEE	✓	DESCRIPTION	CPT-4/MD	FEE
	OFFICE VISIT-NEW PATIENT				**WELL BABY EXAM**				**LABORATORY**		
	Level 1	99201		✓	Intial	99381	50.00		Glucose Blood	82962	
	Level 2	99202			Periodic	99391			Heamatocrit	85013	
	Level 3	99203			**OFFICE PROCEDURES**				Occult Blood	82270	
	Level 4	99204			Anscopy	46600			Urine Dip	81000	
	Level 5	99205			ECG 24-hr	93224			**X-RAY**		
	OFFICE VISIT-ESTAB, PATIENT				Fracture Rpr Foot	28470			Foot - 2 View	73620	
	Level 1	99211			I & D	10060			Forearm - 2 View	73090	
	Level 2	99212			Suture Repair				Nasal Bone - 3	70160	
	Level 3	99213		✓	Circumcision	54150	111.78		Spine LS - 2 view	72100	
	Level 4	99214			**INJECTIONS/VACCINATIONS**						
	Level 5	99215			DPT	90701			**MISCELLANEOUS**		
	OFFICE CONSULT-NP/EST				IM-Antibiotic	90788			Handling of Spec	99000	
	Level 3	99243			OPU-Poliovirus	90712			Supply	99070	
	Level 4	99244			Tetanus	90703			Venipuncture	36415	
	Level 5	99245		✓	Hepatitis B	90744	65.00				

COMMENTS:

Physician: *Pedro Atrics, M.D.*

RETURN APPOINTMENT

___/___ Week(s)   _____ Month(s)

DIAGNOSIS: DESCRIPTION   CODE
Primary: *Circumcision*   *V 50.2*
Secondary: *Well baby check*   *V 20.2*
_____   _____

REC'D BY:
☐ BANK CARD
☒ CASH
☐ CHECK
_____

PREVIOUS BALANCE   -0-
TODAY'S FEE   226.78
AMOUNT REC'D/CO-PAY   10.00
BALANCE   216.78

Figure 8–12

ASSIGNMENT **8–14** ▸ **TRANSMIT AN ELECTRONIC INSURANCE CLAIM FOR A PRIVATE CASE**

Performance Objective

Task: Transmit an electronic insurance claim form and post the information to the patient's financial account record.

Conditions: Use Dennis E. McCoy's encounter form (Figure 8–13), patient's electronic data, and computer.

Standards: Productivity Measurement

                Time: _____ minutes

                Accuracy: _____

                (Note: The time element and accuracy criteria may be given by your instructor.)

Directions:

1. Electronically prepare an insurance claim form by referring to Dennis E. McCoy's encounter form in the *Workbook* and his electronic personal and medical data. Follow the step-by-step general directions for transmission of an insurance claim.

2. Enter the patient's data into the software to obtain the procedural and diagnostic codes and College Clinic fee amounts.

3. Transmit the insurance claim to Federated Health Advocate.

4. Print a hard copy of the insurance claim to hand in to your instructor to receive a score.

5. A Performance Evaluation Checklist may be reproduced from the "Instruction Guide to the Workbook" chapter if your instructor wishes you to submit it to assist with scoring and comments.

   After the instructor has returned your work to you, either make the necessary corrections and place your work in a three-ring notebook for future reference or, if you received a high score, place it in your portfolio for reference when applying for a job.

TAX ID #3664021CC
Medicaid #HSC12345F

College Clinic

4567 Broad Avenue
Woodlands Hills, XY
12345-0001
Tel (555) 486-9002
Fax (555) 487-8976

Doctors No. _____

☒ PRIVATE   ☐ MANAGED CARE   ☐ MEDICAID   ☐ MEDICARE   ☐ TRICARE   ☐ W/C

ACCOUNT #	PATIENT'S LAST NAME	FIRST	INITIAL	TODAY'S DATE
005	Mc Coy	Dennis	E.	3/4/2007

ASSIGNMENT: I hereby assign payment directly to College Clinic of the surgical and/or medical benefits, if any, otherwise payable to me for his/her services as described below.
SIGNED (Patient, or Parent, if Minor)   Dennis E. Mc Coy   DATE: 3/4/2007

✓	DESCRIPTION	CPT-4/MD	FEE	✓	DESCRIPTION	CPT-4/MD	FEE	✓	DESCRIPTION	CPT-4/MD	FEE
	OFFICE VISIT-NEW PATIENT				**WELL BABY EXAM**				**LABORATORY**		
	Level 1	99201			Intial	99381			Glucose Blood	82962	
	Level 2	99202			Periodic	99391			Heamatocrit	85013	
✓	Level 3	99203	70.92		**OFFICE PROCEDURES**				Occult Blood	82270	
	Level 4	99204			Anscopy	46600			Urine Dip	81000	
	Level 5	99205			ECG 24-hr	93224			**X-RAY**		
	OFFICE VISIT-ESTAB, PATIENT				Fracture Rpr Foot	28470			Foot - 2 View	73620	
	Level 1	99211			I & D	10060			Forearm - 2 View	73090	
	Level 2	99212			Suture Repair				Nasal Bone - 3	70160	
	Level 3	99213							Spine LS - 2 view	72100	
	Level 4	99214			**INJECTIONS/VACCINATIONS**			✓	Wrist-2 view	73100	31.61
	Level 5	99215			DPT	90701			**MISCELLANEOUS**		
	OFFICE CONSULT-NP/EST				IM-Antibiotic	90788			Handling of Spec	99000	
	Level 3	99243			OPU-Poliovirus	90712		✓	Supply	99070	25.00
	Level 4	99244			Tetanus	90703			Venipuncture	36415	
	Level 5	99245									

COMMENTS: Wrist splint (supply)
Patient fell at home 3/4/2007
Physician: Raymond Skeleton, M.D.

RETURN APPOINTMENT
6 Week(s) ____ Month(s)

DIAGNOSIS: DESCRIPTION   CODE
Primary: Wrist sprain   842.00
Secondary: _____

REC'D BY:
☐ BANK CARD
☐ CASH
☒ CHECK
692

PREVIOUS BALANCE -0-
TODAY'S FEE 127.53
AMOUNT REC'D/CO-PAY 10.00
BALANCE 117.53

Figure 8–13

HELPFUL HINTS: When Printing a PRINTING AN INSURANCE CLAIMS REPORT

1. From the main menu, select "Reports," then mouse down and click "Print Custom Reports."

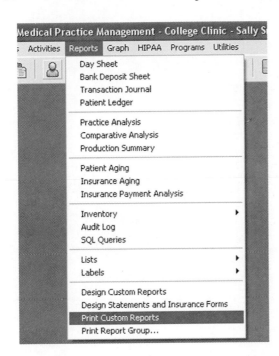

2. In "Print Custom Report" screen at [Report Code field:] click on the magnifying glass and under [Code field] scroll to "INSPRI/Outstanding Claims—Primary."

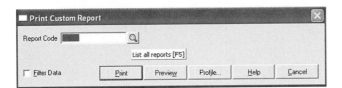

3. Click "OK."

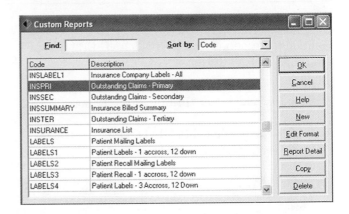

Note: If you wish to save this file as a PDF with your homework assignments after scrolling to "INS PRI" in the "Print Custom Reports" screen rather than selecting "Print," select "Preview." Then, at the bottom of the screen, select "PDF." You will be prompted to indicate where you want to save this file.

ASSIGNMENT **8-15** ▸ **PRINT A BATCH CLAIM REPORT**

General Instructions for VIEWING AND PRINTING
A CLAIM BATCH LIST

1. After generating a batch of claims, click on
"Reports" and select "Print Custom Reports."

2. Find in the [Code field]: "BATCHSUM" (Claim
Batch Summary) and click "OK."

Performance Objective

Task: Print a batch claim report after completing Assignments 8–9, 8–10, 8–11, 8–12, and 8–13.

Conditions: Use electronic data that has been input for Assignments 8–9 through 8–13 and computer.

Standards: Productivity Measurement

Time:_____ minutes

Accuracy:_____

(Note: The time element and accuracy criteria may be given by your instructor.)

Directions:

1. Follow the step-by-step general directions in preparing and printing a batch insurance
claims report.

2. After the instructor has returned your work to you, either make the necessary
corrections and place your work in a three-ring notebook for future reference or, if you
received a high score, place it in your portfolio for reference when applying for a job.

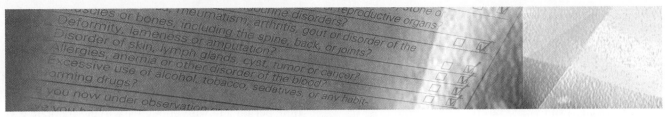

Receiving Payments and Insurance Problem Solving

KEY TERMS

Your instructor may wish to select some specific words pertinent to this chapter for a test. For definitions of the terms, further study, and/or reference, the words, phrases, and abbreviations may be found in the glossary at the end of the Handbook. *Key terms for this chapter follow.*

appeal

delinquent claim

denied paper or electronic claim

explanation of benefits (EOB)

inquiry

lost claim

overpayment

peer review

rebill (resubmit)

rejected claim

remittance advice (RA)

review

suspended claim

suspense

tracer

PERFORMANCE OBJECTIVES

The student will be able to:

■ Define and spell the key terms for this chapter, given the information from the *Handbook* glossary, within a reasonable time period and with enough accuracy to obtain a satisfactory evaluation.

■ After reading the chapter, answer the self-study review questions with enough accuracy to obtain a satisfactory evaluation.

■ Complete the insurance claim tracer form, given a request for an insurance claim trace and the patient's insurance claim, within a reasonable time period and with enough accuracy to obtain a satisfactory evaluation.

■ Locate the errors on each claim, given three returned insurance claims, within a reasonable time period and with enough accuracy to obtain a satisfactory evaluation.

■ Complete form CMS-1965, Request for Hearing, Part B, Medicare Claim, within a reasonable time period and with enough accuracy to obtain a satisfactory evaluation.

■ File an official appeal by composing and typing a letter with envelope, within a reasonable time period and with enough accuracy to obtain a satisfactory evaluation.

■ State observations after viewing a video about medical billing, within a reasonable time period and with enough accuracy to obtain a satisfactory evaluation.

PERFORMANCE OBJECTIVES—cont'd

■ Post electronically to a daysheet from an explanation of benefits document using practice management software and print a patient's financial accounting record, within a reasonable time period and with enough accuracy to obtain a satisfactory evaluation.

■ View a payer response from a clearinghouse using practice management software, within a reasonable time period and with enough accuracy to obtain a satisfactory evaluation.

STUDY OUTLINE

Follow-up after Claim Submission
Claim Policy Provisions
  Insured
  Payment Time Limits
Explanation of Benefits
  Components of an EOB
  Interpretation of an EOB
  Posting an EOB
Claim Management Techniques
  Insurance Claims Register
  Tickler File
  Insurance Company Payment History
Claim Inquiries

Problem Paper and Electronic Claims
  Types of Problems
Rebilling
Review and Appeal Process
Filing an Official Appeal
  Medicare Review and Redetermination Process
  TRICARE Review and Appeal Process
State Insurance Commissioner
  Commission Objectives
  Types of Problems
  Commission Inquiries
Procedure: Trace an Unpaid Insurance Claim
Procedure: File an Official Appeal

 SELF-STUDY **9-1** ▸ **REVIEW QUESTIONS**

    Review the objectives, key terms, and chapter information before completing the following review questions.

1. Name provisions seen in health insurance policies.

  a. _____

  b. _____

  c. _____

  d. _____

2. After an insurance claim is processed by the insurance carrier (paid, suspended,

  rejected, or denied), a document known as a/an _____ is sent to the patient and to the provider of professional medical services.

3. Name other items that indicate the patient's responsibility to pay that may appear on the document explaining the payment and check issued by the insurance carrier.

  a. _____

  b. _____

c. _____

d. _____

e. _____

f. _____

4. After receiving an explanation of benefits (EOB) document and posting insurance

   payment, the copy of the insurance claim form is put into a file marked _____.

5. To locate delinquent insurance claims on an insurance claims register quickly, which

   column should be looked at first? _____

   Would it appear blank or completed? _____

6. Name some of the principal procedures that should be followed in good bookkeeping
   and record-keeping practice when a payment has been received from an insurance company.

   _____

   _____

   _____

7. In good office management, a manual method used to track submitted pending or

   resubmitted insurance claims, a/an _____ is used.

8. Two routine procedures to include in a manual reminder system to track pending claims are:

   a. _____

   b. _____

9. In making an inquiry about a claim by telephone, efficient secretarial procedure would

   be to _____

   _____

   _____

10. Denied paper or electronic claims are those denied because of _____

    _____ or _____

11. State the solution if a claim has been denied because the professional service rendered
    was for an injury that is being considered as compensable under workers' compensation.

    _____

    _____

    _____

12. At the time of his first office visit, Mr. Doi signed an Assignment of Benefits, and Dr. James' office submitted a claim to ABC Insurance Company. Mr. Doi received, in error, a check from the insurance company and cashed it. What steps should be taken by Dr. James' office after this error is discovered?

a. _____

b. _____

c. _____

13. If an appeal of an insurance claim is not successful, the next step to proceed with is a/an

_____.

14. Name the five levels for appealing a Medicare claim.

a. _____

b. _____

c. _____

d. _____

e. _____

15. Medicare reconsideration by the insurance carrier is usually completed within

_____ to _____ days.

16. A Medicare patient has insurance with United American (a Medigap policy), and payment has not been received from the Medigap insurer within a reasonable

length of time. State the action to take in this case. _____

_____

17. A TRICARE EOB is received stating that the allowable charge for Mrs. Dayton's office visit is $30. Is it possible to appeal this for additional payment? Yes or no and why?

_____

18. A state department or agency that helps resolve insurance conflicts and verifies that insurance contracts are carried out in good faith is known as a/an

_____.

When an insurance company consistently pays slowly on insurance claims, it may help

speed up payments if a formal written complaint is made to the _____.

To check your answers to this self-study assignment, see Appendix D.

A S S I G N M E N T   **9 – 2** ▸ **C R I T I C A L   T H I N K I N G :   L O C A T E   A N D   E X P L A I N**
C H O I C E   O F   D I A G N O S T I C   C O D E S

Performance Objective

Task: Locate the correct diagnostic code for the case scenario presented.

Conditions: Use a pen or pencil and the *International Classification of Diagnoses,*
Ninth Revision, Clinical Modification (ICD-9-CM) diagnostic code book.

Standards: Time: _____ minutes

Accuracy: _____

(Note: The time element and accuracy criteria may be given by your instructor.)

Directions: Using your critical thinking skills, answer question after reading the scenario. Record your answer on the blank lines. This question is presented to enhance your skill in critical thinking. Using your diagnostic code book, look up the ICD-9-CM diagnostic code for a patient being treated for a perforated and hemorrhaging gastric ulcer, with no mention of whether it was acute or chronic. To code such a case, what would you do and why?

Checklist

1. Locate the main term or condition in the Alphabetic Index, Volume 2. _____

2. Refer to any notes under the main term. _____

3. Read any notes or terms enclosed in parentheses after the main term. _____

4. Look for appropriate subterm. _____

5. Look for appropriate sub-subterm and follow any cross-reference instructions. _____

6. Write down the code. _____

7. Verify the code number in the Tabular List, Volume 1. _____

8. Read and be guided by any instructional terms in the Tabular List. _____

9. Read complete description and then code to the highest specificity. _____

10. Assign the code. _____

11. Write justification of chosen code(s). _____

ASSIGNMENT **9-3** ▸ **POST TO A FINANCIAL ACCOUNTING RECORD (LEDGER) FROM AN EXPLANATION OF BENEFITS DOCUMENT**

Performance Objective

Task: Post data from an EOB document to a patient's financial accounting record (ledger).

Conditions: Use a blank financial accounting record (ledger) (Figure 9–1), an EOB document (Figure 9–2), and a pen or typewriter.

Standards: Time: _____ minutes

                 Accuracy: _____

                 (Note: The time element and accuracy criteria may be given by your instructor.)

Directions: Post in ink the payment received and preferred provider organization (PPO) discount to a patient's financial accounting record (ledger) (Figure 9–1) by referring to an EOB document (Figure 9–2). An example of financial accounting record (ledger) entries is shown in Figure 3–18 in the *Handbook*. An EOB document is defined in Figure 9–1 in the *Handbook*.

After the instructor has returned your work to you, either make the necessary corrections and place your work in a three-ring notebook for future reference or, if you received a high score, place it in your portfolio for reference when applying for a job.

1. Locate patient's financial accounting record (ledger) and EOB. _____

   Note: Refer to the step-by-step procedures at the end of Chapter 3 in the *Handbook* and graphic examples Figures 3–18, 10–2, and 12–15.

2. Ledger lines: Insert date of service (DOS), reference (CPT code number, check number, or dates of service for posting adjustments or when insurance was billed), description of the transaction, charge amounts, payments, adjustments, and running current balance. The posting date is the actual date the transaction is recorded. If the DOS differs from the posting date, list the DOS in the reference or description column.

   Line 6: _____

   Line 7: _____

   Note: A good bookkeeping practice is to take a red pen and draw a line across the financial accounting record (ledger) from left to right to indicate the last entry billed to the insurance company.

Acct No. __9-3__

STATEMENT
Financial Account
COLLEGE CLINIC
4567 Broad Avenue
Woodland Hills, XY 12345-0001
Tel. 555-486-9002
Fax No. 555-487-8976

Mr. Jabe Bortolussi
989 Moorpark Road
Woodland Hills, XY 12345

Phone No. (H) (555) 230-8870   (W) (555) 349-6689   Birthdate   04-07-71

Primary Insurance Co.   ABC Insurance Company   Policy/Group No. 4206/010

DATE	REFERENCE	DESCRIPTION	CHARGES	CREDITS PYMNTS.	ADJ.	BALANCE
		BALANCE FORWARD ➝				
6-3-xx	99204	E/M NP Level 4	250 00			250 00
6-3-xx	94375	Respiratory flow vol loop	40 00			290 00
6-3-xx	94060	Spirometry	75 00			365 00
6-3-xx	94664	Aerosol inhalation	50 00			415 00
6-3-xx	94760	Pulse oximetry	50 00			465 00

PLEASE PAY LAST AMOUNT IN BALANCE COLUMN ⬆

THIS IS A COPY OF YOUR FINANCIAL ACCOUNT AS IT APPEARS ON OUR RECORDS

Figure 9–1

ABC Insurance Company
P.O. Box 4300
Woodland Hills, XY 12345-0001

Claim No.:	1-00-16987087-00-zmm
Group Name:	COLLEGE CLINIC
Group No.:	010
Employee:	JABE V. BORTOLUSSI
Patient:	JABE V. BORTOLUSSI
SSN:	554-XX-8876
Plan No.:	4206
Prepared by:	M. SMITH
Prepared on:	07/04/20XX

GERALD PRACTON MD
4567 BROAD AVENUE
WOODLAND HILLS XY 12345

Patient Responsibility
Amount not covered:	00
Co-pay amount:	00
Deductible:	00
Co-insurance:	64.61
Patient's total responsibility:	64.61
Other insurance payment:	00

EXPLANATION OF BENEFITS

Treatment Dates	Service Code	CPT Code	Charge Amount	Not Covered	Reason Code	PPO Discount	Covered Amount	Deductible Amount	Co-pay Amount	Paid At	Payment Amount
06/03/xx	200	99204	250.00	00	48	136.00	114.00	00	00	80%	91.20
06/03/xx	540	94375	40.00	00	48	00	40.00	00	00	80%	32.00
06/03/xx	540	94060	75.00	00	48	00	75.00	00	00	80%	60.00
06/03/xx	200	94664	50.00	00	48	1.55	48.45	00	00	80%	38.76
06/03/xx	540	94760	50.00	00	48	4.40	45.60	00	00	80%	36.48
	TOTAL		465.00	00		141.95	123.05	00	00		258.44

Other Insurance Credits or Adjustments   00

CPT Code
99204 OFFICE/OUTPT VISIT E&M NEW MOD-HI SEVERIT
94375 RESPIRATORY FLOW VOLUM LOOP
94060 BRONCHOSPSM EVAL SPIROM PRE & POST BRON
94664 AEROSOL/VAPOR INHALA; INIT DEMO & EVAL
94760 NONINVASIVE EAR/PULSE OXIMETRY-02 SAT

Total Payment Amount   258.44

Reason Code
48 CON DISCOUNT/PT NOT RESPONSIBLE

GC 1234567890

258.44

Participant	Date
GERALD PRACTON MD	07-04-xx
Patient	ID Number
JABE V. BORTOLUSSI	554-XX-8876
Plan Number Patient Number	Office No.
4206	010

PAY TO THE ORDER OF

COLLEGE CLINIC
4567 BROAD AVENUE
WOODLAND HILLS XY 12345

J M Smith
ABC Insurance Company

Figure 9–2

ASSIGNMENT 9-4 ▸ TRACE AN UNPAID INSURANCE CLAIM

Performance Objective

Task: Complete an insurance claim tracer form and attach to this document a photocopy of the claim.

Conditions: Use an Insurance Claim Tracer form (Figure 9–3), an insurance claim form from the *Handbook* (Figure 7–9), and a computer or typewriter.

Standards: Time: _____ minutes

              Accuracy: _____

              (Note: The time element and accuracy criteria may be given by your instructor.)

Directions: You discover that the Medicare claim you submitted to Medicare Blue Shield, 146 Main Street, Woodland Hills, XY 12345, on Bill Hutch 3 months ago was never paid. Complete an insurance claim tracer form (Figure 9–3). Make a photocopy of Bill Hutch's insurance claim form from the *Handbook* in Chapter 7 to attach to the tracer form. Mr. Hutch is retired. Place your name on the tracer form as the person to contact at Dr. Coccidioides' office.

After the instructor has returned your work to you, either make the necessary corrections and place your work in a three-ring notebook for future reference or, if you received a high score, place it in your portfolio for reference when applying for a job.

Checklist

1. Inserted name of insurance company.   _____

2. Dated the form.   _____

3. Inserted the address of the insurance company.   _____

4. Listed the patient's name and insured's name.   _____

5. Inserted the patient's insurance policy and group numbers. _____

6. Inserted information about employment.   _____

7. Listed date of claim submission and amount.   _____

8. Inserted your name as the contact person.   _____

9. Listed the physician's name, address, and telephone number. _____

INSURANCE CLAIM TRACER

INSURANCE COMPANY NAME:_____ DATE:_____

ADDRESS_____

PATIENT NAME:_____ INSURED:_____

POLICY/CERTIFICATE NUMBER:_____ GROUP NAME/NUMBER:_____

EMPLOYER NAME AND ADDRESS:_____

DATE OF INITIAL CLAIM SUBMISSION:_____ AMOUNT:_____

An inordinate amount of time has passed since submission of our original claim as described above. We have not received a request for additional information and still await payment of this assigned claim. Please review the attached duplicate and process for payment within seven (7) days.

If there is any difficulty with this claim, please check one of these below and return this letter to our office.

Claim pending because:_____

Payment of claim in process:_____

Payment made on claim:_____ Date:_____ To Whom:_____

Claim denied: (Reason)_____

Patient notified: Yes_____ No_____

Remarks:_____

_____

Thank you for your assistance in this important matter. Please contact_____ in our office if you have any questions regarding this claim.

Office of:_____ M.D.

Address:_____

_____ TELEPHONE NUMBER:_____

Figure 9–3

ASSIGNMENT 9-5 ► **LOCATE ERRORS ON A RETURNED INSURANCE CLAIM**

Performance Objective

Task: Highlight the blocks on the insurance claim form where errors are discovered.

Conditions: Use an insurance claim form (Figure 9–4) and a highlighter or red pen.

Standards: Time: _____ minutes

                   Accuracy: _____

                   (Note: The time element and accuracy criteria may be given by your instructor.)

Directions: An insurance claim (Figure 9–4) was returned by the Prudential Insurance Company. Highlight or circle in red all blocks on the claim form where errors are discovered.

Option 1:   Retype the claim and either insert the correction if data are available to fix the error or insert the word "NEED" in the block of the claim form.

Option 2:   On a separate sheet of paper, list the blocks from 1 to 33 and state where errors occur.

   A Performance Evaluation Checklist may be reproduced from the "Instruction Guide to the Workbook" chapter if your instructor wishes you to submit it to assist with scoring and comments.
   After the instructor has returned your work to you, either make the necessary corrections and place your work in a three-ring notebook for future reference or, if you received a high score, place it in your portfolio for reference when applying for a job.

PLEASE
DO NOT
STAPLE
IN THIS
AREA

PRUDENTIAL INSURANCE COMPANY
500 SOUTH BEND STREET
WOODLAND HILLS XY 12345

CARRIER →

| | PICA | | | | | | | | **HEALTH INSURANCE CLAIM FORM** | | PICA | | |

| 1. MEDICARE ☐ (Medicare #) | MEDICAID ☐ (Medicaid #) | CHAMPUS ☐ (Sponsor's SSN) | CHAMPVA ☐ (VA File #) | GROUP HEALTH PLAN ☐ (SSN or ID) | FECA BLK LUNG ☐ (S SN) | OTHER ☒ (ID) | 1a. INSURED'S I.D. NUMBER (FOR PROGRAM IN ITEM 1) |

2. PATIENT'S NAME (Last Name, First Name, Middle Initial)
JOHNSON EMILY B.

3. PATIENT'S BIRTH DATE
MM 02 DD 12 YY 1963   SEX M ☐ F ☐

4. INSURED'S NAME (Last Name, First Name, Middle Initial)
JOHNSON ERRON T.

5. PATIENT'S ADDRESS (No., Street)
4391 EVERETT STREET

6. PATIENT RELATIONSHIP TO INSURED
Self ☐ Spouse ☒ Child ☐ Other ☐

7. INSURED'S ADDRESS (No., Street)
SAME

CITY WOODLAND HILLS   STATE XY

8. PATIENT STATUS
Single ☐ Married ☒ Other ☐
Employed ☐ Full-Time Student ☐ Part-Time Student ☐

CITY   STATE

ZIP CODE 12345   TELEPHONE (Include Area Code) ( )

ZIP CODE   TELEPHONE (INCLUDE AREA CODE) ( )

9. OTHER INSURED'S NAME (Last Name, First Name, Middle Initial)

10. IS PATIENT'S CONDITION RELATED TO:

11. INSURED'S POLICY GROUP OR FECA NUMBER

a. OTHER INSURED'S POLICY OR GROUP NUMBER

a. EMPLOYMENT? (CURRENT OR PREVIOUS) ☐ YES ☐ NO

a. INSURED'S DATE OF BIRTH MM DD YY   SEX M ☐ F ☐

b. OTHER INSURED'S DATE OF BIRTH MM DD YY SEX M ☐ F ☐

b. AUTO ACCIDENT? PLACE (State) ☐ YES ☐ NO

b. EMPLOYER'S NAME OR SCHOOL NAME

c. EMPLOYER'S NAME OR SCHOOL NAME

c. OTHER ACCIDENT? ☐ YES ☐ NO

c. INSURANCE PLAN NAME OR PROGRAM NAME

d. INSURANCE PLAN NAME OR PROGRAM NAME

10d. RESERVED FOR LOCAL USE

d. IS THERE ANOTHER HEALTH BENEFIT PLAN?
☐ YES ☒ NO *If yes*, return to and complete item 9 a-d.

READ BACK OF FORM BEFORE COMPLETING & SIGNING THIS FORM.

12. PATIENT'S OR AUTHORIZED PERSON'S SIGNATURE I authorize the release of any medical or other information necessary to process this claim. I also request payment of government benefits either to myself or to the party who accepts assignment below.

SIGNED *Emily B. Johnson*   DATE 01 04 20XX

13. INSURED'S OR AUTHORIZED PERSON'S SIGNATURE I authorize payment of medical benefits to the undersigned physician or supplier for services described below.

SIGNED *Emily B. Johnson*

14. DATE OF CURRENT: MM DD YY ◄ ILLNESS (First symptom) OR INJURY (Accident) OR PREGNANCY(LMP)

15. IF PATIENT HAS HAD SAME OR SIMILAR ILLNESS. GIVE FIRST DATE MM DD YY

16. DATES PATIENT UNABLE TO WORK IN CURRENT OCCUPATION FROM MM DD YY TO MM DD YY

17. NAME OF REFERRING PHYSICIAN OR OTHER SOURCE

17a. I.D. NUMBER OF REFERRING PHYSICIAN
6780502700

18. HOSPITALIZATION DATES RELATED TO CURRENT SERVICES FROM MM DD YY TO MM DD YY

19. RESERVED FOR LOCAL USE

20. OUTSIDE LAB? ☐ YES ☒ NO $ CHARGES

21. DIAGNOSIS OR NATURE OF ILLNESS OR INJURY. (RELATE ITEMS 1,2,3 OR 4 TO ITEM 24E BY LINE)
1. |___|___   3. |___|___
2. |___|___   4. |___|___

22. MEDICAID RESUBMISSION CODE   ORIGINAL REF. NO.

23. PRIOR AUTHORIZATION NUMBER

24. A. DATE(S) OF SERVICE						B. Place of Service	C. Type of Service	D. PROCEDURES, SERVICES, OR SUPPLIES (Explain Unusual Circumstances) CPT/HCPCS	MODIFIER	E. DIAGNOSIS CODE	F. $ CHARGES		G. DAYS OR UNITS	H. EPSDT Family Plan	I. EMG	J. COB	K. RESERVED FOR LOCAL USE
From MM	DD	YY	To MM	DD	YY												
01	04	20XX				11		99213		1	25	00				70	568717XX
01	04	20XX				11		99213		1	25	00					

25. FEDERAL TAX I.D. NUMBER SSN ☐ EIN ☐
71 80561XX

26. PATIENT'S ACCOUNT NO.

27. ACCEPT ASSIGNMENT? (For govt. claims, see back) ☒ YES ☐ NO

28. TOTAL CHARGE $ 60 00

29. AMOUNT PAID $

30. BALANCE DUE $ 60 00

31. SIGNATURE OF PHYSICIAN OR SUPPLIER INCLUDING DEGREES OR CREDENTIALS (I certify that the statements on the reverse apply to this bill and are made a part thereof.)
VERA CUTIS MD
SIGNED *Vera Cutis MD*   DATE 01 06 20XX

32. NAME AND ADDRESS OF FACILITY WHERE SERVICES WERE RENDERED (If other than home or office)

33. PHYSICIAN'S, SUPPLIER'S BILLING NAME, ADDRESS, ZIP CODE & PHONE #
COLLEGE CLINIC
4567 BROAD AVENUE
WOODLAND HILLS XY 12345
555 486 9002
PIN#   GRP# 3664021XX

(APPROVED BY AMA COUNCIL ON MEDICAL SERVICE 8/88) **PLEASE PRINT OR TYPE**

APPROVED OMB-0938-0008 FORM CMS-1500 (12-90), FORM RRB-1500,
APPROVED OMB-1215-0055 FORM OWCP-1500, APPROVED OMB-0720-0001 (CHAMPUS)

PATIENT AND INSURED INFORMATION

PHYSICIAN OR SUPPLIER INFORMATION

Figure 9–4

ASSIGNMENT 9–6 ▸ LOCATE ERRORS ON A RETURNED
INSURANCE CLAIM

Performance Objective

Task: Highlight the blocks on the insurance claim form where errors are discovered.

Conditions: Use an insurance claim form (Figure 9–5) and a highlighter or red pen.

Standards: Time: _____ minutes

                 Accuracy: _____

                 (Note: The time element and accuracy criteria may be given by your instructor.)

Directions: An insurance claim was returned by the Healthtech Insurance Company. Highlight or circle in red all blocks on the claim form where errors are discovered.

Option 1:   Retype the claim and either insert the correction if data are available to fix the error or insert the word "NEED" in the block of the claim form.

Option 2:   On a separate sheet of paper, list the blocks from 1 to 33 and state where errors occur.

A Performance Evaluation Checklist may be reproduced from the "Instruction Guide to the Workbook" chapter if your instructor wishes you to submit it to assist with scoring and comments.

After the instructor has returned your work to you, either make the necessary corrections and place your work in a three-ring notebook for future reference or, if you received a high score, place it in your portfolio for reference when applying for a job.

PLEASE
DO NOT
STAPLE
IN THIS
AREA

HEALTHTECH INSURANCE COMPANY
4821 WESTLAKE AVENUE
WOODLAND HILLS, XY 12345

CARRIER →

HEALTH INSURANCE CLAIM FORM

| | PICA | | | | | | | | PICA | |

1. MEDICARE	MEDICAID	CHAMPUS	CHAMPVA	GROUP HEALTH PLAN (SSN or ID)	FECA BLK LUNG (S SN)	OTHER	1a. INSURED'S I.D. NUMBER	(FOR PROGRAM IN ITEM 1)
☐ (Medicare #)	☒ (Medicaid #)	☒ (Sponsor's SSN)	☐ (VA File #)	☐	☐	☒ (ID)	433129870ANC	

2. PATIENT'S NAME (Last Name, First Name, Middle Initial)	3. PATIENT'S BIRTH DATE MM DD YY	SEX	4. INSURED'S NAME (Last Name, First Name, Middle Initial)
DUGAN CHARLES C	12 24 1968	M ☒ F ☐	SAME

5. PATIENT'S ADDRESS (No., Street)	6. PATIENT RELATIONSHIP TO INSURED	7. INSURED'S ADDRESS (No., Street)
5900 ELM STREET	Self ☒ Spouse ☐ Child ☐ Other ☐	SAME

CITY	STATE	8. PATIENT STATUS	CITY	STATE
WOODLAND HILLS	XY	Single ☐ Married ☒ Other ☐		

ZIP CODE	TELEPHONE (Include Area Code)		ZIP CODE	TELEPHONE (INCLUDE AREA CODE)
12345	(555) 559 3300	Employed ☐ Full-Time Student ☐ Part-Time Student ☐		( )

9. OTHER INSURED'S NAME (Last Name, First Name, Middle Initial)	10. IS PATIENT'S CONDITION RELATED TO:	11. INSURED'S POLICY GROUP OR FECA NUMBER

a. OTHER INSURED'S POLICY OR GROUP NUMBER	a. EMPLOYMENT? (CURRENT OR PREVIOUS) ☐ YES ☒ NO	a. INSURED'S DATE OF BIRTH MM DD YY SEX M ☐ F ☐
b. OTHER INSURED'S DATE OF BIRTH MM DD YY SEX M ☐ F ☐	b. AUTO ACCIDENT? PLACE (State) ☐ YES ☒ NO	b. EMPLOYER'S NAME OR SCHOOL NAME
c. EMPLOYER'S NAME OR SCHOOL NAME	c. OTHER ACCIDENT? ☐ YES ☒ NO	c. INSURANCE PLAN NAME OR PROGRAM NAME
d. INSURANCE PLAN NAME OR PROGRAM NAME	10d. RESERVED FOR LOCAL USE	d. IS THERE ANOTHER HEALTH BENEFIT PLAN? ☐ YES ☐ NO *If yes*, return to and complete item 9 a-d.

READ BACK OF FORM BEFORE COMPLETING & SIGNING THIS FORM.

12. PATIENT'S OR AUTHORIZED PERSON'S SIGNATURE I authorize the release of any medical or other information necessary to process this claim. I also request payment of government benefits either to myself or to the party who accepts assignment below. SIGNED _____ DATE _____	13. INSURED'S OR AUTHORIZED PERSON'S SIGNATURE I authorize payment of medical benefits to the undersigned physician or supplier for services described below. SIGNED _____

14. DATE OF CURRENT: MM DD YY ◀ ILLNESS (First symptom) OR INJURY (Accident) OR PREGNANCY(LMP)	15. IF PATIENT HAS HAD SAME OR SIMILAR ILLNESS. GIVE FIRST DATE MM DD YY	16. DATES PATIENT UNABLE TO WORK IN CURRENT OCCUPATION FROM MM DD YY TO MM DD YY
17. NAME OF REFERRING PHYSICIAN OR OTHER SOURCE	17a. I.D. NUMBER OF REFERRING PHYSICIAN 67805027XX	18. HOSPITALIZATION DATES RELATED TO CURRENT SERVICES FROM MM DD YY TO MM DD YY
19. RESERVED FOR LOCAL USE		20. OUTSIDE LAB? ☐ YES ☒ NO $ CHARGES

21. DIAGNOSIS OR NATURE OF ILLNESS OR INJURY. (RELATE ITEMS 1,2,3 OR 4 TO ITEM 24E BY LINE)

1. ∟ 239 9   3. ∟

2. ∟   4. ∟

22. MEDICAID RESUBMISSION CODE   ORIGINAL REF. NO.
23. PRIOR AUTHORIZATION NUMBER

24. A DATE(S) OF SERVICE From MM DD YY To MM DD YY	B Place of Service	C Type of Service	D PROCEDURES, SERVICES, OR SUPPLIES (Explain Unusual Circumstances) CPT/HCPCS MODIFIER	E DIAGNOSIS CODE	F $ CHARGES	G DAYS OR UNITS	H EPSDT Family Plan	I EMG	J COB	K RESERVED FOR LOCAL USE
1	09 5520 XX	11		99203	1	70 92	1			46	278897XX
2	09 5520 XX	11		12001	1					46	278897XX
3											
4											
5											
6											

25. FEDERAL TAX I.D. NUMBER SSN EIN ☒	26. PATIENT'S ACCOUNT NO.	27. ACCEPT ASSIGNMENT? (For govt. claims, see back) ☒ YES ☐ NO	28. TOTAL CHARGE $	29. AMOUNT PAID $	30. BALANCE DUE $

31. SIGNATURE OF PHYSICIAN OR SUPPLIER INCLUDING DEGREES OR CREDENTIALS (I certify that the statements on the reverse apply to this bill and are made a part thereof.) GERALD PRACTION MD 09 30 20XX SIGNED *Gerald Praction MD* DATE	32. NAME AND ADDRESS OF FACILITY WHERE SERVICES WERE RENDERED (If other than home or office) COLLEGE HOSPITAL 4500 BROAD AVENUE WOODLAND HILLS XY 12345 93 7310XX	33. PHYSICIAN'S, SUPPLIER'S BILLING NAME, ADDRESS, ZIP CODE & PHONE # COLLEGE CLINIC 4567 BROAD AVENUE WOODLAND HILLS XY 12345 555 486 9002 PIN# GRP# 3664021XX

(APPROVED BY AMA COUNCIL ON MEDICAL SERVICE 8/88)   **PLEASE PRINT OR TYPE**   APPROVED OMB-0938-0008 FORM CMS-1500 (12-90), FORM RRB-1500,
APPROVED OMB-1215-0055 FORM OWCP-1500,   APPROVED OMB-0720-0001 (CHAMPUS)

PATIENT AND INSURED INFORMATION

PHYSICIAN OR SUPPLIER INFORMATION

Figure 9–5

ASSIGNMENT 9-7 ▸ **LOCATE ERRORS ON A RETURNED INSURANCE CLAIM**

Performance Objective

Task: Highlight the blocks on the insurance claim form where errors are discovered.

Conditions: Use an insurance claim form (Figure 9–6) and a highlighter or red pen.

Standards: Time: _____ minutes

                  Accuracy: _____

                  (Note: The time element and accuracy criteria may be given by your instructor.)

Directions: An insurance claim (Figure 9–6) was returned by an insurance plan. Highlight or circle in red all blocks on the claim form where errors are discovered.

Option 1:   Retype the claim and either insert the correction if data are available to fix the error or insert the word "NEED" in the block of the claim form.

Option 2:   On a separate sheet of paper, list the blocks from 1 to 33 and state where errors occur.

   A Performance Evaluation Checklist may be reproduced from the "Instruction Guide to the Workbook" chapter if your instructor wishes you to submit it to assist with scoring and comments.
   After the instructor has returned your work to you, either make the necessary corrections and place your work in a three-ring notebook for future reference or, if you received a high score, place it in your portfolio for reference when applying for a job.

PLEASE
DO NOT
STAPLE
IN THIS
AREA

AMERICAN INSURANCE COMPANY
509 MAIN STREET
WOODLAND HILLS XY 12345

CARRIER →

| | PICA | **HEALTH INSURANCE CLAIM FORM** | PICA | | |

1. MEDICARE MEDICAID CHAMPUS CHAMPVA GROUP HEALTH PLAN FECA BLK LUNG OTHER	1a. INSURED'S I.D. NUMBER (FOR PROGRAM IN ITEM 1)
(Medicare #) (Medicaid #) (Sponsor's SSN) (VA File #) (SSN or ID) (SSN) [X] (ID)	

2. PATIENT'S NAME (Last Name, First Name, Middle Initial)	3. PATIENT'S BIRTH DATE MM DD YYYY SEX	4. INSURED'S NAME (Last Name, First Name, Middle Initial)
MARY T AVERY	05 07 1980 M ☐ F ☐	SAME

5. PATIENT'S ADDRESS (No., Street)
4309 MAIN STREET

6. PATIENT RELATIONSHIP TO INSURED
Self [X]   Spouse ☐   Child ☐   Other ☐

7. INSURED'S ADDRESS (No., Street)

CITY: WOODLAND HILLS   STATE: XY

8. PATIENT STATUS
Single ☐   Married ☐   Other ☐
Employed ☐   Full-Time Student ☐   Part-Time Student ☐

CITY   STATE

ZIP CODE: 12345   TELEPHONE (Include Area Code): (555) 450-9899

ZIP CODE   TELEPHONE (include Area Code): ( )

9. OTHER INSURED'S NAME (Last Name, First Name, Middle Initial)

10. IS PATIENT'S CONDITION RELATED TO:

11. INSURED'S POLICY GROUP OR FECA NUMBER

a. OTHER INSURED'S POLICY OR GROUP NUMBER

a. EMPLOYMENT? (CURRENT OR PREVIOUS)
YES ☐   [X] NO

a. INSURED'S DATE OF BIRTH   MM DD YY   SEX   M ☐   F ☐

b. OTHER INSURED'S DATE OF BIRTH   MM DD YY   SEX   M ☐   F ☐

b. AUTO ACCIDENT?   PLACE (State)
YES ☐   [X] NO

b. EMPLOYER'S NAME OR SCHOOL NAME

c. EMPLOYER'S NAME OR SCHOOL NAME

c. OTHER ACCIDENT?
YES ☐   [X] NO

c. INSURANCE PLAN NAME OR PROGRAM NAME

d. INSURANCE PLAN NAME OR PROGRAM NAME

10d. RESERVED FOR LOCAL USE

d. IS THERE ANOTHER HEALTH BENEFIT PLAN?
YES ☐   NO ☐   If yes, return to and complete item 9 a-d.

READ BACK OF FORM BEFORE COMPLETING AND SIGNING THIS FORM.

12. PATIENT'S OR AUTHORIZED PERSON'S SIGNATURE I authorize the release of any medical or other information necessary to process this claim. I also request payment of government benefits either to myself or to the party who accepts assignment below.

SIGNED *Mary T. Avery*   DATE 11 10 20XX

13. INSURED'S OR AUTHORIZED PERSON'S SIGNATURE I authorize payment of medical benefits to the undersigned physician or supplier for services described below.

SIGNED *Mary T. Avery*

14. DATE OF CURRENT: MM DD YY   ◀ ILLNESS (First symptom) OR INJURY (Accident) OR PREGNANCY (LMP)

15. IF PATIENT HAS HAD SAME OR SIMILAR ILLNESS GIVE FIRST DATE   MM DD YY

16. DATES PATIENT UNABLE TO WORK IN CURRENT OCCUPATION
FROM MM DD YY   TO MM DD YY

17. NAME OF REFERRING PHYSICIAN OR OTHER SOURCE
GERALD PRACTON MD

17a. I.D. NUMBER OF REFERRING PHYSICIAN

18. HOSPITALIZATION DATES RELATED TO CURRENT SERVICES
FROM MM 11 DD 11 YY 20XX   TO MM 11 DD 12 YY 20XX

19. RESERVED FOR LOCAL USE

20. OUTSIDE LAB?   YES ☐   [X] NO $ CHARGES

21. DIAGNOSIS OR NATURE OF ILLNESS OR INJURY. (RELATE ITEMS 1,2,3 OR 4 TO ITEM 24E BY LINE)
1. 463
2.
3.
4.

22. MEDICAID RESUBMISSION CODE   ORIGINAL REF. NO.

23. PRIOR AUTHORIZATION NUMBER

24. A. DATE(S) OF SERVICE		B. Place of Service	C. Type of Service	D. PROCEDURES, SERVICES, OR SUPPLIES		E. DIAGNOSIS CODE	F. $ CHARGES		G. DAYS OR UNITS	H. EPSDT Family Plan	I. EMG	J. COB	K. RESERVED FOR LOCAL USE
From MM DD YY	To MM DD YY			CPT/HCPCS	MODIFIER								
11 10 20 XX		11		99203		1	50	00	1			43	050047XX
11 11 20 XX		21		99222		1	120	00	1			43	050047XX
11 11 20 XX		21		42821		1	410	73				43	050047XX
11 12 20 XX		21		99231		1	20	00					

25. FEDERAL TAX I.D. NUMBER   SSN ☐ EIN [X]
71 5737291

26. PATIENT'S ACCOUNT NO.

27. ACCEPT ASSIGNMENT? (For govt. claims, see back)   YES ☐   NO ☐

28. TOTAL CHARGE $

29. AMOUNT PAID $

30. BALANCE DUE $

31. SIGNATURE OF PHYSICIAN OR SUPPLIER INCLUDING DEGREES OR CREDENTIALS (I certify that the statements on the reverse apply to this bill and are made a part thereof.)

SIGNED   DATE 11 15 20XX

32. NAME AND ADDRESS OF FACILITY WHERE SERVICES WERE RENDERED (if other than home or office)
COLLEGE HOSPITAL
4500 BROAD AVENUE
WOODLAND HILLS XY 12345
95 07310XX

33. PHYSICIAN'S, SUPPLIER'S BILLING NAME, ADDRESS, ZIP CODE AND PHONE #
COLLEGE CLINIC
4567 BROAD AVENUE
WOODLAND HILLS XY 12345
555 486 9002
PIN#   GRP# 3664021XX

(APPROVED BY AMA COUNCIL ON MEDICAL SERVICE 8/88)

PLEASE PRINT OR TYPE

APPROVED OMB-0938-0008 FORM CMS-1500 (12-90), FORM RRB-1500,
APPROVED OMB-1215-0055 FORM OWCP-1500, APPROVED OMB-0720-0001 (CHAMPUS)

PATIENT AND INSURED INFORMATION   PHYSICIAN OR SUPPLIER INFORMATION

Figure 9–6

ASSIGNMENT 9-8 ▸ **REQUEST A HEARING ON A PREVIOUSLY APPEALED CLAIM**

Performance Objective

Task: Insert information on a HCFA-1965 Request for Hearing, Part B, Medicare Claim form.

Conditions: Use a Request for Hearing, Part B, Medicare Claim form (Figure 9–7) and a typewriter.

Standards: Time: _____ minutes

                Accuracy: _____

                (Note: The time element and accuracy criteria may be given by your instructor.)

Directions: After Medicare processes the tracer on the insurance claim for Bill Hutch, you receive a Medicare EOB and payment check, but the amount is incorrect because of an excessive reduction in the allowed payment. An appeal was made in September and denied; Dr. Brady Coccidioides believes that a mistake has been made and wishes to request a hearing.

Complete the HCFA-1965 Request for Hearing, Part B, Medicare Claim form for this case (Figure 9–7) by referring to the tracer form completed for Assignment 9–3 (Figure 9–3) and Figure 7–9 in the *Handbook*. As you will learn in the chapter on Medicare, the Health Insurance Claim Number is the patient's Medicare identification number as shown in Figure 7–9, Block 1a. No additional evidence is to be presented, and the doctor does not wish to appear for the hearing. Date the form December 5, 20xx.

After the instructor has returned your work to you, either make the necessary corrections and place your work in a three-ring notebook for future reference or, if you received a high score, place it in your portfolio for reference when applying for a job.

Checklist

1. Located the HCFA-1965 Medicare form   _____

2. Inserted the patient's name   _____

3. Inserted the patient's Medicare number   _____

4. Listed the reason for the appeal   _____

5. Checked the statements   _____

6. Inserted the physician's name, address, and telephone number   _____

7. Inserted the date when the form was completed   _____

8. Obtained the patient's signature   _____

9. Inserted the patient's address and telephone number   _____

10. Inserted the date when the patient's signed the form   _____

DEPARTMENT OF HEALTH AND HUMAN SERVICES
HEALTH CARE FINANCING ADMINISTRATION

Form Approved
OMB No. 0938-0034

REQUEST FOR HEARING — PART B MEDICARE CLAIM

Medical Insurance Benefits – Social Security Act

NOTICE—Anyone who misrepresents or falsifies essential information requested by this form may upon conviction be subject to fine and imprisonment under Federal Law.

Carrier's Name and Address

1 Name of Patient

2 Health Insurance Claim Number

3 I disagree with the review determination on my claim, and request a hearing before a hearing officer of the insurance carrier named above.

MY REASONS ARE: *(Attach a copy of the Review Notice. NOTE—If the review decision was made more than 6 months ago include your reason for not making this request earlier.)*

4 Check one of the following:

☐ I have additional evidence to submit.
(Attach such evidence to this form or forward it to the carrier within 10 days.)

☐ I do not have additional evidence.

Check <u>Only One</u> of the Statements Below:

☐ I wish to appear in person before the Hearing Officer.

☐ I do not wish to appear and hereby request a decision on the evidence before the Hearing Officer.

5 EITHER THE CLAIMANT OR REPRESENTATIVE SHOULD SIGN IN THE APPROPRIATE SPACE BELOW:

Signature or Name of Claimant's Representative
➡

Claimant's Signature
➡

Address

Address

City, State, and ZIP Code

City, State, and ZIP Code

Telephone Number

Date

Telephone Number

Date

(Claimant should not write below this line)

Your request for a hearing was received on _____. You will be notified of the time and place of the hearing at least 10 days before the date of the hearing.

Signed

Date

Form HCFA-1965 (8-79)

CARRIER COPY

Figure 9–7

ASSIGNMENT **9–9** ▸ **FILE AN OFFICIAL APPEAL**

Performance Objective

Task: Compose, format, key, proofread, and print a letter of appeal, and attach to this document photocopies of information to substantiate reimbursement requested.

Conditions: Typewriter or computer, printer, letterhead paper, envelope, attachments, thesaurus, English dictionary, medical dictionary, and pen or pencil.

Standards: Time: _____ minutes

Accuracy: _____

(Note: The time element and accuracy criteria may be given by your instructor.)

Scenario:

After retyping and resubmitting Mary T. Avery's insurance claim in Assignment 9–6, the insurance company sends an EOB/RA (health insurance claim number 123098) with a check in the amount of $300 to the College Clinic for payment of the claim. Dr. Cutler wishes an appeal to be made for an increase of the payment to an additional $100. Note: This patient's marital status is single and the insured's identification number is T45098.

Directions: Use the retyped claim to Assignment 9–6 for Mary T. Avery. Follow these basic step-by-step procedures.

1. Refer to the end of Chapter 4 in the *Handbook* and follow the procedure to compose, format, key, proofread, and print a letter.

2. Include the beneficiary's name, health insurance claim number, dates of service in question, and items or services in question with name, address, and signature of the provider.

3. Compose a letter with an introduction that stresses the medical practice's qualifications, the physician's commitment to complying with regulations and providing appropriate services, and the importance of the practice to the payer's panel of physicians or specialists.

4. Provide a detailed account of the necessity of the treatment given and its relationship to the patient's problems and chief complaint. You might cross reference the medical record and emphasize parts of it that the reviewer may have missed.

5. Explain the reason why the provider does not agree with the payment. Use a blank sheet labeling it "Explanation of Benefits" because you do not have this printed document to attach.

6. Abstract excerpts from the coding resource book if necessary.

7. Direct the correspondence to Mr. Donald Pearson, a claims adjuster at the American Insurance Company.

8. Type an envelope for the letter.

9. Retain copies of all data sent for the physician's files.

ASSIGNMENT 9–10 ▸ OBSERVATIONS OF INSURANCE VIDEO

Performance Objective

Task: View the video "The HCFA Files: A Case for Medical Billing Accuracy." Either insert answers to these questions as you view the video or take notes and then answer questions regarding the remarks of the three insurance billing specialists who lend their comments about the scenarios presented.

Conditions: Use VHS video equipment, paper, and a pencil or pen.

Standards: Time: _____ minutes

                Accuracy: _____

                (Note: The time element and accuracy criteria may be given by your instructor.)

Directions: After or while viewing the video, use your notes to answer the following questions.

1. List types of problems that may cause a claim to be either denied or rejected after receipt by the insurance company. See how many you noted when viewing this video.

   a. _____

   b. _____

   c. _____

   d. _____

   e. _____

   f. _____

   g. _____

   h. _____

   i. _____

   j. _____

   k. _____

   l. _____

   m. _____

   n. _____

   o. _____

   p. _____

q. _____

r. _____

2. Claire Johnson's insurance claim was rejected for payment the first time because

_____

3. On February 10, 2001, the diagnosis code for Claire Johnson was _____ .

4. Claire Johnson also had _____ syndrome.

5. The medical assistant resubmitted an insurance claim, and it was rejected a second time because

_____ .

6. Other errors made on Claire Johnson's submitted insurance claim were as follows:

a. _____

b. _____

c. _____

d. _____

7. When an insurance claim is processed, the _____ information is checked to determine whether the patient has insurance coverage and is eligible to receive medical benefits.

8. On an average, what percentage of submitted insurance claims is rejected? _____ %

9. List some items that must agree or match during the editing process to eliminate the claim being denied or rejected.

a. _____

b. _____

c. _____

d. _____

10. If a coder knowingly codes improperly, is this considered fraud or abuse?

_____

11. An insurance claim must be completed and submitted according to each _____

_____ guidelines.

ASSIGNMENT 9-11 ▸ POST ELECTRONICALLY TO A DAY SHEET FROM AN EXPLANATION OF BENEFITS DOCUMENT AND PRINT A PATIENT'S FINANCIAL ACCOUNTING RECORD

e hint   General Instructions for Entering a SINGLE (LINE ITEM) PAYMENT

1. After finding the patient record in the "Transaction Entry" screen, click on the magnifying glass in the [Bill No.] field.

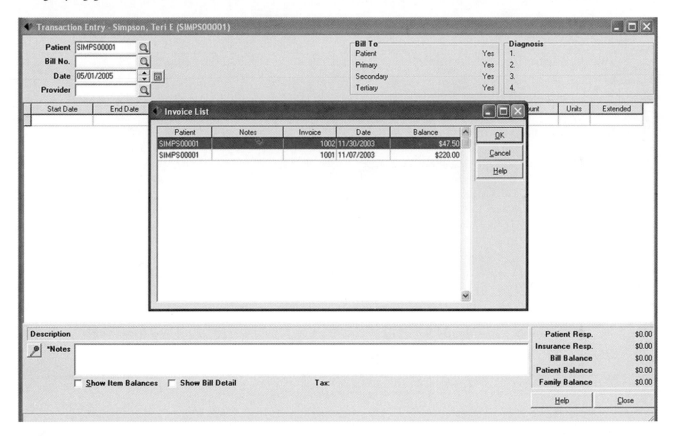

2. The "Invoice List" screen will open. Choose the correct "Date" (indicates the date of service) for which the payment will be applied. Click OK, then click in the middle of the screen so the "Transaction Entry" screen shows all services posted/billed to have payment applied.

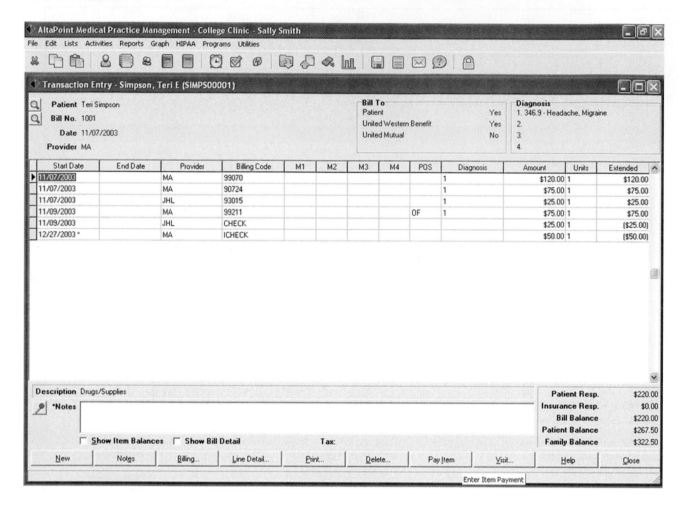

3. To post a payment, look at the EOB and match the line item [Start Date] and [Bill Code] to be sure to apply funds to the correct date of service.

4. Click on "Pay Item" at the bottom of the screen, and the "Apply Item Payment" window will open.

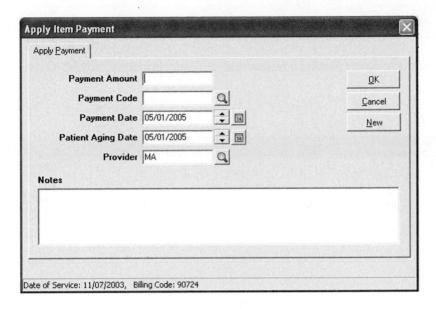

5. [Payment Amount] field: Refer to the EOB and enter the amount being paid.

6. [Payment Code] field: Click the magnifying glass and choose the proper code, depending on the assignment. Click "OK."

7. Verify the exact amount you entered was posted to the record.

8. Depending on your *Workbook* assignment, click "Close" at the bottom of the screen *or* follow the directions for "Printing a Patient Ledger."

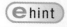 General Instructions for PRINTING A PATIENT LEDGER

1. While in the patient record after posting a transaction, click on "Print" and select "Print Ledger."

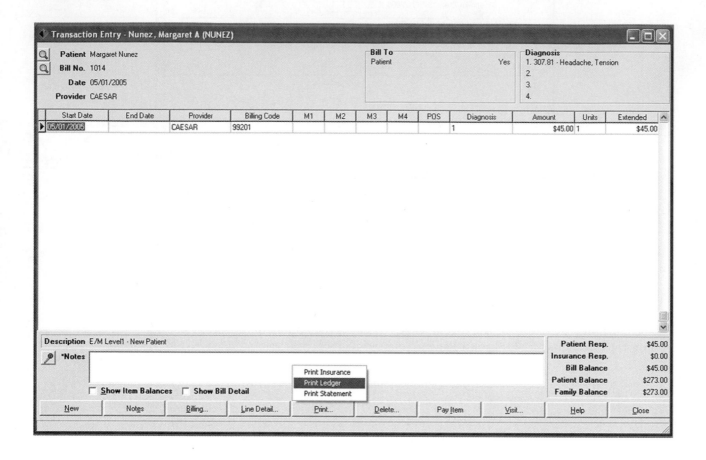

2. Select "Print."

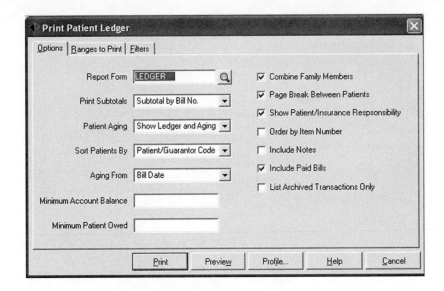

3. Alternatively, from the main menu, click "Reports" and select "Patient Ledger."

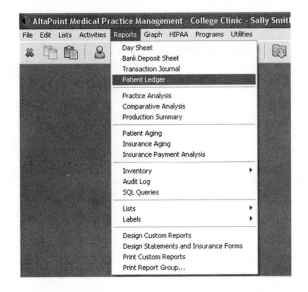

4. Click the "Ranges to Print" tab.

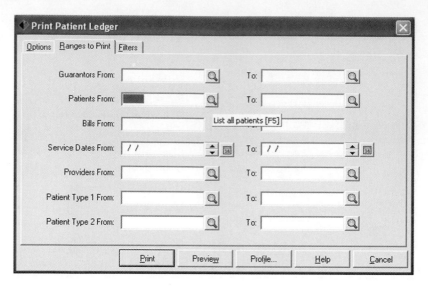

5. [Patients From Field]: Click on the magnifying glass to find the patient and then "Print."

Performance Objective

Task: Post data from an EOB document to a day sheet and print a patient's financial accounting record.

Conditions: EOB document (Workbook Figure 9–2); practice management software; and a computer.

Standards: Productivity Measurement

                   Time: _____ minutes

                   Accuracy: _____

                   (Note: The time element and accuracy criteria may be given by your instructor.)

Directions:

1. Post the payment received and preferred provider organization (PPO) discount to a day sheet by referring to an EOB document (*Workbook* Figure 9–2) for patient Jabe Bortolussi.

2. Follow the step-by-step directions for posting electronically to a financial accounting record.

3. Print the patient's financial accounting record to show the transactions posted.

   After the instructor has returned your work to you, either make the necessary corrections and place your work in a three-ring notebook for future reference or, if you received a high score, place it in your portfolio for reference when applying for a job.

ASSIGNMENT **9–12** ▸ **VIEW A PAYER RESPONSE FROM A CLEARINGHOUSE**

Performance Objective

Task: View electronically a payer response from a clearinghouse.

Conditions: Practice management software and a computer

Standards: Productivity Measurement

Time: _____ minutes

Accuracy: _____

(Note: The time element and accuracy criteria may be given by your instructor.)

Directions:

1. With the software CD in your computer and from the "Start" menu on your computer's desktop, *right* click on "My Computer." Select "Explore."

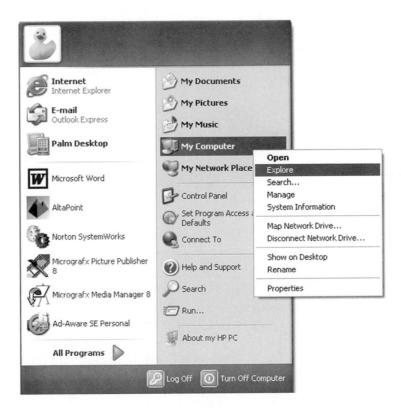

2. Find the correct drive within which the software CD is located and double click on it.

3. Find the "Handouts" folder and click to open.

4. Click on the file titled "Payer Response" to open.

5. Print a hard copy of the Payer Response and hand in to your instructor.

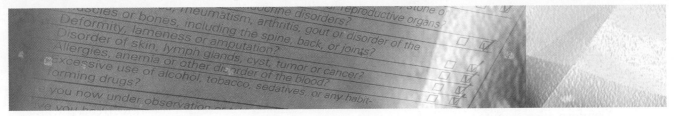

CHAPTER

10

Office and Insurance Collection Strategies

KEY TERMS

Your instructor may wish to select some specific words pertinent to this chapter for a test. For definitions of the terms, further study, and/or reference, the words, phrases, and abbreviations may be found in the glossary at the end of the Handbook. *Key terms for this chapter follow.*

accounts receivable (AR)

age analysis

AMA Code of Medical Ethics

automatic stay

balance

bankruptcy

bonding

cash flow

Code of Medical Ethics

collateral

collection ratio

credit

credit card

creditor

cycle billing

debit card

debit

debtor

discount

dun messages

embezzlement

estate administrator

estate executor

fee schedule

financial accounting record

garnishment

insurance balance billing

itemized statement

lien

manual billing

netback

no charge (NC)

nonexempt assets

professional courtesy

reimbursement

secured debt

skip

statute of limitations

unsecured debt

write-off

PERFORMANCE OBJECTIVES

The student will be able to:

- Define and spell the key terms for this chapter, given the information from the *Handbook* glossary, within a reasonable time period and with enough accuracy to obtain a satisfactory evaluation.
- After reading the chapter, answer the self-study review questions with enough accuracy to obtain a satisfactory evaluation.
- Choose an appropriate dun message for a patient's bill, given a patient's ledger/statement, within a reasonable time period and with enough accuracy to obtain a satisfactory evaluation.
- Post a courtesy adjustment, given a patient's ledger/statement, within a reasonable period of time and with enough accuracy to obtain a satisfactory evaluation.
- Using the Mock Fee Schedule in Appendix A in this *Workbook*, a patient's payment to the ledger/statement within a reasonable time period and with enough accuracy to obtain a satisfactory evaluation.
- Compose a collection letter for a delinquent account, given letterhead stationery, within a reasonable time period and with enough accuracy to obtain a satisfactory evaluation.
- Complete a credit card voucher, given a patient's ledger/statement, within a reasonable time period and with enough accuracy to obtain a satisfactory evaluation.
- Complete a financial agreement, given a patient's ledger/statement, within a reasonable time period and with enough accuracy to obtain a satisfactory evaluation.
- Electronically create and produce a dun message and print a patient statement using practice management software, within a reasonable time period and with enough accuracy to obtain a satisfactory evaluation.
- Electronically post a courtesy adjustment on a self-pay patient's financial accounting record and print a daysheet using practice management software, within a reasonable time period and with enough accuracy to obtain a satisfactory evaluation.
- Electronically print a collection letter using practice management software, within a reasonable time period and with enough accuracy to obtain a satisfactory evaluation.

STUDY OUTLINE

Cash Flow Cycle
  Accounts Receivable
  Patient Education
  Patient Registration Form

Fees
  Fee Schedule
  Fee Adjustments
  Communicating Fees
  Collecting Fees

Credit Arrangements
  Payment Options

Credit and Collection Laws
  Statute of Limitations
  Equal Credit Opportunity Act
  Fair Credit Reporting Act
  Fair Credit Billing Act
  Truth in Lending Act
  Truth in Lending Consumer Credit Cost
    Disclosure
  Fair Debt Collection Practices Act

The Collection Process
  Office Collection Techniques
  Insurance Collection
  Collection Agencies
  Credit Bureaus
  Credit Counseling
  Small Claims Court
  Tracing a Skip
  Special Collection Issues

Procedure: Seven-Step Billing and Collection Guidelines

Procedure: Telephone Collection Plan

Procedure: Create a Financial Agreement With a Patient

Procedure: File a Claim in Small Claims Court

Procedure: File an Estate Claim

S E L F - S T U D Y **10–1** ▸ **R E V I E W   Q U E S T I O N S**

Review the objectives, key terms, chapter information, glossary definitions of key terms, and figures before completing the following review questions.

1. Third-party payers are composed of

   a. _____

   b. _____

   c. _____

   d. _____

2. The unpaid balance due from patients for professional services rendered is known as

   a/an _____.

3. Write the formula for calculating the office accounts receivable (A/R) ratio. _____

   _____

   _____

4. What is the collection rate if a total of $40,300 was collected for the month and the

   total of the accounts receivable is $50,670? _____ %

5. An important document that provides identifying data for each patient and assists

   in billing and collection is called a/an _____.

6. A term preferable to "write-off" when used in a medical practice is

   _____.

7. To verify a check, ask the patient for a/an _____ and _____.

8. The procedure of systematically arranging the accounts receivable, by age, from the

   date of service is called _____.

9. Are physicians' patient accounts single-entry accounts, open-book accounts, or

   written contract accounts? _____

10. Match the terms in the right column with the descriptions, and fill in the blank with the appropriate letter.

_____	Reductions of the normal fee based on a specific amount of money or a percentage of the charge	a. debtor
_____	Phrase to remind a patient about a delinquent account	b. itemized statement
_____	Item that permits bank customers to withdraw cash at any hour from an automated teller machine	c. fee schedule
_____	Individual owing money	d. discounts
_____	Claim on the property of another as security for a debt	e. financial account record (ledger)
_____	Individual record indicating charges, payments, adjustments, and balances owed for services rendered	f. creditor
_____	Detailed summary of all transactions of a creditor's account	g. dun message
_____	Person to whom money is owed	h. debit card
_____	Listing of accepted charges or established allowances for specific medical procedures	i. lien

11. A court order attaching a debtor's property or wages to pay off a debt is known as

_____.

12. Match the following federal acts with their descriptions and fill in the blank with the appropriate letter.

_____	Law stating that a person has 60 days to complain about an error from the date that a statement is mailed	a. Equal Credit Opportunity Act
_____	Consumer protection act that applies to anyone who charges interest or agrees on payment of a bill in more than four installments, excluding a downpayment	b. Fair Credit Reporting Act
_____	Regulates collection practices of third-party debt collectors and attorneys who collect debts for others	c. Fair Credit Billing Act
_____	Federal law prohibiting discrimination in all areas of granting credit	d. Truth in Lending Act
_____	Regulates agencies that issue or use credit reports on consumers	e. Fair Debt Collection Practices Act

13. An individual who owes on an account and moves, leaving no forwarding address,

is called a/an _____.

14. A straight petition in bankruptcy or absolute bankruptcy is also known as a/an

_____.

15. A wage earner's bankruptcy is sometimes referred to as a/an _____.

16. Translate these credit and collection abbreviations.

NSF _____   T _____

WCO _____   SK _____

PIF _____   FN _____

NLE _____   UE _____

17. State three bonding methods.

a. _____

b. _____

c. _____

18. A system of billing accounts at spaced intervals during the month on the basis of a breakdown of accounts by alphabet, account number, insurance type, or date of

service is known as _____.

To check your answers to this self-study assignment, see Appendix D.

ASSIGNMENT **10–2** ▸ **SELECT A DUN MESSAGE**

Performance Objective

Task: Select an appropriate dun message and insert it on a patient's financial accounting record (ledger card).

Conditions: Use the patient's financial accounting record (Figure 10–1) and a typewriter.

Standards: Time: _____ minutes

             Accuracy: _____

             (Note: The time element and accuracy criteria may be given by your instructor.)

Directions: Read the scenario and refer to the patient's financial accounting record (Figure 10–1). Select appropriate dun messages for each month the patient has been billed. You may wish to refer to Figure 10–2 in the *Handbook*.

Scenario: Carrie Jones was on vacation in June and July and did not pay on her account. It is August (current year).

June 1, 20XX Dun message   _____

July 1, 20XX Dun message   _____

August 1, 20XX Dun message   _____

After the instructor has returned your work to you, either make the necessary corrections and place your work in a three-ring notebook for future reference or, if you received a high score, place it in your portfolio for reference when applying for a job.

Acct   No. 10-2

STATEMENT
Financial Account
COLLEGE CLINIC
4567 Broad Avenue
Woodland Hills, XY 12345-0001
Tel. 555-486-9002
Fax No. 555-487-8976

Carrie Jones
15543 Dean Street
Woodland Hills, XY 12345

Phone No. (H)   (555) 439-8800   (W)   (555) 550-8706   Birthdate   05-14-72

Primary Insurance Co.   Prudential Insurance Company   Policy/Group No.   450998

	REFERENCE	DESCRIPTION	CHARGES	CREDITS PYMNTS.	ADJ.	BALANCE	
				BALANCE FORWARD ➧		20	00
4-16–xx	99215	C hx/exam HC DM DX 582				154	99
4-17–xx		Prudential billed (4-16-xx)				154	99
5-27–xx		Rec'd insurance ck #435		30	00	124	99
6-1-xx		Billed pt				124	99
7-1-xx		Billed pt				124	99
8-1-xx		Billed pt				124	99

PLEASE PAY LAST AMOUNT IN BALANCE COLUMN ⬆

THIS IS A COPY OF YOUR FINANCIAL ACCOUNT AS IT APPEARS ON OUR RECORDS

Figure 10–1

ASSIGNMENT **10–3** ▶ **POST A COURTESY ADJUSTMENT**

Performance Objective

Task: Post a courtesy adjustment to a patient's financial accounting record (ledger card).

Conditions: Use the patient's financial accounting record (Figure 10–2) and a pen.

Standards: Time: _____ minutes

                  Accuracy: _____

                  (Note: The time element and accuracy criteria may be given by your instructor.)

Directions: Read the case scenario and refer to the patient's financial accounting record (Figure 10–2). You may wish to refer to Figure 10–2 in the *Handbook*. Post a courtesy adjustment to her financial accounting record.

Scenario: Maria Smith recently lost her job and is raising two children as a single parent. It is September 1 (current year). A discussion with Dr. Gerald Practon leads to a decision to write off the balance on the account.

   September 1, 20XX Financial account posted _____

   After the instructor has returned your work to you, either make the necessary corrections and place your work in a three-ring notebook for future reference or, if you received a high score, place it in your portfolio for reference when applying for a job.

Acct No. 10-3

STATEMENT
Financial Account
COLLEGE CLINIC
4567 Broad Avenue
Woodland Hills, XY 12345-0001
Tel. 555-486-9002
Fax No. 555-487-8976

Ms. Maria Smith
3737 Unser Road
Woodland Hills, XY 12345

Phone No. (H) (555) 430-8877   (W)   (555) 908-1233   Birthdate 06-11-80

Primary Insurance Co.   Metropolitan Insurance Company   Policy/Group No.   4320870

	REFERENCE	DESCRIPTION	CHARGES		CREDITS PYMNTS.	ADJ.	BALANCE	
					BALANCE FORWARD ⟶		20	00
5-19-xx	99214	OV DX 582	61	51			81	51
5-20-xx		Metropolitan billed (5-19-xx)					81	51
6-20-xx		Rec'd ins ck #6778			25	00	56	51
7-1-xx		Pt billed					56	51
8-1-xx		Pt billed					56	51

PLEASE PAY LAST AMOUNT IN BALANCE COLUMN ⟱

THIS IS A COPY OF YOUR FINANCIAL ACCOUNT AS IT APPEARS ON OUR RECORDS

Figure 10–2

ASSIGNMENT **10-4** ▸ **POST A PATIENT'S PAYMENT**

Performance Objective

Task: Post a payment to a patient's financial accounting record (ledger card).

Conditions: Use the patient's financial accounting record (Figure 10–3), the Mock Fee Schedule in Appendix A in this *Workbook*, and a pen.

Standards: Time: _____ minutes

               Accuracy: _____

               (Note: The time element and accuracy criteria may be given by your instructor.)

Directions: Read the case scenario, refer to the patient's financial accounting record (Figure 10–3), and refer to the Mock Fee Schedule in Appendix A in this *Workbook*. You may wish to refer to Figure 10–2 in the *Handbook*. Post the charges for the services rendered and payment to the patient's financial accounting record.

Scenario: On October 12 (current year), new patient Kenneth Brown came in for a Level III office visit and electrocardiogram (ECG). He has no insurance and paid $50 on his account with check number 3421.

   October 12, 20XX Financial account posted _____

   After the instructor has returned your work to you, either make the necessary corrections and place your work in a three-ring notebook for future reference or, if you received a high score, place it in your portfolio for reference when applying for a job.

Acct No.　10-4

STATEMENT
Financial Account
COLLEGE CLINIC
4567 Broad Avenue
Woodland Hills, XY　12345-0001
Tel.　555-486-9002
Fax No. 555-487-8976

Mr. Kenneth Brown
8896 Aster Drive
Woodland Hills, XY　12345

Phone No. (H)　(555) 760-5211　　　(W)　(555) 987-3355　　　Birthdate　01-15-82

Primary Insurance Co.　none　　　　　　　　　　　Policy/Group No.　

REFERENCE	DESCRIPTION	CHARGES	CREDITS PYMNTS.	ADJ.	BALANCE
		BALANCE FORWARD ⟶			

PLEASE PAY LAST AMOUNT IN BALANCE COLUMN

THIS IS A COPY OF YOUR FINANCIAL ACCOUNT AS IT APPEARS ON OUR RECORDS

Figure 10–3

ASSIGNMENT **10–5** ▸ **COMPOSE A COLLECTION LETTER**

Performance Objective

Task: Key a letter for the physician's signature and post the entry on the patient's financial accounting record (ledger card).

Conditions: Use the patient's financial accounting record (Figure 10–4), one sheet of letterhead (Figure 10–5), a number 10 envelope, and a pen.

Standards: Time: _____ minutes

               Accuracy: _____

               (Note: The time element and accuracy criteria may be given by your instructor.)

Directions: Read the case scenario, refer to the patient's financial accounting record (Figure 10–4), and compose a collection letter, using your signature and requesting payment. Type this letter on letterhead stationery in full block format (paragraphs to left margin). Include a paragraph stating that a copy of the delinquent statement is enclosed. You may wish to refer to Figure 10–14 in the *Handbook*. Post an entry on the patient's financial accounting record.

Scenario: It is December 1 (current year), and you have sent Mr. Ron Kelsey two statements with no response. You tried to reach him by telephone without success and have decided to send him a collection letter (Figure 10–5).

Checklist

1. Assemble materials, determine the recipient's address, and decide on modified or full block letter style or format.   _____

2. Turn on the computer and select the word processing program. Open a blank document.   _____

3. Key the date line beginning at least three lines below the letterhead and make certain it is in the proper location for the chosen style.   _____

4. Double-space down and insert the inside address and make certain it is in the proper location for the chosen style.   _____

5. Double-space and key the salutation. Use either open or mixed punctuation.   _____

6. Double-space and key the body (content) of the letter in single-space and make certain the paragraph style is proper for the format chosen. Double-space between paragraphs. Save the letter to the computer hard drive every 15 minutes.   _____

7. Proofread the letter on the computer screen for composition.   _____

8. Proofread the letter on the computer screen for typographical, spelling, grammatical, and mechanical errors. Use the spell-check feature of the word processing program and reference books to check for correct spelling, meaning, or usage.   _____

9. Key a complimentary close and make certain it is in the proper location for the chosen style.   _____

10. Drop down four spaces and key the sender's name and title.   _____

11. Single- or double-space to insert copy ("CC"), or enclosure ("Enclosure" or "Enc"), or attachment notations.   _____

12. Save the file before printing a hard copy and proofread the letter once more. Make corrections, if needed.   _____

13. Print the final copy to be sent and proofread. Make a copy to be retained in the files in case it is needed for future reference.   _____

14. Save the file to a CD-ROM to be stored for future reference.   _____

15. Prepare an envelope and use the format for optical scanning recommended by the United States Postal Service.   _____

16. Clip attachments to the letter and sign.   _____

17. Post entry to the patient's financial accounting record.   _____

After the instructor has returned your work to you, either make the necessary corrections and place your work in a three-ring notebook for future reference or, if you received a high score, place it in your portfolio for reference when applying for a job.

Acct No. 10-5

STATEMENT
Financial Account
COLLEGE CLINIC
4567 Broad Avenue
Woodland Hills, XY 12345-0001
Tel. 555-486-9002
Fax No. 555-487-8976

Mr. Ron Kelsey
6321 Ocean Street
Woodland Hills, XY 12345

Phone No. (H) (555) 540-9800   (W) (555) 890-7766   Birthdate 03-25-75

Primary Insurance Co.   XYZ Insurance Company   Policy/Group No. 8503Y

	REFERENCE	DESCRIPTION	CHARGES	CREDITS PYMNTS.	ADJ.	BALANCE	
				BALANCE FORWARD →			
07-09-xx	99283	ER new pt EPF hx/exam MC DM	66 23			66	23
07-10-xx		XYZ Insurance billed (3-9-xx)				66	23
09-20-xx		EOB rec'd pt has not met deductible				66	23
10-01-xx		Billed pt				66	23
11-01-xx		Billed pt				66	23

PLEASE PAY LAST AMOUNT IN BALANCE COLUMN

THIS IS A COPY OF YOUR FINANCIAL ACCOUNT AS IT APPEARS ON OUR RECORDS

Figure 10–4

COLLEGE CLINIC
4567 Broad Avenue
Woodland Hills, XY 12345-0001
Tel. (555) 486-9002
FAX (555) 487-8976

Figure 10–5

ASSIGNMENT **10–6** ▸ **COMPLETE A CREDIT CARD VOUCHER**

Performance Objective

Task: Complete a credit card voucher and post an entry on the patient's ledger.

Conditions: Use the patient's ledger card (Figure 10–6), a credit card voucher (Figure 10–7), and a pen.

Standards: Time: _____ minutes

                        Accuracy: _____

                        (Note: The time element and accuracy criteria may be give by your instructor.)

Directions: Read the case scenario and refer to the patient's ledger/statement (Figure 10–6). Fill in the credit card voucher (Figure 10–7) and post an appropriate entry on the ledger/statement. You may wish to refer to Figure 10–11 in the *Handbook*.

Scenario: It is November 6 (current year), and you receive a telephone call at the College Clinic. It is Kevin Long, who has an unpaid balance, and it is up to you to discuss this delinquency with Mr. Long and come to an agreement on how the account can be paid. After discussion, Mr. Long decides to pay the total balance due by MasterCard credit card, giving you his authorization and account number: 5676 1342 5437 XXX0 (expiration date, December 31, 20xx). His name is listed on the card as Kevin O. Long. You call the bank, and the authorization number given is 534889.

Checklist

1. Read scenario.   _____

2. Entered the patient's name on the credit card voucher.   _____

3. Entered the credit card account number and expiration date.   _____

4. Inserted a check mark for the verification of the expiration date.   _____

5. Inserted the College Clinic name and address.   _____

6. Completed signature line.   _____

7. Entered the date of the transaction.   _____

8. Entered the authorization number from the bank.   _____

9. Described the physician's services.   _____

10. Listed the charges authorized by the patient.   _____

11. Circled the type of credit card.   _____

12. Entered the total amount authorized by the patient.   _____

13. Inserted your initials on the credit card voucher.   _____

14. Posted to the patient's financial accounting record.   _____

    After the instructor has returned your work to you, either make the necessary corrections and place your work in a three-ring notebook for future reference or, if you received a high score, place it in your portfolio for reference when applying for a job.

Acct No. 10-6

STATEMENT
Financial Account
COLLEGE CLINIC
4567 Broad Avenue
Woodland Hills, XY 12345-0001
Tel. 555-486-9002
Fax No. 555-487-8976

Mr. Kevin O. Long
2443 Davis Street
Woodland Hills, XY 12345

Phone No. (H) (555) 244-5600   (W)   (555) 970-4466   Birthdate 08-15-76

Primary Insurance Co. Blue Cross   Policy/Group No. 130-XX-0987

	REFERENCE	DESCRIPTION	CHARGES		CREDITS PYMNTS.	ADJ.	BALANCE	
			BALANCE FORWARD ⟶					
09-08-xx	99205	OV Level V DX 582	132	28			132	28
09-09-xx		Blue Cross billed (9-8-xx)					132	28
10-12-xx		BC EOB rec'd pt has not met deductible					132	28
10-23-xx		Not covered by insurance. Balance due					132	28

PLEASE PAY LAST AMOUNT IN BALANCE COLUMN ⬆

THIS IS A COPY OF YOUR FINANCIAL ACCOUNT AS IT APPEARS ON OUR RECORDS

Figure 10–6

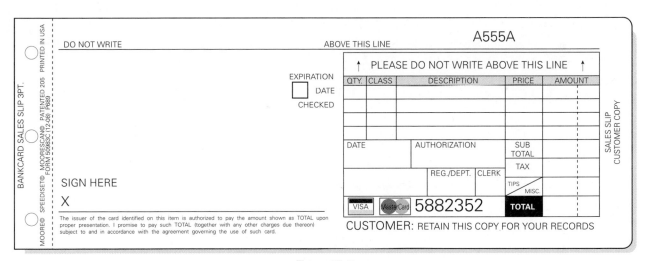

Figure 10–7

ASSIGNMENT **10–7** ▸ **COMPLETE A FINANCIAL AGREEMENT**

Performance Objective

Task: Complete a financial agreement and post an entry on the patient's ledger.

Conditions: Use the patient's ledger card (Figure 10–8), a financial statement form (Figure 10–9), and a pen.

Standards: Time: _____ minutes

                  Accuracy: _____

                  (Note: The time element and accuracy criteria may be given by your instructor.)

Scenario: Mr. Joseph Small has a large balance due. Create a payment plan for this case. You have discussed the installment plan concerning the amount of the total debt, the downpayment, amount and date of each installment, and the date of final payment. On June 1 (current year), Mr. Small is paying $500 cash as a downpayment, and the balance is to be divided into five equal payments, due on the first of each month. There will be no monthly finance charge. Mr. Small's daytime telephone number is 555-760-5502. He is a patient of Dr. Brady Coccidioides.

Directions:

Checklist

1. Read the case scenario.   _____

2. Complete a financial agreement (Figure 10–9) by subtracting the downpayment
   from the total debt.   _____

3. Refer to the patient's ledger/statement (Figure 10–8) and post an appropriate
   entry to the ledger/statement using a pen. You may wish to refer to Figure 10–5
   in the *Handbook*.   _____

4. Review the completed financial agreement with the patient (role played by
   another student).   _____

5. Ask the patient (role played by another student) to sign the financial agreement.   _____

6. Make a photocopy of the form for the patient to retain.   _____

7. File the original financial agreement in the patient's financial files in the office.   _____

   After the instructor has returned your work to you, either make the necessary corrections and place your work in a three-ring notebook for future reference or, if you received a high score, place it in your portfolio for reference when applying for a job.

Acct No. <u>10-7</u>

STATEMENT
Financial Account
COLLEGE CLINIC
4567 Broad Avenue
Woodland Hills, XY 12345-0001
Tel. 555-486-9002
Fax No. 555-487-8976

Mr. Joseph Small
655 Sherry Street
Woodland Hills, XY 12345

Phone No. (H) <u>(555) 320-8801</u>   (W) <u>(555) 760-5502</u>   Birthdate <u>11-04-77</u>

Primary Insurance Co. <u>Blue Shield</u>   Policy/Group No. <u>870-XX-4398</u>

| | REFERENCE | DESCRIPTION | CHARGES | | CREDITS | | | | BALANCE | |
					PYMNTS.		ADJ.			
					BALANCE FORWARD ⟶				20	00
04-19-xx	99215	OV Level	96	97					116	97
04-30-xx	99218	Adm hosp	74	22					191	19
04-30-xx	32440	Pneumonectomy, total	1972	10					2163	29
05-20-xx		Blue Shield billed (1-19 to 30-xx)							2163	29
05-15-xx		BS EOB Pt deductible $2000 rec'd ck #544			163	29			2000	00

PLEASE PAY LAST AMOUNT IN BALANCE COLUMN ⬆

THIS IS A COPY OF YOUR FINANCIAL ACCOUNT AS IT APPEARS ON OUR RECORDS

Figure 10–8

| | | FINANCIAL AGREEMENT | | | SCHEDULE OF PAYMENT | | | | |

FINANCIAL AGREEMENT

For PROFESSIONAL SERVICES rendered or to be rendered to:

Patient _____ Daytime Phone _____

Parent if patient is a minor _____

1. Cash price for services . . . . $ _____
2. Cash down payment . . . . $ _____
3. Charges covered by insurance service plan . . . . $ _____
4. Unpaid balance of cash price. . . . . $ _____
5. Amount financed (the amount of credit provided to you) . . . . $ _____
6. FINANCE CHARGE (the dollar amount the credit will cost you) . . . . . $ _____
7. ANNUAL PERCENTAGE RATE
   (the cost of credit as a yearly rate) . . . . _____ %
8. Total of payments (5 + 6 above-the amount you will have
   paid when you have made all scheduled payments). . . . . $ _____
9. Total sales price (1 + 6 above-sum of cash price, financing
   charge and any other amounts financed by the creditor, not part of
   the finance charge) . . . . $ _____

You have the right at any time to pay the unpaid balance due under this agreement without penalty.
   You have the right at this time to receive an itemization of the amount financed.
   ☐ I want an itemization   ☐ I do not want an itemization

Total of payments (#8 above) is payable to Dr. _____
in _____ monthly installments of $ _____ each and _____ installments of
$ _____ each. The first installment being payable on _____ 20 _____
and subsequent installments on the same day of each consecutive month until paid in full.

NOTICE TO PATIENT
Do not sign this agreement if it contains any blank spaces. You are entitled to an exact copy of any agreement you sign. You have the right at any time to pay the unpaid balance due under this agreement.

The patient (parent or guardian) agrees to be and is fully responsible for total payment of services performed in this office including any amounts not covered by health insurance or prepayment program the responsible party may have. See your contract documents for any additional information about nonpayment, default, any required prepayment in full before the scheduled date and prepayment refunds and penalties.

Signature of patient or one parent if patient is a minor:

X _____

Doctor's Signature _____

Form 1826 • 1982

SCHEDULE OF PAYMENT

No.	Date Due	Amount of Installment	Date Paid	Amount Paid	Balance Owed
		Total Amount			
D.P.					
1					
2					
3					
4					
5					
6					
7					
8					
9					
10					
11					
12					
13					
14					
15					
16					
17					
18					
19					
20					
21					
22					
23					

Figure 10–9

e hint   General Instructions for CREATING A PATIENT STATEMENT DUN MESSAGE

1. From the main menu, click "File" and select "Practice Information."

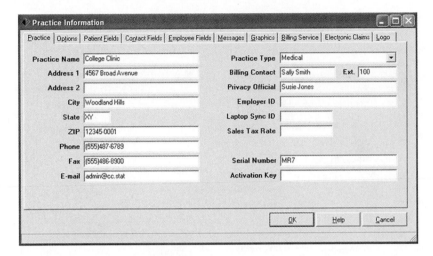

2. Click the "Messages" tab. In each field, type in an appropriate message. Look at the following as an example:

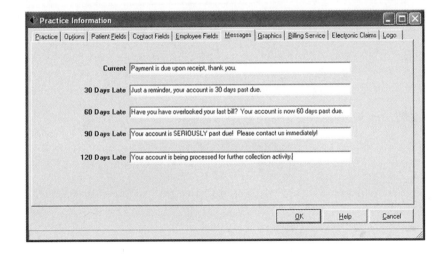

ASSIGNMENT **10–8** ▸ **ELECTRONICALLY CREATE A DUN MESSAGE AND PRINT A PATIENT'S STATEMENT**

e hint General Instructions for PRINTING A PATIENT STATEMENT

1. After posting in Transaction Entry screen, click on "Print" at the bottom of the screen.

Print Statements ✕

Options | Ranges to Print | Filters | Handouts | HIPAA Forms | Electronic Statements

Statement Form	STATEMENT 🔍
Effective Date	05/01/2005
Balance Forward Date	04/01/2005
Minimum Account Balance	0.00
Minimum Patient Owed	0.00
Sort Statements By	Patient/Guarantor Code ▾
Print Paid Bills	Unpaid Bills Only ▾
Print Payments	Include All Payments ▾
Subtotals	Subtotal by Patient ▾
Aging From	Bill Date (Balance Forward) ▾

☐ Balance Forward Format
☑ Combine Family Members
☑ Combine Split Patient Payments
☑ Summarize Patient Payments
☑ Summarize Insurance Payments
☐ Order by Item Number
☑ Show Patient/Insurance Respsonsibility
☑ Show Future Appointments
☑ Show Notes
☑ Show Dunning Messages
☑ Create Billing Log

[Print] [Preview] [Profile...] [Help] [Cancel]

2. Select "Print Statement."

3. In the "Print Statements" screen, change any necessary field data and then click "Print."

Performance Objective

Task: Electronically create a dun message and print a patient's financial account record using software.

Conditions: Use practice management software, patient's electronic data, and computer.

Standards: Productivity Measurement

Time: _____ minutes

Accuracy: _____

(Note: The time element and accuracy criteria may be given by your instructor.)

Directions:

1. Electronically create a dun message.

2. Print Ron Kelsey's financial accounting record.

e hint Follow the previous instructions for PRINTING A PATIENT LEDGER

After the instructor has returned your work to you, either make the necessary corrections and place your work in a three-ring notebook for future reference or, if you received a high score, place it in your portfolio for reference when applying for a job.

ASSIGNMENT **10-9** ▸ **ELECTRONICALLY POST AN INSURANCE ADJUSTMENT ON A PATIENT'S FINANCIAL ACCOUNTING RECORD**

Performance Objective

Task: Electronically post an insurance adjustment on a patient's financial accounting record using software.

Conditions: Use practice management software, patient's electronic data, and computer.

Standards: Productivity Measurement

Time: _____ minutes

Accuracy: _____

(Note: The time element and accuracy criteria may be given by your instructor.)

Directions:

1. Electronically post two separate insurance adjustments, one for $20.00 and one for $36.51, on Maria Smith's financial accounting record.

2. Print Maria Smith's financial accounting record.

After the instructor has returned your work to you, either make the necessary corrections and place your work in a three-ring notebook for future reference or, if you received a high score, place it in your portfolio for reference when applying for a job.

ASSIGNMENT 10–10 ▸ ELECTRONICALLY PRINT A COLLECTION LETTER

ⓔ hint   General Instructions for PRINTING A COLLECTION LETTER

1. From main menu, click "Reports" and select "Print Custom Reports."

2. [Report Code Field]: Find and choose "COLLECTION" (Collection Letter).

3. Press "Print."

Performance Objective

Task: Electronically print a collection letter using software.

Conditions: Use practice management software, patient's electronic data, 8½- by 11-inch white paper, computer, and printer.

Standards: Productivity Measurement

                    Time: _____ minutes

                    Accuracy: _____

                    (Note: The time element and accuracy criteria may be given by your instructor.)

Directions:

1. Electronically prepare a collection letter.

2. Print the collection letter to Ron Kelsey.

   After the instructor has returned your work to you, either make the necessary corrections and place your work in a three-ring notebook for future reference or, if you received a high score, place it in your portfolio for reference when applying for a job.

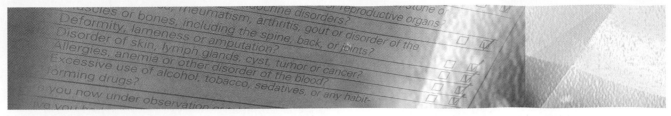

CHAPTER

11

The Blue Plans, Private Insurance, and Managed Care Plans

KEY TERMS

Your instructor may wish to select some specific words pertinent to this chapter for a test. For definitions of the terms, further study, and/or reference, the words, phrases, and abbreviations may be found in the glossary at the end of the Handbook. *Key terms for this chapter follow.*

ancillary services

buffing

capitation

carve outs

churning

claims-review type of foundation

closed panel program

comprehensive type of foundation

copayment (copay)

deductible

direct referral

disenrollment

exclusive provider organization (EPO)

fee-for-service

formal referral

foundation for medical care (FMC)

gatekeeper

health maintenance organization (HMO)

in-area

independent (or individual) practice association (IPA)

managed care organizations (MCOs)

participating physician

per capita

physician provider group (PPG)

point-of-service (POS) plan

preferred provider organization (PPO)

prepaid group practice model

primary care physician (PCP)

self-referral

service area

staff model

stop loss

tertiary care

turfing

utilization review (UR)

verbal referral

withhold

PERFORMANCE OBJECTIVES

The student will be able to:

- Define and spell the key terms for this chapter, given the information from the *Handbook* glossary, within a reasonable time period and with enough accuracy to obtain a satisfactory evaluation.
- After reading the chapter, answer the self-study review questions with enough accuracy to obtain a satisfactory evaluation.
- Complete treatment authorization forms of managed care plans, given completed new patient information forms, within a reasonable time period and with enough accuracy to obtain a satisfactory evaluation.
- Transmit an electronic insurance claims for a private case using practice management software, within a reasonable time period and with enough accuracy to obtain a satisfactory evaluation.
- Print a remaining authorizations report using practice management software, within a reasonable time period and with enough accuracy to obtain a satisfactory evaluation.

STUDY OUTLINE

Private Insurance
  Blue Cross and Blue Shield Plans
Managed Care
  Prepaid Group Practice Health Plans
  Benefits
  Health Care Reform
Managed Care Systems
  Health Maintenance Organizations
  Exclusive Provider Organizations
  Foundations for Medical Care
  Independent Practice Associations
  Preferred Provider Organizations
  Physician Provider Groups
  Point-of-Service Plans
  Triple-Option Health Plans
Medical Review
  Quality Improvement Organization
  Utilization Review of Management

Management of Plans
  Contracts
  Preauthorization of Prior Approval
  Diagnostic Tests
  Managed Care Guide
  Plan Administration
Financial Management
  Payment
  Statement of Remittance
  Accounting
  Fee-for-Service
  Year-End Evaluation
  Bankruptcy
Conclusion

SELF-STUDY **11–1** ▶ **REVIEW QUESTIONS**

Review the objectives, key terms, glossary definitions of key terms, figures, and chapter information before completing the following review questions.

1. If a physician or hospital in a managed care plan is paid a fixed, per capita amount for each patient enrolled regardless of the type and number of services rendered, this is a

payment system known as _____.

2. When a prepaid group practice plan limits the patient's choice of personal physicians,

this is termed a/an _____ program.

3. In a managed care setting, a physician who controls patient access to specialists and

diagnostic testing services is known as a/an _____.

4. Systems that allow for better negotiations for contracts with large employers are

   a. _____

   b. _____

   c. _____

5. The oldest type of the prepaid health plans is _____.

6. Name three types of health maintenance organization (HMO) models.

   a. _____

   b. _____

   c. _____

7. What is a foundation for medical care?

   _____

   _____

   _____

8. Name two types of operations used by foundations for medical care, and explain the main feature of each.

   a. _____

   _____

   b. _____

   _____

9. A health benefit program in which enrollees may choose any physician or hospital for services but obtain a higher level of benefits if preferred providers are used is

   known as a/an _____.

10. HMOs and preferred provider organizations (PPOs) consisting of a network of physicians and hospitals that provide an insurance company or employer with

    discounts on their services are referred to collectively as a/an _____.

11. An organization that reviews medical necessity and completeness of inpatient

    hospital care is called a/an _____.

12. Name at least three responsibilities and/or tasks of a quality improvement organization.

    a. _____

    _____

    b. _____

    _____

    c. _____

    _____

13. To control health care costs, the process of reviewing and establishing medical

    necessity for services and providers' use of medical care resources is termed

    _____.

14. Explain the meaning of a "stop-loss" provision that might appear in a managed

    care contract. _____

    _____

    _____.

15. When a certain percentage of the premium fund is set aside to operate an

    individual practice association, this is known as a/an _____.

16. Mark the following statements as true or false.

    _____ a. An HMO can be sponsored and operated by a foundation.

    _____ b. A quality improvement organization determines the quality and operation of health care.

    _____ c. An employer may offer the services of an HMO clinic if he or she has five or more employees.

    _____ d. Medicare and Medicaid beneficiaries may not join an HMO.

    _____ e. Withheld managed care amounts that are not yet received from the managed care plan by the medical practice should be shown as a write-off in an accounts journal.

To check your answers to this self-study assignment, see Appendix D.

ASSIGNMENT 11–2 ▸ OBTAIN AUTHORIZATION FOR A CONSULTATION FROM A MANAGED CARE PLAN

Performance Objective

Task: Complete a treatment authorization form to obtain permission for an office consultation for a patient covered by a managed care plan.

Conditions: Use a treatment authorization form (Figure 11–1), a new patient information form (Figure 11–2), and a typewriter.

Standards: Time: _____ minutes

Accuracy: _____

(Note: The time element and accuracy criteria may be given by your instructor.)

Directions: Complete a treatment authorization form (Figure 11–1) for Mrs. Cohn's managed care plan to obtain permission for the office consultation, and date it August 2 of the current year. To obtain information, refer to the New Patient Information form completed by Mrs. Cohn when she came into the office for her visit with Dr. Practon (Figure 11–2). Dr. Practon's FHP provider number is FHP C01402X.

Scenario: Meriweather B. Cohn's primary care physician, Dr. Gerald Practon, took her clinical history. Physical examination revealed a normal blood pressure (120/80); however, abnormal heart sounds were heard and a diagnosis of a heart murmur was made. Dr. Practon decided to make a semiurgent request to refer Mrs. Cohn for a cardiac consultation (other service) to Dr. Victor M. Salazar, whose office is located at 20 Excalibur Street, Woodland Hills, XY 12345, and whose office telephone number is 555-625-7344. Dr. Salazar will take a detailed history, perform a detailed examination, and make low-complexity medical decisions to evaluate Mrs. Cohn's heart murmur.

Checklist

1. Read the directions and scenario.   _____

2. Checked the reason for the request.   _____

3. Inserted the patient's name on the authorization form.   _____

4. Inserted the date.   _____

5. Inserted the gender.   _____

6. Inserted the birthdate and/or age.   _____

7. Inserted the managed care plan number.   _____

8. Inserted the patient's telephone number.   _____

9. Inserted the patient's address.   _____

10. Inserted the names of the primary care and referring physicians.   _____

11. Inserted the physicians' provider identification numbers.   _____

12. Inserted to whom and/or where the patient is being referred.   _____

Checklist—cont'd

13. Inserted the referring physician's telephone number.   _____

14. Inserted the diagnosis and diagnosis code(s).   _____

15. Inserted the treatment and/or plan.   _____

16. Inserted the procedure code with description.   _____

17. Inserted the reason for the service.   _____

18. Indicated whether an accident.   _____

19. Checked the facility to be used.   _____

After the instructor has returned your work to you, either make the necessary corrections and place your work in a three-ring notebook for future reference or, if you receive a high score, place it in your portfolio for reference when applying for a job.

FHP® HEALTH CARE

IPA TREATMENT AUTHORIZATION FORM

____ Referral
____ Participating
____ Non-Participating
____ Commercial
____ Senior

For Billing Instructions, Patient and Non-Affiliated Providers, and Consultants please see reverse side for instructions

THIS PORTION COMPLETED BY PHYSICIAN

Patient Name _____   Date ___/___/___

M ___ F ___ Age ___ FHP # _____   Home Phone _____

Address _____

Primary Care MD_____   Primary Care MD's FHP # _____

Referring MD _____   Referring MD's FHP # _____

Referred To _____   Address _____

_____   Office Phone _____

Type of service: ☐ In-Patient ☐ Out-Patient Services ☐ Initial Visit ☐ Return Visit ☐ Other

Clinical History and Findings _____

Diagnosis _____

ICD-9-CM CODE

Evaluation and Treatment to Date _____

Procedure _____

RVS CPT-4 CODE

Reason for Referral/Consultation/Procedure _____

Accident: ☐ Yes ☐ No   Where Occurred: ☐ Home ☐ Work ☐ Auto ☐ Other
☐ Urgent ☐ Semi-Urgent ☐ Elective

Facility To Be Used: _____   Estimated Length of Stay _____
☐ Office ☐ Out-Patient ☐ In-Patient

THIS PORTION COMPLETED BY FHP UR
THIS AUTHORIZATION GOOD FOR 60 DAYS ONLY

Type of Contract: ☐ Capitation ☐ Fee For Service ☐ Per Diem

Projected Cost of Procedure _____   Projected Cost of Facility _____

HMO Verification: Effective _____   Group # _____

Benefits: Co-Pay Per Visit _____   Hospital _____

Limitations: _____

____ Authorized   Date ____ Initials ____ Reason _____ Authorization #_____
____ Deferred   Date ____ Initials ____ Reason _____
____ Denied   Date ____ Initials ____ Reason _____
____ Modified   Date ____ Initials ____ Reason _____

WHITE – UR Copy   CANARY – Hospital Copy   PINK – Physician Copy   GOLDENROD – Claims Copy

Figure 11–1

Welcome To Our Office   **NEW PATIENT INFORMATION**   DATE ___8-2-20xx___

| PATIENT'S NAME (PLEASE PRINT) Meriweather B. Cohn | S.S. # 430-XX-0261 | MARITAL STATUS S [X]N W D SEP | SEX M [X] | BIRTH DATE 11-14-65 | AGE | RELIGION (optional) |

| STREET ADDRESS PERMANENT TEMPORARY 267 Blake Street | CITY AND STATE Woodland Hills XY | ZIP CODE 12345 | HOME PHONE # 555-263-0911 |

| PATIENT'S OR PARENT'S EMPLOYER Sun Corporation | OCCUPATION (INDICATE IF STUDENT) sales representative | HOW LONG EMPLOYED 5 yrs | BUS. PHONE # EXT # 555-263-0099 |

| EMPLOYER'S STREET ADDRESS 74 Rain Street | CITY AND STATE Woodland Hills XY | ZIP CODE 12345 |

| DRUG ALLERGIES, IF ANY Penicillin |

| SPOUSE OR PARENT'S NAME Starkweather L. Cohn | S.S. # 273-XX-9961 | BIRTH DATE 7-9-63 |

| SPOUSE OR PARENT'S EMPLOYER B & L Stormdrain Co. | OCCUPATION (INDICATE IF STUDENT) accountant | HOW LONG EMPLOYED 10 yrs | BUS. PHONE # 555-421-0091 |

| EMPLOYER'S STREET ADDRESS 20 South Wind Road | CITY AND STATE Woodland Hills XY | ZIP CODE 12345 |

| *SPOUSE'S STREET ADDRESS, IF DIVORCED OR SEPARATED | CITY AND STATE | ZIP CODE | HOME PHONE # |

PLEASE READ: ALL CHARGES ARE DUE AT THE TIME OF SERVICES. IF HOSPITALIZATION IS INDICATED, THE PATIENT IS RESPONSIBLE FOR FURNISHING INSURANCE CLAIM FORMS TO THE OFFICE PRIOR TO HOSPITALIZATION.

| PERSON RESPONSIBLE FOR PAYMENT, IF NOT ABOVE | STREET ADDRESS, CITY, STATE | ZIP CODE | HOME PHONE # |

| BLUE SHIELD (GIVE NAME OF POLICYHOLDER) [ ] | EFFECTIVE DATE | CERTIFICATE # | GROUP # | COVERAGE CODE |

| OTHER (WRITE IN NAME OF INSURANCE COMPANY) [ ] FHP Healthcare | EFFECTIVE DATE 1-1-8X | POLICY # FHP # A4932 |

| OTHER (WRITE IN NAME OF INSURANCE COMPANY) [ ] | EFFECTIVE DATE | POLICY # |

| MEDICARE (PLEASE GIVE NUMBER) [ ] | RAILROAD RETIREMENT (PLEASE GIVE NUMBER) [ ] |

| MEDICAID [ ] | EFFECTIVE DATE | PROGRAM # | COUNTY # | CASE # | ACCOUNT # |

| INDUSTRIAL [ ] | WERE YOU INJURED ON THE JOB? [ ] YES [X] NO | DATE OF INJURY | INDUSTRIAL CLAIM # |

| ACCIDENT [ ] | WAS AN AUTOMOBILE INVOLVED? [ ] YES [X] NO | DATE OF ACCIDENT | NAME OF ATTORNEY |

| WERE X-RAYS TAKEN OF THIS INJURY OR PROBLEM? [ ] YES [X] NO | IF YES, WHERE WERE X-RAYS TAKEN? (HOSPITAL, ETC) | DATE X-RAYS TAKEN |

HAS ANY MEMBER OF YOUR IMMEDIATE FAMILY BEEN TREATED BY OUR PHYSICIAN(S) BEFORE? INCLUDE NAME OF PHYSICIAN AND FAMILY MEMBER
No

| REFERRED BY BREEZIE N. CLOUD | STREET ADDRESS, CITY, STATE 521 N. Wind Rd., Woodland Hills XY | ZIP CODE 12345 | PHONE # 555-721-9641 |

ALL PROFESSIONAL SERVICES RENDERED ARE CHARGED TO THE PATIENT. NECESSARY FORMS WILL BE COMPLETED TO HELP EXPEDITE INSURANCE CARRIER PAYMENTS. HOWEVER, THE PATIENT IS RESPONSIBLE FOR ALL FEES, REGARDLESS OF INSURANCE COVERAGE. IT IS ALSO CUSTOMARY TO PAY FOR SERVICES WHEN RENDERED UNLESS OTHER ARRANGEMENTS HAVE BEEN MADE IN ADVANCE WITH OUR OFFICE BOOKKEEPER.

INSURANCE AUTHORIZATION AND ASSIGNMENT

Name of Policy Holder ___Meriweather B. Cohn___   HC Number ___College Clinic___

I request that payment of authorized Medicare/Other Insurance company benefits be made either to me or on my behalf to for any services furnished me by that party who accepts assignment/physcian. Regulations pertaining to Medicare assignment of benefits apply.

I authorize any holder of medical or other information about me to release to the Social Security Administration and Health Care Financing Administration or its intermediaries or carrier or any other insurance company any information needed for this or a related Medicare/Other Insurance company claim.

I understand my signature requests that payment be made and authorizes release of medical information necessary to pay the claim. If item 9 of the HCFA-1500 claim form is completed, my signature authorizes releasing of the information to the insurer or agency shown. In Medicare/Other Insurance company assigned cases, the physician or supplier agrees to accept the charge determination of the Medicare/Other Insurance company as the full charge, and the patient is responsible only for the deductible, coinsurance, and noncovered services. Coinsurance and the deductible are based upon the charge determination of the Medicare/Other Insurance company.

Signature ___Meriweather B. Cohn___   Date ___8-2-20XX___

NEW PATIENT INFORMATION

Figure 11–2

ASSIGNMENT **11–3** ▶ **OBTAIN AUTHORIZATION FOR PHYSICAL THERAPY FROM A MANAGED CARE PLAN**

Performance Objective

Task: Complete a treatment authorization form to obtain permission for physical therapy for a patient covered by a managed care plan.

Conditions: Use a treatment authorization form (Figure 11–3) and a typewriter.

Standards: Time: _____ minutes

                   Accuracy: _____

                   (Note: The time element and accuracy criteria may be given by your instructor.)

Directions: Complete the treatment authorization form for this patient (Figure 11–3), date it July 7 of the current year, and submit it to the managed care plan. Refer to Figure 11–1 in the *Handbook* for visual guidance.

Scenario: Mrs. Rosario Jimenez comes into Dr. Gerald Practon's office complaining of neck pain. Mrs. Jimenez is a member of the managed care program HealthNet, and Dr. Practon is her primary care physician. Mrs. Jimenez lives at 350 South Carib Street, Woodland Hills, XY 12340-0329. Her telephone number is 555-450-9987, and she was born April 6, 1960. Her plan identification number is JIM40896, and the effective date is January 1, 20xx. After taking a history, completing a physical examination, and taking and reviewing radiographs, Dr. Practon makes a diagnosis of cervical radiculitis. He gives Mrs. Jimenez a prescription for some medication and says it is necessary to order outpatient physical therapy (one area, for 15 minutes; therapeutic exercises to develop strength, motion, and flexibility) twice a week for 6 weeks at College Hospital. Authorization must be obtained for this treatment. Dr. Practon's HealthNet provider number is HN C01402X.

Checklist

1. Read the directions and scenario.   _____

2. Checked the managed care plan name.   _____

3. Inserted the managed care plan member number.   _____

4. Inserted the patient's name on the authorization form.   _____

5. Inserted the date.   _____

6. Inserted the gender.   _____

7. Inserted the birthdate and/or age.   _____

8. Inserted the patient's telephone number.   _____

9. Inserted the patient's address.   _____

10. Inserted the names of the primary care and referring physicians.   _____

11. Inserted the physicians' provider identification numbers.   _____

12. Inserted to whom and/or where the patient is being referred.   _____

13. Inserted the referred to telephone number.   _____

14. Inserted the diagnosis and diagnosis code(s).   _____

15. Inserted the treatment and/or plan.   _____

16. Inserted the procedure code with description.   _____

17. Inserted the facility and estimated stay.   _____

18. Checked location.   _____

19. Obtained physician's signature.   _____

20. Stated primary care physician's recommendations.   _____

21. Primary care physician initialed form.   _____

22. Inserted date eligibility checked.   _____

23. Inserted effective date.   _____

After the instructor has returned your work to you, either make the necessary corrections and place your work in a three-ring notebook for future reference or, if you receive a high score, place it in your portfolio for reference when applying for a job.

Clinic Name:		**MANAGED CARE PLAN AUTHORIZATION REQUEST**	☐ Health Net	☐ Met Life
Address:			☐ Pacificare	☐ Travelers
Telephone No.:			☐ Secure Horizons	☐ Pru Care
Fax No.:			☐ Other	
Contact:			Member/Group No.:	

TO BE COMPLETED BY PRIMARY CARE PHYSICIAN OR OUTSIDE PROVIDER

Patient Name:		Date:
☐ Male ☐ Female Birthdate:		Home Telephone Number:
Address:		
Primary Care Physician:		Provider ID #:
Referring Physician:		Provider ID #:
Referred to:		Office Telephone Number:
Address:		
Diagnosis Code:	Description:	
Diagnosis Code:	Description:	
Treatment Plan:		

Authorization requested for: ☐ Consult only   ☐ Treatment only   ☐ Consult/Treatment
☐ Consult/Procedure/Surgery   ☐ Diagnostic Tests

Procedure Code:	Description:
Procedure Code:	Description:

Place of Service: ☐ Office ☐ Outpatient ☐ Inpatient ☐ Other	Number of Visits:
Facility:	Length of Stay:

List of potential future consultants (i.e., anesthetists, surgical assistants or medical/surgical):

Physician's Signature:

TO BE COMPLETED BY PRIMARY CARE PHYSICIAN

PCP Recommendations:	PCP Initials:
Date eligibility checked:	Effective Date:

TO BE COMPLETED BY UTILIZATION MANAGEMENT

Authorized:	Auth. No.:	Not Authorized:
Deferred:		Modified:
Comments:		

Figure 11–3

ASSIGNMENT **11-4** ▸ **OBTAIN AUTHORIZATION FOR DIAGNOSTIC ARTHROSCOPY FOR A MANAGED CARE PLAN**

Performance Objective

Task: Complete a treatment authorization form to obtain permission for diagnostic arthroscopy with débridement for a patient from a managed care plan.

Conditions: Use a treatment authorization form (Figure 11–4) and a typewriter.

Standards: Time: _____ minutes

                 Accuracy: _____

                 (Note: The time element and accuracy criteria may be given by your instructor.)

Directions: Complete the treatment authorization form for this patient (Figure 11–4), date it August 12 of the current year, and submit it to the managed care plan. Refer to Figure 11–1 in the *Handbook* for visual guidance.

Scenario: Daniel Chan has been referred by his primary care physician, Dr. Gerald Practon, to an orthopedic surgeon, Dr. Raymond Skeleton. Both physicians are members of his managed care plan, Metropolitan Life. The patient comes into Dr. Skeleton's office complaining of pain, swelling, and crepitus of the right knee. The patient is having difficulty walking but indicates no recent injury to the knee.

Mr. Chan lives at 226 West Olive Avenue, Woodland Hills, XY 12340-0329, and his telephone number is 555-540-6700. His plan identification number is FTW90876, effective February 1, 20xx, and he was born February 23, 1971.

After taking a history, completing a physical examination, and taking and reviewing radiographs, Dr. Skeleton suspects the patient has a tear of the medial meniscus and may require debridement of articular cartilage. This procedure will be performed on an outpatient basis at College Hospital. Authorization must be obtained for the surgical arthroscopy with debridement of articular cartilage. Dr. Practon's Metropolitan Life provider number is ML C01402X and Dr. Skeleton's Metropolitan Life provider number is ML C4561X.

Checklist

1. Read the directions and scenario.   _____

2. Checked the managed care plan name.   _____

3. Inserted the managed care plan member number.   _____

4. Inserted the patient's name on the authorization form.   _____

5. Inserted the date.   _____

6. Inserted the gender.   _____

7. Inserted the birthdate and/or age.   _____

8. Inserted the patient's telephone number.   _____

9. Inserted the patient's address.   _____

10. Inserted the names of the primary care and referring physicians.   _____

11. Inserted the physicians' provider identification numbers.   _____

12. Inserted to whom and/or where the patient is being referred.   _____

13. Inserted the referred to telephone number.   _____

14. Inserted the diagnoses and diagnosis code(s).   _____

15. Inserted the treatment and/or plan.   _____

16. Inserted the procedure code with description.   _____

17. Inserted the facility and estimated stay.   _____

18. Checked location.   _____

19. Obtained physician's signature.   _____

20. Stated primary care physician's recommendations.   _____

21. Primary care physician's initialed form.   _____

22. Inserted date eligibility checked.   _____

23. Inserted effective date.   _____

After the instructor has returned your work to you, either make the necessary corrections and place your work in a three-ring notebook for future reference or, if you received a high score, place it in your portfolio for reference when applying for a job.

	MANAGED CARE PLAN AUTHORIZATION REQUEST	☐ Health Net ☐ Met Life

Clinic Name:		☐ Health Net	☐ Met Life
Address:	MANAGED CARE	☐ Pacificare	☐ Travelers
Telephone No.:	PLAN	☐ Secure Horizons	☐ Pru Care
Fax No.:	AUTHORIZATION	☐ Other	
Contact:	REQUEST	Member/Group No.:	

TO BE COMPLETED BY PRIMARY CARE PHYSICIAN OR OUTSIDE PROVIDER

Patient Name:		Date:
☐ Male ☐ Female Birthdate:		Home Telephone Number:
Address:		
Primary Care Physician:		Provider ID #:
Referring Physician:		Provider ID #:
Referred to:		Office Telephone Number:
Address:		
Diagnosis Code:	Description:	
Diagnosis Code:	Description:	
Treatment Plan:		

Authorization requested for: ☐ Consult only   ☐ Treatment only   ☐ Consult/Treatment   ☐ Consult/Procedure/Surgery   ☐ Diagnostic Tests

Procedure Code:	Description:
Procedure Code:	Description:

Place of Service: ☐ Office ☐ Outpatient ☐ Inpatient ☐ Other	Number of Visits:
Facility:	Length of Stay:

List of potential future consultants (i.e., anesthetists, surgical assistants or medical/surgical):

Physician's Signature:

TO BE COMPLETED BY PRIMARY CARE PHYSICIAN

PCP Recommendations:	PCP Initials:
Date eligibility checked:	Effective Date:

TO BE COMPLETED BY UTILIZATION MANAGEMENT

Authorized:	Auth. No.:	Not Authorized:
Deferred:		Modified:
Comments:		

Figure 11–4

ASSIGNMENT **11–5** ▶ **OBTAIN AUTHORZATION FOR CONSULTATION FROM A MANAGED CARE PLAN**

Performance Objective

Task: Complete a treatment authorization form to obtain permission for consultation for a patient from a managed care plan.

Conditions: Use a treatment authorization form (Figure 11–5) and a typewriter.

Standards: Time: _____ minutes

                 Accuracy: _____

                 (Note: The time element and accuracy criteria may be given by your instructor.)

Directions: Complete the treatment authorization form for this patient (Figure11–5), date it September 3 of the current year, and submit it to the managed care plan. Refer to Figure 11–1 in the *Handbook* for visual guidance.

Scenario: Frederico Fellini, with a history of getting up four times during the night with a slow urinary stream, was seen by his primary care physician, Dr. Gerald Practon. An intravenous pyelogram yielded negative results except for distention of the urinary bladder. Physical examination of the prostate showed an enlargement. The preliminary diagnosis is benign prostatic hypertrophy (BPH).

  The patient will be referred to Dr. Douglas Lee, a urologist, for consultation (Level 4) and cystoscopy. Transurethral resection of the prostate is possible at a future date. Dr. Lee's address is 4300 Cyber Street, Woodland Hills, XY 12345, and his office telephone number is 555-675-3322.

  Dr. Practon's managed care contract is with PruCare, identification number PC C01402X, of which this patient is a member.

  Mr. Fellini lives at 476 Miner Street, Woodland Hills, XY 12345, and his telephone number is 555-679-0098. His PruCare plan identification number is VRG87655, effective January 1, 20xx. His birthdate is May 24, 1944.

Checklist

1. Read the directions and scenario.   _____

2. Checked the managed care plan name.   _____

3. Inserted the managed care plan member number.   _____

4. Inserted the patient's name on the authorization form.   _____

5. Inserted the date.   _____

6. Inserted the gender.   _____

7. Inserted the birthdate and/or age.   _____

8. Inserted the patient's telephone number.   _____

9. Inserted the patient's address.   _____

10. Inserted the names of the primary care and referring physicians.   _____

Checklist—cont'd

11. Inserted the physicians' provider identification numbers.   _____

12. Inserted to whom and/or where the patient is being referred.   _____

13. Inserted the referred to telephone number.   _____

14. Inserted the diagnosis and diagnosis code(s).   _____

15. Inserted the treatment and/or plan.   _____

16. Inserted the procedure codes with description.   _____

17. Inserted the facility and estimated stay.   _____

18. Checked location.   _____

19. Listed potential consultant.   _____

20. Obtained physician's signature.   _____

21. Stated primary care physician's recommendations.   _____

22. Primary care physician initialed form.   _____

23. Inserted date eligibility checked.   _____

24. Inserted effective date.   _____

After the instructor has returned your work to you, either make the necessary corrections and place your work in a three-ring notebook for future reference or, if you received a high score, place it in your portfolio for reference when applying for a job.

Clinic Name:	**MANAGED CARE PLAN AUTHORIZATION REQUEST**	☐ Health Net ☐ Met Life
Address:		☐ Pacificare ☐ Travelers
Telephone No.:		☐ Secure Horizons ☐ Pru Care
Fax No.:		☐ Other
Contact:		Member/Group No.:

TO BE COMPLETED BY PRIMARY CARE PHYSICIAN OR OUTSIDE PROVIDER

Patient Name:	Date:

☐ Male ☐ Female Birthdate:	Home Telephone Number:

Address:

Primary Care Physician:	Provider ID #:
Referring Physician:	Provider ID #:
Referred to:	Office Telephone Number:

Address:

Diagnosis Code:	Description:
Diagnosis Code:	Description:

Treatment Plan:

Authorization requested for: ☐ Consult only ☐ Treatment only ☐ Consult/Treatment ☐ Consult/Procedure/Surgery ☐ Diagnostic Tests

Procedure Code:	Description:
Procedure Code:	Description:

Place of Service: ☐ Office ☐ Outpatient ☐ Inpatient ☐ Other	Number of Visits:
Facility:	Length of Stay:

List of potential future consultants (i.e., anesthetists, surgical assistants or medical/surgical):

Physician's Signature:

TO BE COMPLETED BY PRIMARY CARE PHYSICIAN

PCP Recommendations:	PCP Initials:
Date eligibility checked:	Effective Date:

TO BE COMPLETED BY UTILIZATION MANAGEMENT

Authorized:	Auth. No.:	Not Authorized:
Deferred:		Modified:

Comments:

Figure 11–5

ASSIGNMENT 11-6 ▸ OBTAIN AUTHORIZATION FOR DIAGNOSTIC BODY SCAN FROM A MANAGED CARE PLAN

Performance Objective

Task: Complete a treatment authorization form to obtain permission for diagnostic complete body bone scan and mammogram for a patient covered by a managed care plan.

Conditions: Use a treatment authorization form (Figure 11–6) and a typewriter.

Standards: Time: _____ minutes

Accuracy: _____

(Note: The time element and accuracy criteria may be given by your instructor.)

Directions: Complete the treatment authorization form for this patient (Figure 11–6), date it October 23 of the current year, and submit it to the managed care plan. Refer to Figure 11–1 in the *Handbook* for visual guidance.

Scenario: A patient, Debbie Dye, sees her primary care physician, Dr. Gerald Practon, for complaint of midback pain. She underwent a lumpectomy 2 years ago for a malignant neoplasm of the lower left breast; thus she has a history of breast cancer. She has been referred by Dr. Practon (PacifiCare identification number PC C01402X) to Dr. Donald Patos, an oncologist, for a complete workup. He finds that her complaint of midback pain warrants the need to refer her to XYZ Radiology for bilateral diagnostic mammography and a complete body bone scan.

Dr. Patos' address is 4466 East Canter Drive, Woodland Hills, XY 12345, and his office telephone number is 555-980-5566. Dr. Patos' PacifiCare identification number is PC 5673X.

Ms. Dye lives at 6700 Flora Road, Woodland Hills, XY 12345, and her telephone number is 555-433-6755. Her PacifiCare plan identification number is SR45380, effective January 1, 20xx. Her birth date is August 6, 1952.

XYZ Radiology's address is 4767 Broad Avenue, Woodland Hills, XY 12345-0001, and the office telephone number is 555-486-9162.

Checklist

1. Read the directions and scenario. _____

2. Checked the managed care plan name. _____

3. Inserted the managed care plan member number. _____

4. Inserted the patient's name on the authorization form. _____

5. Inserted the date. _____

6. Inserted the gender. _____

7. Inserted the birthdate and/or age. _____

8. Inserted the patient's telephone number. _____

9. Inserted the patient's address. _____

10. Inserted the names of the primary care and referring physicians. _____

11. Inserted the physicians' provider identification numbers.   _____

12. Inserted to whom and/or where the patient is being referred.   _____

13. Inserted the referred to telephone number.   _____

14. Inserted the diagnoses and diagnosis code(s).   _____

15. Inserted the treatment and/or plan.   _____

16. Inserted the procedure codes with descriptions.   _____

17. Inserted the facility and estimated stay.   _____

18. Checked location.   _____

19. Obtained physician's signature.   _____

20. Stated primary care physician's recommendations.   _____

21. Primary care physician's initialed form.   _____

22. Inserted date eligibility checked.   _____

23. Inserted effective date.   _____

   After the instructor has returned your work to you, either make the necessary corrections and place your work in a three-ring notebook for future reference or, if you received a high score, place it in your portfolio for reference when applying for a job.

	MANAGED CARE PLAN AUTHORIZATION REQUEST	☐ Health Net	☐ Met Life

Clinic Name:

Address:

Telephone No.:

Fax No.:

Contact:

☐ Health Net ☐ Met Life
☐ Pacificare ☐ Travelers
☐ Secure Horizons ☐ Pru Care
☐ Other

Member/Group No.:

TO BE COMPLETED BY PRIMARY CARE PHYSICIAN OR OUTSIDE PROVIDER

Patient Name: **Date:**

☐ Male   ☐ Female   **Birthdate:**   **Home Telephone Number:**

Address:

Primary Care Physician: **Provider ID #:**

Referring Physician: **Provider ID #:**

Referred to: **Office Telephone Number:**

Address:

Diagnosis Code: **Description:**

Diagnosis Code: **Description:**

Treatment Plan:

Authorization requested for: ☐ Consult only   ☐ Treatment only   ☐ Consult/Treatment
☐ Consult/Procedure/Surgery   ☐ Diagnostic Tests

Procedure Code: **Description:**

Procedure Code: **Description:**

Place of Service: ☐ Office ☐ Outpatient ☐ Inpatient ☐ Other   **Number of Visits:**

Facility: **Length of Stay:**

List of potential future consultants (i.e., anesthetists, surgical assistants or medical/surgical):

Physician's Signature:

TO BE COMPLETED BY PRIMARY CARE PHYSICIAN

PCP Recommendations: **PCP Initials:**

Date eligibility checked: **Effective Date:**

TO BE COMPLETED BY UTILIZATION MANAGEMENT

Authorized: **Auth. No.:**   **Not Authorized:**

Deferred: **Modified:**

Comments:

Figure 11–6

ASSIGNMENT **11–7** ▸ **TRANSMIT AN ELECTRONIC INSURANCE CLAIM FOR A PRIVATE CASE**

(**e hint**)   Follow the General Instructions for TRANSMISSION OF AN ELECTRONIC CLAIM (A SINGLE CLAIM) as given in *Workbook* Chapter 8

Performance Objective

Task: Transmit an electronic insurance claim form and post the information to the patient's financial account record.

Conditions: Use Carey S. Wolford's encounter form (Figures 11–7 and 11–8), patient's electronic data, and computer.

Standards: Productivity Measurement

                     Time: _____ minutes

                     Accuracy: _____

                     (Note: The time element and accuracy criteria may be given by your instructor.)

Directions:

1. Electronically prepare an insurance claim form by referring to Carey S. Wolford's encounter form in this *Workbook* and her electronic personal and medical data. Follow the step-by-step general directions for transmission of an insurance claim.

2. Enter the patient's data into the software to obtain the procedural and diagnostic codes and College Clinic fee amounts.

3. Transmit the insurance claim to Global Insurance Company.

4. Print a hard copy of the insurance claim to hand in to your instructor to receive a score.

5. A Performance Evaluation Checklist may be reproduced from the "Instruction Guide to the Workbook" chapter if your instructor wishes you to submit it to assist with scoring and comments.

After the instructor has returned your work to you, either make the necessary corrections and place your work in a three-ring notebook for future reference or, if you received a high score, place it in your portfolio for reference when applying for a job.

TAX ID #3664021CC
Medicaid #HSC12345F

College Clinic

4567 Broad Avenue
Woodland Hills, XY
12345-0001
Tel (555) 486-9002
Fax (555) 487-8976

Doctor No. _____

☒ PRIVATE   ☐ MANAGED CARE   ☐ MEDICAID   ☐ MEDICARE   ☐ TRICARE   ☐ W/C

ACCOUNT # 006	PATIENT'S LAST NAME Wolford	FIRST Carey	INITIAL S.	TODAY'S DATE 1/27/2007

ASSIGNMENT: I hereby assign payment directly to College Clinic of the surgical and/or medical benefits, if any, otherwise payable to me for his/her services as described below.
SIGNED (Patient, or Parent, if Minor)   *Carey s. Wolford*   DATE: 1/27/2007

✓	DESCRIPTION	CPT-4/MD	FEE	✓	DESCRIPTION	CPT-4/MD	FEE	✓	DESCRIPTION	CPT-4/MD	FEE
	OFFICE VISIT-NEW PATIENT				**WELL BABY EXAM**				**LABORATORY**		
	Level 1	99201			Initial	99381			Glucose Blood	82962	
	Level 2	99202			Periodic	99391			Heamatocrit	85013	
	Level 3	99203			**OFFICE PROCEDURES**				Occult Blood	82270	
	Level 4	99204			Anoscopy	46600			Urine Dip	81000	
	Level 5	99205			ECG 24-hr	93224			**X-RAY**		
	OFFICE VISIT-ESTAB. PATIENT				Fracture Rpr Foot	28470			Foot - 2 View	73620	
	Level 1	99211			I & D	10060			Forearm - 2 View	73090	
	Level 2	99212			Suture Repair				Nasal Bone - 3	70160	
	Level 3	99213							Spine LS - 2 view	72100	
	Level 4	99214			**INJECTIONS/VACCINATIONS**						
	Level 5	99215			DPT	90701			**MISCELLANEOUS**		
	OFFICE CONSULT-NP/EST				IM-Antibiotic	90788			Handling of Spec	99000	
✓	Level 2	99242	80.24		OPU-Poliovirus	90712			Supply	99070	
	Level 4	99244			Tetanus	90703			Venipuncture	36415	
	Level 5	99245									

COMMENTS:

Physician: *Vera Cutis, MD*

RETURN APPOINTMENT

_2_ Week(s)   _____ Month(s)

DIAGNOSIS:	DESCRIPTION	CODE
Primary:	*actinic keratosis*	702.0
Secondary:	*seborrheic keratosis*	702.1

REC'D BY:
☐ BANK CARD
☐ CASH
☐ CHECK
  # _____

PREVIOUS BALANCE	-0-
TODAY'S FEE	80.24
AMOUNT REC'D/CO-PAY	⊖
BALANCE	80.24

Figure 11–7

TAX ID #3664021CC
Medicaid #HSC12345F

College Clinic

4567 Broad Avenue
Woodland Hills, XY
12345-0001
Tel (555) 486-9002
Fax (555) 487-8976

Doctor No. _____

☒ PRIVATE　☐ MANAGED CARE　☐ MEDICAID　☐ MEDICARE　☐ TRICARE　☐ W/C

ACCOUNT # 006	PATIENT'S LAST NAME Wolford	FIRST Carey	INITIAL S.	TODAY'S DATE 2/12/2007

ASSIGNMENT: I hereby assign payment directly to College Clinic of the surgical and/or medical benefits, if any, otherwise payable to me for his/her services as described below.
SIGNED (Patient, or Parent, if Minor)　*Carey s. Wolford*　　DATE: *2/12/2007*

✓	DESCRIPTION	CPT-4/MD	FEE	✓	DESCRIPTION	CPT-4/MD	FEE	✓	DESCRIPTION	CPT-4/MD	FEE
	OFFICE VISIT-NEW PATIENT				**WELL BABY EXAM**				**LABORATORY**		
	Level 1	99201			Initial	99381			Glucose Blood	82962	
	Level 2	99202			Periodic	99391			Heamatocrit	85013	
	Level 3	99203			**OFFICE PROCEDURES**				Occult Blood	82270	
	Level 4	99204			Anoscopy	46600			Urine Dip	81000	
	Level 5	99205			ECG 24-hr	93224			**X-RAY**		
	OFFICE VISIT-ESTAB, PATIENT				Fracture Rpr Foot	28470			Foot - 2 View	73620	
	Level 1	99211			I & D	10060			Forearm - 2 View	73090	
	Level 2	99212		✓	Remove 1 lesion	17000	52.56		Nasal Bone - 3	70160	
	Level 3	99213		✓	Remove 2-4 lesions	17003	15.21		Spine LS - 2 view	72100	
	Level 4	99214			**INJECTIONS/VACCINATIONS**						
	Level 5	99215			DPT	90701			**MISCELLANEOUS**		
	OFFICE CONSULT-NP/EST				IM-Antibiotic	90788			Handling of Spec	99000	
	Level 3	99242			OPU-Poliovirus	90712			Supply	99070	
	Level 4	99244			Tetanus	90703			Venipuncture	36415	
	Level 5	99245									

COMMENTS:

Physician: *Vera Cutis, M.D.*

RETURN APPOINTMENT
PRN
_____ Week(s)　_____ Month(s)

DIAGNOSIS:	DESCRIPTION	CODE
Primary:	*actinic keratosis*	*702.0*
Secondary:	*seborrheic keratosis*	*702.1*

REC'D BY:
☐ BANK CARD
☐ CASH
☐ CHECK
_____

PREVIOUS BALANCE	*80.24*
TODAY'S FEE	*67.77*
AMOUNT REC'D/CO-PAY	*⊖*
BALANCE	*148.01*

Figure 11–8

ASSIGNMENT 11-8 ▸ PRINT A REMAINING AUTHORIZATIONS REPORT

ⓔhint   General Instructions for PRINTING A REMAINING
AUTHORIZATIONS REPORT

Directions:

1. From the main menu, click on "Reports" and select "Print Custom Reports."

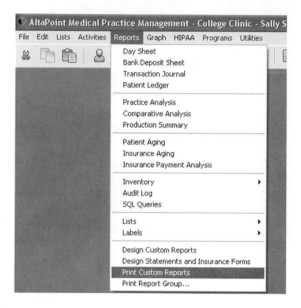

2. [Report Code] Field: Find and choose "AUTHOREM" (Remaining Authorization).

3. Click "Print."

Performance Objective

Task: Print a Remaining Authorizations Report.

Conditions: Use practice management to generate report for all patients with remaining authorizations.

Standards: Productivity Measurement

                Time: _____ minutes

                Accuracy: _____

                (Note: The time element and accuracy criteria may be given by your instructor.)

1. Print out a hard copy of the Remaining Authorizations Report and turn it in to your
   instructor to receive a score.

   After the instructor has returned your work to you, either make the necessary
corrections and place your work in a three-ring notebook for future reference or, if you
received a high score, place it in your portfolio for references when applying for a job.

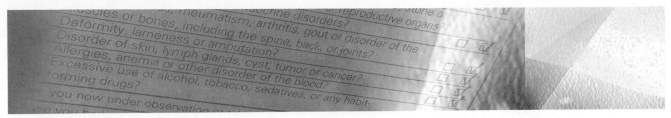

Medicare

KEY TERMS

Your instructor may wish to select some specific words pertinent to this chapter for a test. For definitions of the terms, further study, and/or reference, the words, phrases, and abbreviations may be found in the glossary at the end of the Handbook. *Key terms for this chapter follow.*

advance beneficiary notice (ABN)

approved charges

assignment

benefit period

Centers for Medicare and Medicaid Services (CMS)

Correct Coding Initiative (CCI)

crossover claim

diagnostic cost groups (DCGs)

disabled

end-stage renal disease (ESRD)

fiscal intermediary (FI)

hospice

hospital insurance

intermediate care facilities (ICFs)

limiting charge

medical necessity

Medicare

Medicare Part A

Medicare Part B

Medicare Part C

Medicare/Medicaid (Medi-Medi)

Medicare Secondary Payer (MSP)

Medicare Summary Notice (MSN)

Medigap (MG)

national alphanumeric codes

nonparticipating physician (nonpar)

nursing facility (NF)

participating physician (par)

peer review organization (PRO)

premium

prospective payment system (PPS)

qui tam action

reasonable fee

relative value unit (RVU)

remittance advice (RA)

resource-based relative value scale (RBRVS)

respite care

Supplemental Security Income (SSI)

supplementary medical insurance (SMI)

volume performance standard (VPS)

whistleblowers

PERFORMANCE OBJECTIVES

The student will be able to:

- Define and spell the key terms for this chapter, given the information from the *Handbook* glossary, within a reasonable time period and with enough accuracy to obtain a satisfactory evaluation
- After reading the chapter answer the self-study review questions with enough accuracy to obtain a satisfactory evaluation.
- Fill in the correct meaning of each abbreviation, given a list of common medical abbreviations and symbols that appear in chart notes, within a reasonable time period and with enough accuracy to obtain a satisfactory evaluation.
- Complete each CMS-1500 Health Insurance Claim Form for billing, given the patients' medical chart notes, ledger cards, and blank insurance claim forms, within a reasonable time period and with enough accuracy to obtain a satisfactory evaluation.
- Post payments, adjustments, and balances on the patients' ledger cards, using the Medicare Mock Fee Schedule in Appendix A in this *Workbook*, within a reasonable time period and with enough accuracy to obtain a satisfactory evaluation.
- Compute mathematical calculations, given Medicare problem situations, within a reasonable time period and with enough accuracy to obtain a satisfactory evaluation.
- Using the *Current Procedural Terminology* (CPT) code book or the Mock Fee Schedule in Appendix A in this *Workbook* and the Healthcare Common Procedure Coding System (HCPCS) list of codes in Appendix B in this *Workbook*, select the HCPCS and/or procedural code numbers, given a series of medical services, procedures, or supplies, within a reasonable time period and with enough accuracy to obtain a satisfactory evaluation.
- Transmit electronic insurance claims for Medicare cases using practice management software, within a reasonable time period and with enough accuracy to obtain a satisfactory evaluation.

STUDY OUTLINE

Background

Policies and Regulations
Eligibility Requirements
Health Insurance Card
Enrollment Status
Benefits and Nonbenefits

Additional Insurance Programs
Medicare/Medicaid
Medicare/Medigap
Medicare Secondary Payer
Automobile or Liability Insurance Coverage

Medicare Managed Care Plans
Health Maintenance Organizations
Carrier Dealing Prepayment Organization

Utilization and Quality Control
Quality Improvement Organizations
Federal False Claims Amendment Act

Medicare Billing Compliance Issues
Clinical Laboratory Improvement Amendment

Payment Fundamentals
Provider
Prior Authorization
Waiver of Liability Provision
Elective Surgery Estimate
Prepayment Screens
Correct Coding Initiative

Medicare Reimbursement
Chronology of Payment
Reasonable Fee

Resource-Based Relative Value Scale
Healthcare Common Procedure Coding System
  (HCPCS)

Claim Submission
Local Coverage Determination
Fiscal Intermediaries and Fiscal Agents
Provider Identification Numbers
Patient's Signature Authorization
Time Limit
Paper Claims
Electronic Claims
Medicare/Medicaid Claims
Medicare/Medigap Claims
Medicare/Employer Supplemental Insurance Claims
Medicare/Supplemental and MSP Claims
Deceased Patients Claims
Physician Substitute Coverage

After Claim Submission
Remittance Advice
Medicare Summary Notice

Beneficiary Representative/Representative Payee
Posting Payments
Review and Redetermination Process

Procedure: Determine Whether Medicare is Primary or Secondary and Determine Additional Benefits

Procedure: Complete an Advance Beneficiary Notice (ABN) Form

S E L F - S T U D Y **12–1** ▶ **R E V I E W   Q U E S T I O N S**

Review the objectives, key terms, glossary definitions of key terms, chapter information, and figures before completing the following review questions.

1. An individual becomes eligible for Medicare Parts A and B at age _____.

2. Medicare Part A is _____ coverage, and Medicare Part B is _____ coverage.

3. Name an eligibility requirement that would allow aliens to receive Medicare benefits.

   _____

4. Funding for the Medicare Part A program is obtained from _____

   _____

   and funding for the Medicare Part B program is obtained equally from _____

   _____.

5. Define a Medicare Part A hospital benefit period. _____

   _____

   _____

6. A program designed to provide pain relief, symptom management, and supportive

   services to terminally ill individuals and their families is known as _____

   _____.

7. Short-term inpatient medical care for terminally ill individuals to give temporary

   relief to the caregiver is known as _____.

8. The frequency of Pap tests for Medicare patients is _____, and that

   for mammograms is _____.

9. Some third-party payers offer policies that fall under guidelines issued by the federal
   government and cover prescription costs, Medicare deductibles, and copayments;

   these policies are known as _____ insurance policies.

10. Name two types of health maintenance organization (HMO) plans that may have
    Medicare Part B contracts.

    a. _____

    b. _____

11. The federal laws establishing standards of quality control and safety measures in

    clinical laboratories are known as _____.

12. Acceptance of assignment by a participating physician means that he or she agrees

    to _____ after the $ _____

    deductible has been met.

13. Philip Lenz is seen by Dr. Doe, who schedules an operative procedure in 1 month.

    This type of surgery is known as _____,
    because it does not have to be performed immediately.

14. A Medicare insurance claim form showed a number, J0540, for an injection of

    600,000 U of penicillin G. This number is referred to as a/an _____.

15. Organizations or claims processors under contract to the federal government
    that handle insurance claims and payments for hospitals under Medicare Part A

    are known as _____,
    and those that process claims for physicians and other suppliers of services under

    Medicare Part B are called _____.

16. A Centers for Medicare and Medicaid Services (CMS)–assigned provider

    identification number is known as a/an _____.

    Physicians who supply durable medical equipment must have a/an _____
    number.

17. If circumstances make it impossible to obtain a signature on an insurance claim

    from a Medicare patient, physicians may obtain a/an _____.

18. The time limit for sending in a Medicare insurance claim is _____.

19. Mrs. Davis, a Medicare/Medicaid (Medi-Medi) patient, has a cholecystectomy.
    In completing the insurance claim form, the assignment portion is left blank

    in error. What will happen in this case? _____

    _____

20. If an individual is 65 years of age and is a Medicare beneficiary but is working
    and has a group insurance policy, where is the insurance claim form sent initially?

    _____

21. If a Medicare beneficiary is injured in an automobile accident, the physician

    submits the claim form to _____.

To check your answers to this self-study assignment, see Appendix D.

ASSIGNMENT 12–2 ▸ CALCULATE MATHEMATICAL PROBLEMS

Performance Objective

Task: Calculate and insert the correct amounts for seven Medicare scenarios.

Conditions: Use a pen or pencil, the description of problem, and, for Problem 7, Figures 12–1 and 12–2.

Standards: Time: _____ minutes

                 Accuracy: _____

                 (Note: The time element and accuracy criteria may be given by your instructor.)

Directions: Submitting insurance claims, particularly Medicare claims, involves a bit of arithmetic. Several problems are given here so that you will gain experience with situations encountered daily in your work. The Medicare deductible is always subtracted from the allowed amount first before mathematic computations continue.

Problem 1: Mr. Doolittle has Medicare Part B coverage. He was well during the entire past year. On January 1, Mr. Doolittle is rushed to the hospital, where Dr. Input performs an emergency gastric resection. Medicare is billed for $450, and the doctor agrees to accept assignment. The patient has not paid any deductible. Complete the following statements by putting in the correct amounts.

Original Bill

a. Medicare allows $400. Medicare payment: _____

b. Patient owes Dr. Input: _____

c. Dr. Input's courtesy adjustment: _____

   Mathematical computations:

Problem 2: Mrs. James has Medicare Part B coverage. She met her deductible when she was ill in March of this year. On November 1, Dr. Caesar performs a bilateral salpingo-oophorectomy, for which he bills her $300 and agrees to accept a Medicare assignment.

Original Bill

a. Medicare allows $275. Medicare payment: _____

b. Patient owes Dr. Caesar: _____

c. Dr. Caesar's courtesy adjustment: _____

Mathematical computations for surgeon:

The assistant surgeon charged Mrs. James $60 (the Medicare limiting charge) and does not accept assignment. After receiving her check from Medicare, Mrs. James sends the surgeon his $60. Medicare has allowed $55 for the fee.

a. How much of the money was from Mrs. James' private funds? $_____.

b. How much did Medicare pay? $_____.

Mathematical computations for assistant surgeon:

Problem 3: You work for Dr. Coccidioides. He does not accept assignment. He is treating Mr. Robinson for allergies. Mr. Robinson has Medicare Part A. You send in a bill to Medicare for the $135 that Mr. Robinson owes you. What portion of the bill will Medicare pay?

Problem 4: In June, Mr. Fay has an illness that incurs $89 in medical bills. He asks you to bill Medicare, and the physician does not accept assignment. He has paid the deductible at another physician's office.

a. If Medicare allows the entire amount of your fees, the Medicare check to the patient

   is $_____ (which comes to you).

b. The patient's part of the bill to you is $_____.

Mathematical computations:

Problem 5: Mr. Iba, a Medicare patient with a Medigap insurance policy, is seen for an office visit and the fee is $80. The Medicare-approved amount is $54.44. The patient has met his deductible for the year.

a. The Medicare payment check is $ _____

b. After the claim is submitted to the Medigap insurance, the Medigap payment check is

   $ _____

   (Note: Chapter 11 in the *Handbook* gives details on Medigap coverage guidelines.)

c. To zero out the balance, the Medicare courtesy adjustment is $ _____.

   Mathematical computations:

Problem 6: Mrs. Smith, a Medicare patient, had surgery, and the participating physician's fee is $1250. This patient is working part-time, and her employer group health plan (primary insurance) allowed $1100, applied $500 to the deductible, and paid 80% of $600.

a. Amount paid by this plan: $ _____.

b. The spouse's employer group health plan (secondary insurance) is billed for the balance,

   which is $ _____, and this program also has a $500 deductible. This plan pays 100% of the fee billed, minus the deductible.

c. The spouse's employer group plan makes a payment of $ _____.

   You send copies of remittance advice from the two group health plans and submit a claim to

   Medicare (the third insurance) for $1250. The balance at this point is $ _____.

   Mathematical computations:

Problem 7: In the late 1980s, Medicare's Resource-Based Relative Value System (RBRVS) became the way payment was determined each year. However, since the early 1990s, annual fee schedules have been supplied by local fiscal intermediaries, and so the RBRVS has become more useful in determining practice cost to convert patients to capitation in negotiations of managed care contracts. Because physicians may request determination of fees for certain procedures to discover actual cost and what compensation ratios should be, it is important to know how Medicare fees are determined. Each year the *Federal Register* publishes geographic practice cost indices by Medicare carrier and locality as well as relative value units and related information. This assignment will give you some mathematical practice in using figures for annual conversion factors to determine fees for given procedures in various regions of the United States. Refer to Figures 12–1 and 12–2, which are pages of the *Federal Register*.

a. HCPCS Code 47600: Removal of gallbladder. The medical practice is located in Phoenix, Arizona.

	Work	*Overhead*	*Malpractice*
RVUs	_____	_____	_____
GPCI	× _____	× _____	× _____

+ _____ + _____ + _____ = Total adjusted RVUs _____

2005 Conversion factor $37.8975 × Total adjusted RVUs _____ =

allowed amount $ _____ .

b. HCPCS Code 47715: Excision of bile duct cyst. The medical practice is located in Arkansas.

	Work	*Overhead*	*Malpractice*
RVUs	_____	_____	_____
GPCI	× _____	× _____	× _____

+ _____ + _____ + _____ = Total adjusted RVUs _____

2005 Conversion factor $37.8975 × Total adjusted RVUs _____ = allowed

amount $ _____ .

c. HCPCS Code 48146: Pancreatectomy. The medical practice is located in Fresno, California.

	Work	*Overhead*	*Malpractice*
RVUs	_____	_____	_____
GPCI	× _____	× _____	× _____

+ _____ + _____ + _____ = Total adjusted RVUs _____

2005 Conversion factor $37.8975 × Total adjusted RVUs _____ = allowed

amount $ _____ .

ADDENDUM D.---GEOGRAPHIC PRACTICE COST INDICES BY MEDICARE CARRIER AND LOCALITY						
Carrier number	Locality number	Locality name	Work	Practice expense	Mal-practice	
510	5	Birmingham, AL	0.981	0.913	0.824	
510	4	Mobile, AL	0.964	0.911	0.824	
510	2	North Central AL	0.970	0.867	0.824	
510	1	Northwest AL	0.985	0.869	0.824	
510	6	Rest of AL	0.975	0.851	0.824	
510	3	Southeast AL	0.972	0.869	0.824	
1020	1	Alaska	1.106	1.255	1.042	
1030	5	Flagstaff (city), AZ	0.983	0.911	1.255	
1030	1	Phoenix, AZ	1.003	1.016	1.255	
1030	7	Prescott (city), AZ	0.983	0.911	1.255	
1030	99	Rest of Arizona	0.987	0.943	1.255	
1030	2	Tucson (city), AZ	0.987	0.989	1.255	
1030	8	Yuma (city), AZ	0.983	0.911	1.255	
520	13	Arkansas	0.960	0.856	0.302	
2050	26	Anaheim-Santa Ana, CA	1.046	1.220	1.370	
542	14	Bakersfield, CA	1.028	1.050	1.370	
542	11	Fresno/Madera, CA	1.006	1.009	1.370	
542	13	Kings/Tulare, CA	0.999	1.001	1.370	
2050	18	Los Angeles, CA (1st of 8)	1.060	1.196	1.370	
2050	19	Los Angeles, CA (2nd of 8)	1.060	1.196	1.370	

Figure 12–1

ADDENDUM B.— RELATIVE VALUE UNITS (RVUs) AND RELATED INFORMATION

HCPCS[1]	MOD	Sta-tus	Description	Work RVUs	Practice expense RVUs[2]	Mal-practice RVUs	Total	Global period	Up-date
47399	....	C	Liver surgery procedure	0.00	0.00	0.00	0.00	YYY	S
47400	....	A	Incision of liver duct	19.11	8.62	1.38	29.11	090	S
47420	....	A	Incision of bile duct	15.48	9.59	2.01	27.08	090	S
47425	....	A	Incision of bile duct	14.95	11.84	2.48	29.27	090	S
47440	....	A	Incision of bile duct	18.51	10.61	2.23	31.35	090	S
47460	....	A	Incision of bile duct sphincter................................	14.57	15.71	1.84	32.12	090	N
47480	....	A	Incision of gallbladder	8.14	7.68	1.61	17.43	090	S
47490	....	A	Incision of gallbladder	6.11	3.61	0.38	10.10	090	N
47500	....	A	Injection for liver x-rays	1.98	1.53	0.14	3.65	000	N
47505	....	A	Injection for liver x-rays	0.77	1.34	0.14	2.25	000	N
47510	....	A	Insert catheter, bile duct	7.47	2.90	0.25	10.62	090	N
47511	....	A	Insert bile duct drain	10.02	2.90	0.25	13.17	090	N
47525	....	A	Change bile duct catheter	5.47	1.61	0.16	7.24	010	N
47530	....	A	Revise, reinsert bile tube	5.47	1.53	0.19	7.19	090	N
47550	....	A	Bile duct endoscopy	3.05	1.58	0.35	4.98	000	S
47552	....	A	Biliary endoscopy, thru skin	6.11	1.38	0.21	7.70	000	S
47553	....	A	Biliary endoscopy, thru skin	6.42	3.84	0.63	10.89	000	N
47554	....	A	Biliary endoscopy, thru skin	9.16	3.97	0.68	13.81	000	S
47555	....	A	Biliary endoscopy, thru skin	7.64	2.66	0.30	10.60	000	N
47556	....	A	Biliary endoscopy, thru skin	8.66	2.66	0.30	11.62	000	N
47600	....	A	Removal of gallbladder	10.80	7.61	1.60	20.01	090	S
47605	....	A	Removal of gallbladder	11.66	8.23	1.77	21.66	090	S
47610	....	A	Removal of gallbladder	14.01	9.47	2.02	25.50	090	S
47612	....	A	Removal of gallbladder	14.91	14.39	3.08	32.38	090	S
47620	....	A	Removal of gallbladder	15.97	11.35	2.39	29.71	090	S
47630	....	A	Removal of bile duct stone	8.40	3.79	0.40	12.59	090	N
47700	....	A	Exploration of bile ducts	13.90	7.71	1.60	23.21	090	S
47701	....	A	Bile duct revision	26.87	8.30	1.92	37.09	090	S
47710	....	A	Excision of bile duct tumor	18.64	12.19	2.49	33.32	090	S
47715	....	A	Excision of bile duct cyst	14.66	8.31	1.73	24.70	090	S
47716	....	A	Fusion of bile duct cyst	12.67	6.63	1.55	20.85	090	S
47720	....	A	Fuse gallbladder and bowel	12.03	9.26	1.95	23.34	090	S
47721	....	A	Fuse upper gi structures	14.57	11.55	2.50	28.62	090	S
47740	....	A	Fuse gallbladder and bowel	14.08	10.32	2.16	26.56	090	S
47760	....	A	Fuse bile ducts and bowel	20.15	11.74	2.56	34.45	090	S
47765	....	A	Fuse liver ducts and bowel	19.25	14.77	3.00	37.02	090	S
47780	....	A	Fuse bile ducts and bowel	20.63	13.22	2.76	36.61	090	S
47800	....	A	Reconstruction of bile ducts	17.91	13.37	2.46	33.74	090	S
47801	....	A	Placement, bile duct support	11.41	5.54	0.82	17.77	090	S
47802	....	A	Fuse liver duct and intestine	16.19	10.38	1.77	28.34	090	S
47999	....	C	Bile tract surgery procedure	0.00	0.00	0.00	0.00	YYY	S
48000	....	A	Drainage of abdomen	13.25	7.13	1.42	21.80	090	S
48001	....	A	Placement of drain, pancreas	15.71	8.22	1.91	25.84	090	S
48005	....	A	Resect/debride pancreas	17.77	9.29	2.16	29.22	090	S
48020	....	A	Removal of pancreatic stone	13.12	6.86	1.59	21.57	090	S
48100	....	A	Biopsy of pancreas	10.30	4.26	0.80	15.36	090	S
48102	....	A	Needle biopsy, pancreas	4.48	2.44	0.25	7.17	010	N
48120	....	A	Removal of pancreas lesion	12.93	9.83	2.09	24.85	090	S
48140	....	A	Partial removal of pancreas	18.47	13.44	2.86	34.77	090	S
48145	....	A	Partial removal of pancreas	19.30	15.88	3.20	38.38	090	S
48146	....	A	Pancreatectomy	21.97	16.67	1.94	40.58	090	S
48148	....	A	Removal of pancrearic duct	14.57	8.32	1.70	24.59	090	S
48150	....	A	Partial removal of pancreas	34.55	22.79	4.80	62.14	090	S
48151	....	D	Partial removal of pancreas	0.00	0.00	0.00	0.00	090	0
48152	....	A	Pancreatectomy	31.33	22.79	4.80	58.92	090	S
48153	....	A	Pancreatectomy	34.55	22.79	4.80	62.14	090	S
48154	....	A	Pancreatectomy	31.33	22.79	4.80	58.92	090	S
48155	....	A	Removal of pancreas	19.65	20.63	4.31	44.59	090	S
48160	....	N	Pancreas removal, transplant	0.00	0.00	0.00	0.00	XXX	0
48180	....	A	Fuse pancreas and bowel	21.11	12.74	2.66	36.51	090	S
48400	....	A	Injection, intraoperative	1.97	1.04	0.24	3.25	ZZZ	S
48500	....	A	Surgery of pancreas cyst	12.17	8.62	1.68	22.47	090	S
48510	....	A	Drain pancreatic pseudocyst	11.34	7.62	1.46	20.42	090	S
48520	....	A	Fuse pancreas cyst and bowel................................	13.11	11.43	2.46	27.00	090	S
48540	....	A	Fuse pancreas cyst and bowel	15.95	12.80	2.68	31.43	090	S
48545	....	A	Pancreatorrhaphy	14.81	7.75	1.81	24.37	090	S
48547	....	A	Duodenal exclusion	21.42	11.20	2.61	35.23	090	S

[1] All numeric CPT HCPCS Copyright 1993 American Medical Association.
[2] *Indicates reduction of Practice Expense RVUs as a result of OBRA 1993.

Figure 12–2

ASSIGNMENT **12-3** ▸ **LOCATE HCPCS ALPHANUMERIC CODES**

Performance Objective

Task: Insert the correct HCPCS codes for problems presented.

Conditions: Use a pen or pencil, the CPT code book, and Appendix B in this *Workbook*.

Standards: Time: _____ minutes

                     Accuracy: _____

                     (Note: The time element and accuracy criteria may be given by your instructor.)

Directions: As you have learned from the Handbook, it is necessary to use three levels of codes (CPT, HCPCS, and regional codes) when submitting Medicare claims. Refer to Appendix B in this Workbook to complete this HCPCS coding exercise for Medicare claims.

1. Cellular therapy   _____

2. Injection amygdalin, laetrile, vitamin B_{17} _____

3. Lidocaine (Xylocaine) injection for local anesthetic   _____

4. Splint, wrist   _____

5. Crutches   _____

6. Cervical head harness   _____

7. 1 ml gamma globulin   _____

8. Injection, vitamin B_{12} _____

9. Contraceptives (unclassified drugs)   _____

10. Surgical tray   _____

11. Penicillin, procaine, aqueous, injection   _____

Now get some practice in selecting HCPCS modifiers. For this part of the assignment, in addition to referring to Appendix B in this Workbook, you will need to refer to your CPT code book or Appendix A in this Workbook to complete these Medicare problems.

12. Second surgical opinion by a professional review organization,
     detailed history and examination, low-complexity decision making _____

13. Chiropractic manipulation of spine, one region,
     acute treatment   _____

14. Office visit by a locum tenens physician of established
     patient, problem-focused history and examination
     with straightforward decision making   _____

15. Strapping of thumb of left hand   _____

ASSIGNMENT 12-4 ▸ LOCATE HCPCS PREVENTIVE CARE EXAMINATION CODES

> ### HCPCS Preventive Care Examination Codes
>
> **G0344** Initial preventive physical examination; face-to-face visit, services limited to new beneficiary during the first 6 months of Medicare Part B enrollment. Status indicator "V."
>
> **G0366** Electrocardiogram (ECG), routine ECG with at least 12 leads; performed as a component of the initial preventive physical examination with interpretation and report. Status indicator "B" (bundled into payment for another service that is not specified).
>
> **G0367** Electrocardiogram, tracing only, without interpretation and report, performed as a component of the initial preventive physical examination. Status indicator "S."
>
> **G0368** Electrocardiogram, interpretation and report only, performed as a component of the initial preventative physical examination. Status indicator "A" (paid under physician fee schedule).

Directions: Read the scenarios and refer to the HCPCS Preventive Care Examination codes to assist you in selecting the correct code.

1. Within 6 months after enrollment in Medicare Part B, Mary Sanchez is seen in Dr. Cardi's office for a physical examination and then he sends her over to the College Hospital for the ECG with interpretation.

   Hospital HCPCS Code _____

   Provider who interprets ECG HCPCS Code _____

   Physician's HCPCS Code _____

2. Dr. Donald Smith, a hospital-based clinic physician, does a physical examination and an ECG tracing with report and interpretation on David Bloch within 6 months of his enrollment in Medicare Part B.

   Hospital HCPCS Codes _____ and _____

   Physician's HCPCS Code _____

3. Dr. Gerald Practon performs both the physical examination and the ECG tracing with report and interpretation in his office on Anna Scofield within 6 months of her enrollment in Medicare Part B.

   Physician's HCPCS Codes _____ and _____

Insurance Claim Assignments

Assignments presented in this section are to give you hands-on experience in completing a variety of Medicare insurance cases by using the CMS-1500 claim form. Periodically, newsletters are issued by Medicare fiscal intermediaries relaying new federal policies and guidelines. This may change block requirements on the claim form, codes (procedural and diagnostic) that are covered in the Medicare program, or mean lower reimbursement or denial of reimbursement for a particular code number. Cases shown do not reflect payment policies for a particular procedure or service; this depends on federal guidelines and local medical review policies (LMRPs) at the time of claim submission.

The cases presented in this section are:

Assignment 12–5   Medicare

Assignment 12–6   Medicare/Medicaid (Medi-Medi)

Assignment 12–7   Medicare Secondary Payer (MSP) [advanced]

Assignment 12–8   Medicare/Medigap

Assignment 12–9   Medicare Railroad, Retiree with Advance Beneficiary Notice [advanced]

Assignment 12–10   Medicare/Medicaid (Medi-Medi)

Additional cases presented on the CD-ROM are:

Computer Case 8   Medicare

Computer Case 9   Medicare/Medigap

Computer Case 10   Medicare/Medicaid

ASSIGNMENT 12-5 ▸ COMPLETE A CLAIM FORM FOR A MEDICARE CASE

Performance Objective

Task: Complete a CMS-1500 claim form for a Medicare case, post transactions to the financial accounting record, and define patient record abbreviations.

Conditions: Use the patient's medical record (Figure 12–3) and financial statement (Figure 12–4), one health insurance claim form (Figure 12–5), a typewriter or computer, procedural and diagnostic code books, and Appendices A and B in this *Workbook*.

Standards: Claim Productivity Measurement

Time: _____ minutes

Accuracy: _____

(Note: The time element and accuracy criteria may be given by your instructor.)

Directions:

1. Complete the CMS-1500 claim form, using Office for Civil Rights (OCR) guidelines for a Medicare case, and direct it to your local fiscal intermediary by going to the Web site listed in Internet Resources at the end of Chapter 12 in the *Handbook*. Refer to Elsa M. Mooney's patient record for information. Refer to Appendix A in this *Workbook* to locate the fees to be recorded on the claim and posted to the financial statement. Date the claim December 21. Dr. Cardi is accepting assignment, and Mrs. Mooney has already met her deductible for the year owing to previous medical expenses with another physician.

2. Refer to Chapter 7 (Figure 7–9) of the *Handbook* for instructions on how to complete this claim form and a Medicare template.

3. Use your CPT code book or Appendix A in this *Workbook* to determine the correct five-digit code number and modifiers for each professional service rendered. Use your HCPCS Level II code book or refer to Appendix B in this *Workbook* for HCPCS procedure codes and modifiers.

4. Record all transactions on the financial accounting record and indicate when you have billed Medicare.

5. On January 12, Medicare sent check No. 115620 and paid 80% of the allowed amount for services rendered on December 15, 20xx. Post this amount to the patient's financial account and indicate the balance due from the patient.

6. A Performance Evaluation Checklist may be reproduced from the "Instruction Guide to the Workbook" chapter if your instructor wishes you to submit it to assist with scoring and comments.

   After the instructor has returned your work to you, either make the necessary corrections and place your work in a three-ring notebook for future reference or, if you received a high score, place it in your portfolio for reference when applying for a job.

Abbreviations pertinent to this record:

Pt   _____   LC   _____

N   _____   MDM   _____

EKG   _____   adv   _____

STAT   _____   rtn   _____

CPK   _____   ofc   _____

Dx   _____   echo   _____

ASCVD _____   RTO   _____

Additional Coding and Fee Calculations

1. Refer to Mrs. Mooney's medical record, abstract information, and code procedures that would be billed by outside providers.

Site	Description of Service	Code
a. College Hospital Laboratory	_____	_____
b. College Hospital Physiology	_____	_____
c. College Hospital Physiology	_____	_____
d. College Hospital Radiology	_____	_____

2. Refer to the Mock Fee Schedule shown in Appendix A in this *Workbook* and complete the following questions:

A. If Dr. Cardi is *not* participating in the Medicare program, what is the maximum (limiting charge) he can bill for the professional services rendered?

Office visit $ _____   ECG $ _____

B. In the case of a *nonparticipating* physician, how much will Medicare pay for these services?

Office visit $ _____   ECG $ _____

C. How much is the patient's responsibility for these services?

Office visit $ _____   ECG $ _____

D. How much will the courtesy adjustment be on the patient's financial record?

Office visit $ _____   ECG $ _____

3. Locate a financial accounting record (ledger).   _____

   Note: Refer to the step-by-step procedures at the end of Chapter 3 in
   the *Handbook* and graphic examples Figures 3–18, 10–2, and 12–15.   _____

4. Insert the patient's name and address, including ZIP code in the box.   _____

5. Enter the patient's personal data.   _____

6. Ledger lines: Insert date of service (DOS), reference (CPT code number, check
   number, or dates of service for posting adjustments or when insurance was billed),
   description of the transaction, charge amounts, payments, adjustments, and
   running current balance. The posting date is the actual date the transaction
   is recorded. If the DOS differs from the posting date, list the DOS in the
   reference or description column.

   Line 2:   _____

   Line 3:   _____

   Line 4:   _____

   Line 5:   _____

Note: A good bookkeeping practice is to take a red pen and draw a line across the financial accounting record
(ledger) from left to right to indicate the last entry billed to the insurance company.

PATIENT RECORD NO. 12-5

Mooney	Elsa	M.		02-06-30	F	555-452-4968
LAST NAME	FIRST NAME	MIDDLE NAME		BIRTH DATE	SEX	HOME PHONE

5750 Canyon Road	Woodland Hills	XY	12345
ADDRESS	CITY	STATE	ZIP CODE

555-806-3244			Mooney@wb.net
CELL PHONE	PAGER NO.	FAX NO.	E-MAIL ADDRESS

321-XX-2653	R9865549
PATIENT'S SOC. SEC. NO.	DRIVER'S LICENSE

retired secretary	
PATIENT'S OCCUPATION	NAME OF COMPANY

ADDRESS OF EMPLOYER	PHONE

husband deceased	
SPOUSE OR PARENT	OCCUPATION

EMPLOYER	ADDRESS	PHONE

Medicare	self
NAME OF INSURANCE	INSURED OR SUBSCRIBER

321-XX-2653A	
POLICY/CERTIFICATE NO.	GROUP NO.

REFERRED BY: George Gentle, MD, 1000 N. Main Street, Woodland Hills, XY 12345   NPI# 40213102XX

DATE	PROGRESS NOTES
12-15-xx	New pt referred by Dr. Gentle comes in complaining of chest pain and shortness of
	breath; a detailed history was taken. A detailed examination was essentially N. EKG done
	to rule out myocardial infarction; normal sinus rhythm, no abnormalities noted. Pt sent to
	College Hospital for STAT cardiac enzymes (CPK), 2D echocardiogram
	(transthoracic/real-time with Doppler), and complete chest x-ray.
	Working Dx: angina—ASCVD (LC MDM). Pt adv to rtn to ofc this afternoon for test results.
	PC/llf *Perry Cardi, MD*

Figure 12–3

STATEMENT
Financial Account
COLLEGE CLINIC
4567 Broad Avenue
Woodland Hills, XY 12345-0001
Tel. 555-486-9002
Fax No. 555-487-8976

Acct No. 12-5

Mrs. Elsa M. Mooney
5750 Canyon Road
Woodland Hills, XY 12345-0001

Phone No. (H)   (555) 452-4968   (W) _____   Birthdate ____ 02-06-30 ____

Primary Insurance Co. ____ Medicare _____   Policy/Group No. ____ 321-XX-2653A ____

| REFERENCE | DESCRIPTION | CHARGES | CREDITS | | BALANCE |
			PYMNTS.	ADJ.	
			BALANCE FORWARD ➞		
12-15-xx	Init OV, D hx/exam, LC decision making				
12-15-xx	EKG with interpret & report				

PLEASE PAY LAST AMOUNT IN BALANCE COLUMN ⬆

THIS IS A COPY OF YOUR FINANCIAL ACCOUNT AS IT APPEARS ON OUR RECORDS

Figure 12–4

PLEASE
DO NOT
STAPLE
IN THIS
AREA

CARRIER

HEALTH INSURANCE CLAIM FORM

| | PICA | | PICA | |

1. MEDICARE   MEDICAID   CHAMPUS   CHAMPVA   GROUP HEALTH PLAN (SSN or ID)   FECA BLK LUNG (S SN)   OTHER
☐ (Medicare #) ☐ (Medicaid #) ☐ (Sponsor's SSN) ☐ (VA File #) ☐ (SSN or ID) ☐ (S SN) ☐ (ID)

1a. INSURED'S I.D. NUMBER   (FOR PROGRAM IN ITEM 1)

2. PATIENT'S NAME (Last Name, First Name, Middle Initial)

3. PATIENT'S BIRTH DATE   MM DD YY   SEX   M ☐   F ☐

4. INSURED'S NAME (Last Name, First Name, Middle Initial)

5. PATIENT'S ADDRESS (No., Street)

6. PATIENT RELATIONSHIP TO INSURED
Self ☐   Spouse ☐   Child ☐   Other ☐

7. INSURED'S ADDRESS (No., Street)

CITY   STATE

8. PATIENT STATUS
Single ☐   Married ☐   Other ☐
Employed ☐   Full-Time Student ☐   Part-Time Student ☐

CITY   STATE

ZIP CODE   TELEPHONE (Include Area Code)   (   )

ZIP CODE   TELEPHONE (INCLUDE AREA CODE)

9. OTHER INSURED'S NAME (Last Name, First Name, Middle Initial)

10. IS PATIENT'S CONDITION RELATED TO:

11. INSURED'S POLICY GROUP OR FECA NUMBER

a. OTHER INSURED'S POLICY OR GROUP NUMBER

a. EMPLOYMENT? (CURRENT OR PREVIOUS)
☐ YES   ☐ NO

a. INSURED'S DATE OF BIRTH   MM DD YY   SEX   M ☐   F ☐

b. OTHER INSURED'S DATE OF BIRTH   MM DD YY   SEX   M ☐   F ☐

b. AUTO ACCIDENT?   PLACE (State)
☐ YES   ☐ NO

b. EMPLOYER'S NAME OR SCHOOL NAME

c. EMPLOYER'S NAME OR SCHOOL NAME

c. OTHER ACCIDENT?
☐ YES   ☐ NO

c. INSURANCE PLAN NAME OR PROGRAM NAME

d. INSURANCE PLAN NAME OR PROGRAM NAME

10d. RESERVED FOR LOCAL USE

d. IS THERE ANOTHER HEALTH BENEFIT PLAN?
☐ YES   ☐ NO   **If yes,** return to and complete item 9 a-d.

READ BACK OF FORM BEFORE COMPLETING & SIGNING THIS FORM.
12. PATIENT'S OR AUTHORIZED PERSON'S SIGNATURE I authorize the release of any medical or other information necessary to process this claim. I also request payment of government benefits either to myself or to the party who accepts assignment below.

SIGNED _____   DATE _____

13. INSURED'S OR AUTHORIZED PERSON'S SIGNATURE I authorize payment of medical benefits to the undersigned physician or supplier for services described below.

SIGNED _____

14. DATE OF CURRENT: MM DD YY   ◄ ILLNESS (First symptom) OR INJURY (Accident) OR PREGNANCY(LMP)

15. IF PATIENT HAS HAD SAME OR SIMILAR ILLNESS. GIVE FIRST DATE   MM DD YY

16. DATES PATIENT UNABLE TO WORK IN CURRENT OCCUPATION   FROM MM DD YY   TO MM DD YY

17. NAME OF REFERRING PHYSICIAN OR OTHER SOURCE

17a. I.D. NUMBER OF REFERRING PHYSICIAN

18. HOSPITALIZATION DATES RELATED TO CURRENT SERVICES   FROM MM DD YY   TO MM DD YY

19. RESERVED FOR LOCAL USE

20. OUTSIDE LAB? $ CHARGES
☐ YES   ☐ NO

21. DIAGNOSIS OR NATURE OF ILLNESS OR INJURY. (RELATE ITEMS 1,2,3 OR 4 TO ITEM 24E BY LINE)
1. |____|____   3. |____|____
2. |____|____   4. |____|____

22. MEDICAID RESUBMISSION CODE   ORIGINAL REF. NO.

23. PRIOR AUTHORIZATION NUMBER

24. A DATE(S) OF SERVICE						B Place of Service	C Type of Service	D PROCEDURES, SERVICES, OR SUPPLIES (Explain Unusual Circumstances) CPT/HCPCS	MODIFIER	E DIAGNOSIS CODE	F $ CHARGES	G DAYS OR UNITS	H EPSDT Family Plan	I EMG	J COB	K RESERVED FOR LOCAL USE
From MM	DD	YY	To MM	DD	YY											
1																
2																
3																
4																
5																
6																

25. FEDERAL TAX I.D. NUMBER   SSN ☐ EIN ☐

26. PATIENT'S ACCOUNT NO.

27. ACCEPT ASSIGNMENT? (For govt. claims, see back)   ☐ YES   ☐ NO

28. TOTAL CHARGE $

29. AMOUNT PAID $

30. BALANCE DUE $

31. SIGNATURE OF PHYSICIAN OR SUPPLIER INCLUDING DEGREES OR CREDENTIALS (I certify that the statements on the reverse apply to this bill and are made a part thereof.)

SIGNED _____   DATE _____

32. NAME AND ADDRESS OF FACILITY WHERE SERVICES WERE RENDERED (If other than home or office)

33. PHYSICIAN'S, SUPPLIER'S BILLING NAME, ADDRESS, ZIP CODE & PHONE #

PIN#   GRP#

(APPROVED BY AMA COUNCIL ON MEDICAL SERVICE 8/88)   **PLEASE PRINT OR TYPE**   APPROVED OMB-0938-0008 FORM CMS-1500 (12-90),   FORM RRB-1500, APPROVED OMB-1215-0055 FORM OWCP-1500,   APPROVED OMB-0720-0001 (CHAMPUS)

Figure 12-5

ASSIGNMENT **12-6** ▸ **COMPLETE A CLAIM FORM FOR A MEDICARE/MEDICAID CASE**

Performance Objective

Task: Complete a CMS-1500 claim form for a Medicare/Medicaid case, post transactions to the financial accounting record, and define patient record abbreviations.

Conditions: Use the patient's medical record (Figure 12–6) and financial statement (Figure 12–7), one health insurance claim form (Figure 12–8), a typewriter or computer, procedural and diagnostic code books, and Appendices A and B in this *Workbook*.

Standards: Claim Productivity Measurement

                  Time: _____ minutes

                  Accuracy: _____

                  (Note: The time element and accuracy criteria may be given by your instructor.)

Directions:

1. Complete the CMS-1500 claim form, using OCR guidelines for a Medicare/Medicaid case, and direct it to your local Medicare fiscal intermediary by going to the Web site listed in Internet Resources at the end of Chapter 12 in the *Handbook* (see Appendix A in the text) and on to Medicaid. Refer to Mrs. Helen P. Nolan's patient record for information. Refer to Appendix A in this *Workbook* to locate the fees to be recorded on the claim and posted to the financial statement. Date the claim May 31.
2. Refer to Chapter 7 and Figure 7–10 of the *Handbook* for instructions on how to complete the CMS-1500 claim form.
3. Use your CPT code book or Appendix A in this *Workbook* to determine the correct five-digit code number and modifiers for each professional service rendered. Use your HCPCS Level II code book or refer to Appendix B in this *Workbook* for HCPCS procedure codes and modifiers.
4. Record all transactions on the financial record and indicate the proper information when you have billed Medicare/Medicaid. On July 1, you receive a check (number 107621) from Medicare for $600, and on July 15 you receive a voucher (number 3571) from Medicaid for $200. Record these payments on the account, and show a courtesy adjustment to zero the account.
5. A Performance Evaluation Checklist may be reproduced from the "Instruction Guide to the Workbook" chapter if your instructor wishes you to submit it to assist with scoring and comments.

After the instructor has returned your work to you, either make the necessary corrections and place your work in a three-ring notebook for future reference or, if you received a high score, place it in your portfolio for reference when applying for a job.

Abbreviations pertinent to this record:

Pt	_____	phys	_____
hx	_____	prep	_____
BP	_____	hosp	_____
ext	_____	EPF	_____
Dx	_____	exam	_____

int _____   MC _____

adv _____   MDM _____

pre-op _____   slt _____

adm _____   PF _____

UA _____   SF _____

auto _____   RTO _____

FBS _____   wk _____

micro _____   OV _____

CXR _____   p.r.n. _____

Additional Coding and Fee Calculations

1. Refer to Mrs. Nolan's medical record, abstract information, and code procedures that would be billed by outside providers.

Site	Description of Service	Code
a. College Hospital Laboratory	_____	_____
b. College Hospital Laboratory	_____	_____
c. College Hospital Laboratory	_____	_____
d. College Hospital Radiology	_____	_____

2. Calculate Dr. Cutler's assistant surgeon fee, which is 18.5% of the primary surgeon's fee:

   Hemorrhoidectomy with fistulectomy: $ _____

Checklist

3. Locate a financial accounting record (ledger).   _____

   Note: Refer to the step-by-step procedures at the end of Chapter 3 in the *Handbook* and graphic examples Figures 3–18, 10–2, and 12–15.

4. Insert the patient's name and address, including ZIP code in the box.   _____

5. Enter the patient's personal data.   _____

6. Ledger lines: Insert date of service (DOS), reference (CPT code number, check number, or dates of service for posting adjustments or when insurance was billed), description of the transaction, charge amounts, payments, adjustments, and running current balance. The posting date is the actual date the transaction is recorded. If the DOS differs from the posting date, list the DOS in the reference or description column.

Line 2: _____

Line 3: _____

Line 4: _____

Line 5: _____

Line 6: _____

Line 7: _____

Line 8: _____

Line 9: _____

Line 10: _____

Line 11: _____

Line 12: _____

Note: A good bookkeeping practice is to take a red pen and draw a line across the financial accounting record (ledger) from left to right to indicate the last entry billed to the insurance company.

PATIENT RECORD NO. 12-6

Nolan	Helen	P.	05-10-37	F	555-660-9878
LAST NAME	FIRST NAME	MIDDLE NAME	BIRTH DATE	SEX	HOME PHONE

2588 Cedar Street	Woodland Hills	XY	12345
ADDRESS	CITY	STATE	ZIP CODE

		555-660-9878	Nolan@wb.net
CELL PHONE	PAGER NO.	FAX NO.	E-MAIL ADDRESS

732-XX-1573	J4022876
PATIENT'S SOC. SEC. NO.	DRIVER'S LICENSE

homemaker	
PATIENT'S OCCUPATION	NAME OF COMPANY

ADDRESS OF EMPLOYER	PHONE

James J. Nolan	retired journalist
SPOUSE OR PARENT	OCCUPATION

EMPLOYER	ADDRESS	PHONE

Medicare/Medicaid	husband
NAME OF INSURANCE	INSURED OR SUBSCRIBER

732-XX-1573B	19-60-2358490-1-XX
MEDICARE NO.	MEDICAID NO.

REFERRED BY: James B. Jeffers, MD, 100 S. Broadway, Woodland Hills, XY 12345   NPI# 12345069XX

DATE	PROGRESS NOTES
5-1-xx	New pt comes in complaining of constipation, rectal bleeding, and rectal pain. Detailed
	hx taken, BP 120/80. A detailed exam revealed ext hemorrhoids. Diagnostic proctoscopy
	done to further evaluate the hemorrhoids and control bleeding using bipolar cautery.
	Dx: int & ext bleeding hemorrhoids and anorectal fistula. Adv hospitalization for removal
	of hemorrhoids and fistula repair.
	RR/llf *Rex Rumsey, MD*
5-8-xx	Pre-op testing done prior to adm to College Hospital (UA auto/with micro., hemogram
	auto, FBS quantitative, CXR single frontal view). Admit, phys exam & prep of hospital
	records. Hemorrhoidectomy with fistulectomy performed (authorization no. 7699220012).
	Dr. Clarence Cutler assisted.
	RR/llf *Rex Rumsey, MD*
5-9-xx	Hosp visit (EPF hx/exam MC MDM). Pt comfortable, slt pain.
	RR/llf *Rex Rumsey, MD*
5-10-xx	Hosp visit (PF hx/exam SF MDM). No pain.
	RR/llf *Rex Rumsey, MD*
5-11-xx	Discharged pt to home. RTO in 1 wk.
	RR/llf *Rex Rumsey, MD*
5-17-xx	OV (PF hx/exam SF MDM). Pt doing well, surgical site healed. Return p.r.n.
	RR/llf *Rex Rumsey, MD*

Figure 12–6

STATEMENT
Financial Account
COLLEGE CLINIC
4567 Broad Avenue
Woodland Hills, XY 12345-0001
Tel. 555-486-9002
Fax No. 555-487-8976

Acct. No. __12-6__

Helen P. Nolan
2588 Cedar Street
Woodland Hills, XY 12345

Phone No. (H) ___(555) 660-9878___ (W) _____   Birthdate ____05-10-37____

Primary Insurance Co. ___Medicare/Medicaid_____   Policy/Group No. _732-XX-1573B___

	REFERENCE	DESCRIPTION	CHARGES	CREDITS PYMNTS.	ADJ.	BALANCE	
20XX			BALANCE FORWARD ➙				
05-01-xx		NP OV					
05-01-xx		Proctoscopy					
05-08-xx		Hemorrhoidectomy with fistulectomy					
05-09-xx		HV					
05-10-xx		HV					
05-11-xx		Discharge					
05-17-xx		OV					

PLEASE PAY LAST AMOUNT IN BALANCE COLUMN ⬆

THIS IS A COPY OF YOUR FINANCIAL ACCOUNT AS IT APPEARS ON OUR RECORDS

Figure 12–7

PLEASE
DO NOT
STAPLE
IN THIS
AREA

HEALTH INSURANCE CLAIM FORM

PICA | | | PICA

1. MEDICARE   MEDICAID   CHAMPUS   CHAMPVA   GROUP HEALTH PLAN (SSN or ID)   FECA BLK LUNG (S SN)   OTHER | 1a. INSURED'S I.D. NUMBER   (FOR PROGRAM IN ITEM 1)

☐ (Medicare #) ☐ (Medicaid #) ☐ (Sponsor's SSN) ☐ (VA File #) ☐   ☐   ☐ (ID)

2. PATIENT'S NAME (Last Name, First Name, Middle Initial) | 3. PATIENT'S BIRTH DATE MM DD YY   SEX M☐ F☐ | 4. INSURED'S NAME (Last Name, First Name, Middle Initial)

5. PATIENT'S ADDRESS (No., Street) | 6. PATIENT RELATIONSHIP TO INSURED Self☐ Spouse☐ Child☐ Other☐ | 7. INSURED'S ADDRESS (No., Street)

CITY   STATE | 8. PATIENT STATUS Single☐ Married☐ Other☐ | CITY   STATE

ZIP CODE   TELEPHONE (Include Area Code) ( ) | Employed☐ Full-Time Student☐ Part-Time Student☐ | ZIP CODE   TELEPHONE (INCLUDE AREA CODE)

9. OTHER INSURED'S NAME (Last Name, First Name, Middle Initial) | 10. IS PATIENT'S CONDITION RELATED TO: | 11. INSURED'S POLICY GROUP OR FECA NUMBER

a. OTHER INSURED'S POLICY OR GROUP NUMBER | a. EMPLOYMENT? (CURRENT OR PREVIOUS) ☐ YES ☐ NO | a. INSURED'S DATE OF BIRTH MM DD YY SEX M☐ F☐

b. OTHER INSURED'S DATE OF BIRTH MM DD YY SEX M☐ F☐ | b. AUTO ACCIDENT? PLACE (State) ☐ YES ☐ NO | b. EMPLOYER'S NAME OR SCHOOL NAME

c. EMPLOYER'S NAME OR SCHOOL NAME | c. OTHER ACCIDENT? ☐ YES ☐ NO | c. INSURANCE PLAN NAME OR PROGRAM NAME

d. INSURANCE PLAN NAME OR PROGRAM NAME | 10d. RESERVED FOR LOCAL USE | d. IS THERE ANOTHER HEALTH BENEFIT PLAN? ☐ YES ☐ NO If yes, return to and complete item 9 a-d.

READ BACK OF FORM BEFORE COMPLETING & SIGNING THIS FORM.
12. PATIENT'S OR AUTHORIZED PERSON'S SIGNATURE I authorize the release of any medical or other information necessary to process this claim. I also request payment of government benefits either to myself or to the party who accepts assignment below.
SIGNED_____ DATE_____ | 13. INSURED'S OR AUTHORIZED PERSON'S SIGNATURE I authorize payment of medical benefits to the undersigned physician or supplier for services described below.
SIGNED_____

14. DATE OF CURRENT: MM DD YY ◀ ILLNESS (First symptom) OR INJURY (Accident) OR PREGNANCY(LMP) | 15. IF PATIENT HAS HAD SAME OR SIMILAR ILLNESS. GIVE FIRST DATE MM DD YY | 16. DATES PATIENT UNABLE TO WORK IN CURRENT OCCUPATION MM DD YY FROM TO MM DD YY

17. NAME OF REFERRING PHYSICIAN OR OTHER SOURCE | 17a. I.D. NUMBER OF REFERRING PHYSICIAN | 18. HOSPITALIZATION DATES RELATED TO CURRENT SERVICES MM DD YY FROM TO MM DD YY

19. RESERVED FOR LOCAL USE | | 20. OUTSIDE LAB? $ CHARGES ☐ YES ☐ NO

21. DIAGNOSIS OR NATURE OF ILLNESS OR INJURY. (RELATE ITEMS 1,2,3 OR 4 TO ITEM 24E BY LINE) | 22. MEDICAID RESUBMISSION CODE ORIGINAL REF. NO.
1._____ 3._____ | 23. PRIOR AUTHORIZATION NUMBER
2._____ 4._____ |

24. | A DATE(S) OF SERVICE From MM DD YY To MM DD YY | B Place of Service | C Type of Service | D PROCEDURES, SERVICES, OR SUPPLIES (Explain Unusual Circumstances) CPT/HCPCS MODIFIER | E DIAGNOSIS CODE | F $ CHARGES | G DAYS OR UNITS | H EPSDT Family Plan | I EMG | J COB | K RESERVED FOR LOCAL USE
1 | | | | | | | | | | |
2 | | | | | | | | | | |
3 | | | | | | | | | | |
4 | | | | | | | | | | |
5 | | | | | | | | | | |
6 | | | | | | | | | | |

25. FEDERAL TAX I.D. NUMBER SSN☐ EIN☐ | 26. PATIENT'S ACCOUNT NO. | 27. ACCEPT ASSIGNMENT? (For govt. claims, see back) ☐ YES ☐ NO | 28. TOTAL CHARGE $ | 29. AMOUNT PAID $ | 30. BALANCE DUE $

31. SIGNATURE OF PHYSICIAN OR SUPPLIER INCLUDING DEGREES OR CREDENTIALS (I certify that the statements on the reverse apply to this bill and are made a part thereof.)
SIGNED_____ DATE_____ | 32. NAME AND ADDRESS OF FACILITY WHERE SERVICES WERE RENDERED (If other than home or office) | 33. PHYSICIAN'S, SUPPLIER'S BILLING NAME, ADDRESS, ZIP CODE & PHONE #
PIN#   GRP#

(APPROVED BY AMA COUNCIL ON MEDICAL SERVICE 8/88) **PLEASE PRINT OR TYPE** APPROVED OMB-0938-0008 FORM CMS-1500 (12-90), FORM RRB-1500, APPROVED OMB-1215-0055 FORM OWCP-1500, APPROVED OMB-0720-0001 (CHAMPUS)

CARRIER | PATIENT AND INSURED INFORMATION | PHYSICIAN OR SUPPLIER INFORMATION

Figure 12–8

ASSIGNMENT 12–7 ▸ COMPLETE A CLAIM FORM FOR A MEDICARE/SECONDARY PAYER CASE

Performance Objective

Task: Complete a CMS-1500 claim form, for a MSP case, post transactions to the financial accounting record, and define patient record abbreviations.

Conditions: Use the patient's medical record (Figure 12–9) and financial statement (Figure 12–10), one health insurance claim form (Figure 12–11), a typewriter or computer, procedural and diagnostic code books, and Appendices A and B in this *Workbook*.

Standards: Claim Productivity Measurement

Time: _____ minutes

Accuracy: _____

(Note: The time element and accuracy criteria may be given by your instructor.)

Directions:

1. Complete the CMS-1500 Form, using OCR guidelines for an MSP case, and direct it to the primary insurance carrier. This assignment requires two claim forms, so make a photocopy of the CMS-1500 claim form for the second claim. Refer to Peter F. Donlon's patient record for information. Refer to Appendix A in this *Workbook* to locate the fees to be recorded on the claim and posted to the financial statement. Date the claim May 14. Dr. Antrum is not accepting assignment in this case. For a nonparticipating physician, use the limiting charge column of the mock fee schedule.
2. See Chapter 7 (Figure 7–12) of the *Handbook* for help in completing these forms.
3. Use your CPT code book or Appendix A in this *Workbook* to determine the correct five-digit code number and modifiers for each professional service rendered. Refer to your HCPCS Level II code book or Appendix B in this *Workbook* for HCPCS procedure codes and modifiers.
4. Record all transactions on the financial record and indicate when you have billed the primary insurance carrier.
5. On June 5, Coastal Health Insurance Company paid $800 (check number 45632) on this claim. Post this payment to the patient's financial account and indicate the balance that will be billed to Medicare the following day. Note: The explanation of benefits from Coastal Health would be sent to Medicare with a completed CMS-1500 claim form.
6. A Performance Evaluation Checklist may be reproduced from the "Instruction Guide to the Workbook" chapter if your instructor wishes you to submit it to assist with scoring and comments.

After the instructor has returned your work to you, either make the necessary corrections and place your work in a three-ring notebook for future reference or, if you received a high score, place it in your portfolio for reference when applying for a job.

Abbreviations pertinent to this record:

ER	_____	&	_____
p.m.	_____	adm	_____
EPF	_____	MC	_____
hx	_____	imp	_____
exam	_____	PF	_____
LC	_____	SF	_____
MDM	_____	hosp	_____
est	_____	RTO	_____
pts	_____	OV	_____
cm	_____	surg	_____
consult	_____	sched	_____
c̄	_____	ofc	_____
D	_____	post-op	_____
C	_____	wk	_____
M	_____		
MRI	_____		
px	_____		

Additional Coding and Fee Calculations

1. Refer to Mr. Donlon's medical record, abstract information, and code procedures that would be billed by outside providers.

Site	Description of Service	Code
a. Emergency room (ER) physician	_____	_____
b. ER consult	_____	_____
c. College Hospital Radiology	_____	_____
d. College Hospital Radiology	_____	_____

2. Use your diagnostic code book and code the symptoms that the patient presented with in the ER

        Symptom   *Code*

a. _____   _____

b. _____   _____

c. _____   _____

3. On the septoplasty surgery (May 10, 20xx), assume that Coastal Health Insurance Company paid $459.74.

  a. What would the Medicare payment be? _____

  b. What would the patient responsibility be? _____

  c. What would the courtesy adjustment be? _____

                                                 Checklist

4. Locate a financial accounting record (ledger).   _____

  Note: Refer to the step-by-step procedures at the end of Chapter 3 in the *Handbook* and graphic examples Figures 3–18, 10–2, and 12–15.

5. Insert the patient's name and address, including ZIP code in the box.   _____

6. Enter the patient's personal data.   _____

7. Ledger lines: Insert date of service (DOS), reference (CPT code number, check number, or dates of service for posting adjustments or when insurance was billed), description of the transaction, charge amounts, payments, adjustments, and running current balance. The posting date is the actual date the transaction is recorded. If the DOS differs from the posting date, list the DOS in the reference or description column.

Line 2:   _____

Line 3:   _____

Line 4:   _____

Line 5:   _____

Line 6:   _____

Line 7:   _____

Line 8:   _____

Line 9:   _____

Line 10:   _____

Line 11:   _____

Line 12:   _____

Line 13:   _____

Note: A good bookkeeping practice is to take a red pen and draw a line across the financial accounting record (ledger) from left to right to indicate the last entry billed to the insurance company.

PATIENT RECORD NO. 12-7

Donlon	Peter	F	08-09-38	M	555-762-3580
LAST NAME	FIRST NAME	MIDDLE NAME	BIRTH DATE	SEX	HOME PHONE

1840 East Chevy Chase Drive	Woodland Hills	XY	12345
ADDRESS	CITY	STATE	ZIP CODE

CELL PHONE	PAGER NO.	FAX NO.	E-MAIL ADDRESS

987-XX-4321	Y2100968
PATIENT'S SOC. SEC. NO.	DRIVER'S LICENSE

chef	Harbor Town Eatery
PATIENT'S OCCUPATION	NAME OF COMPANY

1116 Harbor Way, Woodland Hills, XY 12345	555-762-0050
ADDRESS OF EMPLOYER	PHONE

wife deceased	
SPOUSE OR PARENT	OCCUPATION

Coastal Health Insurance Co., 10 N. Main Street, Woodland Hills, XY 12345	555-369-4401
NAME OF PRIMARY INSURANCE	ADDRESS	PHONE

NAME OF INSURANCE	INSURED OR SUBSCRIBER

34276	45A
POLICY/CERTIFICATE NO.	GROUP NO.

Medicare	987-XX-4321A
NAME OF SECONDARY INSURANCE	MEDICARE NO.

REFERRED BY:

DATE	PROGRESS NOTES
5-1-xx	Called to ER on Sunday, 11 p.m. ER physician, Dr. Rene Whitney (NPI # 77 536222XX) performed an EPF hx/exam with LC MDM on one of my est pts who was injured at home while walking across lawn pushing garbage can; tripped and hit his head on curb. Pt complains of acute headache, nausea, and nasal pain caused by impact and skin laceration. Sutured a 2.0 cm simple laceration of nose. Pt vomited twice in ER. Requested ER consult c̄ neurologist, Dr. Parkinson (C hx/exam M MDM), who ordered MRI of brain (without contrast) and complete skull series. I performed a C hx and px & adm pt to College Hospital; MDM MC. Imp: Concussion without skull fracture, no loss of consciousness; nasal laceration; deviated septum which may need reconstruction. CA/llf *Concha Antrum, MD*
5-2-xx	Hospital visit (PF hx/exam LC MDM). CA/llf *Concha Antrum, MD*
5-3-xx	Hospital visit (PF hx/exam SF MDM). CA/llf *Concha Antrum, MD*
5-4-xx	Discharge from hospital. See hosp records for daily notes. RTO in 2 day for suture removal. CA/llf *Concha Antrum, MD*
5-6-xx	OV. Sutures removed; wound healed. Discussed deviated septum and recommended septoplasty. Surg sched for 5/10/xx at College Hospital. CA/llf *Concha Antrum, MD*
5-10-xx	Adm to College Hospital (D hx/exam LC MDM). Performed septoplasty. Pt doing well; moved to recovery room. CA/llf *Concha Antrum, MD*
5-11-xx	Pt doing well, no hemorrhage, discharged home. CA/llf *Concha Antrum, MD*
5-12-xx	Pt comes into ofc with postop anterior nasal hemorrhage. Cauterized rt side. RTO in 1 wk. CA/llf *Concha Antrum, MD*

Figure 12–9

STATEMENT
Financial Account
COLLEGE CLINIC
4567 Broad Avenue
Woodland Hills, XY 12345-0001
Tel. 555-486-9002
Fax No. 555-487-8976

Acct. No. 12-7

Peter F. Donlon
1840 East Chevy Chase Drive
Woodland Hills, XY 12345

Phone No. (H)   (555) 762-3580   (W)   (555)762-0050   Birthdate   08-09-38

Insurance Co.   Coastal Health Insurance Co./Medicare   Policy/Group No.   34276 Grp. 45A
                                                                Medicare No.   987-XX-4321A

| | REFERENCE | DESCRIPTION | CHARGES | CREDITS | | BALANCE |
				PYMNTS.	ADJ.	
20XX			BALANCE FORWARD ⟶			
05-01-xx		Initial hospital care				
05-01-xx		Skin repair				
05-02-xx		HV				
05-03-xx		HV				
05-04-xx		Discharge				
05-06-xx		Suture removal				
05-10-xx		Admit-Septoplasty				
05-11-xx		Discharge				
05-12-xx		Postop OV				

PLEASE PAY LAST AMOUNT IN BALANCE COLUMN

THIS IS A COPY OF YOUR FINANCIAL ACCOUNT AS IT APPEARS ON OUR RECORDS

Figure 12–10

CARRIER

| | | PICA | **HEALTH INSURANCE CLAIM FORM** | | PICA | | |

| PICA | | | | | | HEALTH INSURANCE CLAIM FORM | | | PICA | | |

1. MEDICARE   MEDICAID   CHAMPUS   CHAMPVA   GROUP HEALTH PLAN (SSN or ID)   FECA BLK LUNG (SSN)   OTHER

☐ (Medicare #) ☐ (Medicaid #) ☐ (Sponsor's SSN) ☐ (VA File #) ☐   ☐   ☐ (ID)

1a. INSURED'S I.D. NUMBER   (FOR PROGRAM IN ITEM 1)

2. PATIENT'S NAME (Last Name, First Name, Middle Initial)

3. PATIENT'S BIRTH DATE
MM   DD   YY   SEX
M ☐   F ☐

4. INSURED'S NAME (Last Name, First Name, Middle Initial)

5. PATIENT'S ADDRESS (No., Street)

6. PATIENT RELATIONSHIP TO INSURED
Self ☐   Spouse ☐   Child ☐   Other ☐

7. INSURED'S ADDRESS (No., Street)

CITY   STATE

8. PATIENT STATUS
Single ☐   Married ☐   Other ☐
Employed ☐   Full-Time Student ☐   Part-Time Student ☐

CITY   STATE

ZIP CODE   TELEPHONE (Include Area Code)
)

ZIP CODE   TELEPHONE (INCLUDE AREA CODE)

9. OTHER INSURED'S NAME (Last Name, First Name, Middle Initial)

10. IS PATIENT'S CONDITION RELATED TO:

11. INSURED'S POLICY GROUP OR FECA NUMBER

a. OTHER INSURED'S POLICY OR GROUP NUMBER

a. EMPLOYMENT? (CURRENT OR PREVIOUS)
☐ YES   ☐ NO

a. INSURED'S DATE OF BIRTH
MM   DD   YY   SEX
M ☐   F ☐

b. OTHER INSURED'S DATE OF BIRTH
MM   DD   YY   SEX
M ☐   F ☐

b. AUTO ACCIDENT?   PLACE (State)
☐ YES   ☐ NO

b. EMPLOYER'S NAME OR SCHOOL NAME

c. EMPLOYER'S NAME OR SCHOOL NAME

c. OTHER ACCIDENT?
☐ YES   ☐ NO

c. INSURANCE PLAN NAME OR PROGRAM NAME

d. INSURANCE PLAN NAME OR PROGRAM NAME

10d. RESERVED FOR LOCAL USE

d. IS THERE ANOTHER HEALTH BENEFIT PLAN?
☐ YES   ☐ NO   *If yes*, return to and complete item 9 a-d.

READ BACK OF FORM BEFORE COMPLETING & SIGNING THIS FORM.
12. PATIENT'S OR AUTHORIZED PERSON'S SIGNATURE I authorize the release of any medical or other information necessary to process this claim. I also request payment of government benefits either to myself or to the party who accepts assignment below.

SIGNED _____   DATE _____

13. INSURED'S OR AUTHORIZED PERSON'S SIGNATURE I authorize payment of medical benefits to the undersigned physician or supplier for services described below.

SIGNED _____

PATIENT AND INSURED INFORMATION

14. DATE OF CURRENT: ILLNESS (First symptom) OR INJURY (Accident) OR PREGNANCY(LMP)
MM   DD   YY

15. IF PATIENT HAS HAD SAME OR SIMILAR ILLNESS. GIVE FIRST DATE   MM   DD   YY

16. DATES PATIENT UNABLE TO WORK IN CURRENT OCCUPATION
MM   DD   YY   MM   DD   YY
FROM   TO

17. NAME OF REFERRING PHYSICIAN OR OTHER SOURCE

17a. I.D. NUMBER OF REFERRING PHYSICIAN

18. HOSPITALIZATION DATES RELATED TO CURRENT SERVICES
MM   DD   YY   MM   DD   YY
FROM   TO

19. RESERVED FOR LOCAL USE

20. OUTSIDE LAB? $ CHARGES
☐ YES   ☐ NO

21. DIAGNOSIS OR NATURE OF ILLNESS OR INJURY. (RELATE ITEMS 1,2,3 OR 4 TO ITEM 24E BY LINE)

1. _____   3. _____
2. _____   4. _____

22. MEDICAID RESUBMISSION CODE   ORIGINAL REF. NO.

23. PRIOR AUTHORIZATION NUMBER

EXAMPLE ONLY

24. A						B	C	D		E	F	G	H	I	J	K
DATE(S) OF SERVICE						Place of Service	Type of Service	PROCEDURES, SERVICES, OR SUPPLIES (Explain Unusual Circumstances)		DIAGNOSIS CODE	$ CHARGES	DAYS OR UNITS	EPSDT Family Plan	EMG	COB	RESERVED FOR LOCAL USE
From			To					CPT/HCPCS	MODIFIER							
MM	DD	YY	MM	DD	YY											
1																
2																
3																
4																
5																
6																

25. FEDERAL TAX I.D. NUMBER   SSN EIN ☐

26. PATIENT'S ACCOUNT NO.

27. ACCEPT ASSIGNMENT? (For govt. claims, see back)
☐ YES   ☐ NO

28. TOTAL CHARGE
$

29. AMOUNT PAID
$

30. BALANCE DUE
$

31. SIGNATURE OF PHYSICIAN OR SUPPLIER INCLUDING DEGREES OR CREDENTIALS (I certify that the statements on the reverse apply to this bill and are made a part thereof.)

SIGNED _____   DATE _____

32. NAME AND ADDRESS OF FACILITY WHERE SERVICES WERE RENDERED (If other than home or office)

33. PHYSICIAN'S, SUPPLIER'S BILLING NAME, ADDRESS, ZIP CODE & PHONE #

PIN#   GRP#

PHYSICIAN OR SUPPLIER INFORMATION

(APPROVED BY AMA COUNCIL ON MEDICAL SERVICE 8/88)   **PLEASE PRINT OR TYPE**   APPROVED OMB-0938-0008 FORM CMS-1500 (12-90), FORM RRB-1500,
APPROVED OMB-1215-0055 FORM OWCP-1500,   APPROVED OMB-0720-0001 (CHAMPUS)

PLEASE DO NOT STAPLE IN THIS AREA

Figure 12–11

ASSIGNMENT 12–8 ▸ COMPLETE A CLAIM FOR A MEDICARE/ MEDIGAP CASE

Performance Objective

Task: Complete a CMS-1500 claim form for a Medicare/Medigap case, post transactions to the financial accounting record, and define patient record abbreviations.

Conditions: Use the patient's medical record (Figure 12–12) and financial statement (Figure 12–13), one health insurance claim form (Figure 12–14), a typewriter or computer, procedural and diagnostic code books, and Appendices A and B in this *Workbook*.

Standards: Claim Productivity Measurement

Time: _____ minutes

Accuracy: _____

(Note: The time element and accuracy criteria may be given by your instructor.)

Directions:

1. Complete the CMS-1500 claim form, using Medicare/Medigap OCR guidelines, and direct it to your local fiscal intermediary by going to the Web site listed in Internet Resources at the end of Chapter 12 in the *Handbook*. This case involves a patient who has a Medigap supplemental policy that is secondary payer. Refer to Jeremiah W. Diffenderffer's patient record and financial statement for information. See Medicare participating provider fees in Appendix A in this *Workbook* to locate the fees to be recorded on the claim and posted to the financial statement. Date the claim June 13. Dr. Coccidioides is accepting assignment in this case. Mr. Diffenderffer has met his deductible for the year, owing to previous care by Dr. Coccidioides.
2. Refer to Chapter 7 and Figure 7–11 of the *Handbook* for instructions on how to complete the CMS-1500 claim form.
3. Use your CPT code book or Appendix A in this *Workbook* to determine the correct five-digit code number and modifiers for each professional service rendered. Refer to your HCPCS Level II code book or Appendix B in this *Workbook* for HCPCS procedure codes and modifiers.
4. Record all transactions on the financial record, and indicate the proper information when you have billed Medicare and Medigap.
5. On August 3, Medicare check number 654821 was received in the amount of $270.05, paying 80% of the allowable amount for all services except the medication charge, of which they allowed $10. Post this payment to the patient's financial account, and calculate and post the courtesy adjustment. On August 15, United American Insurance Company check number 3254 was received in the amount of $67.51, paying 20% of the allowable amount for all services, including the $10 allowed amount determined by Medicare for the medication. Post this payment to the patient's financial statement, and indicate the balance due from the patient.
6. A Performance Evaluation Checklist may be reproduced from the "Instruction Guide to the Workbook" chapter if your instructor wishes to submit it to assist with scoring and comments.

After the instructor has returned your work to you, either make the necessary corrections and place your work in a three-ring notebook for future reference or, if you received a high score, place it in your portfolio for reference when applying for a job.

Abbreviations pertinent to this record:

Est	_____	hx	_____
oft	_____	exam	_____
p.m.	_____	HC	_____
SOB	_____	MDM	_____
adv	_____	imp	_____
AP	_____	RTO	_____
lat	_____	wk	_____
tech	_____	c/o	_____
CXR	_____	HCN	_____
ABG	_____	PF	_____
PFT	_____	SF	_____
a.m.	_____	IV	_____
RTO	_____	ml	_____
CPX	_____	appt	_____
C	_____		

Additional Coding

1. Refer to Mr. Diffenderffer's medical record, abstract information, and code procedures that would be billed by outside providers.

Site	Description of Service	Code
a. College Hospital Laboratory	_____	_____
b. College Hospital Respiratory Department	_____	_____

2. Locate a financial accounting record (ledger).

   Note: Refer to the step-by-step procedures at the end of Chapter 3 in the *Handbook* and graphic examples Figures 3–18, 10–2, and 12–15.

3. Insert the patient's name and address, including ZIP code in the box.

4. Enter the patient's personal data.

5. Ledger lines: Insert date of service (DOS), reference (CPT code number, check number, or dates of service for posting adjustments or when insurance was billed), description of the transaction, charge amounts, payments, adjustments, and running current balance. The posting date is the actual date the transaction is recorded. If the DOS differs from the posting date, list the DOS in the reference or description column.

Line 2: _____

Line 3: _____

Line 4: _____

Line 5: _____

Line 6: _____

Line 7: _____

Line 8: _____

Line 9: _____

Line 10: _____

Line 11: _____

Note: A good bookkeeping practice is to take a red pen and draw a line across the financial accounting record (ledger) from left to right to indicate the last entry billed to the insurance company.

PATIENT RECORD NO. 12-8

Diffenderffer	Jeremiah	W		08-24-31	M	555-471 9930
LAST NAME	FIRST NAME	MIDDLE NAME		BIRTH DATE	SEX	HOME PHONE

120 Elm Street	Woodland Hills	XY	12345
ADDRESS	CITY	STATE	ZIP CODE

555-218-0087		555-471-9930	Diffenderffer@wb.net
CELL PHONE	PAGER NO.	FAX NO.	E-MAIL ADDRESS

731-XX-7401	none
PATIENT'S SOC. SEC. NO.	DRIVER'S LICENSE

retired painter	
PATIENT'S OCCUPATION	NAME OF COMPANY

ADDRESS OF EMPLOYER	PHONE

deceased	
SPOUSE OR PARENT	OCCUPATION

Medicare	731-XX-7401T
NAME OF INSURANCE	MEDICARE NO

United American Insurance Company, P.O. Box 810, Dallas, TX 75221		555-328-2841
NAME OF OTHER INSURANCE	ADDRESS	PHONE

007559715	UNITXY003
POLICY/CERTIFICATE NO.	PAYERID NO.

REFERRED BY: John M. Diffenderffer (brother)

DATE	PROGRESS NOTES
6-1-xx	Est pt telephoned ofc this p.m. stating he has been involved in a long painting project in
	his home and when he breathed paint fumes in his kitchen today he experienced
	SOB & coughing. Dr. Coccidioides is out of the ofc this p.m. and was paged. Physician
	adv pt to come into ofc for AP & lat chest x-ray and bilateral bronchogram this afternoon.
	Chest x-ray and bronchogram taken by x-ray tech.
	RH/llf *Rene Holmes, CMA*
6-2-xx	CXR and bronchogram showed pulmonary emphysema. Adv pt by phone to have ABG for
	direct O_2 saturation and PFT (spirometry) at College Hospital this a.m. and RTO for CPX
	this afternoon.
	BC/llf *Brady Coccidioides, MD*
6-2-xx	Pt returns for C hx/exam HC MDM. Imp: emphysema, bronchitis and pneumonitis due to
	inhalation of fumes and vapors. Adv no more painting; bed rest. RTO 1 wk.
	BC/llf *Brady Coccidioides, MD*
6-5-xx	Pt calls as ofc is closing c/o difficulty breathing; he has been ambulating and climbing
	stairs. HCN PF hx/exam SF MDM. Administered Coramine (nikethamide) medication IV
	(unclassified drug, 1.5 ml two ampules $25). Imp: recurrent bronchitis and pneumonitis,
	exertional dyspnea. Adv complete bed rest. RTO for appt on 6-9-xx.
	BC/llf *Brady Coccidioides, MD*

Figure 12–12

STATEMENT
Financial Account
COLLEGE CLINIC
4567 Broad Avenue
Woodland Hills, XY 12345-0001
Tel. 555-486-9002
Fax No. 555-487-8976

Acct. No. _12-8_

Jeremiah W. Diffenderffer
120 Elm Street
Woodland Hills, XY 12345

Phone No. (H) _(555) 471-9930_ (W) _____   Birthdate _08-24-31_

Insurance Co. _Medicare/United American Insurance Co._

Policy/Group No. _007559715_
Medicare No. _731-XX-7401T_

	REFERENCE	DESCRIPTION	CHARGES	PYMNTS.	ADJ.	BALANCE	
20XX				BALANCE FORWARD →		20	00
06-01-xx		Chest x-ray					
06-01-xx		Bronchogram					
06-02-xx		OV					
06-05-xx		HC					
06-05-xx		IV administration					
06-05-xx		Medication					

PLEASE PAY LAST AMOUNT IN BALANCE COLUMN

THIS IS A COPY OF YOUR FINANCIAL ACCOUNT AS IT APPEARS ON OUR RECORDS

Figure 12–13

PLEASE
DO NOT
STAPLE
IN THIS
AREA

| PICA | | **HEALTH INSURANCE CLAIM FORM** | PICA |

1. MEDICARE   MEDICAID   CHAMPUS   CHAMPVA   GROUP HEALTH PLAN   FECA BLK LUNG   OTHER   1a. INSURED'S I.D. NUMBER   (FOR PROGRAM IN ITEM 1)

(Medicare #)   (Medicaid #)   (Sponsor's SSN)   (VA File #)   (SSN or ID)   (S SN)   (ID)

2. PATIENT'S NAME (Last Name, First Name, Middle Initial)   3. PATIENT'S BIRTH DATE MM DD YY   SEX M   F   4. INSURED'S NAME (Last Name, First Name, Middle Initial)

5. PATIENT'S ADDRESS (No., Street)   6. PATIENT RELATIONSHIP TO INSURED   Self   Spouse   Child   Other   7. INSURED'S ADDRESS (No., Street)

CITY   STATE   8. PATIENT STATUS   Single   Married   Other   CITY   STATE

ZIP CODE   TELEPHONE (Include Area Code) ( )   Employed   Full-Time Student   Part-Time Student   ZIP CODE   TELEPHONE (INCLUDE AREA CODE)

9. OTHER INSURED'S NAME (Last Name, First Name, Middle Initial)   10. IS PATIENT'S CONDITION RELATED TO: 11. INSURED'S POLICY GROUP OR FECA NUMBER

a. OTHER INSURED'S POLICY OR GROUP NUMBER   a. EMPLOYMENT? (CURRENT OR PREVIOUS)   YES   NO   a. INSURED'S DATE OF BIRTH MM DD YY   SEX M   F

b. OTHER INSURED'S DATE OF BIRTH MM DD YY   SEX M   F   b. AUTO ACCIDENT?   PLACE (State)   YES   NO   b. EMPLOYER'S NAME OR SCHOOL NAME

c. EMPLOYER'S NAME OR SCHOOL NAME   c. OTHER ACCIDENT?   YES   NO   c. INSURANCE PLAN NAME OR PROGRAM NAME

d. INSURANCE PLAN NAME OR PROGRAM NAME   10d. RESERVED FOR LOCAL USE   d. IS THERE ANOTHER HEALTH BENEFIT PLAN?   YES   NO   If yes, return to and complete item 9 a-d.

READ BACK OF FORM BEFORE COMPLETING & SIGNING THIS FORM.
12. PATIENT'S OR AUTHORIZED PERSON'S SIGNATURE I authorize the release of any medical or other information necessary to process this claim. I also request payment of government benefits either to myself or to the party who accepts assignment below.

SIGNED _____   DATE _____

13. INSURED'S OR AUTHORIZED PERSON'S SIGNATURE I authorize payment of medical benefits to the undersigned physician or supplier for services described below.

SIGNED _____

14. DATE OF CURRENT: MM DD YY   ILLNESS (First symptom) OR INJURY (Accident) OR PREGNANCY(LMP)   15. IF PATIENT HAS HAD SAME OR SIMILAR ILLNESS. GIVE FIRST DATE MM DD YY   16. DATES PATIENT UNABLE TO WORK IN CURRENT OCCUPATION MM DD YY   FROM   TO MM DD YY

17. NAME OF REFERRING PHYSICIAN OR OTHER SOURCE   17a. I.D. NUMBER OF REFERRING PHYSICIAN   18. HOSPITALIZATION DATES RELATED TO CURRENT SERVICES MM DD YY   FROM   TO MM DD YY

19. RESERVED FOR LOCAL USE   20. OUTSIDE LAB?   YES   NO $ CHARGES

21. DIAGNOSIS OR NATURE OF ILLNESS OR INJURY. (RELATE ITEMS 1,2,3 OR 4 TO ITEM 24E BY LINE)

1. ____   3. ____
2. ____   4. ____

22. MEDICAID RESUBMISSION CODE   ORIGINAL REF. NO.

23. PRIOR AUTHORIZATION NUMBER

24. A DATE(S) OF SERVICE From To MM DD YY MM DD YY	B Place of Service	C Type of Service	D PROCEDURES, SERVICES, OR SUPPLIES (Explain Unusual Circumstances) CPT/HCPCS MODIFIER	E DIAGNOSIS CODE	F $ CHARGES	G DAYS OR UNITS	H EPSDT Family Plan	I EMG	J COB	K RESERVED FOR LOCAL USE
1										
2										
3										
4										
5										
6										

25. FEDERAL TAX I.D. NUMBER   SSN   EIN   26. PATIENT'S ACCOUNT NO.   27. ACCEPT ASSIGNMENT? (For govt. claims, see back)   YES   NO   28. TOTAL CHARGE $ 29. AMOUNT PAID $ 30. BALANCE DUE $

31. SIGNATURE OF PHYSICIAN OR SUPPLIER INCLUDING DEGREES OR CREDENTIALS (I certify that the statements on the reverse apply to this bill and are made a part thereof.)

SIGNED _____   DATE _____

32. NAME AND ADDRESS OF FACILITY WHERE SERVICES WERE RENDERED (If other than home or office)

33. PHYSICIAN'S, SUPPLIER'S BILLING NAME, ADDRESS, ZIP CODE & PHONE #

PIN#   GRP#

(APPROVED BY AMA COUNCIL ON MEDICAL SERVICE 8/88)   **PLEASE PRINT OR TYPE**   APPROVED OMB-0938-0008 FORM CMS-1500 (12-90),   FORM RRB-1500, APPROVED OMB-1215-0055 FORM OWCP-1500,   APPROVED OMB-0720-0001 (CHAMPUS)

Figure 12–14

ASSIGNMENT 12–9 ▸ COMPLETE A CLAIM FORM FOR A MEDICARE CASE WITH AN ADVANCE BENEFICIARY NOTICE

Performance Objective

Task: Complete a CMS-1500 claim form for a Medicare case and an advance beneficiary notice, post transactions to the financial accounting record, and define patient record abbreviations.

Conditions: Use the patient's record (Figure 12–15) and financial statement (Figure 12–16), an Advance Beneficiary Notice form (Figure 12–17), two health insurance claim forms (photocopy Figure 12–18), a typewriter or computer, procedural and diagnostic code books, and Appendices A and B in this *Workbook*.

Standards: Claim Productivity Measurement

Time: _____ minutes

Accuracy: _____

(Note: The time element and accuracy criteria may be given by your instructor.)

Directions:

1. Complete a CMS-1500 claim form for a Medicare case, using OCR guidelines, and direct it to your local Medicare Railroad fiscal intermediary by going to the Web site listed in Internet Resources at the end of Chapter 12 in the *Handbook*. This assignment requires two claim forms, so make a photocopy for the second claim. Refer to Raymond D. Fay's patient record for information. Refer to Appendix A in this *Workbook* to locate the fees to be recorded on the claim and posted to the financial statement. Date the claim December 31. Dr. Antrum is accepting assignment in this case.
2. Refer to Figure 7–11 in the *Handbook* for instructions on how to complete the CMS-1500 form.
3. The nystagmus service is disallowed by Medicare, and an Advance Beneficiary Notice needs to be completed. Refer to Figure 12–10 in the *Handbook*. for a completed example of this form. Note: When a noncovered service is provided, a fee will not be listed in the Medicare fee schedule; therefore, list the regular (mock) fee.
4. Use your CPT code book or Appendix A in this *Workbook* to determine the correct five-digit code number and modifiers for each professional service rendered. Use your HCPCS Level II code book or refer to Appendix B in this *Workbook* for HCPCS procedure codes and modifiers.
5. Record all transactions on the financial accounting record, and indicate the proper information when you have billed Medicare.
6. A Performance Evaluation Checklist may be reproduced from the "Instruction Guide to the Workbook" chapter if your instructor wishes you to submit it to assist with scoring and comments.

After the instructor has returned your work to you, either make the necessary corrections and place your work in a three-ring notebook for future reference or, if you received a high score, place it in your portfolio for reference when applying for a job.

Abbreviations pertinent to this record:

Pt _____   RTO _____

D _____   rtn _____

hx _____   OV _____

exam _____   appt(s) _____

retn _____   wk _____

R/O _____   inj. _____

LC _____   Dx _____

MDM _____   PF _____

N _____   SF _____

X _____   sx _____

incl _____   disc _____

Additional Fee Calculations

1. Medicare sent payment on this claim, allowing 80% of the amount after the deductible was met, which was subtracted from the amount of this claim. Medicare denied payment on code 92531 as a noncovered service.

    a. What is the amount of the Medicare check?   _____

    b. What is the amount of the patient responsibility?   _____

    c. Is there a courtesy adjustment?   _____

2. Locate a financial accounting record (ledger).

    Note: Refer to the step-by-step procedures at the end of Chapter 3 in the *Handbook* and graphic examples Figures 3–18, 10–2, and 12–15.

3. Insert the patient's name and address, including ZIP code in the box.

4. Enter the patient's personal data.

5. Ledger lines: Insert date of service (DOS), reference (CPT code number, check number, or dates of service for posting adjustments or when insurance was billed), description of the transaction, charge amounts, payments, adjustments, and running current balance. The posting date is the actual date the transaction is recorded. If the DOS differs from the posting date, list the DOS in the reference or description column.

    Line 2: _____

    Line 3: _____

    Line 4: _____

    Line 5: _____

Line 6: _____

Line 7: _____

Line 8: _____

Line 9: _____

Line 10: _____

Line 11: _____

Line 12: _____

Line 13: _____

Note: A good bookkeeping practice is to take a red pen and draw a line across the financial accounting record (ledger) from left to right to indicate the last entry billed to the insurance company.

Advance Beneficiary Notice

Checklist

1. Inserted patient's name.   _____

2. Inserted patient's Medicare number.   _____

3. Inserted name of service or procedure.   _____

4. Inserted the reason for the service.   _____

5. Checked whether or not the patient wishes to receive the service.   _____

6. Dated the form.   _____

7. Obtained the patient's signature.   _____

PATIENT RECORD NO. 12-9

Fay	Raymond		02-03-32	M	555-788-9090
LAST NAME	FIRST NAME	MIDDLE NAME	BIRTH DATE	SEX	HOME PHONE

33 North Pencil Avenue	Woodland Hills	XY	12345
ADDRESS	CITY	STATE	ZIP CODE

	555-250-4890	555-788-9090		fay@wb.net
CELL PHONE	PAGER NO.	FAX NO.		E-MAIL ADDRESS

887-66-1235	R8966543
PATIENT'S SOC. SEC. NO.	DRIVER'S LICENSE

retired railroad engineer
PATIENT'S OCCUPATION   NAME OF COMPANY

ADDRESS OF EMPLOYER   PHONE

Marilyn B. Fay	homemaker
SPOUSE OR PARENT	OCCUPATION

EMPLOYER   ADDRESS   PHONE

Medicare Railroad	self
NAME OF INSURANCE	INSURED OR SUB SCRIBER

A 887-XX-1235A
MEDICARE NO.

REFERRED BY: George Gentle, MD, 1000 N. Main St., Woodland Hills, XY 12345   NPI# 402131102XX

DATE	PROGRESS NOTES
10-31-xx	New pt presents, a D hx was taken. Pt complains of skin rash and dizziness for 3 days.
	A detailed exam reveals rash on chest and arms. Retn in 4 days for tests to R/O eye/ear
	causes for dizziness and food allergies (LC MDM).
	CA/llf *Concha Antrum, MD*
11-4-xx	Comprehensive audiometric threshold evaluation (with speech)—N. 10 intradermal
	allergy tests; delayed reaction. Bilateral mastoid X (complete)—N. Spontaneous nystagmus
	test, incl. gaze—N. RTO in 3 days for skin test results.
	CA/llf *Concha Antrum, MD*
11-7-xx	Rtn OV for allergy skin test results—positive for 3 substances. Pt to purchase allergen
	extract and make sequential appts next wk for daily immunotherapy inj. Dx: food allergies.
	CA/llf *Concha Antrum, MD*
11-14-xx thru 11-18-xx	Immunotherapy; 3 inj. per/day
	CA/llf *Concha Antrum, MD*
11-21-xx thru 11-25-xx	Immunotherapy; 3 inj. per/day
	CA/llf *Concha Antrum, MD*
11-28-xx thru 12-2-xx	Immunotherapy; 3 inj. per/day
	CA/llf *Concha Antrum, MD*
12-5-xx thru 12-8-xx	Immunotherapy; 3 inj. per/day
	CA/llf *Concha Antrum, MD*
12-9-xx	OV (PF hx/exam SF MDM) Pt. sx improved. Received final inj and evaluated for disch.
	CA/llf *Concha Antrum, MD*

Figure 12–15

Acct No. 12-9

STATEMENT
Financial Account
COLLEGE CLINIC
4567 Broad Avenue
Woodland Hills, XY 12345-0001
Tel. 555-486-9002
Fax No. 555-487-8976

Raymond Fay
33 North Pencil Avenue
Woodland Hills, XY 12345

Phone No. (H) (555) 788-9090   (W) _____   Birthdate 02-03-32

Primary Insurance Co. Medicare Railroad _____ Policy/Group No. A 887-XX 1235A

Secondary Insurance Co. N/A _____ Policy/Group No. _____

| DATE | REF-ERENCE | DESCRIPTION | CHARGES | CREDITS | | BALANCE |
				PYMNTS.	ADJ.	
20xx				BALANCE FORWARD →		
10-31-xx		OV				
11-4-xx		Audiometry evaluation				
11-4-xx		Intradermal allergy tests				
11-4-xx		Bilateral mastoid x-rays				
11-4-xx		Spontaneous nystagmus test				
11-7-xx		Allergy test results				
11-14 to 11-18-xx		Immunotherapy inj. (3/day X 5)				
11-21 to 11-25-xx		Immunotherapy inj. (3/day X 5)				
11-28 to 12-2-xx		Immunotherapy inj. (3/day X 5)				
12-5 to 12-9-xx		Immunotherapy inj. (3/day X 5)				
12-9-xx		OV				

PLEASE PAY LAST AMOUNT IN BALANCE COLUMN ⬆

THIS IS A COPY OF YOUR FINANCIAL ACCOUNT AS IT APPEARS ON OUR RECORDS

Figure 12–16

College Clinic
4567 Broad Avenue
Woodland Hills, XY 12345-0001

Patient's Name: _____ Medicare # (HICN): _____

ADVANCE BENEFICIARY NOTICE (ABN)

NOTE: You need to make a choice about receiving these health care items or services.

We expect that Medicare will not pay for the item(s) or service(s) that are described below. Medicare does not pay for all of your health care costs. Medicare only pays for covered items and services when Medicare rules are met. The fact that Medicare may not pay for a particular item or service does not mean that you should not receive it. There may be a good reason your doctor recommended it. Right now, in your case, **Medicare probably will not pay for –**

Items or Services:
Because:

The purpose of this form is to help you make an informed choice about whether or not you want to receive these items or services, knowing that you might have to pay for them yourself. Before you make a decision about your options, you should **read this entire notice carefully.**
• Ask us to explain, if you don't understand why Medicare probably won't pay.
• Ask us how much these items or services will cost you **(Estimated cost: $_____)**, in case you have to pay for them yourself or through other insurance.

PLEASE CHOOSE **ONE** OPTION. CHECK **ONE** BOX. **SIGN & DATE** YOUR CHOICE.

☐ **Option 1. YES. I want to receive these items or services.**

I understand that Medicare will not decide whether to pay unless I receive these items or services. Please submit my claim to Medicare. I understand that you may bill me for items or services and that I may have to pay the bill while Medicare is making its decision. If Medicare does pay, you will refund to me any payments I made to you that are due to me. If Medicare denies payment, I agree to be personally and fully responsible for payment. That is, I will pay personally, either out of pocket or through any other insurance that I have. I understand I can appeal Medicare's decision.

☐ **Option 2. NO. I have decided not to receive these items or services.**

I will not receive these items or services. I understand that you will not be able to submit a claim to Medicare and that I will not be able to appeal your opinion that Medicare won't pay.

_____   _____
Date   **Signature of patient or person acting on patient's behalf**

NOTE: Your health information will be kept confidential. Any information that we collect about you on this form will be kept confidential in our offices. If a claim is submitted to Medicare, your health information on this form may be shared with Medicare. Your health information which Medicare sees will be kept confidential by Medicare.

OMB Approval No. 0938-0566   Form No. CMS-R-131-G   (June 2002)

Figure 12–17

PLEASE
DO NOT
STAPLE
IN THIS
AREA

CARRIER

HEALTH INSURANCE CLAIM FORM

| | PICA | | | | | PICA | | |

1. MEDICARE (Medicare #) **MEDICAID** (Medicaid #) **CHAMPUS** (Sponsor's SSN) **CHAMPVA** (VA File #) **GROUP HEALTH PLAN** (SSN or ID) **FECA BLK LUNG** (S SN) **OTHER** (ID)   **1a. INSURED'S I.D. NUMBER** (FOR PROGRAM IN ITEM 1)

2. PATIENT'S NAME (Last Name, First Name, Middle Initial)   **3. PATIENT'S BIRTH DATE** MM DD YY **SEX** M F   **4. INSURED'S NAME** (Last Name, First Name, Middle Initial)

5. PATIENT'S ADDRESS (No., Street)   **6. PATIENT RELATIONSHIP TO INSURED** Self Spouse Child Other   **7. INSURED'S ADDRESS** (No., Street)

CITY   STATE   **8. PATIENT STATUS** Single Married Other   CITY   STATE

ZIP CODE   TELEPHONE (Include Area Code) ( )   Employed Full-Time Student Part-Time Student   ZIP CODE   TELEPHONE (INCLUDE AREA CODE)

9. OTHER INSURED'S NAME (Last Name, First Name, Middle Initial)   **10. IS PATIENT'S CONDITION RELATED TO:**   **11. INSURED'S POLICY GROUP OR FECA NUMBER**

a. OTHER INSURED'S POLICY OR GROUP NUMBER   **a. EMPLOYMENT?** (CURRENT OR PREVIOUS) YES NO   **a. INSURED'S DATE OF BIRTH** MM DD YY **SEX** M F

b. OTHER INSURED'S DATE OF BIRTH MM DD YY **SEX** M F   **b. AUTO ACCIDENT?** PLACE (State) YES NO   **b. EMPLOYER'S NAME OR SCHOOL NAME**

c. EMPLOYER'S NAME OR SCHOOL NAME   **c. OTHER ACCIDENT?** YES NO   **c. INSURANCE PLAN NAME OR PROGRAM NAME**

d. INSURANCE PLAN NAME OR PROGRAM NAME   **10d. RESERVED FOR LOCAL USE**   **d. IS THERE ANOTHER HEALTH BENEFIT PLAN?** YES NO *If yes*, return to and complete item 9 a-d.

READ BACK OF FORM BEFORE COMPLETING & SIGNING THIS FORM.
12. PATIENT'S OR AUTHORIZED PERSON'S SIGNATURE I authorize the release of any medical or other information necessary to process this claim. I also request payment of government benefits either to myself or to the party who accepts assignment below.

SIGNED _____ DATE _____

13. INSURED'S OR AUTHORIZED PERSON'S SIGNATURE I authorize payment of medical benefits to the undersigned physician or supplier for services described below.

SIGNED _____

14. DATE OF CURRENT: ILLNESS (First symptom) OR INJURY (Accident) OR PREGNANCY(LMP) MM DD YY   **15. IF PATIENT HAS HAD SAME OR SIMILAR ILLNESS. GIVE FIRST DATE** MM DD YY   **16. DATES PATIENT UNABLE TO WORK IN CURRENT OCCUPATION** FROM MM DD YY TO MM DD YY

17. NAME OF REFERRING PHYSICIAN OR OTHER SOURCE   **17a. I.D. NUMBER OF REFERRING PHYSICIAN**   **18. HOSPITALIZATION DATES RELATED TO CURRENT SERVICES** FROM MM DD YY TO MM DD YY

19. RESERVED FOR LOCAL USE   **20. OUTSIDE LAB?** YES NO **$ CHARGES**

21. DIAGNOSIS OR NATURE OF ILLNESS OR INJURY. (RELATE ITEMS 1,2,3 OR 4 TO ITEM 24E BY LINE)
1. ____ 3. ____
2. ____ 4. ____

22. MEDICAID RESUBMISSION CODE **ORIGINAL REF. NO.**

23. PRIOR AUTHORIZATION NUMBER

24. A						B	C	D		E	F	G	H	I	J	K
DATE(S) OF SERVICE						Place of Service	Type of Service	PROCEDURES, SERVICES, OR SUPPLIES (Explain Unusual Circumstances)		DIAGNOSIS CODE	$ CHARGES	DAYS OR UNITS	EPSDT Family Plan	EMG	COB	RESERVED FOR LOCAL USE
From MM	DD	YY	To MM	DD	YY			CPT/HCPCS	MODIFIER							
1																
2																
3																
4																
5																
6																

25. FEDERAL TAX I.D. NUMBER SSN EIN   **26. PATIENT'S ACCOUNT NO.**   **27. ACCEPT ASSIGNMENT?** (For govt. claims, see back) YES NO   **28. TOTAL CHARGE** $ **29. AMOUNT PAID** $ **30. BALANCE DUE** $

31. SIGNATURE OF PHYSICIAN OR SUPPLIER INCLUDING DEGREES OR CREDENTIALS (I certify that the statements on the reverse apply to this bill and are made a part thereof.)

SIGNED _____ DATE _____

32. NAME AND ADDRESS OF FACILITY WHERE SERVICES WERE RENDERED (If other than home or office)

33. PHYSICIAN'S, SUPPLIER'S BILLING NAME, ADDRESS, ZIP CODE & PHONE #

PIN# GRP#

(APPROVED BY AMA COUNCIL ON MEDICAL SERVICE 8/88)   ***PLEASE PRINT OR TYPE***   APPROVED OMB-0938-0008 FORM CMS-1500 (12-90), FORM RRB-1500,
APPROVED OMB-1215-0055 FORM OWCP-1500, APPROVED OMB-0720-0001 (CHAMPUS)

PATIENT AND INSURED INFORMATION

PHYSICIAN OR SUPPLIER INFORMATION

EXAMPLE ONLY

Figure 12–18

ASSIGNMENT **12-10** ▸ **COMPLETE A CLAIM FORM FOR**
A MEDICARE/MEDICAID CASE

Performance Objective

Task: Complete a CMS-1500 claim form for a Medicare/Medicare case, post transactions to the
financial accounting record, and define patient record abbreviations.

Conditions: Use the patient's medical record (Figure 12–19) and financial statement (Figure 12–20), one
health insurance claim form (Figure 12–21), a typewriter or computer, procedural and diagnostic
code books, and Appendices A and B in this *Workbook*.

Standards: Claim Productivity Measurement

Time: _____ minutes

Accuracy: _____

(Note: The time element and accuracy criteria may be given by your instructor.)

Directions:

1. Complete the CMS-1500 claim form, using OCR guidelines for a Medicare/Medicaid case, directing it to both
   your local Medicare fiscal intermediary by going to the Web site listed in Internet Resources at the end of
   Chapter 12 in the *Handbook* and Medicaid. Refer to Mr. Harris Fremont's patient record for information.
   Refer to Appendix A in this *Workbook* to locate the fees to be recorded on the claim and posted to the financial
   statement. Date the claim October 31.
2. Refer to Chapter 7 and Figure 7–10 of the *Handbook* for instructions on how to complete the CMS-1500
   claim form.
3. Use your CPT code book or Appendix A in this *Workbook* to determine the correct five-digit code number
   and modifiers for each professional service rendered. Use your HCPCS Level II code book or refer to
   Appendix B in this *Workbook* for HCPCS procedure codes and modifiers.
4. Record all transactions on the financial account and indicate the proper information when you have billed
   Medicare/Medicaid.
5. On December 12, Medicare paid $125 (check number 281362) on this claim. Post this payment to the patient's
   financial account. On December 29, you receive a voucher number 7234 from Medicaid for $45. Post this
   payment to the patient's financial account and show the courtesy adjustment.
6. A Performance Evaluation Checklist may be reproduced from the "Instruction Guide to the Workbook" chapter
   if your instructor wishes you to submit it to assist with scoring and comments.

   After the instructor has returned your work to you, either make the necessary corrections and place your work in
a three-ring notebook for future reference or, if you received a high score, place it in your portfolio for reference
when applying for a job.

Abbreviations pertinent to this record:

NP	_____	pt	_____
c/o	_____	lab	_____
hx	_____	CBC	_____
R	_____	auto	_____
L	_____	diff	_____
N	_____	ESR	_____
Rx	_____	R/O	_____
adv	_____	PF	_____
rtn	_____	SF	_____
LC	_____	prn	_____
MDM	_____	imp	_____

Additional Coding

1. Refer to Mr. Fremont's medical record, abstract information, and code procedures that would be billed by outside providers.

Site	Description of Service	Code
a. ABC Laboratory	_____	_____
b. ABC Laboratory	_____	_____
c. ABC Laboratory	_____	_____
d. ABC Laboratory	_____	_____

2. Use your diagnostic code book and code the symptoms of which the patient complained.

Symptom	Code
a. _____	_____
b. _____	_____

3. Locate a financial accounting record (ledger).

Note: Refer to the step-by-step procedures at the end of Chapter 3 in the *Handbook* and graphic examples Figures 3–18, 10–2, and 12–15.

4. Insert the patient's name and address, including ZIP code in the box.

5. Enter the patient's personal data.

6. Ledger lines: Insert date of service (DOS), reference (CPT code number, check number, or dates of service for posting adjustments or when insurance was billed), description of the transaction, charge amounts, payments, adjustments, and running current balance. The posting date is the actual date the transaction is recorded. If the DOS differs from the posting date, list the DOS in the reference or description column.

Line 2: _____

Line 3: _____

Line 4: _____

Line 5: _____

Line 6: _____

Line 7: _____

Line 8: _____

Line 9: _____

Note: A good bookkeeping practice is to take a red pen and draw a line across the financial accounting record (ledger) from left to right to indicate the last entry billed to the insurance company.

PATIENT RECORD NO. 12-10

Fremont	Harris		07-10-23	M	555-899-0109
LAST NAME	FIRST NAME	MIDDLE NAME	BIRTH DATE	SEX	HOME PHONE

735 North Center Street	Woodland Hills,	XY	12345
ADDRESS	CITY	STATE	ZIP CODE

CELL PHONE	PAGER NO.	FAX NO.	E-MAIL ADDRESS

454-XX-9569	none	
PATIENT'S SOC. SEC. NO.	DRIVER'S LICENSE	

retired baseball coach	
PATIENT'S OCCUPATION	NAME OF COMPANY

ADDRESS OF EMPLOYER	PHONE

Emily B. Fremont	homemaker
SPOUSE OR PARENT	OCCUPATION

EMPLOYER	ADDRESS	PHONE

Medicare/Medicaid	
NAME OF INSURANCE	INSURED OR SUBSCRIBER

454-XX-9569A	56-10-0020205-0-XX
MEDICARE NO.	MEDICAID NO.

REFERRED BY: Raymond Skeleton, MD

DATE	PROGRESS NOTES
10-2-xx	NP referred by Dr. Skeleton. He comes in c/o discomfort around toes of both feet and
	has difficulty walking. Pt states he dropped shelf on feet about a month ago. A detailed
	hx reveals gout and mycotic nails. X-ray R and L feet (2 views) N. Detailed exam reveals
	bilateral mycotic nails & ingrown nail on great R toe. Rx: Electrically débride and trimmed
	overgrowth of all nails and adv to rtn if pain continues in great R toe (LC MDM). Gave pt
	order to have lab work done at ABC Laboratory (CBC w/auto diff., ESR, uric acid level)
	R/O gout. Imp: Mycotic nails; difficulty walking.
	NP/llf *Nick Pedro, DPM*
10-18-xx	Pt returns c/o ingrown nail on R great toe (PF hx/exam SF MDM). Lab work done on
	10/2/xx showed no signs of gout. Performed wedge excision of skin/nail fold.
	Rtn prn. Imp: Ingrown nail – great R toe; toe pain.
	NP/llf *Nick Pedro, DPM*

Figure 12–19

Acct No. 12-10

STATEMENT
Financial Account
COLLEGE CLINIC
4567 Broad Avenue
Woodland Hills, XY 12345-0001
Tel. 555-486-9002
Fax No. 555-487-8976

Harris Fremont
735 North Center Street
Woodland Hills, XY 12345

Phone No. (H) ___555-899-0109___ (W) _____ Birthdate ___7/10/23___

Primary Insurance Co. ___Medicare_____ Policy/Group No. ___454XX9569A___

Secondary Insurance Co. ___Medicaid_____ Policy/Group No. ___561000202050XX___

DATE	REF-ERENCE	DESCRIPTION	CHARGES	PYMNTS.	ADJ.	BALANCE
20xx			BALANCE FORWARD ➔			
10-2-xx		NP OV				
10-2-xx		X-rays R/L feet				
10-2-xx		Débridement nails				
10-18-xx		OV				
10-18-xx		Wedge excision R. great toe				

PLEASE PAY LAST AMOUNT IN BALANCE COLUMN ⬆

THIS IS A COPY OF YOUR FINANCIAL ACCOUNT AS IT APPEARS ON OUR RECORDS

Figure 12–20

HEALTH INSURANCE CLAIM FORM

PICA ☐☐☐   PICA ☐☐☐

1. MEDICARE	MEDICAID	CHAMPUS	CHAMPVA	GROUP HEALTH PLAN	FECA BLK LUNG	OTHER	1a. INSURED'S I.D. NUMBER	(FOR PROGRAM IN ITEM 1)
☐ (Medicare #)	☐ (Medicaid #)	☐ (Sponsor's SSN)	☐ (VA File #)	☐ (SSN or ID)	☐ (S SN)	☐ (ID)		

2. PATIENT'S NAME (Last Name, First Name, Middle Initial)

3. PATIENT'S BIRTH DATE MM DD YY   SEX M ☐ F ☐

4. INSURED'S NAME (Last Name, First Name, Middle Initial)

5. PATIENT'S ADDRESS (No., Street)

6. PATIENT RELATIONSHIP TO INSURED   Self ☐ Spouse ☐ Child ☐ Other ☐

7. INSURED'S ADDRESS (No., Street)

CITY   STATE

8. PATIENT STATUS   Single ☐ Married ☐ Other ☐

Employed ☐ Full-Time Student ☐ Part-Time Student ☐

CITY   STATE

ZIP CODE   TELEPHONE (Include Area Code) ( )

ZIP CODE   TELEPHONE (INCLUDE AREA CODE)

9. OTHER INSURED'S NAME (Last Name, First Name, Middle Initial)

10. IS PATIENT'S CONDITION RELATED TO:

11. INSURED'S POLICY GROUP OR FECA NUMBER

a. OTHER INSURED'S POLICY OR GROUP NUMBER

a. EMPLOYMENT? (CURRENT OR PREVIOUS) ☐ YES ☐ NO

a. INSURED'S DATE OF BIRTH MM DD YY   SEX M ☐ F ☐

b. OTHER INSURED'S DATE OF BIRTH MM DD YY   SEX M ☐ F ☐

b. AUTO ACCIDENT?   PLACE (State) ☐ YES ☐ NO

b. EMPLOYER'S NAME OR SCHOOL NAME

c. EMPLOYER'S NAME OR SCHOOL NAME

c. OTHER ACCIDENT? ☐ YES ☐ NO

c. INSURANCE PLAN NAME OR PROGRAM NAME

d. INSURANCE PLAN NAME OR PROGRAM NAME

10d. RESERVED FOR LOCAL USE

d. IS THERE ANOTHER HEALTH BENEFIT PLAN? ☐ YES ☐ NO   *If yes*, return to and complete item 9 a-d.

READ BACK OF FORM BEFORE COMPLETING & SIGNING THIS FORM.

12. PATIENT'S OR AUTHORIZED PERSON'S SIGNATURE I authorize the release of any medical or other information necessary to process this claim. I also request payment of government benefits either to myself or to the party who accepts assignment below.

SIGNED _____   DATE _____

13. INSURED'S OR AUTHORIZED PERSON'S SIGNATURE I authorize payment of medical benefits to the undersigned physician or supplier for services described below.

SIGNED _____

14. DATE OF CURRENT: ◄ ILLNESS (First symptom) OR INJURY (Accident) OR PREGNANCY(LMP) MM DD YY

15. IF PATIENT HAS HAD SAME OR SIMILAR ILLNESS. GIVE FIRST DATE MM DD YY

16. DATES PATIENT UNABLE TO WORK IN CURRENT OCCUPATION FROM MM DD YY TO MM DD YY

17. NAME OF REFERRING PHYSICIAN OR OTHER SOURCE

17a. I.D. NUMBER OF REFERRING PHYSICIAN

18. HOSPITALIZATION DATES RELATED TO CURRENT SERVICES FROM MM DD YY TO MM DD YY

19. RESERVED FOR LOCAL USE

20. OUTSIDE LAB? ☐ YES ☐ NO $ CHARGES

21. DIAGNOSIS OR NATURE OF ILLNESS OR INJURY. (RELATE ITEMS 1,2,3 OR 4 TO ITEM 24E BY LINE)

1. |_____   3. |_____

2. |_____   4. |_____

22. MEDICAID RESUBMISSION CODE   ORIGINAL REF. NO.

23. PRIOR AUTHORIZATION NUMBER

24.	A DATE(S) OF SERVICE					B Place of Service	C Type of Service	D PROCEDURES, SERVICES, OR SUPPLIES (Explain Unusual Circumstances) CPT/HCPCS MODIFIER	E DIAGNOSIS CODE	F $ CHARGES	G DAYS OR UNITS	H EPSDT Family Plan	I EMG	J COB	K RESERVED FOR LOCAL USE
	From MM DD YY			To MM DD YY											
1															
2															
3															
4															
5															
6															

25. FEDERAL TAX I.D. NUMBER   SSN ☐ EIN ☐

26. PATIENT'S ACCOUNT NO.

27. ACCEPT ASSIGNMENT? (For govt. claims, see back) ☐ YES ☐ NO

28. TOTAL CHARGE $

29. AMOUNT PAID $

30. BALANCE DUE $

31. SIGNATURE OF PHYSICIAN OR SUPPLIER INCLUDING DEGREES OR CREDENTIALS (I certify that the statements on the reverse apply to this bill and are made a part thereof.)

SIGNED _____   DATE _____

32. NAME AND ADDRESS OF FACILITY WHERE SERVICES WERE RENDERED (If other than home or office)

33. PHYSICIAN'S, SUPPLIER'S BILLING NAME, ADDRESS, ZIP CODE & PHONE #

PIN#   GRP#

(APPROVED BY AMA COUNCIL ON MEDICAL SERVICE 8/88)   ***PLEASE PRINT OR TYPE***   APPROVED OMB-0938-0008 FORM CMS-1500 (12-90), FORM RRB-1500, APPROVED OMB-1215-0055 FORM OWCP-1500,   APPROVED OMB-0720-0001 (CHAMPUS)

CARRIER

PATIENT AND INSURED INFORMATION

PHYSICIAN OR SUPPLIER INFORMATION

Figure 12–21

ASSIGNMENT **12-11** ▸ **TRANSMIT AN ELECTRONIC INSURANCE CLAIM**
FOR A MEDICARE CASE

(**e hint**)   Follow the General Instructions for TRANSMISSION OF AN
ELECTRONIC CLAIM (A SINGLE CLAIM) as given in Chapter 8.

Performance Objective

Task: Transmit an electronic insurance claim form and post the information to the patient's financial
account record.

Conditions: Use John R. Martin's encounter form (Figure 12–22), patient's electronic data, and computer.

Standards: Productivity Measurement

Time: _____ minutes

Accuracy: _____

(Note: The time element and accuracy criteria may be given by your instructor.)

Directions:

1. Electronically prepare an insurance claim form by referring to John R. Martin's encounter form in the *Workbook*
and his electronic personal and medical data. Follow the step-by-step general directions for transmission of an
insurance claim.

2. Enter the patient's data into the software to obtain the procedural and diagnostic codes and College Clinic fee
amounts.

3. Transmit the insurance claim to Medicare Health Systems Corporation.

4. Print a hard copy of the insurance claim to hand in to your instructor to receive a score.

5. A Performance Evaluation Checklist may be reproduced from the "Instruction Guide to the Workbook" chapter
if your instructor wishes you to submit it to assist with scoring and comments.

    After the instructor has returned your work to you, either make the necessary corrections and place your work in
a three-ring notebook for future reference or, if you received a high score, place it in your portfolio for reference
when applying for a job.

TAX ID #3664021CC
Medicaid #HSC12345F

College Clinic

4567 Broad Avenue
Woodlands Hills, XY
12345-0001
Tel (555) 486-9002
Fax (555) 487-8976

Doctors No. _____

☐ PRIVATE   ☐ MANAGED CARE   ☐ MEDICAID   ☒ MEDICARE   ☐ TRICARE   ☐ W/C

ACCOUNT #	PATIENT'S LAST NAME	FIRST	INITIAL	TODAY'S DATE
008	Martin	John	R.	5/18/2007

ASSIGNMENT: I hereby assign payment directly to College Clinic of the surgical and/or medical benefits, if any, otherwise payable to me for his/her services as described below.

SIGNED (Patient, or Parent, if Minor)   John R. Martin   DATE: 5/18/2007

✓	DESCRIPTION	CPT-4/MD	FEE	✓	DESCRIPTION	CPT-4/MD	FEE	✓	DESCRIPTION	CPT-4/MD	FEE
	OFFICE VISIT-NEW PATIENT				**WELL BABY EXAM**				**LABORATORY**		
	Level 1	99201			Intial	99381			Glucose Blood	82962	
	Level 2	99202			Periodic	99391			Heamatocrit	85013	
✓	Level 3	99203	70.92		**OFFICE PROCEDURES**				Occult Blood	82270	
	Level 4	99204			Anscopy	46600			Urine Dip	81000	
	Level 5	99205			ECG 24-hr	93224			**X-RAY**		
	OFFICE VISIT-ESTAB, PATIENT				Fracture Rpr Foot	28470		✓	2-X-rays tibia fibula	73590	33.35
	Level 1	99211			I & D	10060			Forearm - 2 View	73090	
	Level 2	99212			Suture Repair				Nasal Bone - 3	70160	
	Level 3	99213		✓	Closed tibial fx	27530	344.24		Spine LS - 2 view	72100	
	Level 4	99214			**INJECTIONS/VACCINATIONS**			✓	X-ray hip unilateral	73500	31.56
	Level 5	99215			DPT	90701			**MISCELLANEOUS**		
	OFFICE CONSULT-NP/EST				IM-Antibiotic	90788			Handling of Spec	99000	
	Level 3	99243			OPU-Poliovirus	90712		✓	Cast material	A 4590	25.00
	Level 4	99244			Tetanus	90703			Venipuncture	36415	
	Level 5	99245						✓	dressing, gauze	A 4202	25.00

COMMENTS:

Physician: Raymond Skeleton, M.D.

RETURN APPOINTMENT

___3___ Week(s)   _____ Month(s)

DIAGNOSIS:

	DESCRIPTION	CODE
Primary:	Fracture tibia upper end closed	823.00
Secondary:	Contusion hip	924.01
	Contusion upper limb	923.09

REC'D BY:
☐ BANK CARD
☐ CASH
☐ CHECK
_____

PREVIOUS BALANCE	149.86
TODAY'S FEE	530.07
AMOUNT REC'D/CO-PAY	⊖
BALANCE	679.93

Figure 12–22

ASSIGNMENT 12–12 ▸ TRANSMIT AN ELECTRONIC INSURANCE CLAIM FOR A MEDICARE AND MEDIGAP CASE

e hint Follow the General Instructions for TRANSMISSION OF AN ELECTRONIC CLAIM (A SINGLE CLAIM) as given in Chapter 8.

Performance Objective

Task: Transmit an electronic insurance claim form and post the information to the patient's financial account record using AltaPoint software.

Conditions: Use Clinton A. Helms's encounter forms (Figures 12–23 through 12–26), patient's electronic data, and computer.

Standards: Productivity Measurement

Time: _____ minutes

Accuracy: _____

(Note: The time element and accuracy criteria may be given by your instructor.)

Directions:

1. Electronically prepare an insurance claim form by referring to Clinton A. Helm's three encounter forms and Doctor's Daily Schedule slip in the *Workbook* and his electronic personal and medical data. Follow the step-by-step general directions for transmission of an insurance claim.

2. Enter the patient's data into the software to obtain the procedural and diagnostic codes and College Clinic fee amounts.

3. Transmit the insurance claim to Medicare Health Systems Corporation.

4. Print a hard copy of the insurance claim to hand in to your instructor to receive a score.

5. A Performance Evaluation Checklist may be reproduced from the "Instruction Guide to the Workbook" chapter if your instructor wishes you to submit it to assist with scoring and comments.

   After the instructor has returned your work to you, either make the necessary corrections and place your work in a three-ring notebook for future reference or, if you received a high score, place it in your portfolio for reference when applying for a job.

TAX ID #3664021CC
Medicaid #HSC12345F

College Clinic

4567 Broad Avenue
Woodlands Hills, XY
12345-0001
Tel (555) 486-9002
Fax (555) 487-8976

Doctors No. _____

☐ PRIVATE   ☐ MANAGED CARE   ☐ MEDICAID   ☒ MEDICARE   ☐ TRICARE   ☐ W/C

ACCOUNT #	PATIENT'S LAST NAME	FIRST	INITIAL	TODAY'S DATE
009	Helms,	Clinton	A.	10/6/2007

ASSIGNMENT: I hereby assign payment directly to College Clinic of the surgical and/or medical benefits, if any, otherwise payable to me for his/her services as described below.
SIGNED (Patient, or Parent, if Minor)   Clinton a. Helms   DATE: 10/6/2007

✓	DESCRIPTION	CPT-4/MD	FEE	✓	DESCRIPTION	CPT-4/MD	FEE	✓	DESCRIPTION	CPT-4/MD	FEE
	OFFICE VISIT-NEW PATIENT				**WELL BABY EXAM**				**LABORATORY**		
	Level 1	99201			Intial	99381			Glucose Blood	82962	
	Level 2	99202			Periodic	99391			Heamatocrit	85013	
	Level 3	99203			**OFFICE PROCEDURES**				Occult Blood	82270	
	Level 4	99204			Anscopy	46600			Urine Dip	81000	
	Level 5	99205			ECG 24-hr	93224			**X-RAY**		
	OFFICE VISIT-ESTAB, PATIENT				Fracture Rpr Foot	28470			Foot - 2 View	73620	
	Level 1	99211			I & D	10060			Forearm - 2 View	73090	
	Level 2	99212			Suture Repair				Nasal Bone - 3	70160	
	Level 3	99213							Spine LS - 2 view	72100	
	Level 4	99214			**INJECTIONS/VACCINATIONS**						
	Level 5	99215			DPT	90701			**MISCELLANEOUS**		
	OFFICE CONSULT-NP/EST				IM-Antibiotic	90788			Handling of Spec	99000	
	Level 3	99243			OPU-Poliovirus	90712			Supply	99070	
✓	Level 4	99244	145.05		Tetanus	90703			Venipuncture	36415	
	Level 5	99245									

COMMENTS:

Physician: Concha Antrum, M.D.

RETURN APPOINTMENT	2 days
_____ Week(s) _____ Month(s)	

DIAGNOSIS:
Primary: Dyshonia hoarseness   CODE 784.49
Secondary: Other disease of vocal cords   478.5

REC'D BY:
☐ BANK CARD
☐ CASH
☐ CHECK
_____

PREVIOUS BALANCE	33.25
TODAY'S FEE	145.05
AMOUNT REC'D/CO-PAY	⊖
BALANCE	178.30

Figure 12–23

TAX ID #3664021CC
Medicaid #HSC12345F

College Clinic
4567 Broad Avenue
Woodlands Hills, XY
12345-0001
Tel (555) 486-9002
Fax (555) 487-8976

Doctors No. _____

☐ PRIVATE   ☐ MANAGED CARE   ☐ MEDICAID   ☒ MEDICARE   ☐ TRICARE   ☐ W/C

ACCOUNT #	PATIENT'S LAST NAME	FIRST	INITIAL	TODAY'S DATE
009	Helms,	Clinton	A.	10/8/2007

ASSIGNMENT: I hereby assign payment directly to College Clinic of the surgical and/or medical benefits, if any, otherwise payable to me for his/her services as described below.
SIGNED (Patient, or Parent, if Minor)   *Clinton A. Helms*   DATE: *10/8/2007*

✓	DESCRIPTION	CPT-4/MD	FEE	✓	DESCRIPTION	CPT-4/MD	FEE	✓	DESCRIPTION	CPT-4/MD	FEE
	OFFICE VISIT-NEW PATIENT				**WELL BABY EXAM**				**LABORATORY**		
	Level 1	99201			Intial	99381			Glucose Blood	82962	
	Level 2	99202			Periodic	99391			Heamatocrit	85013	
	Level 3	99203			**OFFICE PROCEDURES**				Occult Blood	82270	
	Level 4	99204			Anscopy	46600			Urine Dip	81000	
	Level 5	99205			ECG 24-hr	93224			**X-RAY**		
	OFFICE VISIT-ESTAB, PATIENT				Fracture Rpr Foot	28470			Foot - 2 View	73620	
	Level 1	99211			I & D	10060			Forearm - 2 View	73090	
	Level 2	99212			Suture Repair				Nasal Bone - 3	70160	
	Level 3	99213		✓	laryngoscopy	31575	138.48		Spine LS - 2 view	72100	
	Level 4	99214			**INJECTIONS/VACCINATIONS**						
	Level 5	99215			DPT	90701			**MISCELLANEOUS**		
	OFFICE CONSULT-NP/EST				IM-Antibiotic	90788			Handling of Spec	99000	
	Level 3	99243			OPU-Poliovirus	90712			Supply	99070	
	Level 4	99244			Tetanus	90703			Venipuncture	36415	
	Level 5	99245									

COMMENTS:

Physician: *Concha Antrum, M.D.*

RETURN APPOINTMENT

_____ Week(s)   _____ Month(s)

DIAGNOSIS:	DESCRIPTION	CODE
Primary:	dysphonia hoarseness	784.49
Secondary:	other disease of vocal cords	478.5

REC'D BY:
☐ BANK CARD
☐ CASH
☐ CHECK
_____

PREVIOUS BALANCE	178.30
TODAY'S FEE	138.48
AMOUNT REC'D/CO-PAY	⊖
BALANCE	316.78

Figure 12–24

College Clinic

Doctor's Daily Schedule

Physician : *Concha Antrum, M.D.*   **Hospital:** *College Hospital*

Date: *10/15/2007*

Patient Name	Room No.	DX Code	CPT Code & Description of Service
Clinton A. Helms	450	784.49	31541 Laryngoscopy with
		478.5	operating microscopy $428.33

Figure 12–25

TAX ID #3664021CC
Medicaid #HSC12345F

College Clinic

4567 Broad Avenue
Woodlands Hills, XY
12345-0001
Tel (555) 486-9002
Fax (555) 487-8976

Doctors No. _____

☒ PRIVATE   ☐ MANAGED CARE   ☐ MEDICAID   ☒ MEDICARE   ☐ TRICARE   ☐ W/C

ACCOUNT # 009	PATIENT'S LAST NAME *Helms,*	FIRST *Clinton*	INITIAL *A.*	TODAY'S DATE *10/22/2007*

ASSIGNMENT: I hereby assign payment directly to College Clinic of the surgical and/or medical benefits, if any, otherwise
payable to me for his/her services as described below.
SIGNED (Patient, or Parent, if Minor)   *Clinton A. Helms*   DATE: *10/22/2007*

✓	DESCRIPTION	CPT-4/MD	FEE	✓	DESCRIPTION	CPT-4/MD	FEE	✓	DESCRIPTION	CPT-4/MD	FEE
	OFFICE VISIT-NEW PATIENT				**WELL BABY EXAM**				**LABORATORY**		
	Level 1	99201			Intial	99381			Glucose Blood	82962	
	Level 2	99202			Periodic	99391			Heamatocrit	85013	
	Level 3	99203			**OFFICE PROCEDURES**				Occult Blood	82270	
	Level 4	99204			Anscopy	46600			Urine Dip	81000	
	Level 5	99205			ECG 24-hr	93224			**X-RAY**		
	OFFICE VISIT-ESTAB, PATIENT				Fracture Rpr Foot	28470			Foot - 2 View	73620	
	Level 1	99211			I & D	10060			Forearm - 2 View	73090	
✓	Level 2	99212	28.55		Suture Repair				Nasal Bone - 3	70160	
	Level 3	99213							Spine LS - 2 view	72100	
	Level 4	99214			**INJECTIONS/VACCINATIONS**						
	Level 5	99215			DPT	90701			**MISCELLANEOUS**		
	OFFICE CONSULT-NP/EST				IM-Antibiotic	90788			Handling of Spec	99000	
	Level 3	99243			OPU-Poliovirus	90712			Supply	99070	
	Level 4	99244			Tetanus	90703			Venipuncture	36415	
	Level 5	99245									

COMMENTS:

Physician: *Concha Antrum, M.D.*

RETURN APPOINTMENT
                    PRN
__/__ Week(s)   _____ Month(s)

DIAGNOSIS: DESCRIPTION   CODE
Primary: *dysphonia hoarseness*   *784.49*
Secondary: *other disease of*
            vocal cords   *478.5*

REC'D BY:
☐ BANK CARD
☐ CASH
☐ CHECK
_____

PREVIOUS BALANCE   *745.11*
TODAY'S FEE   *28.55*
AMOUNT REC'D/CO-PAY
BALANCE   *773.66*

Figure 12–26

ASSIGNMENT 12–13 ▸ TRANSMIT AN ELECTRONIC INSURANCE CLAIM FOR A MEDICARE AND MEDICAID CASE

e hint Follow the General Instructions for TRANSMISSION OF AN ELECTRONIC CLAIM (A SINGLE CLAIM) as given in Chapter 8.

Performance Objective

Task: Transmit an electronic insurance claim form and post the information to the patient's financial account record.

Conditions: Use Brianna G. Moreno's encounter form (Figure 12–27), patient's electronic data, and computer.

Standards: Productivity Measurement

                Time: _____ minutes

                Accuracy: _____

                (Note: The time element and accuracy criteria may be given by your instructor.)

Directions:

1. Electronically prepare an insurance claim form by referring to Brianna G. Moreno's encounter form in the *Workbook* and her electronic personal and medical data. Follow the step-by-step general directions for transmission of an insurance claim.

2. Enter the patient's data into the software to obtain the procedural and diagnostic codes and College Clinic fee amounts.

3. Transmit the insurance claim to Medicare Health Systems Corporation.

4. Print a hard copy of the insurance claim to hand in to your instructor to receive a score.

5. A Performance Evaluation Checklist may be reproduced from the "Instruction Guide to the Workbook" chapter if your instructor wishes you to submit it to assist with scoring and comments.

After the instructor has returned your work to you, either make the necessary corrections and place your work in a three-ring notebook for future reference or, if you received a high score, place it in your portfolio for reference when applying for a job.

TAX ID #3664021CC
Medicaid #HSC12345F

College Clinic
4567 Broad Avenue
Woodlands Hills, XY
12345-0001
Tel (555) 486-9002
Fax (555) 487-8976

Doctors No. _____

☒ PRIVATE ☐ MANAGED CARE ☐ MEDICAID ☒ MEDICARE ☐ TRICARE ☐ W/C

ACCOUNT #	PATIENT'S LAST NAME	FIRST	INITIAL	TODAY'S DATE
010	Moreno	Brianna.	G.	11/16/2007

ASSIGNMENT: I hereby assign payment directly to College Clinic of the surgical and/or medical benefits, if any, otherwise payable to me for his/her services as described below.
SIGNED (Patient, or Parent, if Minor) *Brianna G. Moreno*   DATE: *11/16/2007*

✓	DESCRIPTION	CPT-4/MD	FEE	✓	DESCRIPTION	CPT-4/MD	FEE	✓	DESCRIPTION	CPT-4/MD	FEE
	OFFICE VISIT-NEW PATIENT				**WELL BABY EXAM**				**LABORATORY**		
	Level 1	99201			Intial	99381		✓	Glucose *Quantitative*	82947	15.00
	Level 2	99202			Periodic	99391			Heamatocrit	85013	
	Level 3	99203			**OFFICE PROCEDURES**			✓	Occult Blood	82270	4.05
	Level 4	99204			Anscopy	46600			Urine Dip	81000	
✓	Level 5	99205	132-28	✓	ECG	93000	34.26		**X-RAY**		
	OFFICE VISIT-ESTAB, PATIENT				Fracture Rpr Foot	28470			Foot - 2 View	73620	
	Level 1	99211			I & D	10060			Forearm - 2 View	73090	
	Level 2	99212			Suture Repair				Nasal Bone - 3	70160	
	Level 3	99213							Spine LS - 2 view	72100	
	Level 4	99214			**INJECTIONS/VACCINATIONS**						
	Level 5	99215			DPT	90701			**MISCELLANEOUS**		
	OFFICE CONSULT-NP/EST				IM-Antibiotic	90788			Handling of Spec	99000	
	Level 3	99243			OPU-Poliovirus	90712			Supply	99070	
	Level 4	99244			Tetanus	90703			Venipuncture	36415	
	Level 5	99245						✓	TB skin test	86580	11.34

COMMENTS:

Physician: *Perry Cardi, M.D.*

RETURN APPOINTMENT *3 days*
____ Week(s) ____ Month(s)

DIAGNOSIS:
DESCRIPTION / CODE
Primary: *diabetes mellitus type II* 250.00
Secondary: *Abnormal ECG* 794.31
Cough 786.2
Abnormal feces 787.7

REC'D BY:
☐ BANK CARD
☐ CASH
☐ CHECK
_____

PREVIOUS BALANCE -0-
TODAY'S FEE 196.93
AMOUNT REC'D/CO-PAY ⊖
BALANCE 196.93

Figure 12–27

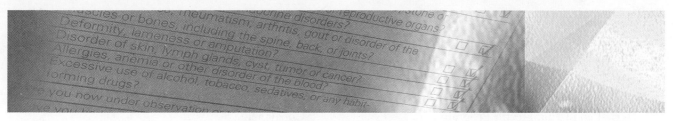

Medicaid and Other State Programs

KEY TERMS

Your instructor may wish to select some specific words pertinent to this chapter for a test. For definitions of the terms, further study, and/or reference, the words, phrases, and abbreviations may be found in the glossary at the end of the Handbook. *Key terms for this chapter follow.*

categorically needy

covered services

Early and Periodic Screening, Diagnosis, and Treatment (EPSDT)

fiscal agent

Maternal and Child Health Program (MCHP)

Medicaid (MCD)

Medi-Cal

medically needy (MN)

prior approval

recipient

share of cost

State Children's Health Insurance Program (SCHIP)

Supplemental Security Income (SSI)

PERFORMANCE OBJECTIVES

The student will be able to:

- Define and spell the key terms for this chapter, given the information from the *Handbook* glossary, within a reasonable time period and with enough accuracy to obtain a satisfactory evaluation.
- After reading the chapter, answer the self-study review questions with enough accuracy to obtain a satisfactory evaluation.
- Fill in the correct meaning of each abbreviation, given a list of common medical abbreviations and symbols that appear in chart notes, within a reasonable time period and with enough accuracy to obtain a satisfactory evaluation.

- Given the patient's medical chart notes, ledger cards, and blank insurance claim forms, complete each CMS-1500 Health Insurance Claim Form for billing within a reasonable time period and with enough accuracy to obtain a satisfactory evaluation.
- Correctly post payments, adjustments, and balances on the patient's ledger cards, using the Mock Fee Schedule in Appendix A in this *Workbook*, within a reasonable time period and with enough accuracy to obtain a satisfactory evaluation.

STUDY OUTLINE

History

Medicaid Programs
Maternal and Child Health Program
Low-Income Medicare Recipients

Medicaid Eligibility
Verifying Eligibility
Categorically Needy
Medically Needy

Maternal and Child Health Program Eligibility
Accepting Medicaid Patients
Identification Card
Point-of-Service Machine
Retroactive Eligibility

Medicaid Benefits
Covered Services
Disallowed Services

Medicaid Managed Care

Claim Procedure
Copayment
Prior Approval
Time Limit
Reciprocity
Claim Form

After Claim Submission
Remittance Advice
Appeals

Medicaid Fraud Control

SELF-STUDY 13–1 ► REVIEW QUESTIONS*

Review the objectives, key terms, glossary definitions of key terms, chapter information, and figures before completing the following review questions.

1. Medicaid is administered by _____ with partial _____ funding.

2. Medicaid is not an insurance program. It is a/an _____ program.

3. In all other states the program is known as Medicaid, but in California the program

   is called _____ .

4. Because the federal government sets minimum requirements, states are free to enhance the Medicaid program. Name two ways in which Medicaid programs vary from state to state.

   a. _____

   b. _____

5. SCHIP means _____

   and MCHP means _____

   and covers children of what age group? _____

---

*Review questions for Medi-Cal are provided in Appendix B in this *Workbook*.

6. What people might be eligible for Medicaid?

   a. _____

   b. _____

   c. _____

   d. _____

   e. _____

7. Name two broad classifications of people eligible for Medicaid assistance.

   a. _____

   b. _____

8. When professional services are rendered, the Medicaid identification card or electronic verification must show eligibility for (circle one)

   a. day of service   b. year of service

   c. month of service   d. week of service

9. The name of the program for the prevention, early detection, and treatment of

   conditions of children receiving welfare is known as _____.

   It is abbreviated as _____.

10. Define the following abbreviations.

    a. MCD _____

    b. SSI _____

    c. AFDC _____

    d. MI _____

11. Your Medicaid patient seen today needs long-term hemodialysis services. You telephone for authorization to get verbal approval. Four important items to obtain are:

    a. _____

    b. _____

    c. _____

    d. _____

12. The time limit for submitting a Medicaid claim varies from _____

    to _____ from the date the service is rendered. In your state,

    the time limit is _____.

13. The insurance claim form for submitting Medicaid claims in all states is

_____.

14. Your Medicaid patient also has TRICARE. What billing procedure do you follow?
Be exact in your steps for a dependent of an active military person.

a. _____

b. _____

15. When a Medicaid patient is injured in an automobile accident and the car has
liability insurance, the insurance claim is sent to the (circle one)

a. Patient

b. Automobile insurance carrier

c. Medicaid fiscal agent

16. Five categories of adjudicated claims that may appear on a Medicaid remittance
advice document are:

a. _____

b. _____

c. _____

d. _____

e. _____

17. Name three levels of Medicaid appeals.

a. _____

b. _____

c. _____

To check your answers to this self-study assignment, see Appendix D.

ASSIGNMENT **13-2** ▸ *CRITICAL THINKING*

Performance Objective

Task: After reading the scenario, answer questions, using critical thinking skills.

Conditions: Use a pen or pencil.

Standards: Time: _____ minutes

                    Accuracy: _____

                    (Note: The time element and accuracy criteria may be given by your instructor.)

Directions: After reading the scenario, answer questions, using your critical thinking skills. Record your answers on the blank lines.

Scenario: Mrs. Ho suddenly experiences a pain in her right lower abdominal area and rushes to a local hospital for emergency care. Laboratory work verifies that she has a ruptured appendix, and immediate surgery is recommended. Is prior authorization required in a bonafide emergency

situation like this? _____

Which two blocks on the CMS-1500 claim form need to be completed for emergency

services? _____

ASSIGNMENT **13-3** ▶ **COMPLETE A CLAIM FORM FOR A MEDICAID CASE**

Performance Objective

Task: Complete a CMS-1500 claim form, post transactions to the financial accounting record, and define patient record abbreviations.

Conditions: Use the patient's record (Figure 13–1) and financial statement (Figure 13–2), one health insurance claim form (Figure 13–3), a typewriter or computer, procedural and diagnostic code books, and Appendices A and B in this *Workbook*.

Standards: Claim Productivity Measurement

Time: _____ minutes

Accuracy: _____

(Note: The time element and accuracy criteria may be given by your instructor.)

Directions:

1. Using OCR guidelines, complete the Health Insurance Claim Form and direct it to Medicaid for Rose Clarkson by referring to her patient record. Date the claim September 6. Refer to Appendix A in this *Workbook* to locate the fees to record on the claim and post them to the financial statement. Obtain the address of your Medicaid fiscal agent by going to the Web site listed in Internet Resources at the end of Chapter 13 in the Handbook. To complete the CMS-1500 Claim Form for the Medi-Cal program, see Appendix C in this *Workbook*.

2. Refer to Chapter 7 (Figure 7–8) in the *Handbook* for instructions on how to complete this claim form and a Medicaid template.

3. Use your *Current Procedural Terminology* (CPT) code book or Appendix A in this *Workbook* to determine the correct five-digit code number and modifiers for each professional service rendered. Use your Healthcare Common Procedure Coding System (HCPCS) Level II code book or refer to Appendix B in this *Workbook* for HCPCS procedure codes and modifiers.

4. Record all transactions on the financial account, and indicate the date when you have billed Medicaid.

5. Refer to Appendix A in this *Workbook* for the clinic and hospital provider numbers that are needed for completing Medicaid forms.

6. A Performance Evaluation Checklist may be reproduced from the "Instruction Guide to the Workbook" chapter if your instructor wishes you to submit it to assist with scoring and comments.

Text continued on p. 371.

PATIENT RECORD NO. 13-3

Clarkson	Rose		03-09-44	F	555-487-2209
LAST NAME	FIRST NAME	MIDDLE NAME	BIRTH DATE	SEX	HOME PHONE

3408 Jackson Street	Hempstead	XY	11551-0300
ADDRESS	CITY	STATE	ZIP CODE

	555-340-2200		
CELL PHONE	PAGER NO.	FAX NO.	E-MAIL ADDRESS

030-XX-9543	R3207897
PATIENT'S SOC. SEC. NO.	DRIVER'S LICENSE

unemployed	
PATIENT'S OCCUPATION	NAME OF COMPANY

ADDRESS OF EMPLOYER	PHONE

SPOUSE OR PARENT	OCCUPATION

EMPLOYER	ADDRESS	PHONE

Medicaid	self
NAME OF INSURANCE	INSURED OR SUBSCRIBER

CC99756329346X	
MEDICAID NO.	GROUP NO.

REFERRED BY: James Jackson, MD, 100 North Main Street, Hempstead, XY 11551   NPI# 72011337XX

DATE	PROGRESS NOTES
9-4-xx	New pt presents complaining of cough & SOB. A detailed hx was taken which revealed
	mitral valve prolapse. A D exam was done indicating elevated cardiac and respiratory rates,
	diminished breath sounds, distended neck veins, and edema of both ankles. 12 lead ECG
	performed; normal sinus rhythm and elevated heart rate. Echocardiogram done
	(2D, complete with Doppler) to evaluate mitral valve, cardiac chamber size, and ventricular
	function; presence of mitral valve regurgitation. Single view chest x-ray indicated presence
	of fluid in lungs. Primary diagnosis: congestive heart disease and mitral valve prolapse
	(LC MDM). Pt given Rx for diuretic, digitalis, and vasodilator. Restrict fluid and sodium
	intake. Retn in 2 wks.
	PC/llf *Perry Cardi, MD*

Figure 13–1

Acct No. __13-3__

STATEMENT
Financial Account
COLLEGE CLINIC
4567 Broad Avenue
Woodland Hills, XY 12345-0001
Tel. 555-486-9002
Fax No. 555-487-8976

Rose Clarkson
3408 Jackson Street
Hempstead, XY 11551-0300

Phone No. (H) ___(555) 487-2209___ (W) _____   Birthdate ___3-9-44___

Primary Insurance Co. ___Medicaid_____   Policy/Group No. ___C99756E___

Secondary Insurance Co. ___None_____   Policy/Group No. _____

DATE	REFERENCE	DESCRIPTION	CHARGES	CREDITS PYMNTS.	ADJ.	BALANCE	
20xx			BALANCE FORWARD ➤				
9-4-xx		OV NP					
9-4-xx		12 lead ECG					
9-4-xx		Echocardiogram					
9-4-xx		Doppler echo					
9-4-xx		Chest x-ray					

PLEASE PAY LAST AMOUNT IN BALANCE COLUMN ⬆

THIS IS A COPY OF YOUR FINANCIAL ACCOUNT AS IT APPEARS ON OUR RECORDS

Figure 13–2

PLEASE
DO NOT
STAPLE
IN THIS
AREA

CARRIER

| | PICA | | | | | | | | HEALTH INSURANCE CLAIM FORM | PICA | |

| 1. MEDICARE | MEDICAID | CHAMPUS | CHAMPVA | GROUP HEALTH PLAN | FECA BLK LUNG | OTHER | 1a. INSURED'S I.D. NUMBER | (FOR PROGRAM IN ITEM 1) |
| (Medicare #) | (Medicaid #) | (Sponsor's SSN) | (VA File #) | (SSN or ID) | (S SN) | (ID) | | |

2. PATIENT'S NAME (Last Name, First Name, Middle Initial)

3. PATIENT'S BIRTH DATE MM DD YY SEX M F

4. INSURED'S NAME (Last Name, First Name, Middle Initial)

5. PATIENT'S ADDRESS (No., Street)

6. PATIENT RELATIONSHIP TO INSURED Self Spouse Child Other

7. INSURED'S ADDRESS (No., Street)

CITY STATE

8. PATIENT STATUS Single Married Other

Employed Full-Time Student Part-Time Student

CITY STATE

ZIP CODE TELEPHONE (Include Area Code) ( )

ZIP CODE TELEPHONE (INCLUDE AREA CODE)

9. OTHER INSURED'S NAME (Last Name, First Name, Middle Initial)

10. IS PATIENT'S CONDITION RELATED TO:

11. INSURED'S POLICY GROUP OR FECA NUMBER

a. OTHER INSURED'S POLICY OR GROUP NUMBER

a. EMPLOYMENT? (CURRENT OR PREVIOUS) YES NO

a. INSURED'S DATE OF BIRTH MM DD YY SEX M F

b. OTHER INSURED'S DATE OF BIRTH MM DD YY SEX M F

b. AUTO ACCIDENT? PLACE (State) YES NO

b. EMPLOYER'S NAME OR SCHOOL NAME

c. EMPLOYER'S NAME OR SCHOOL NAME

c. OTHER ACCIDENT? YES NO

c. INSURANCE PLAN NAME OR PROGRAM NAME

d. INSURANCE PLAN NAME OR PROGRAM NAME

10d. RESERVED FOR LOCAL USE

d. IS THERE ANOTHER HEALTH BENEFIT PLAN? YES NO *If yes*, return to and complete item 9 a-d.

READ BACK OF FORM BEFORE COMPLETING & SIGNING THIS FORM.
12. PATIENT'S OR AUTHORIZED PERSON'S SIGNATURE I authorize the release of any medical or other information necessary to process this claim. I also request payment of government benefits either to myself or to the party who accepts assignment below.

SIGNED _____ DATE _____

13. INSURED'S OR AUTHORIZED PERSON'S SIGNATURE I authorize payment of medical benefits to the undersigned physician or supplier for services described below.

SIGNED _____

14. DATE OF CURRENT: ILLNESS (First symptom) OR INJURY (Accident) OR PREGNANCY(LMP) MM DD YY

15. IF PATIENT HAS HAD SAME OR SIMILAR ILLNESS. GIVE FIRST DATE MM DD YY

16. DATES PATIENT UNABLE TO WORK IN CURRENT OCCUPATION FROM MM DD YY TO MM DD YY

17. NAME OF REFERRING PHYSICIAN OR OTHER SOURCE

17a. I.D. NUMBER OF REFERRING PHYSICIAN

18. HOSPITALIZATION DATES RELATED TO CURRENT SERVICES FROM MM DD YY TO MM DD YY

19. RESERVED FOR LOCAL USE

20. OUTSIDE LAB? YES NO $ CHARGES

21. DIAGNOSIS OR NATURE OF ILLNESS OR INJURY. (RELATE ITEMS 1,2,3 OR 4 TO ITEM 24E BY LINE)

1. _____ 3. _____

2. _____ 4. _____

22. MEDICAID RESUBMISSION CODE ORIGINAL REF. NO.

23. PRIOR AUTHORIZATION NUMBER

24. A						B	C	D		E	F	G	H	I	J	K
	DATE(S) OF SERVICE					Place of Service	Type of Service	PROCEDURES, SERVICES, OR SUPPLIES (Explain Unusual Circumstances)		DIAGNOSIS CODE	$ CHARGES	DAYS OR UNITS	EPSDT Family Plan	EMG	COB	RESERVED FOR LOCAL USE
From			To					CPT/HCPCS	MODIFIER							
MM	DD	YY	MM	DD	YY											
1																
2																
3																
4																
5																
6																

25. FEDERAL TAX I.D. NUMBER SSN EIN

26. PATIENT'S ACCOUNT NO.

27. ACCEPT ASSIGNMENT? (For govt. claims, see back) YES NO

28. TOTAL CHARGE $

29. AMOUNT PAID $

30. BALANCE DUE $

31. SIGNATURE OF PHYSICIAN OR SUPPLIER INCLUDING DEGREES OR CREDENTIALS (I certify that the statements on the reverse apply to this bill and are made a part thereof.)

SIGNED _____ DATE _____

32. NAME AND ADDRESS OF FACILITY WHERE SERVICES WERE RENDERED (If other than home or office)

33. PHYSICIAN'S, SUPPLIER'S BILLING NAME, ADDRESS, ZIP CODE & PHONE #

PIN# GRP#

PATIENT AND INSURED INFORMATION

PHYSICIAN OR SUPPLIER INFORMATION

(APPROVED BY AMA COUNCIL ON MEDICAL SERVICE 8/88)   **PLEASE PRINT OR TYPE**   APPROVED OMB-0938-0008 FORM CMS-1500 (12-90), FORM RRB-1500, APPROVED OMB-1215-0055 FORM OWCP-1500, APPROVED OMB-0720-0001 (CHAMPUS)

Figure 13–3

After the instructor has returned your work to you, either make the necessary corrections and place your work in a three-ring notebook for future reference or, if you received a high score, place it in your portfolio for reference when applying for a job.

Abbreviations pertinent to this record:

Pt   _____   LC   _____

SOB   _____   MDM   _____

hx   _____   Rx   _____

D   _____   retn   _____

ECG _____   wks   _____

Checklist

1. Locate a financial accounting record (ledger).   _____

   Note: Refer to the step-by-step procedures at the end of Chapter 3 in the *Handbook* and graphic examples Figures 3–18, 10–2, and 12–15.   _____

2. Insert the patient's name and address, including ZIP code in the box.   _____

3. Enter the patient's personal data.   _____

4. Ledger lines: Insert date of service (DOS), reference (CPT code number, check number, or dates of service for posting adjustments or when insurance was billed), description of the transaction, charge amounts, payments, adjustments, and running current balance. The posting date is the actual date the transaction is recorded. If the DOS differs from the posting date, list the DOS in the reference or description column.   _____

   Line 2:   _____

   Line 3:   _____

   Line 4:   _____

   Line 5:   _____

   Line 6:   _____

   Line 7:   _____

Note: A good bookkeeping practice is to take a red pen and draw a line across the financial accounting record (ledger) from left to right to indicate the last entry billed to the insurance company.

ASSIGNMENT 13-4 ▸ COMPLETE A CLAIM FORM FOR A MEDICAID CASE

Performance Objective

Task: Complete a CMS-1500 claim form for a Medicaid case, post
             transactions to the financial accounting record, and define patient record
             abbreviations.

Conditions: Use the patient's record (Figure 13–4) and financial statement
             (Figure 13–5), one health insurance claim form (Figure 13–6),
             a typewriter or computer, procedural and diagnostic code books,
             and Appendices A and B in this *Workbook*.

Standards: Claim Productivity Measurement

             Time: _____ minutes

             Accuracy: _____

             (Note: The time element and accuracy criteria may be given by your
             instructor.)

Directions:

1. Using OCR guidelines, complete the Health Insurance Claim Form and direct it to
   Medicaid for Stephen M. Drake by referring to his patient record. Refer to Appendix A
   in this *Workbook* to locate the fees to record on the claim, and post them to the financial
   statement. On May 1, the fee for the injection of Bicillin is $10. Date the claim
   May 26. Obtain the address of your Medicaid fiscal agent by going to the Web site
   listed in Internet Resources at the end of Chapter 13 in the *Handbook*. To complete the
   CMS-1500 claim form for the Medi-Cal program, see Appendix C in the *Handbook*.

   Do not list services not charged for (NC) on the claim form; however, do list postoperative follow-up visits during the global period on the financial statement. Locate the
   correct code number in the CPT Medicine section.

   Remember that the physician must always sign all forms on Medicaid cases; stamped
   signatures are not allowed.

2. Refer to Chapter 7 (Figure 7–8) in the *Handbook* for instructions on how to complete
   this claim form and a Medicaid template.

3. Use your CPT code book or Appendix A in this *Workbook* to determine the correct
   five-digit code number and modifiers for each professional service rendered. Use your
   HCPCS Level II code book or refer to Appendix B in this Workbook for HCPCS
   procedure codes and modifiers.

4. Record all transactions of the financial account and indicate the date when you have
   billed Medicaid.

5. Refer to Appendix A in this *Workbook* for the clinic and hospital provider numbers that
   are needed for completing Medicaid forms.

PATIENT RECORD NO. 13-4

Drake	Stephen	M	04-03-91	M	555-277-5831
LAST NAME	FIRST NAME	MIDDLE NAME	BIRTH DATE	SEX	HOME PHONE

2317 Charnwood Avenue	Woodland Hills	XY	12345
ADDRESS	CITY	STATE	ZIP CODE

CELL PHONE	PAGER NO.	FAX NO.	E-MAIL ADDRESS

566-XX-0081	
PATIENT'S SOC. SEC. NO.	DRIVER'S LICENSE

full time student	
PATIENT'S OCCUPATION	NAME OF COMPANY

ADDRESS OF EMPLOYER   PHONE

Mrs. Virginia B. Drake (mother)	none-family on welfare
SPOUSE OR PARENT	OCCUPATION

EMPLOYER ADDRESS	PHONE

Medicaid	
NAME OF INSURANCE	INSURED OR SUBSCRIBER

Child's identification number	19-37-1524033-16X
POLICY/CERTIFICATE NO.	GROUP NO.

REFERRED BY: James B. Jeffers, MD, 100 S. Broadway, Woodland Hills, XY 12345   Provider No. 12345069XX

DATE	PROGRESS NOTES
5-1-xx	NP comes in complaining of severe sore throat since April 4. A detailed hx was taken.
	Mother states Stephen has had many bouts of tonsillitis since age 4. He has missed
	school on three occasions this year due to throat infections. Did complete phys exam (D)
	which showed enlargement & inflam of tonsils. Temp 101.2. Strep culture done
	(screening) with a preliminary report; positive for strep. Administered penicillin G (Bicillin)
	1.2 million units IM and wrote Rx to start AB and continue x 10 d. Imp: Acute tonsillitis
	(LC MDM). RTO 1 week.
	GP/llf *Gerald Practon, MD*
5-8-xx	Pt returns; sore throat improved but still swollen. Tonsils are 4+ hypertrophic. Received
	medical records from past primary physician which indicated hx of 5 bouts of strep over
	last 3 yrs. Adv. tonsillectomy and adenoidectomy. Phoned for prior authorization 3 p.m.,
	Auth. No. 45042, given by Mrs. Jane Michaels. Pt to be admitted tomorrow for one day
	surgery (PF HX/PX SF MDM).
	GP/llf *Gerald Practon, MD*
5-9-xx	Admit to College Hospital. Tonsillectomy and adenoidectomy performed. Pt doing well,
	discharged 4:00 P.M. RTC 1 week.
	GP/llf *Gerald Practon, MD*
5-17-xx	PO visit. No complaints. Temp 98.1. Retn if necessary (PF HX/PX SF MDM).
	GP/llf *Gerald Practon, MD*

Figure 13–4

Acct No. __13-4__

STATEMENT
Financial Account
COLLEGE CLINIC
4567 Broad Avenue
Woodland Hills, XY 12345-0001
Tel. 555-486-9002
Fax No. 555-487-8976

Stephen M. Drake
c/o Virginia B.Drake
2317 Charnwood Avenue
Woodland Hills, XY 12345

Phone No. (H) ___(555) 277-5831___   (W) _____   Birthdate ___4-3-91___

Primary Insurance Co. ___Medicaid___   Policy/Group No. ___19-37-1524033-16X___

Secondary Insurance Co. ___N/A___   Policy/Group No. _____

DATE	REFERENCE	DESCRIPTION	CHARGES	CREDITS PYMNTS.	ADJ.	BALANCE
20xx		BALANCE FORWARD				
5-1-xx		NP OV				
5-1-xx		Strep culture				
5-1-xx		Injection AB				
5-1-xx		Bicillin				
5-8-xx		OV				
5-9-xx		T & A				
5-17-xx		PO OV				

PLEASE PAY LAST AMOUNT IN BALANCE COLUMN

THIS IS A COPY OF YOUR FINANCIAL ACCOUNT AS IT APPEARS ON OUR RECORDS

Figure 13–5

PLEASE
DO NOT
STAPLE
IN THIS
AREA

CARRIER

HEALTH INSURANCE CLAIM FORM

PICA   PICA

1. MEDICARE	MEDICAID	CHAMPUS	CHAMPVA	GROUP HEALTH PLAN	FECA BLK LUNG	OTHER	1a. INSURED'S I.D. NUMBER (FOR PROGRAM IN ITEM 1)
☐ (Medicare #)	☐ (Medicaid #)	☐ (Sponsor's SSN)	☐ (VA File #)	☐ (SSN or ID)	☐ (S SN)	☐ (ID)	

2. PATIENT'S NAME (Last Name, First Name, Middle Initial)

3. PATIENT'S BIRTH DATE
MM   DD   YY   SEX   M ☐   F ☐

4. INSURED'S NAME (Last Name, First Name, Middle Initial)

5. PATIENT'S ADDRESS (No., Street)

6. PATIENT RELATIONSHIP TO INSURED
Self ☐   Spouse ☐   Child ☐   Other ☐

7. INSURED'S ADDRESS (No., Street)

CITY   STATE

8. PATIENT STATUS
Single ☐   Married ☐   Other ☐
Employed ☐   Full-Time Student ☐   Part-Time Student ☐

CITY   STATE

ZIP CODE   TELEPHONE (Include Area Code)
)

ZIP CODE   TELEPHONE (INCLUDE AREA CODE)

9. OTHER INSURED'S NAME (Last Name, First Name, Middle Initial)

10. IS PATIENT'S CONDITION RELATED TO:

11. INSURED'S POLICY GROUP OR FECA NUMBER

a. OTHER INSURED'S POLICY OR GROUP NUMBER

a. EMPLOYMENT? (CURRENT OR PREVIOUS)
☐ YES   ☐ NO

a. INSURED'S DATE OF BIRTH
MM   DD   YY   SEX   M ☐   F ☐

b. OTHER INSURED'S DATE OF BIRTH
MM   DD   YY   SEX   M ☐   F ☐

b. AUTO ACCIDENT?   PLACE (State)
☐ YES   ☐ NO

b. EMPLOYER'S NAME OR SCHOOL NAME

c. EMPLOYER'S NAME OR SCHOOL NAME

c. OTHER ACCIDENT?
☐ YES   ☐ NO

c. INSURANCE PLAN NAME OR PROGRAM NAME

d. INSURANCE PLAN NAME OR PROGRAM NAME

10d. RESERVED FOR LOCAL USE

d. IS THERE ANOTHER HEALTH BENEFIT PLAN?
☐ YES   ☐ NO   **If yes**, return to and complete item 9 a-d.

PATIENT AND INSURED INFORMATION

READ BACK OF FORM BEFORE COMPLETING & SIGNING THIS FORM.
12. PATIENT'S OR AUTHORIZED PERSON'S SIGNATURE I authorize the release of any medical or other information necessary to process this claim. I also request payment of government benefits either to myself or to the party who accepts assignment below.

SIGNED _____ DATE _____

13. INSURED'S OR AUTHORIZED PERSON'S SIGNATURE I authorize payment of medical benefits to the undersigned physician or supplier for services described below.

SIGNED _____

14. DATE OF CURRENT:
MM   DD   YY   ◀ ILLNESS (First symptom) OR INJURY (Accident) OR PREGNANCY(LMP)

15. IF PATIENT HAS HAD SAME OR SIMILAR ILLNESS. GIVE FIRST DATE   MM   DD   YY

16. DATES PATIENT UNABLE TO WORK IN CURRENT OCCUPATION
MM   DD   YY   MM   DD   YY
FROM _____ TO _____

17. NAME OF REFERRING PHYSICIAN OR OTHER SOURCE

17a. I.D. NUMBER OF REFERRING PHYSICIAN

18. HOSPITALIZATION DATES RELATED TO CURRENT SERVICES
MM   DD   YY   MM   DD   YY
FROM _____ TO _____

19. RESERVED FOR LOCAL USE

20. OUTSIDE LAB? $ CHARGES
☐ YES   ☐ NO

21. DIAGNOSIS OR NATURE OF ILLNESS OR INJURY. (RELATE ITEMS 1,2,3 OR 4 TO ITEM 24E BY LINE)

1. |_____
2. |_____
3. |_____
4. |_____

22. MEDICAID RESUBMISSION CODE   ORIGINAL REF. NO.

23. PRIOR AUTHORIZATION NUMBER

EXAMPLE ONLY

24. A DATE(S) OF SERVICE						B Place of Service	C Type of Service	D PROCEDURES, SERVICES, OR SUPPLIES (Explain Unusual Circumstances) CPT/HCPCS MODIFIER	E DIAGNOSIS CODE	F $ CHARGES	G DAYS OR UNITS	H EPSDT Family Plan	I EMG	J COB	K RESERVED FOR LOCAL USE
From MM	DD	YY	To MM	DD	YY										
1															
2															
3															
4															
5															
6															

25. FEDERAL TAX I.D. NUMBER   SSN ☐ EIN ☐

26. PATIENT'S ACCOUNT NO.

27. ACCEPT ASSIGNMENT? (For govt. claims, see back)
☐ YES   ☐ NO

28. TOTAL CHARGE $

29. AMOUNT PAID $

30. BALANCE DUE $

31. SIGNATURE OF PHYSICIAN OR SUPPLIER INCLUDING DEGREES OR CREDENTIALS (I certify that the statements on the reverse apply to this bill and are made a part thereof.)

SIGNED _____ DATE _____

32. NAME AND ADDRESS OF FACILITY WHERE SERVICES WERE RENDERED (If other than home or office)

33. PHYSICIAN'S, SUPPLIER'S BILLING NAME, ADDRESS, ZIP CODE & PHONE #

PIN#   GRP#

PHYSICIAN OR SUPPLIER INFORMATION

(APPROVED BY AMA COUNCIL ON MEDICAL SERVICE 8/88)   **PLEASE PRINT OR TYPE**   APPROVED OMB-0938-0008 FORM CMS-1500 (12-90),   FORM RRB-1500,
APPROVED OMB-1215-0055 FORM OWCP-1500,   APPROVED OMB-0720-0001 (CHAMPUS)

Figure 13–6

6. On July 1, Medicaid paid $200 on this claim. Post this payment (warrant number 766504) to the patient's financial account and adjust the balance, using the same line.

7. A Performance Evaluation Checklist may be reproduced from the "Instruction Guide to the Workbook" chapter if your instructor wishes you to submit it to assist with scoring and comments.

    After the instructor has returned your work to you, either make the necessary corrections and place your work in a three-ring notebook for future reference or, if you received a high score, place it in your portfolio for reference when applying for a job.

Abbreviations pertinent to this record:

NP	_____	imp	_____
hx	_____	LC	_____
phys	_____	MDM	_____
D	_____	RTO	_____
inflam	_____	yrs	_____
temp	_____	adv	_____
strep	_____	PF	_____
IM	_____	SF	_____
Rx	_____	RTC	_____
AB	_____	PO	_____
X	_____	retn	_____
d	_____		

Additional Coding

1. Using your diagnostic code book, code the symptoms that the patient presented with on May 1, 20xx.

	Symptom	*Code*
a.	_____	_____
b.	_____	_____
c.	_____	_____

2. Locate a financial accounting record (ledger).

Note: Refer to the step-by-step procedures at the end of Chapter 3 in the *Handbook* and graphic examples Figures 3–18, 10–2, and 12–15.

3. Insert the patient's name and address, including ZIP code in the box.

4. Enter the patient's personal data.

5. Ledger lines: Insert date of service (DOS), reference (CPT code number, check number, or dates of service for posting adjustments or when insurance was billed), description of the transaction, charge amounts, payments, adjustments, and running current balance. The posting date is the actual date the transaction is recorded. If the DOS differs from the posting date, list the DOS in the reference or description column.

Line 2: _____

Line 3: _____

Line 4: _____

Line 5: _____

Line 6: _____

Line 7: _____

Line 8: _____

Line 9: _____

Line 10: _____

Note: A good bookkeeping practice is to take a red pen and draw a line across the financial accounting record (ledger) from left to right to indicate the last entry billed to the insurance company.

ASSIGNMENT **13–5 ▸ COMPLETE A CLAIM FORM FOR A MEDICAID CASE**

Performance Objective

Task: Complete a CMS-1500 claim form for a Medicaid case, post transactions to the financial accounting record, and define patient record abbreviations.

Conditions: Use the patient's record (Figure 13–7) and financial statement (Figure 13–8), one health insurance claim form (Figure 13–9), a typewriter or computer, procedural and diagnostic code books, and Appendices A and B in this *Workbook*.

Standards: Claim Productivity Measurement

Time: _____ minutes

Accuracy: _____

(Note: The time element and accuracy criteria may be given by your instructor.)

Directions:

1. Using OCR guidelines, complete the Health Insurance Claim Form and direct it to Medicaid for Barry L. Brooke by referring to his patient record. Refer to Appendix A in this *Workbook* to locate the fees to record on the claim, and post them to the financial statement. The financial statement should be sent in care of (c/o) the patient's parents because he is a minor. Date the claim May 31. Obtain the address of your Medicaid fiscal agent by going to the Web site listed in Internet Resources at the end of Chapter 13 in the *Handbook*. To complete the CMS-1500 Claim Form for the Medi-Cal program, see Appendix C in this *Workbook*.

2. Refer to Chapter 7 (Figure 7–8) in the *Handbook* for instructions on how to complete this claim form and a Medicaid template.

3. Use your CPT code book or Appendix A in this *Workbook* to determine the diagnostic codes and the correct five-digit code number and modifiers for each professional service rendered. Use your HCPCS Level II code book or refer to Appendix B in this *Workbook* for HCPCS procedure codes and modifiers.

4. Record all transactions on the financial account and indicate the date when you have billed Medicaid.

5. Refer to Appendix A in this *Workbook* for the clinic and hospital provider numbers that are needed for completing Medicaid forms.

6. On July 1, Medicaid paid $75 (warrant number 329670) on this claim. Post this payment to the patient's financial statement and adjust the balance.

7. A Performance Evaluation Checklist may be reproduced from the "Instruction Guide to the Workbook" chapter if your instructor wishes you to submit it to assist with scoring and comments.

Text continued on p. 385.

PATIENT RECORD NO. 13-5

Brooke	Barry	L	02-03-90	M	555-487-9770
LAST NAME	FIRST NAME	MIDDLE NAME	BIRTH DATE	SEX	HOME PHONE

3821 Ocean Drive	Woodland Hills	XY	12345
ADDRESS	CITY	STATE	ZIP CODE

brooke@wb.net
CELL PHONE   PAGER NO.   FAX NO.   E-MAIL ADDRESS

776-XX-1931
PATIENT'S SOC. SEC. NO.   DRIVER'S LICENSE

child—full time student
PATIENT'S OCCUPATION   NAME OF COMPANY

ADDRESS OF EMPLOYER   PHONE

Robert D. Brooke (father)   none—family on welfare (father totally disabled)
SPOUSE OR PARENT   OCCUPATION

EMPLOYER   ADDRESS   PHONE

Medicaid   Barry
NAME OF INSURANCE   INSURED OR SUB SCRIBER

54-32-7681533-10X
MEDICAID NO.

REFERRED BY: Virginia B. Drake (friend)

DATE	PROGRESS NOTES
5-28-xx	Sunday evening, new pt seen in ER at College Hospital. Pt twisted L knee while playing
	baseball at Grove Park. X-rays (3 views of L knee) were ordered –N for fx. Imp: effusion
	and ligament strain lt knee. Tx: aspirated lt knee and removed 5 cc bloody fluid.
	Discussion is held with mother and son; bracing versus casting. Mother insists on a cast
	because she states he is noncompliant and thinks he will remove the brace and injure his
	leg further. Barry agrees to have cast. Applied long leg fiberglass walking cast. Pt to be
	seen in office in 2 wks (D HX/PX M MDM).
	RS/llf *Raymond Skeleton, MD*
6-10-xx	Pt returns c/o continued knee pain and wants cast removed. He is in tears and says he
	has been miserable. Mother agrees to have cast is removed; leg examined. Fitted pt with
	orthotic device for his knee (straight-leg canvas immobilizer, longitudinal, prefabricated $85).
	Ordered MRI of L knee to be done at College Hospital Radiology. Pt given directions and
	precautions regarding ambulation with brace (EPF HX/PX LC MDM). RTO 2 wks.
	RS/llf *Raymond Skeleton, MD*

Figure 13–7

Acct No. 13-5

STATEMENT
Financial Account
COLLEGE CLINIC
4567 Broad Avenue
Woodland Hills, XY 12345-0001
Tel. 555-486-9002
Fax No. 555-487-8976

Barry L Brook
c/o Robert D. Brook
3821 Ocean Drive
Woodland Hills, XY 12345

Phone No. (H) _____ (555) 487-9770 _____ (W) _____   Birthdate _____ 2-3-90 _____

Primary Insurance Co. _____ Medicaid _____   Policy/Group No. _____ 5432768153310X _____

Secondary Insurance Co. _____   Policy/Group No. _____

DATE	REFERENCE	DESCRIPTION	CHARGES	CREDITS PYMNTS.	ADJ.	BALANCE
20xx			BALANCE FORWARD ➝			
5-28-xx		ER				
5-28-xx		Aspiration L knee				
5-28-xx		Cast application				
6-10-xx		L Knee immobilizer				

PLEASE PAY LAST AMOUNT IN BALANCE COLUMN ⬆

THIS IS A COPY OF YOUR FINANCIAL ACCOUNT AS IT APPEARS ON OUR RECORDS

Figure 13–8

PLEASE
DO NOT
STAPLE
IN THIS
AREA

HEALTH INSURANCE CLAIM FORM

PICA   PICA

1. MEDICARE   MEDICAID   CHAMPUS   CHAMPVA   GROUP   FECA   OTHER   1a. INSURED'S I.D. NUMBER   (FOR PROGRAM IN ITEM 1)
   (Medicare #) (Medicaid #) (Sponsor's SSN) (VA File #) HEALTH PLAN BLK LUNG
                                                 (SSN or ID) (S SN) (ID)

2. PATIENT'S NAME (Last Name, First Name, Middle Initial)   3. PATIENT'S BIRTH DATE MM DD YY SEX M F   4. INSURED'S NAME (Last Name, First Name, Middle Initial)

5. PATIENT'S ADDRESS (No., Street)   6. PATIENT RELATIONSHIP TO INSURED Self Spouse Child Other   7. INSURED'S ADDRESS (No., Street)

CITY   STATE   8. PATIENT STATUS Single Married Other   CITY   STATE

ZIP CODE   TELEPHONE (Include Area Code)   Employed Full-Time Student Part-Time Student   ZIP CODE   TELEPHONE (INCLUDE AREA CODE)

9. OTHER INSURED'S NAME (Last Name, First Name, Middle Initial)   10. IS PATIENT'S CONDITION RELATED TO: 11. INSURED'S POLICY GROUP OR FECA NUMBER

a. OTHER INSURED'S POLICY OR GROUP NUMBER   a. EMPLOYMENT? (CURRENT OR PREVIOUS) YES NO   a. INSURED'S DATE OF BIRTH MM DD YY SEX M F

b. OTHER INSURED'S DATE OF BIRTH MM DD YY SEX M F   b. AUTO ACCIDENT? PLACE (State) YES NO   b. EMPLOYER'S NAME OR SCHOOL NAME

c. EMPLOYER'S NAME OR SCHOOL NAME   c. OTHER ACCIDENT? YES NO   c. INSURANCE PLAN NAME OR PROGRAM NAME

d. INSURANCE PLAN NAME OR PROGRAM NAME   10d. RESERVED FOR LOCAL USE   d. IS THERE ANOTHER HEALTH BENEFIT PLAN? YES NO If yes, return to and complete item 9 a-d.

READ BACK OF FORM BEFORE COMPLETING & SIGNING THIS FORM.
12. PATIENT'S OR AUTHORIZED PERSON'S SIGNATURE I authorize the release of any medical or other information necessary to process this claim. I also request payment of government benefits either to myself or to the party who accepts assignment below.
SIGNED ___ DATE ___
13. INSURED'S OR AUTHORIZED PERSON'S SIGNATURE I authorize payment of medical benefits to the undersigned physician or supplier for services described below.
SIGNED ___

14. DATE OF CURRENT: ILLNESS (First symptom) OR INJURY (Accident) OR PREGNANCY(LMP) MM DD YY   15. IF PATIENT HAS HAD SAME OR SIMILAR ILLNESS. GIVE FIRST DATE MM DD YY   16. DATES PATIENT UNABLE TO WORK IN CURRENT OCCUPATION FROM MM DD YY TO MM DD YY

17. NAME OF REFERRING PHYSICIAN OR OTHER SOURCE   17a. I.D. NUMBER OF REFERRING PHYSICIAN   18. HOSPITALIZATION DATES RELATED TO CURRENT SERVICES FROM MM DD YY TO MM DD YY

19. RESERVED FOR LOCAL USE   20. OUTSIDE LAB? YES NO $ CHARGES

21. DIAGNOSIS OR NATURE OF ILLNESS OR INJURY. (RELATE ITEMS 1,2,3 OR 4 TO ITEM 24E BY LINE)
1. ___ 3. ___
2. ___ 4. ___
22. MEDICAID RESUBMISSION CODE ORIGINAL REF. NO.
23. PRIOR AUTHORIZATION NUMBER

24. | A DATE(S) OF SERVICE From / To (MM DD YY) | B Place of Service | C Type of Service | D PROCEDURES, SERVICES, OR SUPPLIES (Explain Unusual Circumstances) CPT/HCPCS / MODIFIER | E DIAGNOSIS CODE | F $ CHARGES | G DAYS OR UNITS | H EPSDT Family Plan | I EMG | J COB | K RESERVED FOR LOCAL USE |
|---|---|---|---|---|---|---|---|---|---|---|
| 1 | | | | | | | | | | |
| 2 | | | | | | | | | | |
| 3 | | | | | | | | | | |
| 4 | | | | | | | | | | |
| 5 | | | | | | | | | | |
| 6 | | | | | | | | | | |

25. FEDERAL TAX I.D. NUMBER SSN EIN   26. PATIENT'S ACCOUNT NO.   27. ACCEPT ASSIGNMENT? (For govt. claims, see back) YES NO   28. TOTAL CHARGE $ 29. AMOUNT PAID $ 30. BALANCE DUE $

31. SIGNATURE OF PHYSICIAN OR SUPPLIER INCLUDING DEGREES OR CREDENTIALS (I certify that the statements on the reverse apply to this bill and are made a part thereof.)
SIGNED ___ DATE ___
32. NAME AND ADDRESS OF FACILITY WHERE SERVICES WERE RENDERED (If other than home or office)
33. PHYSICIAN'S, SUPPLIER'S BILLING NAME, ADDRESS, ZIP CODE & PHONE #
PIN#   GRP#

(APPROVED BY AMA COUNCIL ON MEDICAL SERVICE 8/88) **PLEASE PRINT OR TYPE** APPROVED OMB-0938-0008 FORM CMS-1500 (12-90), FORM RRB-1500, APPROVED OMB-1215-0055 FORM OWCP-1500, APPROVED OMB-0720-0001 (CHAMPUS)

CARRIER / PATIENT AND INSURED INFORMATION / PHYSICIAN OR SUPPLIER INFORMATION

Figure 13–9

After the instructor has returned your work to you, either make the necessary corrections and place your work in a three-ring notebook for future reference or, if you received a high score, place it in your portfolio for reference when applying for a job.

Abbreviations pertinent to this record:

Pt	_____	lt	_____
ER	_____	tx	_____
L	_____	cc	_____
N	_____	MRI	_____
fx	_____	RTO	_____
imp	_____	wks	_____

Additional Coding

1. Refer to Barry Brook's medical record, abstract information, and code procedures that would be billed by outside providers.

Site	*Description of Service*	*Code*
a. College Hospital Radiology	_____	_____
b. College Hospital Central Supply	_____	_____
c. College Hospital Radiology	_____	_____

2. Locate a financial accounting record (ledger).

   Note: Refer to the step-by-step procedures at the end of Chapter 3 in the *Handbook* and graphic examples Figures 3–18, 10–2, and 12–15.

3. Insert the patient's name and address, including ZIP code in the box.

4. Enter the patient's personal data.

5. Ledger lines: Insert date of service (DOS), reference (CPT code number, check number, or dates of service for posting adjustments or when insurance was billed), description of the transaction, charge amounts, payments, adjustments, and running current balance. The posting date is the actual date the transaction is recorded. If the DOS differs from the posting date, list the DOS in the reference or description column.

   Line 2: _____

   Line 3: _____

   Line 4: _____

   Line 5: _____

Line 6: _____

Line 7: _____

Line 8: _____

Note: A good bookkeeping practice is to take a red pen and draw a line across the financial accounting record (ledger) from left to right to indicate the last entry billed to the insurance company.

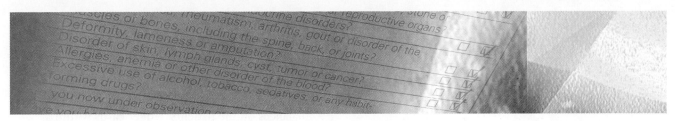

TRICARE and CHAMPVA

KEY TERMS

Your instructor may wish to select some specific words pertinent to this chapter for a test. For definitions of the terms, further study, and/or reference, the words, phrases, and abbreviations may be found in the glossary at the end of the Handbook. *Key terms for this chapter follow.*

active duty service member (ADSM)

allowable charge

authorized provider

beneficiary

catastrophic cap

catchment area

cooperative care

coordination of benefits

cost-share

Defense Enrollment Eligibility Reporting System (DEERS)

emergency

fiscal intermediary (FI)

health benefits advisor (HBA)

Health Care Finder (HCF)

medically (or psychologically) necessary

military treatment facility (MTF)

nonparticipating provider (nonpar)

other health insurance (OHI)

participating provider (par)

partnership program

point-of-service (POS) option

preauthorization

primary care manager (PCM)

quality assurance program

service benefit program

service-connected injury

service retiree (military retiree)

sponsor

summary payment voucher

The Civilian Health and Medical Program of the Department of Veterans Affairs (CHAMPVA)

total, permanent, service-connected disability

TRICARE Extra

TRICARE for life (TFL)

TRICARE Prime

TRICARE service center (TSC)

urgent care

veteran

PERFORMANCE OBJECTIVES

The student will be able to:

■ Define and spell the key terms for this chapter, given the information from the *Handbook* glossary, within a reasonable time period and with enough accuracy to obtain a satisfactory evaluation.

■ After reading the chapter, answer the self-study review questions with enough accuracy to obtain a satisfactory evaluation.

■ Fill in the correct meaning of each abbreviation, given a list of common medical abbreviations and symbols that appear in chart notes, within a reasonable time period and with enough accuracy to obtain a satisfactory evaluation.

■ Given the patient's medical chart notes, ledger cards, and blank insurance claim forms, complete each CMS-1500 Health Insurance Claim Form for billing within a reasonable time period and with enough accuracy to obtain a satisfactory evaluation.

■ Using the Mock Fee Schedule in Appendix A in this *Workbook*, correctly post payments, adjustments, and balances on the patients' ledger cards within a reasonable time period and with enough accuracy to obtain a satisfactory evaluation.

■ Compute mathematical calculations, given TRICARE problem situations, within a reasonable time period and with enough accuracy to obtain a satisfactory evaluation.

■ Transmit an electronic insurance claim for a TRICARE case using practice management software, within a reasonable time period and with enough accuracy to obtain a satisfactory evaluation.

■ View and print an insurance aging report using practice management software, within a reasonable time period and with enough accuracy to obtain a satisfactory evaluation.

STUDY OUTLINE

History of TRICARE

TRICARE Programs
 Eligibility
 Nonavailability Statement

TRICARE Standard
 Enrollment
 Identification Card
 Benefits
 Fiscal Year
 Authorized Providers of Health Care
 Preauthorization
 Payment

TRICARE Extra
 Enrollment
 Identification Card
 Benefits
 Network Provider
 Preauthorization
 Payments

TRICARE Prime
 Enrollment
 Identification Card
 Benefits
 Primary Care Manager
 Preauthorization
 Payments

TRICARE For Life
 Enrollment
 Identification Card
 Benefits

 Referral and Preauthorization
 Payment

TRICARE Plus
 Enrollment
 Identification Card
 Benefits
 Payment

TRICARE Prime Remote Program
 Enrollment
 Identification Card
 Benefits
 Referral and Preauthorization
 Payments

Supplemental Health Care Program
 Enrollment
 Identification Card
 Benefits
 Referral and Preauthorization
 Payments

TRICARE Hospice Program

TRICARE and HMO Coverage

CHAMPVA Program
 Eligibility
 Enrollment
 Identification Card
 Benefits
 Provider
 Preauthorization

Medical Record Access
 Privacy Act of 1974

Computer Matching and Privacy Protection Act
of 1988
Claims Procedure
Fiscal Intermediary
TRICARE Standard and CHAMPVA
TRICARE Extra and TRICARE Prime
TRICARE Prime Remote and Supplemental
Health Care Program
TRICARE for Life
TRICARE/CHAMPVA and Other Insurance
Medicaid and TRICARE/CHAMPVA
Medicare and TRICARE
Medicare and CHAMPVA

Dual or Double Coverage
Third-Party Liability
Workers' Compensation
After Claim Submission
TRICARE Summary Payment Voucher
CHAMPVA Explanation of Benefits Document
Quality Assurance
Claims Inquiries and Appeals
Procedure: Completing a CHAMPVA Claim Form

 SELF-STUDY **14–1** ▸ **REVIEW QUESTIONS**

Review the objectives, key terms, glossary definitions of key terms, chapter information, and figures before completing the following review questions.

1. CHAMPUS, the acronym for Civilian Health and Medical Program of the Uniformed

Services, is now called _____ and was organized to control escalating medical costs and to standardize benefits for active-duty families and military retirees.

2. An active duty service member is known as a/an _____; once retired,

this former member is called a/an _____.

3. Individuals who qualify for TRICARE are known as _____.

4. A system for verifying an individual's TRICARE eligibility is called _____

_____.

5. Mrs. Hancock, a TRICARE beneficiary, lives 2 miles from a Uniformed Services Medical Treatment Facility but needs to be hospitalized for mental healthcare services at Orlando Medical Center, a civilian hospital. What type of authorization does she require?

_____

6. TRICARE Standard and CHAMPVA beneficiary identification cards are issued to

_____ and _____. Information must be obtained from

_____ and _____ of the card and placed on the health insurance claim form.

7. Programs that allow TRICARE Standard beneficiaries to receive treatment, services,

or supplies from civilian providers are called _____ and _____.

8. The TRICARE Standard deductible for outpatient care is how much per patient?

_____ Per family? _____

9. What percentage does TRICARE Standard pay on outpatient services after the

deductible has been met for dependents of active duty members? _____

For retired members or their dependents? _____

10. For retired members or their dependents on TRICARE Standard, what is their

responsibility for outpatient services? _____

11. A voluntary TRICARE health maintenance organization type of option is known as

_____

12. CHAMPVA is the acronym for _____, now

known as the _____.

13. Those individuals who serve in the United States Armed Forces, finish their

service, and are honorably discharged are known as _____.

14. CHAMPVA is not an insurance program but is considered as a/an _____

_____ program.

15. Which individuals are entitled to CHAMPVA medical benefits?

a. _____

b. _____

c. _____

16. The public law establishing a person's right to review and contest inaccuracies in

personal medical records is known as _____.

17. An organization that contracts with the government to process TRICARE and

CHAMPVA health insurance claims is known as a/an _____.

18. The time limit for submitting a TRICARE Standard or CHAMPVA claim

for outpatient service is _____;

for inpatient service, it is _____.

To check your answers to this self-study assignment, see Appendix D.

A S S I G N M E N T   **14-2** ▸ **CRITICAL THINKING**

Performance Objective

Task: After reading the scenarios, answer questions, using critical thinking
                    skills.

Conditions: Use a pen or pencil.

Standards: Time: _____ minutes

                    Accuracy: _____

                    (Note: The time element and accuracy criteria may be given by your
                    instructor.)

Directions: After reading the scenarios, answer questions, using your critical thinking skills. Record your answers
on the blank lines.

1. If Bertha Evans is seen for an office visit and has other insurance besides TRICARE,
   and she is the dependent of an active military person, whom do you bill first?

   _____

2. If Jason Williams, a TRICARE beneficiary who became disabled at age 10 years and
   who is also receiving Medicare Part A benefits, is seen for a consultation, whom do you

   bill first? _____

3. If Tanner Vine, a CHAMPVA and Medicaid beneficiary, is seen on an emergency basis

   in the office, whom do you bill first? _____

ASSIGNMENT **14–3** ▸ **CALCULATE MATHEMATICAL PROBLEMS**

Performance Objective

Task: Calculate and insert the correct amounts for three TRICARE scenarios.

Conditions: Use a pen or pencil, the description of the problem, and calculation.

Standards: Time: _____ minutes

                 Accuracy: _____

                 (Note: The time element and accuracy criteria may be given by your
                 instructor.)

Directions: Calculate and insert the correct amounts for the following scenarios.

Problem 1: On October 1, in consultation, Dr. Caesar sees the wife of a Navy man who is stationed at Port Hueneme. Dr. Caesar orders her to the hospital because of a suspected ectopic pregnancy. She undergoes a laparotomy and salpingectomy. Here are her bills. Indicate what TRICARE Standard will pay.

Outpatient Services: *TRICARE Standard*

	Bill/Allowable	**TRICARE payment**	**Patient Owes**
Consultation	$75	$_____	$_____

Inpatient services:

Salpingectomy	$600		
Assistant surgeon	$120		
Anesthesiologist	$400		
3-day stay (drugs, laboratory tests, operating room)	$2500		
Total	$_____	$_____	

Problem 2: This is the same situation as in Problem 1, except that the patient is the wife of a retired military man and has TRICARE Standard.

Outpatient Services: *TRICARE Standard*

	Bill/Allowable	**TRICARE payment**	**Patient Owes**
Consultation	$75	$_____	$_____

Inpatient services with separately billed professional charges

	Bill/Allowable	TRICARE Payment	Patient Owes
Salpingectomy	$600	$_____	$_____
Assistant surgeon	$120	$_____	$_____
Anesthesiologist	$400	$_____	$_____

Inpatient services billed by hospital

| 3-day stay (drugs, laboratory tests, operating room) | $2500 | $_____ | |
| Total payment owed by patient to Dr. Caesar | | | $_____ |

Problem 3: A TRICARE patient asks Dr. Caesar to accept assignment on her medical care, and Dr. Caesar agrees. She has not met her deductible. She is the wife of an active duty man. She has TRICARE Extra.

Dr. Caesar's bill:

Consultation	$50	Allowable:	$50
Complete blood cell count	20		20
Urinalysis	5		5
Blood serology and complement fixation	25		25
Posteroanterior and lateral chest radiograph	40		40
Electrocardiogram	35		30
Spirometry	40		40
Total	$215		$210

How much is Dr. Caesar's check from TRICARE Extra? $_____. The patient owes the doctor

$_____. Dr. Caesar's courtesy adjustment is $ _____.

ASSIGNMENT **14-4** ▸ **COMPLETE A CLAIM FORM FOR A TRICARE STANDARD CASE**

Performance Objective

Task: Complete a CMS-1500 claim form for a TRICARE Standard case, post transactions to the financial accounting record, and define patient record abbreviations.

Conditions: Use the patient's record (Figure 14–1) and financial statement (Figure 14–2), one health insurance claim form (Figure 14–3), a typewriter or computer, procedural and diagnostic code books, and Appendices A and B in this *Workbook*.

Standards: Claim Productivity Measurement

Time: _____ minutes

Accuracy: _____

(Note: The time element and accuracy criteria may be given by your instructor.)

Directions:

1. Using optical character reader (OCR) guidelines, complete the CMS-1500 Claim Form and direct it to your local TRICARE fiscal intermediary. To locate your local fiscal intermediary, go to Web site http://www.tricare.osd.mil. Click on the area of the map you are residing in and then choose a state to access claims information for that state. Refer to Miss Rosa M. Sandoval's patient record for information and Appendix A to locate the fees to record on the claim and post to the financial statement. Date the claim May 31. Dr. Atrics is not accepting assignment on this TRICARE Standard case but is completing the claim for the patient's convenience. The family of this patient has not previously met its deductible.

2. Refer to Chapter 7 (Figure 7–13) of the *Handbook* for instructions on how to complete this claim form and to view a TRICARE template.

3. Use your *Current Procedural Terminology* (CPT) code book or Appendix A in this *Workbook* to determine the correct five-digit code number and modifiers for each professional service rendered. Use your Healthcare Common Procedure Coding System (HCPCS) Level II code book or refer to Appendix B in this *Workbook* for HCPCS procedure codes and modifiers.

4. On May 8, Miss Sandoval makes a partial payment of $20 by check (No. 4013). Record the proper information on the financial record and claim form, and note the date you have billed TRICARE (May 31).

5. A Performance Evaluation Checklist may be reproduced from the "Instruction Guide to the Workbook" chapter if your instructor wishes you to submit it to assist with scoring and comments.

After the instructor has returned your work to you, either make the necessary corrections and place your work in a three-ring notebook for future reference or, if you received a high score, place it in your portfolio for reference when applying for a job.

Abbreviations pertinent to this record:

pt _____	ofc _____
rt _____	FU _____
EPF _____	retn _____
yr(s) _____	PO _____
temp _____	PF _____
adv _____	HX _____
SF _____	PX _____
MDM_____	wk _____
c̄ _____	T _____

1. Locate a financial accounting record (ledger).

   Note: Refer to the step-by-step procedures at the end of Chapter 3 in the *Handbook* and graphic examples Figures 3–18, 10–2, and 12–15.

2. Insert the patient's name and address, including ZIP code in the box.

3. Enter the patient's personal data.

4. Ledger lines: Insert date of service (DOS), reference (CPT code number, check number, or dates of service for posting adjustments or when insurance was billed), description of the transaction, charge amounts, payments, adjustments, and running current balance. The posting date is the actual date the transaction is recorded. If the DOS differs from the posting date, list the DOS in the reference or description column.

   Line 2: _____

   Line 3: _____

   Line 4: _____

   Line 5: _____

   Line 6: _____

   Line 7: _____

   Note: A good bookkeeping practice is to take a red pen and draw a line across the financial accounting record (ledger) from left to right to indicate the last entry billed to the insurance company.

PATIENT RECORD NO. 14-4

Sandoval	Rosa	M	11-01-91	F	555-456-3322
LAST NAME	FIRST NAME	MIDDLE NAME	BIRTH DATE	SEX	HOME PHONE

209 West Maple Street	Woodland Hills	XY	12345
ADDRESS	CITY	STATE	ZIP CODE

CELL PHONE	PAGER NO.	FAX NO.	E-MAIL ADDRESS

994-XX-1164
PATIENT'S SOC. SEC. NO.   DRIVER'S LICENSE

Child—full time student (lives with mother)
PATIENT'S OCCUPATION   NAME OF COMPANY

ADDRESS OF EMPLOYER   PHONE

Hernan J. Sandoval (father)   Staff Sargeant – Grade 9 (active duty)
SPOUSE OR PARENT   OCCUPATION

United States Army   HHC 3rd Batt, 25th Infantry, APO New York, New York, 10030
EMPLOYER   ADDRESS   PHONE

TRICARE Standard   father (DOB 2/10/70)
NAME OF INSURANCE   INSURED OR SUBSCRIBER

886-XX-0999
POLICY/CERTIFICATE NO.   GROUP NO.

REFERRED BY: Maria Sandoval (mother)

DATE	PROGRESS NOTES
5-1-xx	New pt comes in complaining of pain in rt ear for 3 days. An EPF history was taken which revealed several ear infections (suppurative) over the past 3 yrs. An EPF exam revealed fluid and pus in rt ear. Temp 101°. Adv mother a myringotomy was necessary. Scheduled outpatient surg at College Hospital this afternoon. Imp: Acute rt suppurative otitis media (SF MDM).
	PA/llf *Pedro Atrics, MD*
5-1-xx	Pt admitted to outpatient surgery (College Hospital). Rt myringotomy c̄ aspiration performed. Pt did well. To be seen in ofc for FU in 2 days.
	PA/llf *Pedro Atrics, MD*
5-3-xx	Pt retns PO (PF HX/PX SF MDM). No pain rt ear. Pt progressing well. Retn in 1 wk.
	PA/llf *Pedro Atrics, MD*
5-8-xx	Pt retns PO (PF HX/PX SF MDM). T 98°, no fluid or pus in rt ear. No pain. Pt discharged, retn prn.
	PA/llf *Pedro Atrics, MD*

Figure 14–1

Acct No. 14-4

STATEMENT
Financial Account
COLLEGE CLINIC
4567 Broad Avenue
Woodland Hills, XY 12345-0001
Tel. 555-486-9002
Fax No. 555-487-8976

Rosa M. Sandoval
c/o Maria Sandoval
209 West Maple Street
Woodland Hills, XY 12345-0001

Phone No. (H) (555) 456-3322 (W) _____ Birthdate 11-9-91

Primary Insurance Co. TRICARE Standard   Policy/Group No. 886-XX-0999

Secondary Insurance Co. _____ Policy/Group No. _____

DATE	REFERENCE	DESCRIPTION	CHARGES	CREDITS PYMNTS.	ADJ.	BALANCE
20xx		BALANCE FORWARD →				
5-1-xx		NP OV				
5-1-xx		Myringotomy				
5-3-xx		PO OV				
5-8-xx		PO OV				

PLEASE PAY LAST AMOUNT IN BALANCE COLUMN ⬆

THIS IS A COPY OF YOUR FINANCIAL ACCOUNT AS IT APPEARS ON OUR RECORDS

Figure 14–2

PLEASE
DO NOT
STAPLE
IN THIS
AREA

CARRIER

| | PICA | | | **HEALTH INSURANCE CLAIM FORM** | | | PICA | | |

1. MEDICARE	MEDICAID	CHAMPUS	CHAMPVA	GROUP HEALTH PLAN	FECA BLK LUNG	OTHER	1a. INSURED'S I.D. NUMBER	(FOR PROGRAM IN ITEM 1)
☐ (Medicare #)	☐ (Medicaid #)	☐ (Sponsor's SSN)	☐ (VA File #)	☐ (SSN or ID)	☐ (S SN)	☐ (ID)		

2. PATIENT'S NAME (Last Name, First Name, Middle Initial)	3. PATIENT'S BIRTH DATE / SEX	4. INSURED'S NAME (Last Name, First Name, Middle Initial)
	MM DD YY M ☐ F ☐	

5. PATIENT'S ADDRESS (No., Street)	6. PATIENT RELATIONSHIP TO INSURED	7. INSURED'S ADDRESS (No., Street)
	Self ☐ Spouse ☐ Child ☐ Other ☐	
CITY / STATE	8. PATIENT STATUS	CITY / STATE
	Single ☐ Married ☐ Other ☐	
ZIP CODE / TELEPHONE (Include Area Code)	Employed ☐ Full-Time Student ☐ Part-Time Student ☐	ZIP CODE / TELEPHONE (INCLUDE AREA CODE)

9. OTHER INSURED'S NAME (Last Name, First Name, Middle Initial)	10. IS PATIENT'S CONDITION RELATED TO:	11. INSURED'S POLICY GROUP OR FECA NUMBER
a. OTHER INSURED'S POLICY OR GROUP NUMBER	a. EMPLOYMENT? (CURRENT OR PREVIOUS) ☐ YES ☐ NO	a. INSURED'S DATE OF BIRTH MM DD YY SEX M ☐ F ☐
b. OTHER INSURED'S DATE OF BIRTH MM DD YY SEX M ☐ F ☐	b. AUTO ACCIDENT? PLACE (State) ☐ YES ☐ NO	b. EMPLOYER'S NAME OR SCHOOL NAME
c. EMPLOYER'S NAME OR SCHOOL NAME	c. OTHER ACCIDENT? ☐ YES ☐ NO	c. INSURANCE PLAN NAME OR PROGRAM NAME
d. INSURANCE PLAN NAME OR PROGRAM NAME	10d. RESERVED FOR LOCAL USE	d. IS THERE ANOTHER HEALTH BENEFIT PLAN? ☐ YES ☐ NO If yes, return to and complete item 9 a-d.

READ BACK OF FORM BEFORE COMPLETING & SIGNING THIS FORM.

12. PATIENT'S OR AUTHORIZED PERSON'S SIGNATURE I authorize the release of any medical or other information necessary to process this claim. I also request payment of government benefits either to myself or to the party who accepts assignment below.

SIGNED _____   DATE _____

13. INSURED'S OR AUTHORIZED PERSON'S SIGNATURE I authorize payment of medical benefits to the undersigned physician or supplier for services described below.

SIGNED _____

PATIENT AND INSURED INFORMATION

14. DATE OF CURRENT: ◄ ILLNESS (First symptom) OR INJURY (Accident) OR PREGNANCY(LMP) MM DD YY	15. IF PATIENT HAS HAD SAME OR SIMILAR ILLNESS. GIVE FIRST DATE MM DD YY	16. DATES PATIENT UNABLE TO WORK IN CURRENT OCCUPATION FROM MM DD YY TO MM DD YY
17. NAME OF REFERRING PHYSICIAN OR OTHER SOURCE	17a. I.D. NUMBER OF REFERRING PHYSICIAN	18. HOSPITALIZATION DATES RELATED TO CURRENT SERVICES FROM MM DD YY TO MM DD YY
19. RESERVED FOR LOCAL USE		20. OUTSIDE LAB? $ CHARGES ☐ YES ☐ NO

21. DIAGNOSIS OR NATURE OF ILLNESS OR INJURY. (RELATE ITEMS 1,2,3 OR 4 TO ITEM 24E BY LINE)

1. └___   3. └___

2. └___   4. └___

22. MEDICAID RESUBMISSION CODE   ORIGINAL REF. NO.

23. PRIOR AUTHORIZATION NUMBER

24.	A DATE(S) OF SERVICE					B Place of Service	C Type of Service	D PROCEDURES, SERVICES, OR SUPPLIES (Explain Unusual Circumstances) CPT/HCPCS	MODIFIER	E DIAGNOSIS CODE	F $ CHARGES	G DAYS OR UNITS	H EPSDT Family Plan	I EMG	J COB	K RESERVED FOR LOCAL USE
	From MM DD YY			To MM DD YY												
1																
2																
3																
4																
5																
6																

25. FEDERAL TAX I.D. NUMBER SSN ☐ EIN ☐	26. PATIENT'S ACCOUNT NO.	27. ACCEPT ASSIGNMENT? (For govt. claims, see back) ☐ YES ☐ NO	28. TOTAL CHARGE $	29. AMOUNT PAID $	30. BALANCE DUE $

31. SIGNATURE OF PHYSICIAN OR SUPPLIER INCLUDING DEGREES OR CREDENTIALS (I certify that the statements on the reverse apply to this bill and are made a part thereof.) SIGNED _____ DATE _____	32. NAME AND ADDRESS OF FACILITY WHERE SERVICES WERE RENDERED (If other than home or office)	33. PHYSICIAN'S, SUPPLIER'S BILLING NAME, ADDRESS, ZIP CODE & PHONE # PIN# GRP#

PHYSICIAN OR SUPPLIER INFORMATION

(APPROVED BY AMA COUNCIL ON MEDICAL SERVICE 8/88)   **PLEASE PRINT OR TYPE**   APPROVED OMB-0938-0008 FORM CMS-1500 (12-90), FORM RRB-1500, APPROVED OMB-1215-0055 FORM OWCP-1500, APPROVED OMB-0720-0001 (CHAMPUS)

Figure 14-3

ASSIGNMENT **14–5** ▸ **COMPLETE A CLAIM FORM FOR A TRICARE EXTRA CASE**

Performance Objective

Task: Complete a CMS-1500 claim form for a TRICARE Extra case, post transactions to the financial accounting record, and define patient record abbreviations.

Conditions: Use the patient's record (Figure 14–4) and financial statement (Figure 14–5), one health insurance claim form (Figure 14–6), a typewriter or computer, procedural and diagnostic code books, and Appendices A and B in this *Workbook*.

Standards: Claim Productivity Measurement

                      Time: _____ minutes

                      Accuracy: _____

                      (Note: The time element and accuracy criteria may be given by your instructor.)

Directions:

1. Using OCR guidelines, complete the CMS-1500 Claim Form and direct it to your local TRICARE fiscal intermediary. To locate your local fiscal intermediary, go to Web site http://www.tricare.osd.mil. Click on the area of the map you are residing in and then choose a state to access claims information for that state. Refer to Mrs. Darlene B. Drew's patient record for information and Appendix A to locate the fees to record on the claim and post to the financial statement. Date the claim February 3. Assume that the Nonavailability Statement (NAS) has been transmitted electronically so that the physician can treat the patient at College Hospital. Dr. Ulibarri is accepting assignment on this TRICARE Extra case. This patient met her deductible last November when seen by a previous physician.

2. Refer to Chapter 7 (Figure 7–13) of the *Handbook* for instructions on how to complete this claim form and to view a TRICARE template.

3. Use your CPT code book or Appendix A in this *Workbook* to determine the correct five-digit code number and modifiers for each professional service rendered. Use your HCPCS Level II code book or refer to Appendix B in this *Workbook* for HCPCS procedure codes and modifiers.

4. Record the proper information on the financial record and claim form and note the date when you have billed TRICARE Extra.

5. A Performance Evaluation Checklist may be reproduced from the "Instruction Guide to the Workbook" chapter if your instructor wishes you to submit it to assist with scoring and comments.

After the instructor has returned your work to you, either make the necessary corrections and place your work in a three-ring notebook for future reference or, if you received a high score, place it in your portfolio for reference when applying for a job.

Abbreviations pertinent to this record:

Pt _____   LC _____

D _____   MDM _____

HX _____   PF _____

PX _____   rec _____

UA _____   SF _____

WBC _____   C _____

RBC _____   M _____

cc _____   surg _____

lab _____   ofc _____

Rx _____   PO _____

caps _____   OV _____

t.i.d. _____   rtn _____

Retn _____   PRN _____

Dx _____

1. Locate a financial accounting record (ledger).

   Note: Refer to the step-by-step procedures at the end of Chapter 3 in the *Handbook* and graphic examples Figures 3–18, 10–2, and 12–15.

2. Insert the patient's name and address, including ZIP code in the box.

3. Enter the patient's personal data.

4. Ledger lines: Insert date of service (DOS), reference (CPT code number, check number, or dates of service for posting adjustments or when insurance was billed), description of the transaction, charge amounts, payments, adjustments, and running current balance. The posting date is the actual date the transaction is recorded. If the DOS differs from the posting date, list the DOS in the reference or description column.

   Line 2: _____

   Line 3: _____

   Line 4: _____

Line 5: _____

Line 6: _____

Line 7: _____

Note: A good bookkeeping practice is to take a red pen and draw a line across the financial accounting record (ledger) from left to right to indicate the last entry billed to the insurance company.

PATIENT RECORD NO. 14-5

Drew	Darlene	B	12-22-41	F	555-466-1002
LAST NAME	FIRST NAME	MIDDLE NAME	BIRTH DATE	SEX	HOME PHONE

720 Ganley Street,   Woodland Hills,   XY   12345
ADDRESS   CITY   STATE   ZIP CODE

555-320-9988   555-210-9400   555-466-1002   drew@wb.net
CELL PHONE   PAGER NO.   FAX NO.   E-MAIL ADDRESS

450-XX-3762   H0492188
PATIENT'S SOC. SEC. NO. DRIVER'S LICENSE

Seamstress   J. B. Talon Company
PATIENT'S OCCUPATION   NAME OF COMPANY

2111 Ventura Road, Merck, XY 12346   555-733-0156
ADDRESS OF EMPLOYER   PHONE

Harry M. Drew   U.S. Navy Lieutenant Commander (L/C), Active Status
SPOUSE OR PARENT   OCCUPATION

Service #221-XX-0711   Social Security No. 221-XX-0711   Grade12   4-15-37
                                                                                BIRTH DATE

P.O. Box 2927, A.P.O., New York, New York 09194
ADDRESS

TRICARE Extra   67531   01-01-80
NAME OF INSURANCE   TRICARE EXTRA I.D. CARD NO.   EFFECTIVE DATE

REFERRED BY: James B. Jeffers, MD, 100 S. Broadway, Woodland Hills, XY 12345   Tax ID#77621074X

DATE	PROGRESS NOTES
1-13-xx	New pt comes in complaining of large sore in vagina causing extreme pain. Performed a
	D HX/PX. UA (non-automated with microscopy) loaded with WBCs and RBCs. Upon pelvic
	examination, a very tender mass is located in the paraurethral area (Skene's gland).
	I incised and drained the abscess and obtained 10 cc greenish pus; took culture and sent
	to lab. Pt feels much better. Rx Terramycin 30 caps 1 t.i.d. Retn in 5 days. Dx: Paraurethral
	abscess (LC/MDM).
	GU/llf *Gene Ulibarri, MD*
1-18-xx	Pt returns and a PF HX/PX performed. Abscess is filled with fluid again, opened, and a
	wick of Iodoform gauze placed to help with drainage. Rec daily sitz baths and outpatient
	hospitalization to remove gland. Culture results show pseudomonas organism.
	Arrangements made for surgery on the 24th, admit at 5:30 a.m., surgery at 7:30 a.m.
	(SF MDM).
	GU/llf *Gene Ulibarri, MD*
1-24-xx	Admit to College Hospital outpatient facility (C HX/PX M MDM). Surg: Excision of Skene's
	gland. To be seen in ofc next week for PO exam. Renewed Rx Terramycin.
	GU/llf *Gene Ulibarri, MD*
1-27-xx	PO OV (PF HX/PX SF/MDM). Pt doing well. No pain, urethral tissue and perineum looks
	healthy, healing well. Rtn PRN.
	GU/llf *Gene Ulibarri, MD*

Figure 14-4

Acct No. 14-5

STATEMENT
Financial Account
COLLEGE CLINIC
4567 Broad Avenue
Woodland Hills, XY 12345-0001
Tel. 555-486-9002
Fax No. 555-487-8976

Darlene B. Drew
720 Ganley Street
Woodland Hills, XY 12345

Phone No. (H)____555-466-1002_____   (W)____555-733-0156_____   Birthdate_____12-22-41_____

Primary Insurance Co._____TRICARE Extra_____   Policy/Group No.____221-XX-0711____

Secondary Insurance Co._____   Policy/Group No._____

DATE	REFERENCE	DESCRIPTION	CHARGES	CREDITS PYMNTS.	ADJ.	BALANCE	
20xx			BALANCE FORWARD →				
1-13-xx		NP OV					
1-13-xx		UA					
1-13-xx		Drainage of Skene's gland abscess					
1-13-xx		Handling/Transport culture specimen					
1-18-xx		OV					
1-24-xx		Excision Skene's gland					
1-27-xx		PO OV					

PLEASE PAY LAST AMOUNT IN BALANCE COLUMN ⬆

THIS IS A COPY OF YOUR FINANCIAL ACCOUNT AS IT APPEARS ON OUR RECORDS

Figure 14–5

PLEASE
DO NOT
STAPLE
IN THIS
AREA

CARRIER

HEALTH INSURANCE CLAIM FORM

| | PICA | | | | | | | | | | | | | | PICA | | |

1. MEDICARE   MEDICAID   CHAMPUS   CHAMPVA   GROUP HEALTH PLAN   FECA BLK LUNG   OTHER   1a. INSURED'S I.D. NUMBER   (FOR PROGRAM IN ITEM 1)

☐ (Medicare #)   ☐ (Medicaid #)   ☐ (Sponsor's SSN)   ☐ (VA File #)   ☐ (SSN or ID)   ☐ (S SN)   ☐ (ID)

2. PATIENT'S NAME (Last Name, First Name, Middle Initial)

3. PATIENT'S BIRTH DATE   MM   DD   YY   SEX   M ☐   F ☐

4. INSURED'S NAME (Last Name, First Name, Middle Initial)

5. PATIENT'S ADDRESS (No., Street)

6. PATIENT RELATIONSHIP TO INSURED   Self ☐   Spouse ☐   Child ☐   Other ☐

7. INSURED'S ADDRESS (No., Street)

CITY   STATE

8. PATIENT STATUS   Single ☐   Married ☐   Other ☐

CITY   STATE

ZIP CODE   TELEPHONE (Include Area Code)   )

Employed ☐   Full-Time Student ☐   Part-Time Student ☐

ZIP CODE   TELEPHONE (INCLUDE AREA CODE)

9. OTHER INSURED'S NAME (Last Name, First Name, Middle Initial)

10. IS PATIENT'S CONDITION RELATED TO:

11. INSURED'S POLICY GROUP OR FECA NUMBER

a. OTHER INSURED'S POLICY OR GROUP NUMBER

a. EMPLOYMENT? (CURRENT OR PREVIOUS)   ☐ YES   ☐ NO

a. INSURED'S DATE OF BIRTH   MM   DD   YY   SEX   M ☐   F ☐

b. OTHER INSURED'S DATE OF BIRTH   MM   DD   YY   SEX   M ☐   F ☐

b. AUTO ACCIDENT?   PLACE (State)   ☐ YES   ☐ NO

b. EMPLOYER'S NAME OR SCHOOL NAME

c. EMPLOYER'S NAME OR SCHOOL NAME

c. OTHER ACCIDENT?   ☐ YES   ☐ NO

c. INSURANCE PLAN NAME OR PROGRAM NAME

d. INSURANCE PLAN NAME OR PROGRAM NAME

10d. RESERVED FOR LOCAL USE

d. IS THERE ANOTHER HEALTH BENEFIT PLAN?   ☐ YES   ☐ NO   *If yes*, return to and complete item 9 a-d.

READ BACK OF FORM BEFORE COMPLETING & SIGNING THIS FORM.

12. PATIENT'S OR AUTHORIZED PERSON'S SIGNATURE I authorize the release of any medical or other information necessary to process this claim. I also request payment of government benefits either to myself or to the party who accepts assignment below.

SIGNED _____   DATE _____

13. INSURED'S OR AUTHORIZED PERSON'S SIGNATURE I authorize payment of medical benefits to the undersigned physician or supplier for services described below.

SIGNED _____

PATIENT AND INSURED INFORMATION

14. DATE OF CURRENT: MM   DD   YY   ILLNESS (First symptom) OR INJURY (Accident) OR PREGNANCY(LMP)

15. IF PATIENT HAS HAD SAME OR SIMILAR ILLNESS. GIVE FIRST DATE   MM   DD   YY

16. DATES PATIENT UNABLE TO WORK IN CURRENT OCCUPATION   MM   DD   YY   FROM   TO   MM   DD   YY

17. NAME OF REFERRING PHYSICIAN OR OTHER SOURCE

17a. I.D. NUMBER OF REFERRING PHYSICIAN

18. HOSPITALIZATION DATES RELATED TO CURRENT SERVICES   MM   DD   YY   FROM   TO   MM   DD   YY

19. RESERVED FOR LOCAL USE

20. OUTSIDE LAB? $ CHARGES   ☐ YES   ☐ NO

21. DIAGNOSIS OR NATURE OF ILLNESS OR INJURY. (RELATE ITEMS 1,2,3 OR 4 TO ITEM 24E BY LINE)

1. L_____   3. L_____

2. L_____   4. L_____

22. MEDICAID RESUBMISSION CODE   ORIGINAL REF. NO.

23. PRIOR AUTHORIZATION NUMBER

24. A DATE(S) OF SERVICE						B Place of Service	C Type of Service	D PROCEDURES, SERVICES, OR SUPPLIES (Explain Unusual Circumstances) CPT/HCPCS	MODIFIER	E DIAGNOSIS CODE	F $ CHARGES	G DAYS OR UNITS	H EPSDT Family Plan	I EMG	J COB	K RESERVED FOR LOCAL USE
From MM	DD	YY	To MM	DD	YY											
1																
2																
3																
4																
5																
6																

25. FEDERAL TAX I.D. NUMBER   SSN ☐ EIN ☐

26. PATIENT'S ACCOUNT NO.

27. ACCEPT ASSIGNMENT? (For govt. claims, see back)   ☐ YES   ☐ NO

28. TOTAL CHARGE $

29. AMOUNT PAID $

30. BALANCE DUE $

31. SIGNATURE OF PHYSICIAN OR SUPPLIER INCLUDING DEGREES OR CREDENTIALS (I certify that the statements on the reverse apply to this bill and are made a part thereof.)

SIGNED _____   DATE _____

32. NAME AND ADDRESS OF FACILITY WHERE SERVICES WERE RENDERED (If other than home or office)

33. PHYSICIAN'S, SUPPLIER'S BILLING NAME, ADDRESS, ZIP CODE & PHONE #

PIN#   GRP#

PHYSICIAN OR SUPPLIER INFORMATION

(APPROVED BY AMA COUNCIL ON MEDICAL SERVICE 8/88)   *PLEASE PRINT OR TYPE*   APPROVED OMB-0938-0008 FORM CMS-1500 (12-90),   FORM RRB-1500, APPROVED OMB-1215-0055 FORM OWCP-1500,   APPROVED OMB-0720-0001 (CHAMPUS)

Figure 14–6

ASSIGNMENT **14-6** ▸ **COMPLETE THREE CLAIM FORMS FOR A TRICARE STANDARD CASE**

Performance Objective

Task: Complete three CMS-1500 claim forms for a TRICARE Standard case, post transactions to the financial accounting record, and define patient record abbreviations.

Conditions: Use the patient's record (Figure 14–7) and financial statement (Figure 14–8), health insurance claim forms (Figures 14–9, 14–10, and 14–11), a typewriter or computer, procedural and diagnostic code books, and Appendices A and B in this *Workbook*.

Standards: Claim Productivity Measurement

Time: _____ minutes

Accuracy: _____

(Note: The time element and accuracy criteria may be given by your instructor.)

Directions:

1. This case requires three claim forms. Make photocopies of a CMS-1500 claim form or use Figures 14–9, 14–10, and 14–11 in this *Workbook*. Using OCR guidelines, complete the CMS-1500 claim forms and direct them to your local TRICARE fiscal intermediary. To locate your local fiscal intermediary, go to Web site http://www.tricare.osd.mil. Click on the area of the map you are residing in and then choose a state to access claims information for that state. Refer to Mrs. Mae I. Abbreviate's patient record for information and Appendix A in this *Workbook* to locate the fees to record on the claim, and post them to the financial statement. Date the claims January 31. Dr. Coccidioides is not accepting assignment on this TRICARE Standard case but is completing the claim for the patient's convenience.

2. Refer to Chapter 7 (Figure 7–13) of the *Handbook* for instructions on how to complete these claim forms and to view a TRICARE template.

3. Use your CPT code book or Appendix A in this *Workbook* to determine the correct five-digit code number and modifiers for each professional service rendered. Use your HCPCS Level II code book or refer to Appendix B in this *Workbook* for HCPCS procedure codes and modifiers.

4. Record the proper information on the financial record and note the date when you have billed TRICARE.

5. A Performance Evaluation Checklist may be reproduced from the "Instruction Guide to the Workbook" chapter if your instructor wishes you to submit it to assist with scoring and comments.

   After the instructor has returned your work to you, either make the necessary corrections and place your work in a three-ring notebook for future reference or, if you received a high score, place it in your portfolio for reference when applying for a job.

Abbreviations pertinent to this record:

NP _____   F _____

W _____   P _____

F _____   R _____

PE _____   EENT _____

CC _____   GGE _____

wk _____   HC _____

X _____   MDM _____

pt _____   STAT _____

PH _____   CBC _____

UCHD _____   diff _____

T & A _____   WBC _____

aet _____   RTO _____

Grav _____   RTW _____

Para1 _____   CT _____

D & C _____   dx _____

DUB _____   a.m. _____

LMP _____   D _____

surg _____   HX _____

OS _____   MC _____

yr _____   cm _____

FH _____   lt _____

CA _____   C & S _____

L & W _____   gm _____

GB _____   mg _____

SH _____   IM _____

PX _____   retn _____

ht _____   ofc _____

wt _____   OV _____

lbs _____   PF _____

BP _____   SF _____

T _____   HC _____

Additional Coding

1. Refer to Mrs. Abbreviate's medical record, abstract information, and code procedures that would be billed by outside providers.

Site	*Description of Service*	*Code*
a. College Hospital Radiology	_____	_____
b. College Hospital Laboratory	_____	_____
c. College Hospital Laboratory	_____	_____
d. College Hospital Radiology	_____	_____
e. College Hospital Microbiology	_____	_____
f. College Hospital Radiology	_____	_____

2. Use your diagnostic code book and code the symptoms that the patient complained of on January 14, 20xx.

Symptom	*Code*
a. _____	_____
b. _____	_____
c. _____	_____
d. _____	_____

3. Locate a financial accounting record (ledger).

   Note: Refer to the step-by-step procedures at the end of Chapter 3 in the *Handbook* and graphic examples Figures 3–18, 10–2, and 12–15.

4. Insert the patient's name and address, including ZIP code in the box.

5. Enter the patient's personal data.

6. Ledger lines: Insert date of service (DOS), reference (CPT code number, check number, or dates of service for posting adjustments or when insurance was billed), description of the transaction, charge amounts, payments, adjustments, and running current balance. The posting date is the actual date the transaction is recorded. If the DOS differs from the posting date, list the DOS in the reference or description column.

Line 2: _____

Line 3: _____

Line 4: _____

Line 5: _____

Line 6: _____

Line 7: _____

Line 8: _____

Line 9: _____

Line 10: _____

Line 11: _____

Line 12: _____

Line 13: _____

Line 14: _____

Line 15: _____

Line 16: _____

Line 17: _____

Note: A good bookkeeping practice is to take a red pen and draw a line across the financial accounting record (ledger) from left to right to indicate the last entry billed to the insurance company.

PATIENT RECORD NO. 14-6

Abbreviate	Mae	I	01-02-42	F	555-986-7667
LAST NAME	FIRST NAME	MIDDLE NAME	BIRTH DATE	SEX	HOME PHONE

4667 Symbol Road	Woodland Hills	XY	12345
ADDRESS	CITY	STATE	ZIP CODE

555-740-3300		555-986-7667	abbreviate@wb.net
CELL PHONE	PAGER NO.	FAX NO.	E-MAIL ADDRESS

865-XX-2311	E0598247
PATIENT'S SOC. SEC. NO.	DRIVER'S LICENSE

administrative assistant	U. R. Wright Company
PATIENT'S OCCUPATION	NAME OF COMPANY

6789 Abridge Road, Woodland Hills, XY 12346	555-988-7540
ADDRESS OF EMPLOYER	PHONE

Shorty S. Abbreviate	Staff Sargeant, Grade 12 (Active Duty)
SPOUSE OR PARENT	OCCUPATION

United States Army	HHC, 2nd Batt., 27th Infantry, APO New York, New York, 10030	
EMPLOYER	ADDRESS	PHONE

TRICARE Standard	husband (DOB 3/25/40)
NAME OF INSURANCE	INSURED OR SUBSCRIBER

023-XX-7866	
POLICY/CERTIFICATE NO.	GROUP NO.

REFERRED BY: Jane B. Accurate (friend)

Figure 14–7a

DATE	PROGRESS NOTES No. 14-6
1-14-xx	NP, 45-year-old W F in for complete PE. CC: Recent onset of flu-like symptoms of
	approximate 2 wk duration, including cough; chest pain X 2 days. Pt states beginning to
	cough up moderate amounts of greenish sputum with blood streaks, fatigue, fever, and chills.
	Comprehensive history includes PH: UCHD, T & A aet 6, Grav 1 Para 1, D & C aet 41 for
	DUB, LMP 12-18-XX, surg on OS after accident last yr. FH: Father expired of kidney CA aet
	63; mother L & W after GB surg in 1999; no siblings. SH: Pt admits to past alcohol abuse,
	denies alcohol use in last 6 months. No smoking, denies drug abuse. Comprehensive PX:
	Ht 5' 7", wt 150 lbs, BP 150/80, T 100.5 F, P 88, R 18; EENT ō except OS opaque;
	chest, rales scattered bilaterally, pt is dyspneic. Abdomen soft, nontender.
	GGE (HC MDM). Pt would like to avoid hospitalization if at all possible. Sent to College
	Hospital for STAT chest x-ray (2 views) and laboratory tests (electrolyte panel and complete
	CBC, automated with diff WBC. RTO tomorrow morning for test results.
	Completed disability form for work; estimated RTW, 2 weeks.
	BC/llf *Brady Coccicioides, MD*
1-14-xx	Call received from hospital radiology department: Chest x-rays revealed probable lung
	abscess in left lower lobe; inconclusive. Ordered STAT CT of thorax without contrast for
	more definitive dx. Contacted pt and recommended she have CT done this evening.
	RTO tomorrow a.m.
	BC/llf *Brady Coccicioides, MD*
1-15-xx	Pt returns to office for test results (D HX/PX MC/MDM). CT reveals lung abscess of
	3.0 cm in lt lower lobe. Pt able to produce sputum for C & S (Gram stain smear), sent to
~	College Hospital laboratory, microbiology department. Rocephin (Ceftriaxone sodium)
	1 gm ($5 per 250 mg/1000 mg = 1 gm) given IM in office, instructed pt to retn to ofc daily
	for Rocephin injections; reevaluate on Friday.
	BC/llf *Brady Coccicioides, MD*
1-16-xx	Rocephin 1 gm IM ordered by Dr. Coccicioides; administered by medical assistant in left
	gluteus maximus.
	BC/llf *Ali Marie Hobkins, CMA*
1-17-xx	Rocephin 1 gm IM ordered by Dr. Coccicioides; administered by medical assistant in right
	gluteus maximus.
	BC/llf *Ali Marie Hobkins, CMA*
1-18-xx	Pt returns for reevaluation (OV PF HX/PX SF MDM). Culture revealed streptococcal
	pneumoniae. Administered Rocephin 1 gm IM. Will continue daily injections.
	Arrangements made for house call over weekend.
	BC/llf *Brady Coccicioides, MD*
1-19-xx	HC Saturday (PF HX/PX SF MDM). Rocephin 1 gm IM. Pt states she is feeling much
	better, fatigue gone, cough decreased, afebrile. Ordered repeat chest x-ray (2 views) at
	College Hospital Monday. RTO Monday afternoon.
	BC/llf *Brady Coccicioides, MD*
1-21-xx	OV (PF HX/PX SF MDM). Repeat chest x-ray negative except few residual shadows.
	No injection today, start oral antibiotics. Pt to return in 1 wk for f/u or call sooner if
	symptoms reappear. Estimated RTW, 1/28/XX.
	BC/llf *Brady Coccicioides, MD*

Figure 14–7b

Acct No. 14-6

STATEMENT
Financial Account
COLLEGE CLINIC
4567 Broad Avenue
Woodland Hills, XY 12345-0001
Tel. 555-486-9002
Fax No. 555-487-8976

Mae I. Abbreviate
4667 Symbol Road
Woodland Hills, XY 12345

Phone No. (H)____555-986-7667_____ (W)_____555-988-7540_____   Birthdate__01/02/42_____

Primary Insurance Co.____TRICARE Standard_____   Policy/Group No. 023-XX-7866____

Secondary Insurance Co._____   Policy/Group No._____

DATE	REFERENCE	DESCRIPTION	CHARGES	CREDITS		BALANCE
				PYMNTS.	**ADJ.**	
20xx				BALANCE FORWARD ➡		
1-14-xx		NP OV				
1-15-xx		OV				
1-15-xx		Injection AB				
1-15-xx		Rocefin 1 gm				
1-16-xx		Injection AB				
1-16-xx		Rocefin 1 gm				
1-17-xx		Injection AB				
1-17-xx		Rocefin 1 gm				
1-18-xx		OV				
1-18-xx		Injection AB				
1-18-xx		Rocefin 1 gm				
1-19-xx		HC				
1-19-xx		Injection AB				
1-19-xx		Rocefin 1 gm				
1-21-xx		OV				

PLEASE PAY LAST AMOUNT IN BALANCE COLUMN ⇧

THIS IS A COPY OF YOUR FINANCIAL ACCOUNT AS IT APPEARS ON OUR RECORDS

Figure 14–8

HEALTH INSURANCE CLAIM FORM

PLEASE
DO NOT
STAPLE
IN THIS
AREA

PICA

| | | | PICA |

1. MEDICARE   MEDICAID   CHAMPUS   CHAMPVA   GROUP HEALTH PLAN   FECA BLK LUNG   OTHER

(Medicare #) (Medicaid #) (Sponsor's SSN) (VA File #) (SSN or ID) (S SN) (ID)

1a. INSURED'S I.D. NUMBER   (FOR PROGRAM IN ITEM 1)

2. PATIENT'S NAME (Last Name, First Name, Middle Initial)

3. PATIENT'S BIRTH DATE   MM DD YY   SEX M F

4. INSURED'S NAME (Last Name, First Name, Middle Initial)

5. PATIENT'S ADDRESS (No., Street)

6. PATIENT RELATIONSHIP TO INSURED   Self Spouse Child Other

7. INSURED'S ADDRESS (No., Street)

CITY   STATE

8. PATIENT STATUS   Single Married Other   Employed Full-Time Student Part-Time Student

CITY   STATE

ZIP CODE   TELEPHONE (Include Area Code)

ZIP CODE   TELEPHONE (INCLUDE AREA CODE)

9. OTHER INSURED'S NAME (Last Name, First Name, Middle Initial)

10. IS PATIENT'S CONDITION RELATED TO:

11. INSURED'S POLICY GROUP OR FECA NUMBER

a. OTHER INSURED'S POLICY OR GROUP NUMBER

a. EMPLOYMENT? (CURRENT OR PREVIOUS) YES NO

a. INSURED'S DATE OF BIRTH MM DD YY SEX M F

b. OTHER INSURED'S DATE OF BIRTH MM DD YY SEX M F

b. AUTO ACCIDENT? PLACE (State) YES NO

b. EMPLOYER'S NAME OR SCHOOL NAME

c. EMPLOYER'S NAME OR SCHOOL NAME

c. OTHER ACCIDENT? YES NO

c. INSURANCE PLAN NAME OR PROGRAM NAME

d. INSURANCE PLAN NAME OR PROGRAM NAME

10d. RESERVED FOR LOCAL USE

d. IS THERE ANOTHER HEALTH BENEFIT PLAN? YES NO If yes, return to and complete item 9 a-d.

READ BACK OF FORM BEFORE COMPLETING & SIGNING THIS FORM.
12. PATIENT'S OR AUTHORIZED PERSON'S SIGNATURE I authorize the release of any medical or other information necessary to process this claim. I also request payment of government benefits either to myself or to the party who accepts assignment below.

SIGNED _____ DATE _____

13. INSURED'S OR AUTHORIZED PERSON'S SIGNATURE I authorize payment of medical benefits to the undersigned physician or supplier for services described below.

SIGNED _____

14. DATE OF CURRENT: ILLNESS (First symptom) OR INJURY (Accident) OR PREGNANCY(LMP) MM DD YY

15. IF PATIENT HAS HAD SAME OR SIMILAR ILLNESS. GIVE FIRST DATE MM DD YY

16. DATES PATIENT UNABLE TO WORK IN CURRENT OCCUPATION FROM MM DD YY TO MM DD YY

17. NAME OF REFERRING PHYSICIAN OR OTHER SOURCE

17a. I.D. NUMBER OF REFERRING PHYSICIAN

18. HOSPITALIZATION DATES RELATED TO CURRENT SERVICES FROM MM DD YY TO MM DD YY

19. RESERVED FOR LOCAL USE

20. OUTSIDE LAB? $ CHARGES YES NO

21. DIAGNOSIS OR NATURE OF ILLNESS OR INJURY. (RELATE ITEMS 1,2,3 OR 4 TO ITEM 24E BY LINE)
1. ___ 2. ___ 3. ___ 4. ___

22. MEDICAID RESUBMISSION CODE   ORIGINAL REF. NO.

23. PRIOR AUTHORIZATION NUMBER

24. A DATE(S) OF SERVICE From MM DD YY To MM DD YY	B Place of Service	C Type of Service	D PROCEDURES, SERVICES, OR SUPPLIES (Explain Unusual Circumstances) CPT/HCPCS MODIFIER	E DIAGNOSIS CODE	F $ CHARGES	G DAYS OR UNITS	H EPSDT Family Plan	I EMG	J COB	K RESERVED FOR LOCAL USE
1										
2										
3										
4										
5										
6										

25. FEDERAL TAX I.D. NUMBER SSN EIN

26. PATIENT'S ACCOUNT NO.

27. ACCEPT ASSIGNMENT? (For govt. claims, see back) YES NO

28. TOTAL CHARGE $

29. AMOUNT PAID $

30. BALANCE DUE $

31. SIGNATURE OF PHYSICIAN OR SUPPLIER INCLUDING DEGREES OR CREDENTIALS (I certify that the statements on the reverse apply to this bill and are made a part thereof.)

SIGNED _____ DATE _____

32. NAME AND ADDRESS OF FACILITY WHERE SERVICES WERE RENDERED (If other than home or office)

33. PHYSICIAN'S, SUPPLIER'S BILLING NAME, ADDRESS, ZIP CODE & PHONE #

PIN#   GRP#

(APPROVED BY AMA COUNCIL ON MEDICAL SERVICE 8/88)   PLEASE PRINT OR TYPE   APPROVED OMB-0938-0008 FORM CMS-1500 (12-90),   FORM RRB-1500, APPROVED OMB-1215-0055 FORM OWCP-1500,   APPROVED OMB-0720-0001 (CHAMPUS)

CARRIER

PATIENT AND INSURED INFORMATION

PHYSICIAN OR SUPPLIER INFORMATION

Figure 14–9

14. DATE OF CURRENT: ILLNESS (First symptom) OR INJURY (Accident) OR PREGNANCY(LMP) MM DD YY	15. IF PATIENT HAS HAD SAME OR SIMILAR ILLNESS. GIVE FIRST DATE MM DD YY	16. DATES PATIENT UNABLE TO WORK IN CURRENT OCCUPATION FROM MM DD YY TO MM DD YY
17. NAME OF REFERRING PHYSICIAN OR OTHER SOURCE	17a. I.D. NUMBER OF REFERRING PHYSICIAN	18. HOSPITALIZATION DATES RELATED TO CURRENT SERVICES FROM MM DD YY TO MM DD YY
19. RESERVED FOR LOCAL USE		20. OUTSIDE LAB? $ CHARGES ☐ YES ☐ NO

21. DIAGNOSIS OR NATURE OF ILLNESS OR INJURY. (RELATE ITEMS 1,2,3 OR 4 TO ITEM 24E BY LINE)

1. ___   3. ___
2. ___   4. ___

22. MEDICAID RESUBMISSION CODE   ORIGINAL REF. NO.

23. PRIOR AUTHORIZATION NUMBER

24.

A DATE(S) OF SERVICE From MM DD YY To MM DD YY	B Place of Service	C Type of Service	D PROCEDURES, SERVICES, OR SUPPLIES (Explain Unusual Circumstances) CPT/HCPCS	MODIFIER	E DIAGNOSIS CODE	F $ CHARGES	G DAYS OR UNITS	H EPSDT Family Plan	I EMG	J COB	K RESERVED FOR LOCAL USE
1											
2											
3											
4											
5											
6											

25. FEDERAL TAX I.D. NUMBER SSN EIN ☐ ☐	26. PATIENT'S ACCOUNT NO.	27. ACCEPT ASSIGNMENT? (For govt. claims, see back) ☐ YES ☐ NO	28. TOTAL CHARGE $	29. AMOUNT PAID $	30. BALANCE DUE $
31. SIGNATURE OF PHYSICIAN OR SUPPLIER INCLUDING DEGREES OR CREDENTIALS (I certify that the statements on the reverse apply to this bill and are made a part thereof.) SIGNED DATE	32. NAME AND ADDRESS OF FACILITY WHERE SERVICES WERE RENDERED (If other than home or office)		33. PHYSICIAN'S, SUPPLIER'S BILLING NAME, ADDRESS, ZIP CODE & PHONE # PIN# GRP#		

PHYSICIAN OR SUPPLIER INFORMATION

EXAMPLE ONLY

(APPROVED BY AMA COUNCIL ON MEDICAL SERVICE 8/88)   **PLEASE PRINT OR TYPE**   APPROVED OMB-0938-0008 FORM CMS-1500 (12-90),   FORM RRB-1500,
APPROVED OMB-1215-0055 FORM OWCP-1500,   APPROVED OMB-0720-0001 (CHAMPUS)

Figure 14–10

14. DATE OF CURRENT: ILLNESS (First symptom) OR INJURY (Accident) OR PREGNANCY(LMP) MM DD YY	15. IF PATIENT HAS HAD SAME OR SIMILAR ILLNESS. GIVE FIRST DATE MM DD YY	16. DATES PATIENT UNABLE TO WORK IN CURRENT OCCUPATION FROM MM DD YY TO MM DD YY
17. NAME OF REFERRING PHYSICIAN OR OTHER SOURCE	17a. I.D. NUMBER OF REFERRING PHYSICIAN	18. HOSPITALIZATION DATES RELATED TO CURRENT SERVICES FROM MM DD YY TO MM DD YY
19. RESERVED FOR LOCAL USE		20. OUTSIDE LAB? $ CHARGES ☐ YES ☐ NO

21. DIAGNOSIS OR NATURE OF ILLNESS OR INJURY. (RELATE ITEMS 1,2,3 OR 4 TO ITEM 24E BY LINE)

1. ⌞___ 3. ⌞___
2. ⌞___ 4. ⌞___

22. MEDICAID RESUBMISSION CODE   ORIGINAL REF. NO.

23. PRIOR AUTHORIZATION NUMBER

24. A DATE(S) OF SERVICE From / To MM DD YY MM DD YY	B Place of Service	C Type of Service	D PROCEDURES, SERVICES, OR SUPPLIES (Explain Unusual Circumstances) CPT/HCPCS MODIFIER	E DIAGNOSIS CODE	F $ CHARGES	G DAYS OR UNITS	H EPSDT Family Plan	I EMG	J COB	K RESERVED FOR LOCAL USE
1										
2										
3										
4										
5										
6										

25. FEDERAL TAX I.D. NUMBER SSN ☐ EIN ☐	26. PATIENT'S ACCOUNT NO.	27. ACCEPT ASSIGNMENT? (For govt. claims, see back) ☐ YES ☐ NO	28. TOTAL CHARGE $	29. AMOUNT PAID $	30. BALANCE DUE $
31. SIGNATURE OF PHYSICIAN OR SUPPLIER INCLUDING DEGREES OR CREDENTIALS (I certify that the statements on the reverse apply to this bill and are made a part thereof.) SIGNED DATE	32. NAME AND ADDRESS OF FACILITY WHERE SERVICES WERE RENDERED (If other than home or office)	33. PHYSICIAN'S, SUPPLIER'S BILLING NAME, ADDRESS, ZIP CODE & PHONE # PIN# GRP#

PHYSICIAN OR SUPPLIER INFORMATION

(APPROVED BY AMA COUNCIL ON MEDICAL SERVICE 8/88) **PLEASE PRINT OR TYPE** APPROVED OMB-0938-0008 FORM CMS-1500 (12-90), FORM RRB-1500, APPROVED OMB-1215-0055 FORM OWCP-1500, APPROVED OMB-0720-0001 (CHAMPUS)

Figure 14–11

ASSIGNMENT 14–7 ▸ TRANSMIT AN ELECTRONIC INSURANCE CLAIM
FOR A TRICARE CASE

(e hint) Follow the General Instructions for TRANSMISSION OF AN ELEC-
TRONIC CLAIM (A SINGLE CLAIM) as given in Chapter 8.

Performance Objective

Task: Transmit an electronic insurance claim form and post the information to the patient's financial account record.

Conditions: Use Crystal L. Blackwood's encounter form (Figure 14–12), patient's electronic data, and computer.

Standards: Productivity Measurement

Time: _____ minutes

Accuracy: _____

(Note: The time element and accuracy criteria may be given by your instructor.)

Directions:

1. Electronically prepare an insurance claim form by referring to Crystal L. Blackwood's encounter form in the *Workbook* and her electronic personal and medical data. Follow the step-by-step general directions for transmission of an insurance claim.

2. Enter the patient's data into the software to obtain the procedural and diagnostic codes and College Clinic fee amounts.

3. Transmit the insurance claim to TRICARE.

4. Print a hard copy of the insurance claim to hand in to your instructor to receive a score.

5. A Performance Evaluation Checklist may be reproduced from the "Instruction Guide to the Workbook" chapter if your instructor wishes you to submit it to assist with scoring and comments.

After the instructor has returned your work to you, either make the necessary corrections and place your work in a three-ring notebook for future reference or, if you received a high score, place it in your portfolio for reference when applying for a job.

TAX ID #3664021CC
Medicaid #HSC12345F

College Clinic

4567 Broad Avenue
Woodlands Hills, XY
12345-0001
Tel (555) 486-9002
Fax (555) 487-8976

Doctors No. _____

☐ PRIVATE   ☐ MANAGED CARE   ☐ MEDICAID   ☐ MEDICARE   ☒ TRICARE   ☐ W/C

ACCOUNT #	PATIENT'S LAST NAME	FIRST	INITIAL	TODAY'S DATE
007	Blackwood	Crystal	L.	3/28/2007

ASSIGNMENT: I hereby assign payment directly to College Clinic of the surgical and/or medical benefits, if any, otherwise payable to me for his/her services as described below.
SIGNED (Patient, or Parent, if Minor)   *Crystal L. Blackwood*   DATE: *3/28/2007*

✓	DESCRIPTION	CPT-4/MD	FEE	✓	DESCRIPTION	CPT-4/MD	FEE	✓	DESCRIPTION	CPT-4/MD	FEE
	OFFICE VISIT-NEW PATIENT				**WELL BABY EXAM**				**LABORATORY**		
	Level 1	99201			Intial	99381		✓	Gonadotropin chorion	84702	20.00
	Level 2	99202			Periodic	99391			Heamatocrit	85013	
	Level 3	99203			**OFFICE PROCEDURES**				Occult Blood	82270	
✓	Level 4	99204	106.11		Anscopy	46600		✓	Urine Dip	81000	8.00
	Level 5	99205			ECG 24-hr	93224			**X-RAY**		
	OFFICE VISIT-ESTAB. PATIENT				Fracture Rpr Foot	28470			Foot - 2 View	73620	
	Level 1	99211			I & D	10060			Forearm - 2 View	73090	
	Level 2	99212			Suture Repair				Nasal Bone - 3	70160	
	Level 3	99213							Spine LS - 2 view	72100	
	Level 4	99214			**INJECTIONS/VACCINATIONS**						
	Level 5	99215			DPT	90701			**MISCELLANEOUS**		
	OFFICE CONSULT-NP/EST				IM-Antibiotic	90788		✓	Handling of Spec	99000	5.00
	Level 3	99243			OPU-Poliovirus	90712		✓	Supply	99070	25.00
	Level 4	99244			Tetanus	90703			Venipuncture	36415	
	Level 5	99245									

COMMENTS:

Physician: *Bertha Caesar, M.D.*

	RETURN APPOINTMENT
	___/___ Week(s) _____ Month(s)

DIAGNOSIS:	DESCRIPTION	CODE	REC'D BY:		
Primary:	Pregnancy exam	V72.4	☐ BANK CARD	PREVIOUS BALANCE	16.07
Secondary:	antepartium hemorrhage		☐ CASH	TODAY'S FEE	164.11
	pregnancy complication	640.93	☐ CHECK	AMOUNT REC'D/CO-PAY	⊖
			# _____	BALANCE	180.18

Figure 14–12

ASSIGNMENT **14–8** ▸ **VIEW AND PRINT AN INSURANCE AGING REPORT**

ⓔhint General Instructions for PRINTING AN INSURANCE AGING REPORT

1. From the main menu, click "Reports" and select "Insurance Aging."

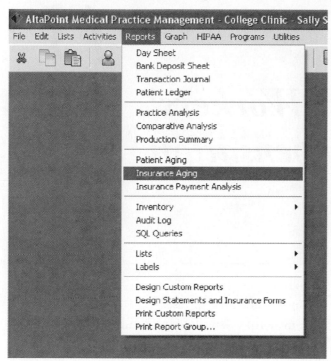

2. Review the "Options" window and change any field information to fit applicable dates, patients, etc. Then click "Print."

3. Additionally, in the "Ranges to Print" menu, you can select various options from the menu, including insurance payers and patients.

Performance Objective

Task: View electronically an insurance aging report and print a hard copy.

Conditions: Practice management software and a computer

Standards: Productivity Measurement

                 Time: _____ minutes

                 Accuracy: _____

                 (Note: The time element and accuracy criteria may be given by your instructor.)

Directions:

1. Print out a hard copy of the Insurance Aging Report and turn it in to your instructor to receive a score.

   After the instructor has returned your work to you, either make the necessary corrections and place your work in a three-ring notebook for future reference or, if you received a high score, place it in your portfolio for reference when applying for a job.

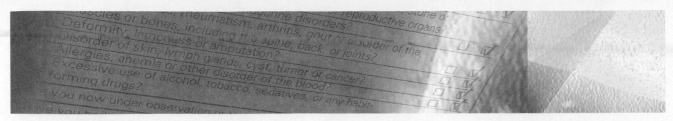

Workers' Compensation

KEY TERMS

Your instructor may wish to select some specific words pertinent to this chapter for a test. For definitions of the terms, further study, and/or reference, the words, phrases, and abbreviations may be found in the glossary at the end of the Handbook. *Key terms for this chapter follow.*

accident

adjudication

by report (BR)

claims examiner

compromise and release (C and R)

deposition

ergonomic

extraterritorial

Federal Employees' Compensation Act (FECA)

fee schedule

injury

insurance adjuster

lien

medical service order

nondisability (ND) claim

occupational illness (or disease)

Occupational Safety and Health Administration (OSHA)

permanent and stationary (P and S)

permanent disability (PD)

petition

second-injury fund

sequelae

sub rosa films

subsequent-injury fund (SIF)

temporary disability (TD)

third-party liability

third-party subrogation

waiting period (WP)

work hardening

Workers' Compensation Appeals Board (WCAB)

workers' compensation (WC) insurance

PERFORMANCE OBJECTIVES

The student will be able to:

▦ Define and spell the key terms for this chapter, given the information from the Handbook glossary, within a reasonable time period and with enough accuracy to obtain a satisfactory evaluation.

▦ After reading the chapter, answer the self-study review questions with enough accuracy to obtain a satisfactory evaluation.

▦ Given a list of common medical abbreviations and symbols that appear in chart notes, fill in the correct meaning of each abbreviation within a reasonable time period and with enough accuracy to obtain a satisfactory evaluation.

▦ Given the patients' medical chart notes, ledger cards, and blank insurance forms, complete each

workers' compensation form for billing, within a reasonable time period and with enough accuracy to obtain a satisfactory evaluation.

▦ Given the patients' medical chart notes, ledger cards, and blank insurance claim forms, complete each CMS-1500 Health Insurance Claim Form for submission to a workers' compensation insurance company within a reasonable time period and with enough accuracy to obtain a satisfactory evaluation.

▦ Using the Mock Fee Schedule in Appendix A in this Workbook, correctly post payments, adjustments, and balances on the patients' ledger cards within a reasonable time period and with enough accuracy to obtain a satisfactory evaluation.

STUDY OUTLINE

History
Workers' Compensation Statutes
Workers' Compensation Reform

Workers' Compensation Laws and Insurance
Purposes of Workers' Compensation Laws
Self-Insurance
Managed Care

Eligibility
Industrial Accident
Occupational Illness

Coverage
Federal Laws
State Laws
State Disability and Workers' Compensation

Benefits

Types of State Claims
Nondisability Claim
Temporary Disability Claim
Permanent Disability Claim

Fraud and Abuse

Occupational Safety and Health Administration Act of 1970
Background
Coverage
Regulations
Filing a Complaint
Inspection
Record Keeping and Reporting

Legal Situations
Medical Evaluator
Depositions
Medical Testimony
Liens
Third-Party Subrogation

Medical Reports
Privacy and Confidentiality
Documentation
Health Information Record Keeping
Terminology

Reporting Requirements
Employer's Report
Medical Service Order
Physician's First Report
Progress or Supplemental Report
Final Report

Claim Submission
Financial Responsibility
Fee Schedules
Helpful Billing Tips
Billing Claims
Out-of-State Claims
Delinquent or Slow Pay Claims

Procedure: Completing the Doctor's First Report of Occupational Injury or Illness

SELF-STUDY 15-1 ▶ REVIEW QUESTIONS

Review the objectives, key terms, glossary definitions of key terms, chapter information, and figures before completing the following review questions.

1. Name two kinds of statutes under workers' compensation.

   a. _____

   b. _____

2. An unexpected, unintended event that occurs at a particular time and place, causing injury to an individual not of his or her own making, is called a/an

   _____.

3. Maria Cardoza works in a plastics manufacturing company and inhales some fumes that cause bronchitis. Because this condition is associated with her employment, it is called

   a/an _____.

4. Name the federal workers' compensation acts that cover workers.

   a. _____

   b. _____

   c. _____

   d. _____

5. State compensation laws that require each employer to accept its provisions and provide for specialized benefits for employees who are injured at work are

   called _____.

6. State compensation laws that may be accepted or rejected by the employer are known

   as _____.

7. State five methods used for funding workers' compensation.

   a. _____

   b. _____

   c. _____

   d. _____

   e. _____

8. Who pays the workers' compensation insurance premiums? _____

9. What is the time limit in your state for submitting the employers' and/or physicians'

   report on an industrial accident? _____

10. When an employee with a preexisting condition is injured at work and the injury
    produces a disability greater than what would have been caused by the second injury

    alone, the benefits are derived from a/an _____.

11. Name jobs that may not be covered by workers' compensation insurance.

    a. _____   d. _____

    b. _____   e. _____

    c. _____   f. _____

12. What is the minimum number of employees per business needed in your state for

    workers' compensation statutes to become effective? _____

13. What waiting period must elapse in your state before workers' compensation

    payments begin? _____

14. List five types of workers' compensation benefits.

    a. _____

    b. _____

    c. _____

    d. _____

    e. _____

15. Who can treat an industrial injury? _____

    _____

16. What are three types of workers' compensation claims and the differences among
    them?

    a. _____

    b. _____

    c. _____

17. After suffering an industrial injury, Mr. Fields is in a treatment program in which he is
    given real work tasks for building strength and endurance. This form of therapy is

    called _____.

18. Define the following abbreviations:

  a. TD _____   b. PD _____

  c. P & S _____   d. C & R _____

19. Weekly temporary disability payments are based on _____

  _____.

20. When an industrial case reaches the time for rating the disability, this is accomplished by

  _____.

21. May an injured person appeal his or her case if he or she is not satisfied with the

  rating? If so, to whom does he or she appeal? _____

  or _____.

22. When fraud or abuse is suspected in a workers' compensation case, the physician

  should report the situation to _____.

23. Employers are required to meet health and safety standards for their employees

  under federal and state statutes known as the _____

  _____.

24. A man takes his girlfriend to a roofing job, and she is injured. Is she covered under

  workers' compensation insurance? _____.

25. A proceeding during which an attorney questions a witness who answers under oath

  but not in open court is called a/an _____.

26. The legal promise of a patient to satisfy a debt to the physician from proceeds

  received from a litigated case is termed a/an _____.

27. The process of carrying on a lawsuit is called _____.

28. Explain third-party subrogation _____.

29. What is the first thing an employee should do after he or she is injured on the job?

  _____.

30. When an individual suffers a work-related injury or illness, the employer must

  complete and send a form called a/an _____ to the
  insurance company and workers' compensation state offices, and if the employee is
  sent to a physician's office for medical care, the employer must complete a form

  called a/an _____ that authorizes the physician to treat the employee.

31. If the physician believes the injured employee is capable of returning to work

    after having been on temporary disability, what does the physician do? _____

    _____.

32. In a workers' compensation case, bills should be submitted or _____,

    and a claim becomes delinquent after a time frame of _____.

33. If an individual seeks medical care for a workers' compensation injury from

    another state, which state's regulations are followed? _____.

34. When a physician treats an industrial injury, he or she must complete

    a/an _____ and send it to the following:

    a. _____

    b. _____

    c. _____

    d. _____

    Is a stamped physician's signature acceptable on the form? Explain.

    _____

To check your answers to this self-study assignment, see Appendix D.

ASSIGNMENT 15–2 ► COMPLETE A DOCTOR'S FIRST REPORT
OF OCCUPATIONAL INJURY OR ILLNESS FORM
FOR A WORKERS' COMPENSATION CASE

Performance Objective

Task: Complete a Doctor's First Report of Occupational Injury or Illness form
               and define patient record abbreviations.

Conditions: Use the patient's record (Figure 15–1), a Doctor's First Report of Occupational
               Injury or Illness form (Figure 15–2), and a typewriter or computer.

Standards: Claim Productivity Measurement

               Time: _____ minutes

               Accuracy: _____

               (Note: The time element and accuracy criteria may be given by your
               instructor.)

Directions:

1. Complete the Doctor's First Report of Occupational Injury or Illness form
   (Figure 15–2) for this nondisability type of claim.

2. Define abbreviations found in the patient's medical record.

   After the instructor has returned your work to you, either make the necessary
corrections and place your work in a three-ring notebook for future reference or, if you
received a high score, place it in your portfolio for reference when applying for a job.

Abbreviations pertinent to this record:

Apt	_____	CT	_____
Lt	_____	Neg	_____
pt	_____	MC	_____
ED	_____	MDM	_____
Hosp	_____	DC	_____
ER	_____	PD	_____
C	_____	FU	_____
HX	_____	Wks	_____
PX	_____	Approx	_____
c/o	_____	RTW	_____
L	_____	WC	_____

PATIENT RECORD NO. 15-2-3

Hiranuma	Glen	M	12-24-45	M	555-467-3383
LAST NAME	FIRST NAME	MIDDLE NAME	BIRTH DATE	SEX	HOME PHONE

4372 Hanley Avenue	Woodland Hills	XY	12345
ADDRESS	CITY	STATE	ZIP CODE

555-908-3433		555-467-3383	hiranuma@wb.net
CELL PHONE	PAGER NO.	FAX NO.	E-MAIL ADDRESS

558-XX-9960	U3402189
PATIENT'S SOC. SEC. NO.	DRIVER'S LICENSE

house painter	Pittsburgh Paint Company (commercial painting company)
PATIENT'S OCCUPATION	NAME OF COMPANY

3725 Bonfeld Avenue, Woodland Hills, XY 12345	555-486-9070
ADDRESS OF EMPLOYER	PHONE

Esme M. Hiranuma	homemaker
SPOUSE OR PARENT	OCCUPATION

EMPLOYER	ADDRESS	PHONE

State Compensation Insurance Fund, 14156 Magnolia Boulevard, Torres, XY 12349
NAME OF INSURANCE

016-2432-211	
POLICY/CERTIFICATE NO.	GROUP NO.

REFERRED BY: Pittsburgh Paint Company

DATE	PROGRESS NOTES
5-22-xx	At 9:30 a.m. this ♂ house painter was painting an apt ceiling (apt located at 3540 W. 87th Street, Woodland Hills,
	XY 12345, County of Woodland Hills) when he slipped and fell from a tall ladder landing on his head and lt side of
	body; brief unconsciousness for approximately 15 minutes. Employer was notified by coworker and pt was sent
	to College Hosp ED. I was called to the hosp at request of employer and saw pt in ER at 5 p.m. (performed a C
	HX/PX). Pt c/o L shoulder pain and swelling; L leg and hip pain; neck and head pain. X-rays were taken of lt hip
	(complete), lt femur (2 views), and cervical spine (3 views) as well as CT of brain (without contrast)—all neg. I
	admitted pt for overnight stay in hosp for concussion. Applied sling for L shoulder sprain. Cleaned and dressed L
	hip and leg abrasions (MC/MDM). Plan to DC 5/23/xx. No PD expected. Pt to FU in 2 wks. Approx. RTW 6/6 xx.
	Prepared WC report.
	GP/llf *Gerald Practon, MD*
5-23-xx	Pt's HA gone. Vital signs normal. Discharged home. RTO 1 wk.
	GP/llf *Gerald Practon, MD*

Figure 15–1

DOCTOR'S FIRST REPORT OF OCCUPATIONAL INJURY OR ILLNESS

Within 5 days of initial examination, for every occupational injury or illness, send 2 copies of this report to the employers' workers' compensation insurance carrier or the self-insured employer. Failure to file a timely doctor's report may result in assessment of a civil penalty. In the case of diagnosed or suspected pesticide poisoning, send a copy of this report to Division of Labor Statistics and Research.

1. **INSURER NAME AND ADDRESS**

2. **EMPLOYER NAME**

   Policy No.

3. Address　　No. and Street　　City　　Zip

4. Nature of business(e.g., food manufacturing, building construction, retailer of women's clothes)

5. **PATIENT NAME** (first, middle initial, last name)	6. Sex ☐Male ☐Female	7. Date of Birth	Mo.	Day	Yr.

8. Address　　No. and Street　　City　　Zip ｜ 9. Telephone Number

10. Occupation (Specific job title) ｜ 11. Social Security Number

12. Injured at:　　No. and Street　　City　　County

13. Date and hour of injury or onset or illness	Mo.	Day	Yr.	Hour ____a.m____p.m	14. Date last worked	Mo.	Day	Yr.

15. Date and hour of first examination or treatment	Mo.	Day	Yr.	Hour ____a.m____p.m	16. Have you (or your office) previously treated patient? ☐Yes ☐No

Patient please complete this portion, if able to do so. Otherwise, doctor please complete immediately. Inability or failure of a patient to complete this portion shall not affect his/her rights to workers' compensation under the Labor Code.
17. DESCRIBE HOW THE ACCIDENT OR EXPOSURE HAPPENED (Give specific object, machinery or chemical.)

18. **SUBJECTIVE COMPLAINTS** (Describe fully.)

19. **OBJECTIVE FINDINGS**

   A. Physical examination

   B. X-ray and laboratory results (State if none or pending.)

20. **DIAGNOSIS** (If occupational illness specify etiologic agent and duration of exposure.) Chemical or toxic compound involved?　　ICD - 9 Code　　☐Yes ☐No

21. Are your findings and diagnosis consistent with patient's account of injury or onset of illness?　　☐Yes ☐No If "no" please explain

22. Is there any other current condition that will impede or delay patient's recovery?　　☐ Yes　☐ No　If "yes" please explain

23. **TREATMENT REQUIRED**

24. If further treatment required, specify treatment plan/estimated duration.

25. If hospitalized as inpatient, give hospital name and location　　Date admitted　Mo.　Day　Yr.　　Estimated stay

26. **WORK STATUS** --Is patient able to perfom usual work?　　☐ Yes　☐ No

   If "no," date when patient can return to: Regular work____/____/

   　　　　　　　　　　　　　　　　Modified work____/____/　　Specify restrictions

Doctor's Signature _____　License Number _____

Doctor's Name and Degree _____　IRS Number _____

Address _____　Telephone Number _____

Figure 15–2

ASSIGNMENT **15–3** ▸ **COMPLETE A CLAIM FORM FOR A WORKERS' COMPENSATION CASE**

Performance Objectives

Task: Complete a CMS-1500 claim form for a workers' compensation case and post transactions to the financial accounting record.

Conditions: Use the patient's record (Figure 15–1) and financial statement (Figure 15–3), a CMS-1500 claim form (Figure 15–4), a typewriter or computer, procedural and diagnostic code books, and Appendix A in this *Workbook*.

Standards: Claim Productivity Measurement

Time: _____ minutes

Accuracy: _____

(Note: The time element and accuracy criteria may be given by your instructor.)

Directions:

1. Using optical character reader (OCR) guidelines, complete a CMS-1500 claim form and direct it to the proper workers' compensation carrier. Refer to Mr. Glen M. Hiranuma's patient record for information and Appendix A in this *Workbook* to locate the fees to record on the claim, and post them to the financial statement. Date the claim May 24 of the current year.
2. Refer to Chapter 7 (Figure 7–15) of the *Handbook* for instructions on how to complete this claim form and a workers' compensation template.
3. Use your CPT code book or Appendix A in this *Workbook* to determine the correct five-digit code number and modifiers for each professional service rendered. Use your HCPCS Level II code book or refer to Appendix B in this *Workbook* for HCPCS procedure codes and modifiers. Note: In your state, a workers' compensation fee schedule may be available with this information.
4. Record the proper information on the financial record and claim form, and note the date you have billed the workers' compensation.
5. A Performance Evaluation Checklist may be reproduced from the "Instruction Guide to the Workbook" chapter if your instructor wishes you to submit it to assist with scoring and comments.

After the instructor has returned your work to you, either make the necessary corrections and place your work in a three-ring notebook for future reference or, if you received a high score, place it in your portfolio for reference when applying for a job.

Additional Coding

1. Refer to Mr. Glen M. Hiranuma's medical record, abstract information, and code procedures that would be billed by outside providers.

Site	Description of Service	Code
a. College Hospital Radiology	_____	_____
b. College Hospital Radiology	_____	_____
c. College Hospital Radiology	_____	_____
d. College Hospital Radiology	_____	_____

2. Locate a financial accounting record (ledger).

   Note: Refer to the step-by-step procedures at the end of Chapter 3 in the Handbook and graphic examples Figures 3–18, 10–2, and 12–15.

3. Insert the patient's name and address, including ZIP code in the box.

4. Enter the patient's personal data.

5. Ledger lines: Insert date of service (DOS), reference (CPT code number, check number, or dates of service for posting adjustments or when insurance was billed), description of the transaction, charge amounts, payments, adjustments, and running current balance. The posting date is the actual date the transaction is recorded. If the DOS differs from the posting date, list the DOS in the reference or description column.

   Line 2: _____

   Line 3: _____

   Line 4: _____

   Line 5: _____

Note: A good bookkeeping practice is to take a red pen and draw a line across the financial accounting record (ledger) from left to right to indicate the last entry billed to the insurance company.

Acct No. 15-2-3

STATEMENT
Financial Account
COLLEGE CLINIC
4567 Broad Avenue
Woodland Hills, XY 12345-0001
Tel. 555-486-9002
Fax No. 555-487-8976

Workers' Compensation

State Compensation Insurance Fund
14156 Magnolia Boulevard
Torres, CY 12349-0218

Patient's Name   Glen M. Hiranuma

Social Security No. 558-XX-9960

Date of Injury   5-22-xx   Employer   Pittsburgh Paint Company

Policy No.   016-2432-211

Phone No. (H) 555-467-3383   Phone No. (W)   555-486-9070

Claim No.   unassigned

DATE	REFERENCE	DESCRIPTION	CHARGES	CREDITS PYMNTS.	ADJ.	BALANCE
20xx			BALANCE FORWARD →			
5-22-xx		Hospital Admit				
5-22-xx		WC Report				
5-22-xx		Discharge				

PLEASE PAY LAST AMOUNT IN BALANCE COLUMN

THIS IS A COPY OF YOUR FINANCIAL ACCOUNT AS IT APPEARS ON OUR RECORDS

Figure 15–3

PLEASE
DO NOT
STAPLE
IN THIS
AREA

CARRIER

HEALTH INSURANCE CLAIM FORM

| | PICA | | | | | | | | PICA | |

1. MEDICARE MEDICAID CHAMPUS CHAMPVA GROUP HEALTH PLAN FECA BLK LUNG OTHER
(Medicare #) (Medicaid #) (Sponsor's SSN) (VA File #) (SSN or ID) (S SN) (ID)

1a. INSURED'S I.D. NUMBER   (FOR PROGRAM IN ITEM 1)

2. PATIENT'S NAME (Last Name, First Name, Middle Initial)

3. PATIENT'S BIRTH DATE MM DD YY   SEX M F

4. INSURED'S NAME (Last Name, First Name, Middle Initial)

5. PATIENT'S ADDRESS (No., Street)

6. PATIENT RELATIONSHIP TO INSURED Self Spouse Child Other

7. INSURED'S ADDRESS (No., Street)

CITY STATE

8. PATIENT STATUS Single Married Other
Employed Full-Time Student Part-Time Student

CITY STATE

ZIP CODE TELEPHONE (Include Area Code)

ZIP CODE TELEPHONE (INCLUDE AREA CODE)

9. OTHER INSURED'S NAME (Last Name, First Name, Middle Initial)

10. IS PATIENT'S CONDITION RELATED TO:

11. INSURED'S POLICY GROUP OR FECA NUMBER

a. OTHER INSURED'S POLICY OR GROUP NUMBER

a. EMPLOYMENT? (CURRENT OR PREVIOUS) YES NO

a. INSURED'S DATE OF BIRTH MM DD YY SEX M F

b. OTHER INSURED'S DATE OF BIRTH MM DD YY SEX M F

b. AUTO ACCIDENT? PLACE (State) YES NO

b. EMPLOYER'S NAME OR SCHOOL NAME

c. EMPLOYER'S NAME OR SCHOOL NAME

c. OTHER ACCIDENT? YES NO

c. INSURANCE PLAN NAME OR PROGRAM NAME

d. INSURANCE PLAN NAME OR PROGRAM NAME

10d. RESERVED FOR LOCAL USE

d. IS THERE ANOTHER HEALTH BENEFIT PLAN? YES NO *If yes*, return to and complete item 9 a-d.

READ BACK OF FORM BEFORE COMPLETING & SIGNING THIS FORM.
12. PATIENT'S OR AUTHORIZED PERSON'S SIGNATURE I authorize the release of any medical or other information necessary to process this claim. I also request payment of government benefits either to myself or to the party who accepts assignment below.
SIGNED _____ DATE _____

13. INSURED'S OR AUTHORIZED PERSON'S SIGNATURE I authorize payment of medical benefits to the undersigned physician or supplier for services described below.
SIGNED _____

14. DATE OF CURRENT: ILLNESS (First symptom) OR INJURY (Accident) OR PREGNANCY(LMP) MM DD YY

15. IF PATIENT HAS HAD SAME OR SIMILAR ILLNESS. GIVE FIRST DATE MM DD YY

16. DATES PATIENT UNABLE TO WORK IN CURRENT OCCUPATION FROM MM DD YY TO MM DD YY

17. NAME OF REFERRING PHYSICIAN OR OTHER SOURCE

17a. I.D. NUMBER OF REFERRING PHYSICIAN

18. HOSPITALIZATION DATES RELATED TO CURRENT SERVICES FROM MM DD YY TO MM DD YY

19. RESERVED FOR LOCAL USE

20. OUTSIDE LAB? $ CHARGES YES NO

21. DIAGNOSIS OR NATURE OF ILLNESS OR INJURY. (RELATE ITEMS 1,2,3 OR 4 TO ITEM 24E BY LINE)
1. ___ 3. ___
2. ___ 4. ___

22. MEDICAID RESUBMISSION CODE ORIGINAL REF. NO.

23. PRIOR AUTHORIZATION NUMBER

24. A DATE(S) OF SERVICE From To MM DD YY MM DD YY	B Place of Service	C Type of Service	D PROCEDURES, SERVICES, OR SUPPLIES (Explain Unusual Circumstances) CPT/HCPCS	MODIFIER	E DIAGNOSIS CODE	F $ CHARGES	G DAYS OR UNITS	H EPSDT Family Plan	I EMG	J COB	K RESERVED FOR LOCAL USE
1											
2											
3											
4											
5											
6											

25. FEDERAL TAX I.D. NUMBER SSN EIN

26. PATIENT'S ACCOUNT NO.

27. ACCEPT ASSIGNMENT? (For govt. claims, see back) YES NO

28. TOTAL CHARGE $

29. AMOUNT PAID $

30. BALANCE DUE $

31. SIGNATURE OF PHYSICIAN OR SUPPLIER INCLUDING DEGREES OR CREDENTIALS (I certify that the statements on the reverse apply to this bill and are made a part thereof.)
SIGNED _____ DATE _____

32. NAME AND ADDRESS OF FACILITY WHERE SERVICES WERE RENDERED (If other than home or office)

33. PHYSICIAN'S, SUPPLIER'S BILLING NAME, ADDRESS, ZIP CODE & PHONE #
PIN# GRP#

(APPROVED BY AMA COUNCIL ON MEDICAL SERVICE 8/88) *PLEASE PRINT OR TYPE* APPROVED OMB-0938-0008 FORM CMS-1500 (12-90), FORM RRB-1500, APPROVED OMB-1215-0055 FORM OWCP-1500, APPROVED OMB-0720-0001 (CHAMPUS)

PATIENT AND INSURED INFORMATION / PHYSICIAN OR SUPPLIER INFORMATION

EXAMPLE ONLY

Figure 15-4

ASSIGNMENT 15-4 ▸ COMPLETE A DOCTOR'S FIRST REPORT
OF OCCUPATIONAL INJURY OR ILLNESS FORM
FOR A WORKERS' COMPENSATION CASE

Performance Objective

Task: Complete a Doctor's First Report of Occupational Injury or Illness form
             and define patient record abbreviations.

Conditions: Use the patient's record (Figure 15–5), a Doctor's First Report of
             Occupational Injury or Illness form (Figure 15–6), and a typewriter or
             computer.

Standards: Claim Productivity Measurement

             Time: _____ minutes

             Accuracy: _____

             (Note: The time element and accuracy criteria may be given by your
             instructor.)

Directions:

1. Complete the Doctor's First Report of Occupational Injury or Illness form for this
   temporary disability type of claim. Refer to Carlos A. Giovanni's patient record for
   November 11 through November 15.

2. Define abbreviations found in the patient's medical record.

   After the instructor has returned your work to you, either make the necessary
corrections and place your work in a three-ring notebook for future reference or, if you
received a high score, place it in your portfolio for reference when applying for a job.

Abbreviations pertinent to this record:

pt	_____	H	_____
ER	_____	MDM	_____
C	_____	TD	_____
HX	_____	RTW	_____
PX	_____	approx	_____
CT	_____	HV	_____
R	_____	EPF	_____
tr	_____	M	_____
adm	_____	PO	_____

DC	_____	PF	_____
Hosp	_____	SF	_____
OV	_____	X	_____
LC	_____	adv	_____
HA	_____	trt	_____
BP	_____	reg	_____
RTO	_____	W	_____
Wks	_____	Cons	_____

PATIENT RECORD NO. 15-4-5

Giovanni	Carlos	A	10-24-45	F	555-677-3485
LAST NAME	FIRST NAME	MIDDLE NAME	BIRTH DATE	SEX	HOME PHONE

89 Beaumont Court	Woodland Hills	XY	12345
ADDRESS	CITY	STATE	ZIP CODE

	555-230-7788	555-677-3485		giovannic@wb.net
CELL PHONE	PAGER NO.	FAX NO.		E-MAIL ADDRESS

556-XX-9699	Y0394876
PATIENT'S SOC. SEC. NO.	DRIVER'S LICENSE

TV repairman	Giant Television Co. (TV repair company)
PATIENT'S OCCUPATION	NAME OF COMPANY

8764 Ocean Avenue, Woodland Hills, XY 12345	555-647-8851
ADDRESS OF EMPLOYER	PHONE

Maria B. Giovanni	homemaker
SPOUSE OR PARENT	OCCUPATION

EMPLOYER	ADDRESS	PHONE

State Compensation Insurance Fund, 600 S. Lafayette Park Place, Ehrlich, XY 12350
NAME OF INSURANCE

57780
POLICY/CERTIFICATE NO.   GROUP NO.

REFERRED BY: Giant Television Company

Figure 15–5

DATE	PROGRESS NOTES
	Patient: Giovanni, Carlos A. Patient Record No. 15-04-05
11-11-xx	Pt referred to College Hospital ER by employer for workers' compensation injury. I was called in as on-call
	neurosurgeon to evaluate the pt. Pt states that today at 2 p.m. he fell from the roof of a private home while
	installing an antenna at 2231 Duarte St., Woodland Hills, XY 12345 in Woodland Hills County. He describes the
	incident as follows: "When I was attaching the base of an antenna, the weight of the antenna shifted and knocked
	me off the roof." Pt complains of head pain and indicates brief loss of consciousness. I performed a C HX/PX.
	Complete skull x-rays showed fractured skull. CT of head/brain (without contrast) indicates well-defined R.
	subdural hematoma. Pt suffering from cerebral concussion; no open wound. Tr plan: Adm pt to College
	Hospital (5 p.m.) and schedule R infratentorial craniotomy to evacuate hematoma. (H/MDM). Obtained
	authorization and prepared Dr.'s First Report.
	AP/llf *Astro Parkinson, MD*
11-12-xx	Performed R infratentorial craniotomy and evacuated subdural hematoma. Pt stable and returned to room; will be
	seen daily. TD: Estimated RTW 1-15-xx. Possible cranial defect & head disfigurement resulting. Pt to be
	hospitalized for approx 2 weeks.
	AP/llf *Astro Parkinson, MD*
11-13-xx	HV (EPF HX/PX M/MDM). Pt improving; recommend consult with Dr. Graff for cranial defect. Authorization
	obtained from adjuster (Steve Burroughs) at State Comp.
	AP/llf *Astro Parkinson, MD*
11-14-xx	Pt seen in cons by Dr. Cosmo Graff who stated he does not recommend correcting PO cranial defect. Both
	Dr. Graff and I explained how the defect resulted from the injury; there may be some improvement over time.
	Pt states he is grateful to be alive (EPF HX/PX M/MDM).
	AP/llf *Astro Parkinson, MD*
11-15-xx	Daily HV (EPF HX/PX M/MDM). Pt progressing appropriately; no complications have occurred.
thru	
11-29-xx	AP/llf *Astro Parkinson, MD*
11-30-xx	DC from hosp. Permanent cranial defect resulting from fracture and surgery. RTO 1 wk.
	AP/llf *Astro Parkinson, MD*
12-7-xx	OV (EPF HX/PX LC/MDM) Pt doing very well. No HA or visual disturbances, BP 120/80, alert and oriented.
	He is anxious to return to work. Pt cautioned about maintaining low activity level until released. RTO 2 wks.
	AP/llf *Astro Parkinson, MD*
12-21-xx	OV (PF HX/PX SF/MDM). Pt continues to improve. Suggested he start a walking program 3 x wk and monitor
	symptoms. May do light activity and lifting (10 lbs). Adv to call if any symptoms return. RTO 10 days.
	AP/llf *Astro Parkinson, MD*
12-29-xx	OV (PF HX/PX SF/MDM). Pt did not experience any symptoms with increased activity. No further trt necessary.
	Pt will increase activity and call if any problems occur. Pt scheduled to resume reg W on 1-15-xx. Final report
	submitted to workers' compensation carrier.
	AP/llf *Astro Parkinson, MD*

Figure 15–5, cont'd

DOCTOR'S FIRST REPORT OF OCCUPATIONAL INJURY OR ILLNESS

Within 5 days of initial examination, for every occupational injury or illness, send 2 copies of this report to the employers' workers' compensation insurance carrier or the self-insured employer. Failure to file a timely doctor's report may result in assessment of a civil penalty. In the case of diagnosed or suspected pesticide poisoning, send a copy of this report to Division of Labor Statistics and Research.

1. **INSURER NAME AND ADDRESS**

2. **EMPLOYER NAME**

Policy No.

3. Address   No. and Street   City   Zip

4. Nature of business(e.g., food manufacturing, building construction, retailer of woman's clothes)

5. **PATIENT NAME** (first, middle initial, last name) | 6. Sex ☐Male ☐Female | 7. Date of Birth   mo.   Day   Yr.

8. Address   No. and Street   City   Zip | 9. Telephone Number

10. Occupation (Specific job title) | 11. Social Security Number

12. Injured at: No. and Street   City   County

13. Date and hour of injury or onset or illness   Mo.   Day   Yr.   Hour ____a.m ____p.m | 14. Date last worked   Mo.   Day   Yr.

15. Date and hour of first examination or treatment   Mo.   Day   Yr.   Hour ____a.m ____p.m | 16. Have you (or your office) previously treated patient?   ☐ Yes   ☐ No

Patient please complete this portion, if able to do so. Otherwise, doctor please complete immediately. Inability or failure of a patient to complete this portion shall not affect his/her rights to workers' compensation under the Labor Code.
17. DESCRIBE HOW THE ACCIDENT OR EXPOSURE HAPPENED (Give specific object, machinery or chemical.)

18. **SUBJECTIVE COMPLAINTS** (Describe fully.)

19. **OBJECTIVE FINDINGS**

   A. Physical examination

   B. X-ray and laboratory results (State if none or pending.)

20. **DIAGNOSIS** (if occupational illness specify etiologic agent and duration of exposure.) Chemical or toxic compound involved?   ICD - 9 Code   ☐Yes ☐No

21. Are your findings and diagnosis consistent with patient's account of injury or onset of illness?   ☐Yes ☐No If "no" please explain

22. Is there any other current condition that will impede or delay patient's recovery?   ☐ Yes   ☐ No   If "yes" please explain

23. **TREATMENT REQUIRED**

24. If further treatment required, specify treatment plan/estimated duration.

25. If hospitalized as inpatient, give hospital name and location   Date admitted   Mo.   Day   Yr.   Estimated stay

26. **WORK STATUS** –is patient able to perfom usual work?   ☐ Yes   ☐ No
   If "no," date when patient can return to: Regular work___/___/
   Modified work___/___/   Specify restrictions

Doctor's Signature _____ License Number _____
Doctor's Name and Degree_____ IRS Number_____
Address_____ Telephone Number _____

Figure 15–6

ASSIGNMENT **15–5** ▸ **COMPLETE A CLAIM FORM FOR A WORKERS' COMPENSATION CASE**

Performance Objective

Task: Complete a CMS-1500 claim form for a workers' compensation case and post transactions to the financial accounting record.

Conditions: Use the patient's record (Figure 15–5) and financial statement (Figure 15–7), a CMS-1500 claim form (Figure 15–8), a typewriter or computer, procedural and diagnostic code books, and Appendix A in this *Workbook*.

Standards: Claim Productivity Measurement

Time: _____ minutes

Accuracy: _____

(Note: The time element and accuracy criteria may be given by your instructor.)

Directions:

1. Using OCR guidelines, complete a CMS-1500 claim form for November dates of service and direct it to the correct workers' compensation carrier for this temporary disability workers' compensation claim. Refer to Mr. Carlos A. Giovanni's patient record for information and Appendix A in this *Workbook* to locate the fees to record on the claim and post to the financial statement. Date the claim November 30 of the current year. **NOTE:** A progress report is being submitted with this claim; services for December will be billed on a separate claim (see Assignment 15–6).
2. Refer to Chapter 7 (Figure 7–15) of the *Handbook* for instructions on how to complete this claim form and a workers' compensation template.
3. Use your CPT code book or Appendix A in this *Workbook* to determine the correct five-digit code number and modifiers for each professional service rendered. Use your HCPCS Level II code book or refer to Appendix B in this *Workbook* for HCPCS procedure codes and modifiers.
4. Record the proper information on the financial record and claim form, and note the date you have billed the workers' compensation insurance carrier.
5. A Performance Evaluation Checklist may be reproduced from the "Instruction Guide to the Workbook" chapter if your instructor wishes you to submit it to assist with scoring and comments.

After the instructor has returned your work to you, either make the necessary corrections and place your work in a three-ring notebook for future reference or, if you received a high score, place it in your portfolio for reference when applying for a job.

Additional Coding

1. Refer to Mr. Giovanni's medical record, abstract information, and code procedures that would be billed by outside providers.

Site	Description of Service	Code
a. College Hospital Radiology	_____	_____
b. College Hospital Radiology	_____	_____

2. Locate a financial accounting record (ledger).

Note: Refer to the step-by-step procedures at the end of Chapter 3. in the *Handbook* and graphic examples Figures 3–18, 10–2, and 12–15.

3. Insert the patient's name and address, including ZIP code in the box.

4. Enter the patient's personal data.

5. Ledger lines: Insert date of service (DOS), reference (CPT code number, check number, or dates of service for posting adjustments or when insurance was billed), description of the transaction, charge amounts, payments, adjustments, and running current balance. The posting date is the actual date the transaction is recorded. If the DOS differs from the posting date, list the DOS in the reference or description column.

Line 2: _____

Line 3: _____

Line 4: _____

Line 5: _____

Line 6: _____

Line 7: _____

Note: A good bookkeeping practice is to take a red pen and draw a line across the financial accounting record (ledger) from left to right to indicate the last entry billed to the insurance company.

Acct No. 15-5

STATEMENT
Financial Account
COLLEGE CLINIC
4567 Broad Avenue
Woodland Hills, XY 12345-0001
Tel. 555-486-9002
Fax No. 555-487-8976

Workers' Compensation

State Compensation Insurance Fund
14156 Magnolia Boulevard
Torres, CY 12349-0218

Patient's Name   Carlos A. Giovanni   Social Security No.   556-XX9699

Date of Injury   11-11-20xx   Employer   Giant Television Company   Policy No.   57780

Phone No. (H) 555-677-3485   Phone No. (W)   555-647-8851   Claim No.   unassigned

| DATE | REFERENCE | DESCRIPTION | CHARGES | CREDITS | | BALANCE |
				PYMNTS.	ADJ.	
20xx		BALANCE FORWARD				
11-11-xx		Hospital admit				
11-11-xx		WC Report				
11-12-xx		Craniotomy				
11-13 to 11-29-xx		HV				
11-30-xx		Discharge				
12-7-xx		OV				
12-21-xx		OV				
12-29-xx		OV				
12-29-xx		Medical Report				

PLEASE PAY LAST AMOUNT IN BALANCE COLUMN

THIS IS A COPY OF YOUR FINANCIAL ACCOUNT AS IT APPEARS ON OUR RECORDS

Figure 15–7

PLEASE
DO NOT
STAPLE
IN THIS
AREA

HEALTH INSURANCE CLAIM FORM

PICA

PICA

1. MEDICARE	MEDICAID	CHAMPUS	CHAMPVA	GROUP HEALTH PLAN	FECA BLK LUNG	OTHER	1a. INSURED'S I.D. NUMBER	(FOR PROGRAM IN ITEM 1)
(Medicare #)	(Medicaid #)	(Sponsor's SSN)	(VA File #)	(SSN or ID)	(S SN)	(ID)		

2. PATIENT'S NAME (Last Name, First Name, Middle Initial)

3. PATIENT'S BIRTH DATE
MM   DD   YY   SEX
M ☐   F ☐

4. INSURED'S NAME (Last Name, First Name, Middle Initial)

5. PATIENT'S ADDRESS (No., Street)

6. PATIENT RELATIONSHIP TO INSURED
Self ☐   Spouse ☐   Child ☐   Other ☐

7. INSURED'S ADDRESS (No., Street)

CITY   STATE

8. PATIENT STATUS
Single ☐   Married ☐   Other ☐
Employed ☐   Full-Time Student ☐   Part-Time Student ☐

CITY   STATE

ZIP CODE   TELEPHONE (Include Area Code)
)

ZIP CODE   TELEPHONE (INCLUDE AREA CODE)

9. OTHER INSURED'S NAME (Last Name, First Name, Middle Initial)

10. IS PATIENT'S CONDITION RELATED TO:

11. INSURED'S POLICY GROUP OR FECA NUMBER

a. OTHER INSURED'S POLICY OR GROUP NUMBER

a. EMPLOYMENT? (CURRENT OR PREVIOUS)
☐ YES   ☐ NO

a. INSURED'S DATE OF BIRTH
MM   DD   YY   SEX
M ☐   F ☐

b. OTHER INSURED'S DATE OF BIRTH
MM   DD   YY   SEX
M ☐   F ☐

b. AUTO ACCIDENT?   PLACE (State)
☐ YES   ☐ NO

b. EMPLOYER'S NAME OR SCHOOL NAME

c. EMPLOYER'S NAME OR SCHOOL NAME

c. OTHER ACCIDENT?
☐ YES   ☐ NO

c. INSURANCE PLAN NAME OR PROGRAM NAME

d. INSURANCE PLAN NAME OR PROGRAM NAME

10d. RESERVED FOR LOCAL USE

d. IS THERE ANOTHER HEALTH BENEFIT PLAN?
☐ YES   ☐ NO   If yes, return to and complete item 9 a-d.

READ BACK OF FORM BEFORE COMPLETING & SIGNING THIS FORM.

12. PATIENT'S OR AUTHORIZED PERSON'S SIGNATURE I authorize the release of any medical or other information necessary to process this claim. I also request payment of government benefits either to myself or to the party who accepts assignment below.

SIGNED _____   DATE _____

13. INSURED'S OR AUTHORIZED PERSON'S SIGNATURE I authorize payment of medical benefits to the undersigned physician or supplier for services described below.

SIGNED _____

14. DATE OF CURRENT: ◄ ILLNESS (First symptom) OR
MM   DD   YY   INJURY (Accident) OR
                          PREGNANCY(LMP)

15. IF PATIENT HAS HAD SAME OR SIMILAR ILLNESS. GIVE FIRST DATE   MM   DD   YY

16. DATES PATIENT UNABLE TO WORK IN CURRENT OCCUPATION
MM   DD   YY   MM   DD   YY
FROM _____ TO _____

17. NAME OF REFERRING PHYSICIAN OR OTHER SOURCE

17a. I.D. NUMBER OF REFERRING PHYSICIAN

18. HOSPITALIZATION DATES RELATED TO CURRENT SERVICES
MM   DD   YY   MM   DD   YY
FROM _____ TO _____

19. RESERVED FOR LOCAL USE

20. OUTSIDE LAB? $ CHARGES
☐ YES   ☐ NO

21. DIAGNOSIS OR NATURE OF ILLNESS OR INJURY. (RELATE ITEMS 1,2,3 OR 4 TO ITEM 24E BY LINE)

1. ∟____   3. ∟____

2. ∟____   4. ∟____

22. MEDICAID RESUBMISSION CODE   ORIGINAL REF. NO.

23. PRIOR AUTHORIZATION NUMBER

24. A				B	C	D		E	F	G	H	I	J	K
DATE(S) OF SERVICE				Place of Service	Type of Service	PROCEDURES, SERVICES, OR SUPPLIES (Explain Unusual Circumstances)		DIAGNOSIS CODE	$ CHARGES	DAYS OR UNITS	EPSDT Family Plan	EMG	COB	RESERVED FOR LOCAL USE
From		To				CPT/HCPCS	MODIFIER							
MM	DD	YY	MM	DD	YY									
1														
2														
3														
4														
5														
6														

25. FEDERAL TAX I.D. NUMBER   SSN ☐ EIN ☐

26. PATIENT'S ACCOUNT NO.

27. ACCEPT ASSIGNMENT? (For govt. claims, see back)
☐ YES   ☐ NO

28. TOTAL CHARGE
$

29. AMOUNT PAID
$

30. BALANCE DUE
$

31. SIGNATURE OF PHYSICIAN OR SUPPLIER INCLUDING DEGREES OR CREDENTIALS
(I certify that the statements on the reverse apply to this bill and are made a part thereof.)

SIGNED _____   DATE _____

32. NAME AND ADDRESS OF FACILITY WHERE SERVICES WERE RENDERED (If other than home or office)

33. PHYSICIAN'S, SUPPLIER'S BILLING NAME, ADDRESS, ZIP CODE & PHONE #

PIN#   GRP#

(APPROVED BY AMA COUNCIL ON MEDICAL SERVICE 8/88)   **PLEASE PRINT OR TYPE**

APPROVED OMB-0938-0008 FORM CMS-1500 (12-90),   FORM RRB-1500,
APPROVED OMB-1215-0055 FORM OWCP-1500,   APPROVED OMB-0720-0001 (CHAMPUS)

Figure 15–8

ASSIGNMENT **15-6** ▸ **COMPLETE A CLAIM FORM FOR A WORKERS'
COMPENSATION CASE**

Performance Objective

Task: Complete a CMS-1500 claim form for a workers' compensation case and post transactions to the financial accounting record.

Conditions: Use the patient's record (Figure 15–5) and financial statement (Figure 15–7), a CMS-1500 claim form (Figure 15–9), a typewriter or computer, procedural and diagnostic code books, and Appendix A in this *Workbook*.

Standards: Claim Productivity Measurement

Time: _____ minutes

Accuracy:

(Note: The time element and accuracy criteria may be given by your instructor.)

Directions:

1. Using OCR guidelines, complete a CMS-1500 claim form for December services and direct it to the correct workers' compensation carrier for this temporary disability workers' compensation claim. Refer to Mr. Carlos A. Giovanni's patient record for information and Appendix A in this *Workbook* to locate the fees to record on the claim, and post them to the financial statement. Date the claim December 29 of the current year.
2. Refer to Chapter 7 (Figure 7–15) of the *Handbook* for instructions on how to complete this claim form and a workers' compensation template.
3. Use your CPT code book or Appendix A in this *Workbook* to determine the correct five-digit code number and modifiers for each professional service rendered. Use your HCPCS Level II code book or refer to Appendix B in this *Workbook* for HCPCS procedure codes and modifiers.
4. Record the proper information on the financial record and claim form, and note the date you have billed the workers' compensation insurance carrier.
5. A Performance Evaluation Checklist may be reproduced from the "Instruction Guide to the Workbook" chapter if your instructor wishes you to submit it to assist with scoring and comments.

   After the instructor has returned your work to you, either make the necessary corrections and place your work in a three-ring notebook for future reference or, if you received a high score, place it in your portfolio for reference when applying for a job.

6. Ledger lines: Insert date of service (DOS), reference (CPT code number, check number, or dates of service for posting adjustments or when insurance was billed), description of the transaction, charge amounts, payments, adjustments, and running current balance. The posting date is the actual date the transaction is recorded. If the DOS differs from the posting date, list the DOS in the reference or description column.

Line 8: _____

Line 9: _____

Line 10: _____

Line 11: _____

Line 12: _____

Note: A good bookkeeping practice is to take a red pen and draw a line across the financial accounting record (ledger) from left to right to indicate the last entry billed to the insurance company.

PLEASE
DO NOT
STAPLE
IN THIS
AREA

CARRIER →

| | PICA | | | HEALTH INSURANCE CLAIM FORM | PICA | | |

HEALTH INSURANCE CLAIM FORM

1. MEDICARE   MEDICAID   CHAMPUS   CHAMPVA   GROUP HEALTH PLAN   FECA BLK LUNG   OTHER   1a. INSURED'S I.D. NUMBER   (FOR PROGRAM IN ITEM 1)
   ☐ (Medicare #)   ☐ (Medicaid #)   ☐ (Sponsor's SSN)   ☐ (VA File #)   ☐ (SSN or ID)   ☐ (S SN)   ☐ (ID)

2. PATIENT'S NAME (Last Name, First Name, Middle Initial)

3. PATIENT'S BIRTH DATE   MM   DD   YY   SEX   M ☐   F ☐

4. INSURED'S NAME (Last Name, First Name, Middle Initial)

5. PATIENT'S ADDRESS (No., Street)

6. PATIENT RELATIONSHIP TO INSURED   Self ☐   Spouse ☐   Child ☐   Other ☐

7. INSURED'S ADDRESS (No., Street)

CITY   STATE
8. PATIENT STATUS   Single ☐   Married ☐   Other ☐
CITY   STATE

ZIP CODE   TELEPHONE (Include Area Code)
                Employed ☐   Full-Time Student ☐   Part-Time Student ☐
ZIP CODE   TELEPHONE (INCLUDE AREA CODE)

9. OTHER INSURED'S NAME (Last Name, First Name, Middle Initial)

10. IS PATIENT'S CONDITION RELATED TO:

11. INSURED'S POLICY GROUP OR FECA NUMBER

a. OTHER INSURED'S POLICY OR GROUP NUMBER

a. EMPLOYMENT? (CURRENT OR PREVIOUS)   ☐ YES   ☐ NO

a. INSURED'S DATE OF BIRTH   MM   DD   YY   SEX   M ☐   F ☐

b. OTHER INSURED'S DATE OF BIRTH   MM   DD   YY   SEX   M ☐   F ☐

b. AUTO ACCIDENT?   PLACE (State)   ☐ YES   ☐ NO

b. EMPLOYER'S NAME OR SCHOOL NAME

c. EMPLOYER'S NAME OR SCHOOL NAME

c. OTHER ACCIDENT?   ☐ YES   ☐ NO

c. INSURANCE PLAN NAME OR PROGRAM NAME

d. INSURANCE PLAN NAME OR PROGRAM NAME

10d. RESERVED FOR LOCAL USE

d. IS THERE ANOTHER HEALTH BENEFIT PLAN?   ☐ YES   ☐ NO   If yes, return to and complete item 9 a-d.

READ BACK OF FORM BEFORE COMPLETING & SIGNING THIS FORM.

12. PATIENT'S OR AUTHORIZED PERSON'S SIGNATURE I authorize the release of any medical or other information necessary to process this claim. I also request payment of government benefits either to myself or to the party who accepts assignment below.

SIGNED _____   DATE _____

13. INSURED'S OR AUTHORIZED PERSON'S SIGNATURE I authorize payment of medical benefits to the undersigned physician or supplier for services described below.

SIGNED _____

14. DATE OF CURRENT: MM   DD   YY   ◄ ILLNESS (First symptom) OR INJURY (Accident) OR PREGNANCY(LMP)

15. IF PATIENT HAS HAD SAME OR SIMILAR ILLNESS. GIVE FIRST DATE   MM   DD   YY

16. DATES PATIENT UNABLE TO WORK IN CURRENT OCCUPATION   FROM   MM   DD   YY   TO   MM   DD   YY

17. NAME OF REFERRING PHYSICIAN OR OTHER SOURCE

17a. I.D. NUMBER OF REFERRING PHYSICIAN

18. HOSPITALIZATION DATES RELATED TO CURRENT SERVICES   FROM   MM   DD   YY   TO   MM   DD   YY

19. RESERVED FOR LOCAL USE

20. OUTSIDE LAB?   ☐ YES   ☐ NO $ CHARGES

21. DIAGNOSIS OR NATURE OF ILLNESS OR INJURY. (RELATE ITEMS 1,2,3 OR 4 TO ITEM 24E BY LINE)

1. L_____
2. L_____
3. L_____
4. L_____

22. MEDICAID RESUBMISSION CODE   ORIGINAL REF. NO.

23. PRIOR AUTHORIZATION NUMBER

24.	A DATE(S) OF SERVICE						B Place of Service	C Type of Service	D PROCEDURES, SERVICES, OR SUPPLIES (Explain Unusual Circumstances) CPT/HCPCS MODIFIER	E DIAGNOSIS CODE	F $ CHARGES	G DAYS OR UNITS	H EPSDT Family Plan	I EMG	J COB	K RESERVED FOR LOCAL USE
	From MM	DD	YY	To MM	DD	YY										
1																
2																
3																
4																
5																
6																

25. FEDERAL TAX I.D. NUMBER   SSN   EIN   ☐ ☐

26. PATIENT'S ACCOUNT NO.

27. ACCEPT ASSIGNMENT? (For govt. claims, see back)   ☐ YES   ☐ NO

28. TOTAL CHARGE $

29. AMOUNT PAID $

30. BALANCE DUE $

31. SIGNATURE OF PHYSICIAN OR SUPPLIER INCLUDING DEGREES OR CREDENTIALS (I certify that the statements on the reverse apply to this bill and are made a part thereof.)

SIGNED _____   DATE _____

32. NAME AND ADDRESS OF FACILITY WHERE SERVICES WERE RENDERED (If other than home or office)

33. PHYSICIAN'S, SUPPLIER'S BILLING NAME, ADDRESS, ZIP CODE & PHONE #

PIN#   GRP#

PATIENT AND INSURED INFORMATION

PHYSICIAN OR SUPPLIER INFORMATION

(APPROVED BY AMA COUNCIL ON MEDICAL SERVICE 8/88)   **PLEASE PRINT OR TYPE**   APPROVED OMB-0938-0008 FORM CMS-1500 (12-90),   FORM RRB-1500,
APPROVED OMB-1215-0055 FORM OWCP-1500,   APPROVED OMB-0720-0001 (CHAMPUS)

Figure 15–9

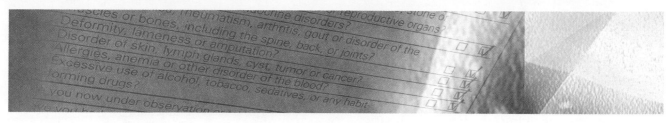

Disability Income Insurance and Disability Benefits Programs

KEY TERMS

Your instructor may wish to select some specific words pertinent to this chapter for a test. For definitions of the terms, further study, and/or reference, the words, phrases, and abbreviations may be found in the glossary at the end of the Handbook. *Key terms for this chapter follow. Some of the insurance terms presented in this chapter are shown marked with an asterisk (*) and may seem familiar from previous chapters. However, their meanings may or may not have a slightly different connotation when referring to disability income insurance. Key terms for this chapter follow.*

accidental death and dismemberment

Armed Services Disability

benefit period*

Civil Service Retirement System (CSRS)

consultative examiner (CE)

cost-of-living adjustment

Disability Determination Services (DDS)

disability income insurance

double indemnity

exclusions*

Federal Employees Retirement System (FERS)

future purchase option

guaranteed renewable*

hearing

long-term disability insurance

noncancelable clause*

partial disability*

reconsideration

regional office (RO)

residual benefits*

residual disability

short-term disability insurance

Social Security Administration (SSA)

Social Security Disability Insurance (SSDI) program

State Disability Insurance (SDI)

supplemental benefits

Supplemental Security Income (SSI)

temporary disability*

temporary disability insurance (TDI)

total disability*

unemployment compensation disability (UCD)

Veterans Affairs (VA) disability program

Veterans Affairs (VA) outpatient clinic

voluntary disability insurance

waiting period*

waiver of premium*

PERFORMANCE OBJECTIVES

The student will be able to:

■ Define and spell the key terms for this chapter, given the information from the *Handbook* glossary, within a reasonable time period, and with enough accuracy to obtain a satisfactory evaluation.

■ After reading the chapter, answer the self-study review questions with enough accuracy to obtain a satisfactory evaluation.

■ Fill in the correct meaning of each abbreviation, given a list of common medical abbreviations and

symbols that appear in chart notes, within a reasonable time period and with enough accuracy to obtain a satisfactory evaluation.

■ Complete each state disability form, given the patients' medical chart notes and blank state disability forms, within a reasonable time period and with enough accuracy to obtain a satisfactory evaluation.

STUDY OUTLINE

Disability Claims

History

Disability Income Insurance
   Individual
   Group

Federal Disability Programs
   Workers' Compensation
   Disability Benefit Programs

State Disability Insurance
   Background
   State Programs

   Funding
   Eligibility
   Benefits
   Time Limits
   Medical Examinations
   Restrictions

Voluntary Disability Insurance

Claims Submission
   Disability Income Claims

Conclusion

 SELF-STUDY **16–1** ▸ **REVIEW QUESTIONS**

Review the objectives, key terms, glossary definitions of key terms, chapter information, tables, and figures before completing the following review questions.

1. Health insurance that provides monthly or weekly income when an individual is

   unable to work because of a nonindustrial illness or injury is called _____.

2. Another insurance term for benefits is _____.

3. Some insurance contracts that pay twice the face amount of the policy if accidental

   death occurs may have a provision titled _____.

4. When an individual who is insured under a disability income insurance policy cannot

   perform one or more of his or her regular job duties, this is known as _____

   or _____ disability.

5. When a person insured under a disability income insurance policy cannot, for a limited period of time, perform all functions of his or her regular job

   duties, this is known as _____ disability.

6. When the purchase of insurance is investigated, the word/words to look for in the insurance contract that mean the premium cannot be increased at renewal time is/are

   _____.

7. When an individual becomes permanently disabled and cannot pay the insurance

   premium, a desirable provision in an insurance contract is _____.

8. Provisions that limit the scope of insurance coverage are known as _____.

9. Ezra Jackson has disability income insurance under a group policy paid for by his employer. One evening he goes inline skating and suffers a complex fracture of the patella, which necessitates several months off work. Are his monthly disability benefits taxable?

   _____ Why or why not? _____

   _____

10. Two federal programs for individuals younger than 65 years of age who have a severe disability are

    a. _____

    b. _____

11. To be eligible to apply for disability benefits under Social Security, an individual

    must be unable to perform any type of work for a period of _____.

12. The Social Security Administration may hire a physician to evaluate an applicant's disability. A physician's role may be any one of the following:

    a. _____

    b. _____

    c. _____

13. A Social Security Administration division that determines an individual's eligibility

    to be placed under the federal disability program is called _____.

14. Jamie Woods, a Navy petty officer, suffers an accident aboard the USS Denebola just before his honorable discharge. To receive veteran's benefits for this injury,

    the time limit in which a claim must be filed is _____.

15. Name the states and the territory that have nonindustrial state disability programs.

    a. _____

    b. _____

    c. _____

    d. _____

    e. _____

    f. _____

16. List two states in which hospital benefits may be paid for nonoccupational illness or injury under a state's temporary disability benefit program.

    a. _____

    b. _____

17. Temporary disability insurance claims must be filed within how many days in your state?

    _____

18. How long can a person continue to draw temporary disability insurance benefits?

    _____

19. After a claim begins, when do basic state disability benefits become payable if the

    patient is confined to his or her home? _____

    If the patient is hospitalized? _____

20. Nick Tyson has recovered since a previous illness ended and becomes ill again

    with the same ailment. Is he entitled to state disability benefits? _____

21. John S. Thatcher stubbed his toe as he was leaving work. Because the injury was only slightly uncomfortable, he thought no more about it. The next morning he found that his foot was too swollen to fit in his shoe, so he stayed home. When the swelling did not subside after 3 days, John went to the doctor. Radiographs showed a broken toe, which kept John home for 2 weeks. After 1 week he applied for temporary state

    disability benefits. Will he be paid? _____ Why or why not? _____

22. Peggy Jonson has an ectopic pregnancy and is unable to work because of complications of this condition. Can she receive state temporary disability benefits?

    _____

23. If a woman has an abnormal condition that arises from her pregnancy (such as diabetes or varicose veins) and is unable to work because of the condition, can she

    receive state disability benefits? _____

Four states that allow for maternity benefits in normal pregnancy are

a. _____   c. _____

b. _____   d. _____

24. Betty T. Kraft had to stay home from her job because her 10-year-old daughter had

measles. She applied for temporary state disability benefits. Will she be paid? _____

Why or why not? _____

25. Vincent P. Michael was ill with a bad cold for 1 week. Will he receive temporary state

disability benefits? _____

Why or why not? _____

26. Betsy C. Palm had an emergency appendectomy and was hospitalized for 3 days.

Will she receive state disability benefits? _____

Why or why not? _____

27. Frank E. Thompson is a box boy at a supermarket on Saturdays and Sundays while
a full-time student at college. He broke his leg while skiing and cannot work at
the market, but he is able to attend classes with his leg in a cast. Can he collect state

disability benefits for his part-time job? _____

Why or why not? _____

28. Jerry L. Slate is out of a job and is receiving unemployment insurance benefits. He is
now suffering from severe intestinal flu. The employment office calls him to interview
for a job, but he is too ill to go. Can he collect temporary state disability benefits for

this illness when he might have been given a job? _____

Why or why not? _____

29. Joan T. Corman has diabetes, which sometimes makes her so weak that she has to leave
work early in the afternoon. She loses pay for each hour she cannot work. Can she

collect temporary state disability benefits? _____

Why or why not? _____

30. While walking the picket line with other employees on strike, Gene J. Berry came
down with pneumonia and was ill for 2 weeks. Can he collect temporary state

disability benefits? _____

Why or why not? _____

Gene went back to work for 3 weeks and then developed a slight cold and cough, which again was diagnosed as pneumonia. The doctor told him to stay home from work. Would he be able to collect temporary disability benefits again?

_____

Why or why not? _____

31. A month after he retired, Roger Reagan had a gallbladder operation. Can he receive

temporary state disability benefits? _____

Why or why not? _____

32. Jane M. Lambert fell in the back yard of her home and fractured her left ankle. She had a nonunion fracture and could not work for 28 weeks. For how long will

she collect temporary state disability benefits? _____

33. Dr. Kay examines Ben Yates and completes a claim form for state disability income because of a prolonged illness. On receiving the information, the insurance adjuster notices some conflicting data. Name other documents that may be requested to justify payment of benefits.

a. _____

b. _____

c. _____

34. Trent Walters, a permanently disabled individual, applies for federal disability benefits. To establish eligibility for benefits under this program, data allowed

must be_____ year/years old.

35. A Veterans Affairs patient is seen on an emergency basis by Dr. Onion. Name the two methods or options for billing this case.

a. _____

b. _____

36. When a claim form is submitted for a patient applying for state disability benefits, the

most important item required on the form is _____.

To check your answers to this self-study assignment, see Appendix D.

ASSIGNMENT **16-2** ▸ **COMPLETE TWO STATE DISABILITY INSURANCE FORMS**

Performance Objective

Task: Complete two state disability insurance forms and define patient record abbreviations.

Conditions: Use the patient's record (Figure 16–1), a Claim Statement of Employee form (Figure 16–2), a Doctor's Certificate form (Figure 16–3), and a typewriter or computer.

Standards: Time: _____ minutes

                 Accuracy: _____

                 (Note: The time element and accuracy criteria may be given by your instructor.)

Directions:

1. To familiarize you with what information the employee must furnish, this assignment will encompass completing both the Claim Statement of Employee (Figure 16–2) and the Doctor's Certificate (Figure 16–3). Mr. Broussard (Figure 16–1) is applying for state disability benefits, and he does not receive sick leave pay from his employer. Date the Claim Statement of Employee November 5, and date the Doctor's Certificate November 10. Remember that this is not a claim for payment to the physician, and so no ledger card has been furnished for this patient.

2. Refer to Chapter 16 and Figures 16–3 and 16–4 of the *Handbook* to assist you in completing this form.

   After the instructor has returned your work to you, either make the necessary corrections and place your work in a three-ring notebook for future reference or, if you received a high score, place it in your portfolio for reference when applying for a job.

Abbreviations pertinent to this record:

NP _____	SLR _____
c/o _____	rt _____
LBP _____	WNL _____
pt _____	STAT _____
lt _____	MRI _____
wk _____	RTO _____
reg _____	imp _____
exam _____	retn _____

PATIENT RECORD NO. 16-2

Broussard	Jeff	L	03-09-52	M	555-466-2490
LAST NAME	FIRST NAME	MIDDLE NAME	BIRTH DATE	SEX	HOME PHONE

3577 Plain Street	Woodland Hills	XY	12345
ADDRESS	CITY	STATE	ZIP CODE

555-667-7654	555-399-5903	555-466-2490	broussard@wb.net
CELL PHONE	PAGER NO.	FAX NO.	E-MAIL ADDRESS

566-XX-0090	F0394588
PATIENT'S SOC. SEC. NO.	DRIVER'S LICENSE

carpenter Payroll #2156	Ace Construction Company
PATIENT'S OCCUPATION	NAME OF COMPANY

4556 West Eighth Street, Dorland, XY 12347	555-447-8900
ADDRESS OF EMPLOYER	PHONE

Harriet M. Broussard	secretary
SPOUSE OR PARENT	OCCUPATION

Merit Accounting Company, 6743 Main Street, Woodland Hills, XY 12345	555-478-0980
EMPLOYER ADDRESS	PHONE

Blue Cross	Jeff L. Broussard
NAME OF INSURANCE	INSURED OR SUBSCRIBER

466-XX-9979	6131
POLICY/CERTIFICATE NO.	GROUP NO.

REFERRED BY: Harold B. Hartburn (friend)

DATE	PROGRESS NOTES
10-21-xx	8:30 a.m. NP seen c/o ongoing LBP. On 8-15-XX after swinging a golf club, pt had sudden onset of severe pain in low back with radiation to lt side. Pt unable to work 8-16 but resumed wk on 8-17 and has been working full time but doing no lifting while working. Pain is exacerbating affecting his work and reg duties. Exam showed SLR strongly positive on lt, on rt causes pain into lt side. Neurological exam WNL. Ordered STAT MRI. Off work. RTO.
	RS/mtf *Raymond Skeleton, MD*
10-23-xx	Pt returns for test results. MRI showed huge defect of L4-5. Imp: acute herniated disc L4-5 with spinal stenosis. Recommended laminotomy, foraminotomy, and diskectomy L4-5.
	RS/mtf *Raymond Skeleton, MD*
11-1-xx	Admit to College Hospital. Operation: Lumbar laminotomy with exploration and decompression of spinal cord without diskectomy L4-5; lumbar anteriorarthrodesis. Pt seen daily in hosp.
	RS/mtf *Raymond Skeleton, MD*
11-5-xx	At 3 p.m. pt discharged to home. Will retn to wk 12-15-XX.
	RS/mtf *Raymond Skeleton, MD*

Figure 16–1

CLAIM STATEMENT OF EMPLOYEE
COMPLETE ALL ITEMS. IF INCOMPLETE, THIS FORM WILL BE RETURNED, CAUSING A DELAY IN BENEFIT PAYMENTS

Do you need assistance in a language other than English? ☐ No ☐ Yes   **If yes, write language here.**
¿Prefiere Ud. formularios escritos en Español? ☐ No ☐ Sí

1. Print your full name: FIRST   INITIAL   LAST

   Other Names (including maiden, married and ethnic surnames) Used:

   Your Mailing Address:
   STREET ADDRESS, P.O. BOX OR RFD   APT. NO.   CITY OR TOWN   STATE AND ZIP CODE

   Your Home Address: (if different from mailing address)
   STREET ADDRESS, OR SPECIFIC DIRECTIONS TO YOUR HOME IF P.O. BOX OR RFD.

2. **IMPORTANT: Enter your Social Security Account Number**
   ☐☐☐ ☐☐ ☐☐☐☐

   2A. If you have used another Social Security number, enter that number here.
   _ _ _ _ _ _ _ _ _

3. What was the first day you were too sick to perform all the duties of your regular or customary work, even if it was a Saturday, Sunday, holiday or normal day off?

   MONTH [   ]   DAY [   ]   YEAR [   ]

MALE ☐   FEMALE ☐   Birthdate Mo. [ ] Day [ ] Yr. [ ]

4. What was the last day you worked?
   MONTH [   ]   DAY [   ]   YEAR [   ]

5. Employer's Business Name: Telephone Number (   )
   Employer's Business Address: NUMBER AND STREET   CITY   STATE AND ZIP CODE

6. Your occupation with this employer: Your Badge or Payroll number:

7. What is your usual occupation?

8. Are you self-employed?   Yes ☐   No ☐

9. Did you lose any time from work because of this illness or injury during the two weeks before the last day you worked as shown in item (4) above?   Yes ☐   No ☐

10. Did you stop work because of sickness, injury or pregnancy?
    If "No," please give reason: Yes ☐   No ☐

11. Have you filed for or received UNEMPLOYMENT INSURANCE benefits between the last day you worked and the first day you became disabled?   Yes ☐   No ☐

12. a. Has, or will your employer continue your pay by means of sick leave, vacation, pension, gift or other means?   Yes ☐   No ☐
    b. Do you authorize the Employment Development Department to disclose benefit eligibility information to your employer to be used only for the purpose of integrating your employer's wage continuation/ sick leave program with your benefits? (This information is limited to the claim effective date; the weekly and maximum benefit amounts; and the periods covered by benefit payments.)   Yes ☐   No ☐

13. Was this disability or any other disability during this claim period caused by your work?   Yes ☐   No ☐
    If "Yes," please provide the name and address of any insurance carrier from whom you are claiming or receiving Workers' Compensation Benefits:

14. Have you recovered from your disability?
    If "Yes," enter date of recovery: Yes ☐   No ☐

15. Have you returned to work for any day, part-time or full-time after the beginning date of your disability as shown in item (3) above?
    If "Yes," please enter such dates: Yes ☐   No ☐

16. Were you, as a result of an arrest, confined to a jail, detention center, prison, medical center or other correctional institution or any other place at any time during your disability? If "Yes," give dates: Yes ☐   No ☐

I hereby claim benefits and certify that for the period covered by this claim I was unemployed and disabled, that the foregoing statements including any accompanying statements are to the best of my knowledge and belief true, correct and complete. I hereby authorize my attending physician, practitioner, hospital and employer to furnish and disclose all facts concerning my disability and wages or earnings that are within their knowledge and to allow inspection of and provide copies of any hospital records concerning my disability that are under their control. I understand that authorizations contained in this claim statement are granted for a period of 18 months from the date of my signature or the effective date of the claim, whichever is later. I agree that a photocopy of this release shall be as valid as the original.

Claim signed on: MONTH   DAY   YEAR | Claimant's signature: (DO NOT PRINT) | Telephone Number (   )

Under Section 2101 of the California Unemployment Insurance Code, it is a violation to willfully make a false statement or knowingly conceal a material fact in order to obtain the payment of any benefits, such violation being punishable by imprisonment and/or a fine not exceeding $20,000 or both.

If your signature is made by mark (X) it must be attested by two witnesses with their addresses.
SIGNATURE-WITNESS   SIGNATURE-WITNESS

ADDRESS   ADDRESS

If an authorized agent is filing for benefits for an INCAPACITATED or DECEASED claimant, or a spouse is filing for a MENTALLY INCAPACITATED individual, contact the office below for the required forms and instructions.

Figure 16–2

DOCTOR'S CERTIFICATE
Certification may be made by a licensed medical or osteopathic physician and surgeon, chiropractor, dentist, optometrist, designated psychologist or an authorized medical officer of a United States Government facility. Certification may also be made by a licensed nurse-midwife or nurse practitioner for the purposes of disability related to normal pregnancy or childbirth. All items on this sheet must be completed legibly.

Patient File No.	Name	Social Security Number

17. I attended the patient for the present medical problem from: MONTH DAY YEAR   MONTH DAY YEAR
    To   At intervals of:

18. Are you completing this form for the sole purpose of referral or recommendation to an alcoholic recovery home or drug-free residential facility?
Yes☐ No☐   If yes, please enter facility name and address in item #28.

19. History: Findings (state nature, severity and bodily extent of the incapacitating disease or injury):

    Diagnosis:

ICD Disease Code, Primary: (REQUIRED)	ICD Disease Code, Secondary:

    Type of treatment and/or medication rendered to patient:

20. Diagnosis confirmed by: **(Specify type of test or X-ray)**

21. Is this patient now pregnant or has she been pregnant since the date of treatment as reported above?   Yes☐ No☐   If "Yes," date pregnancy terminated or future EDC.
    Is the pregnancy normal?   Yes☐ No☐   If "No," state the abnormal and involuntary complication causing maternal disability:

22. Operation: Date performed or to be performed _____   Type of Operation: ICD Procedure Code: (REQUIRED)

23. Has the patient at any time during your attendance for this medical problem, been incapable of performing his or her regular work?   Yes☐ No☐   If "Yes" the disability commenced on:

24. APPROXIMATE date, based on your examination of patient, disability (if any) should end or has ended sufficiently to permit the patient to resume regular or customary work. Even if considerable question exists, make SOME "estimate." This is a requirement of the Code, and the claim will be delayed if such date is not entered. Such answers as "Indefinite" or "don't know" will not suffice.   (ENTER DATE) _____

25. Based on your examination of patient, is this disability the result of "occupation" either as an "industrial accident" or as an "occupational disease"?

    Yes☐ No☐ (This should include aggravation of pre-existing conditions by occupation.)

26. Have you reported this OR A CONCURRENT DISABILITY to any insurance carrier as a Workers' Compensation Claim?
    Yes☐ No☐   If "Yes," to whom?
    (Name of carrier or firm)

27. Was patient in a hospital surgical unit, surgical unit, ambulatory surgical center certified to participate in the federal Medicare program or a postsurgical recovery care unit as designated by section 1250.9 of the Health and Safety Code?   Yes☐ No☐
    If "Yes," please provide name and address:

28. Was or is patient a resident in an alcoholic recovery home or drug-free residential facility?   Yes☐ No☐
    If "Yes," please provide name and address:

29. Was or is patient confined as a registered bed patient in a hospital?   Yes☐ No☐
    If "Yes," please provide name and address:

    Date and hour entered as a registered bed patient and discharged pursuant to your orders:

ENTERED		STILL CONFINED	DISCHARGED	
on , 20 , at	A.M. P.M.	on , 20	on , 20 , at	A.M. P.M.

30. Would the disclosure of this information to your patient be medically or psychologically detrimental to the patient?
    Yes☐ No☐

I hereby certify that, based on my examination, the above statements truly describe the patient's disability (if any) and the estimated duration thereof, and that I am a _____ licensed to practice by the State of _____
(TYPE OF DOCTOR)

▶ _____
    PRINT OR TYPE DOCTOR'S NAME AS SHOWN ON LICENSE

▶ _____
    SIGNATURE OF ATTENDING DOCTOR

▶ _____
    NO. AND STREET   CITY   ZIP CODE   STATE LICENSE NUMBER

▶ (   )
    TELEPHONE NO.   DATE OF SIGNING THIS FORM

"Under Section 2116 of the California Unemployment Insurance Code, it is a violation for any individual who, with the intent to defraud, falsely certifies the medical condition of any person in order to obtain disability insurance benefits, whether for the maker or for any other person, and is punishable by imprisonment and/or a fine not exceeding twenty thousand dollars.

Figure 16–3

A S S I G N M E N T **16–3 ► COMPLETE TWO STATE DISABILITY INSURANCE FORMS**

Performance Objective

Task: Complete two state disability insurance forms and define patient record abbreviations.

Conditions: Use the patient's record (Figure 16–4), a Doctor's Certificate form (Figure 16–5), a Physician's Supplementary Certificate form (Figure 16–6), and a typewriter or computer.

Standards: Time: _____ minutes

Accuracy: _____

(Note: The time element and accuracy criteria may be given by your instructor.)

Directions:

1. Assume that the Claim Statement of Employee has been completed satisfactorily by Mr. Fred E. Thorndike (Figure 16–4). Complete the Doctor's Certificate form (Figure 16–5) and date it December 2. In completing this portion of the assignment, look at the first entry made by Dr. Practon on November 25 only.

2. Mr. Thorndike returns to see Dr. Practon on December 7, at which time his disability leave needs to be extended. Complete the Physician's Supplementary Certificate form (Figure 16–6) by referring to the entry made during the second visit, and date the certificate December 7. Remember that this is not a claim for payment to the physician, and so no ledger card has been furnished for this patient.

3. Refer to Chapter 16 and Figures 16–4 and 16–5 of the *Handbook* to assist you in completing these forms.

After the instructor has returned your work to you, either make the necessary corrections and place your work in a three-ring notebook for future reference or, if you received a high score, place it in your portfolio for reference when applying for a job.

Abbreviations pertinent to this record:

pt _____   wk _____

SDI _____   est _____

PE _____   FU _____

wks _____   c̄ _____

dx _____   CXR _____

Cont _____   reg _____

RTO _____

PATIENT RECORD NO. 16-3

Thorndike	Fred	E	02-17-44	M	555-465-7820
LAST NAME	FIRST NAME	MIDDLE NAME	BIRTH DATE	SEX	HOME PHONE

5784 Helen Street	Woodland Hills	XY	12345
ADDRESS	CITY	STATE	ZIP CODE

555-432-7744	555-320-5500	555-466-7820		thorndike@wb.net
CELL PHONE	PAGER NO.	FAX NO.		E-MAIL ADDRESS

549-XX-8721	M00430548
PATIENT'S SOC. SEC. NO.	DRIVER'S LICENSE

salesman Payoll No. 6852	Easy on Paint Company
PATIENT'S OCCUPATION	NAME OF COMPANY

4586 West 20th Street, Woodland Hills, XY 12345	555-467-8898
ADDRESS OF EMPLOYER	PHONE

Jennifer B. Thorndike	homemaker
SPOUSE OR PARENT	OCCUPATION

EMPLOYER	ADDRESS	PHONE

Pacific Mutual Insurance Company,120 South Main Street, Merck, XY 12346
NAME OF INSURANCE

	6709	Fred E. Thorndike
POLICY/CERTIFICATE NO.	GROUP NO.	INSURED OR SUBSCRIBER

REFERRED BY: John Diehl (Friend)

DATE	PROGRESS NOTES
11-25-xx	On or about 11-3-xx, pt began to have chest pain and much coughing. On 11-24-xx, pt too ill to work and
	decided to file for SDI benefits. Pt states illness is not work connected and he does not receive sick pay.
	PE: Pt examined and complained of productive cough of 3 wks duration and chest pain. Chest x-rays
	confirmed dx-mucopurulent chronic bronchitis. Cont home rest and prescribed antibiotic medication. RTO
	12-7-xx. Pt will be capable of returning to wk 12-8-xx.
	GP/mtf *Gerald Practon, MD*
12-07-xx	Est pt returns for F/U c̄ bronchitis. Chest pain improved. Still running low grade temp c̄ productive cough.
	F/U CXR shows clearing. Recommended bed rest x 7d. Will extend disability to 12-15-xx at which time pt
	can resume reg work. No complications anticipated.
	GP/mtf *Gerald Practon, MD*

Figure 16–4

DOCTOR'S CERTIFICATE
Certification may be made by a licensed medical or osteopathic physician and surgeon, chiropractor, dentist, optometrist, designated psychologist or an authorized medical officer of a United States Government facility. Certification may also be made by a licensed nurse-midwife or nurse practitioner for the purposes of disability related to normal pregnancy or childbirth. All items on this sheet must be completed legibly.

Patient File No.   Name   Social Security Number

17. I attended the patient for the present medical problem from: MONTH DAY YEAR   MONTH DAY YEAR   To   At intervals of:

18. Are you completing this form for the sole purpose of referral or recommendation to an alcoholic recovery home or drug-free residential facility? Yes☐ No☐ If yes, please enter facility name and address in item #28.

19. History: Findings (state nature, severity and bodily extent of the incapacitating disease or injury):

Diagnosis:

ICD Disease Code, Primary: (REQUIRED)   ICD Disease Code, Secondary:

Type of treatment and/or medication rendered to patient:

20. Diagnosis confirmed by: **(Specify type of test or X-ray)**

21. Is this patient now pregnant or has she been pregnant since the date of treatment as reported above? Yes☐ No☐ Is the pregnancy normal? Yes☐ No☐   If "Yes," date pregnancy terminated or future EDC. If "No," state the abnormal and involuntary complication causing maternal disability:

22. Operation: Date performed or to be performed   Type of Operation: ICD Procedure Code: (REQUIRED)

23. Has the patient at any time during your attendance for this medical problem, been incapable of performing his or her regular work? Yes☐ No☐   If "Yes" the disability commenced on:

24. APPROXIMATE date, based on your examination of patient, disability (if any) should end or has ended sufficiently to permit the patient to resume regular or customary work. Even if considerable question exists, make SOME "estimate." This is a requirement of the Code, and the claim will be delayed if such date is not entered. Such answers as "Indefinite" or "don't know" will not suffice.   (ENTER DATE)

25. Based on your examination of patient, is this disability the result of "occupation" either as an "industrial accident" or as an "occupational disease"? Yes☐ No☐ (This should include aggravation of pre-existing conditions by occupation.)

26. Have you reported this OR A CONCURRENT DISABILITY to any insurance carrier as a Workers' Compensation Claim? Yes☐ No☐ If "Yes," to whom? (Name of carrier or firm)

27. Was patient in a hospital surgical unit, surgical unit, ambulatory surgical center certified to participate in the federal Medicare program or a postsurgical recovery care unit as designated by section 1250.9 of the Health and Safety Code? Yes☐ No☐ If "Yes," please provide name and address:

28. Was or is patient a resident in an alcoholic recovery home or drug-free residential facility? Yes☐ No☐ If "Yes," please provide name and address:

29. Was or is patient confined as a registered bed patient in a hospital? Yes☐ No☐ If "Yes," please provide name and address:

Date and hour entered as a registered bed patient and discharged pursuant to your orders:

ENTERED	STILL CONFINED	DISCHARGED
on , 20 , at A.M. P.M.	on , 20	on , 20 , at A.M. P.M.

30. Would the disclosure of this information to your patient be medically or psychologically detrimental to the patient? Yes☐ No☐

I hereby certify that, based on my examination, the above statements truly describe the patient's disability (if any) and the estimated duration thereof, and that I am a _____ (TYPE OF DOCTOR) licensed to practice by the State of _____

▶ PRINT OR TYPE DOCTOR'S NAME AS SHOWN ON LICENSE   ▶ SIGNATURE OF ATTENDING DOCTOR

▶ NO. AND STREET   CITY   ZIP CODE   ▶ STATE LICENSE NUMBER   ( ) TELEPHONE NO.   DATE OF SIGNING THIS FORM

"Under Section 2116 of the California Unemployment Insurance Code, it is a violation for any individual who, with the intent to defraud, falsely certifies the medical condition of any person in order to obtain disability insurance benefits, whether for the maker or for any other person, and is punishable by imprisonment and/or a fine not exceeding twenty thousand dollars.

Figure 16–5

NOTICE OF FINAL PAYMENT

The information contained in your claim for Disability Insurance indicates that you are now able to work, therefore, this is the final check that you will receive on this claim.

IF YOU ARE **STILL** DISABLED: You should complete the Claimant's Certification portion of this form and contact your doctor immediately to have him/her complete the Physician's Supplementary Certificate below.

IF YOU BECOME DISABLED **AGAIN:** File a new Disability Insurance claim form.

IF YOU ARE UNEMPLOYED AND AVAILABLE FOR WORK: Report to the nearest Unemployment Insurance office of the Department for assistance in finding work and to determine your entitlement to Unemployment Insurance Benefits.

This determination is final unless you file an appeal within twenty (20) days from the date of the mailing of this notification. You may appeal by giving a detailed statement as to why you believe the determination is in error. All communications regarding this Disability Insurance claim should include your Social Security Account Number and be addressed to the office shown.

- -

CLAIMANT'S CERTIFICATION

I certify that I continue to be disabled and incapable of doing my regular work, and that I have reported all wages, Worker's Compensation benefits and other monies received during the claim period to the Employment Development Department.

ENTER YOUR SOCIAL SECURITY NUMBER __549__ __XX__ __8721__

**Sign
Your Name**_____   **Date
Signed**_____
Fred E. Thorndike   December 6, 20XX

PHYSICIAN'S SUPPLEMENTARY CERTIFICATE

Department Use Only	

1. Are you still treating patient?_____ Date of last treatment_____, 20___.
2. What present condition continues to make the patient disabled?
_____
_____
_____

3. Date patient recovered, or will recover sufficiently (even if under treatment) to be able to perform his/her regular and customary work_____, 20_____. Please enter a specific or estimated recovery date.
4. Would the disclosure of this information to your patient be medically or psychologically detrimental to the patient?
Yes ☐   No ☐

I hereby certify that the above statements in my opinion truly describe the claimant's condition and the estimated duration thereof.

_____, 20____
Date

Doctor's Signature_____

Phone Number_____

DE 2525XX Rev. 13 (3-86)   – Versión en español en el dorso –

Figure 16–6

ASSIGNMENT **16-4** ▸ **COMPLETE A STATE DISABILITY INSURANCE FORM**

Performance Objective

Task: Complete a state disability insurance form and define patient record abbreviations.

Conditions: Use the patient's record (Figure 16–7), a Doctor's Certificate form (Figure 16–8), and a typewriter or computer.

Standards: Time: _____ minutes

Accuracy: _____

(Note: The time element and accuracy criteria may be given by your instructor.)

Directions:

1. Assume that the Claim Statement of Employee has been completed satisfactorily by Mr. James T. Fujita (Figure 16–7). Complete the Doctor's Certificate form (Figure 16–8) and date it December 15. Remember that this is not a claim for payment to the physician, and so no ledger card has been furnished for this patient.

2. Refer to Chapter 16 and Figure 16–4 of the *Handbook* to assist you in completing this form.

After the instructor has returned your work to you, either make the necessary corrections and place your work in a three-ring notebook for future reference or, if you received a high score, place it in your portfolio for reference when applying for a job.

Abbreviations pertinent to this record:

pt _____   imp _____

exam _____   wk _____

hx _____   SDI _____

neg _____   wk _____

WBC _____

PATIENT RECORD NO. 16-4

Fujita	James	T	03-27-34	M	555-677-2881
LAST NAME	FIRST NAME	MIDDLE NAME	BIRTH DATE	SEX	HOME PHONE

3538 South A Street	Woodland Hills	XY		12345
ADDRESS	CITY	STATE		ZIP CODE

555-499-6556	555-988-4100	555-677-2881	fujita@wb.net
CELL PHONE	PAGER NO.	FAX NO.	E-MAIL ADDRESS

567-XX-8898	M4387931
PATIENT'S SOC. SEC. NO.	DRIVER'S LICENSE

electrician Payoll No. 8834	Macy Electric Company
PATIENT'S OCCUPATION	NAME OF COMPANY

2671 North C Street, Woodland Hills, XY 12345	555-677-2346
ADDRESS OF EMPLOYER	PHONE

Mary J. Fujita	homemaker
SPOUSE OR PARENT	OCCUPATION

EMPLOYER	ADDRESS	PHONE

Atlantic Mutual Insurance Company, 111 South Main Street, Woodland Hills, XY 12345
NAME OF INSURANCE

F20015		James T. Fujita
POLICY/CERTIFICATE NO.	GROUP NO.	INSURED OR SUBSCRIBER

REFERRED BY: Cherry Hotta (aunt)

DATE	PROGRESS NOTES
12-07-XX	Today pt could not go to work and came for exam complaining of pain in abdomen, nausea, and no vomiting. Pt has hx of mesentery adenopathy. Exam neg except abdomen showed tenderness all over with voluntary guarding. WBC 10,000. Imp: Mesenteric adenitis. Advised strict bed rest at home and bland diet. To return in 1 wk. Will file for SDI benefits. Pt states illness is not work connected and he receives sick leave pay of $150/wk.
	GI/mtf *Gaston Input, MD*
12-15-xx	Exam showed normal nontender abdomen. No nausea. Pt tolerating food well. WBC 7,500. Pt will be capable of returning to work 12-22-xx.
	GI/mtf *Gaston Input, MD*

Figure 16–7

DOCTOR'S CERTIFICATE

Certification may be made by a licensed medical or osteopathic physician and surgeon, chiropractor, dentist, optometrist, designated psychologist or an authorized medical officer of a United States Government facility. Certification may also be made by a licensed nurse-midwife or nurse practitioner for the purposes of disability related to normal pregnancy or childbirth. All items on this sheet must be completed legibly.

Patient File No.	Name	Social Security Number

17. I attended the patient for the present medical problem
MONTH DAY YEAR MONTH DAY YEAR
from: To At intervals of:

18. Are you completing this form for the sole purpose of referral or recommendation to an alcoholic recovery home or drug-free residential facility? Yes☐ No☐ If yes, please enter facility name and address in item #28.

19. History:

Diagnosis:

Findings (state nature, severity and bodily extent of the incapacitating disease or injury):

ICD Disease Code, Primary: (REQUIRED)

ICD Disease Code, Secondary:

Type of treatment and/or medication rendered to patient:

20. Diagnosis confirmed by: **(Specify type of test or X-ray)**

21. Is this patient now pregnant or has she been pregnant since the date of treatment as reported above? Yes☐ No☐
Is the pregnancy normal? Yes☐ No☐
If "Yes," date pregnancy terminated or future EDC.
If "No," state the abnormal and involuntary complication causing maternal disability:

22. Operation: Date performed or to be performed Type of Operation: ICD Procedure Code: (REQUIRED)

23. Has the patient at any time during your attendance for this medical problem, been incapable of performing his or her regular work? Yes☐ No☐ If "Yes" the disability commenced on:

24. APPROXIMATE date, based on your examination of patient, disability (if any) should end or has ended sufficiently to permit the patient to resume regular or customary work. Even if considerable question exists, make SOME "estimate." This is a requirement of the Code, and the claim will be delayed if such date is not entered. Such answers as "Indefinite" or "don't know" will not suffice. (ENTER DATE)

25. Based on your examination of patient, is this disability the result of "occupation" either as an "industrial accident" or as an "occuaptional disease"? Yes☐ No☐ (This should include aggravation of pre-existing conditions by occupation.)

26. Have you reported this OR A CONCURRENT DISABILITY to any insurance carrier as a Workers' Compensation Claim? Yes☐ No☐ If "Yes," to whom? (Name of carrier or firm)

27. Was patient in a hospital surgical unit, surgical unit, ambulatory surgical center certified to participate in the federal Medicare program or a postsurgical recovery care unit as designated by section 1250.9 of the Health and Safety Code? Yes☐ No☐ If "Yes," please provide name and address:

28. Was or is patient a resident in an alcoholic recovery home or drug-free residential facility? Yes☐ No☐ If "Yes," please provide name and address:

29. Was or is patient confined as a registered bed patient in a hospital? Yes☐ No☐ If "Yes," please provide name and address:

Date and hour entered as a registered bed patient and discharged pursuant to your orders:

ENTERED		STILL CONFINED	DISCHARGED	
on , 20 , at	A.M. P.M.	on , 20	on , 20 , at	A.M. P.M.

30. Would the disclosure of this information to your patient be medically or psychologically detrimental to the patient? Yes☐ No☐

I hereby certify that, based on my examination, the above statements truly descibe the patient's disability (if any) and the estimated duration thereof, and that I am a _____ (TYPE OF DOCTOR) licensed to practice by the State of _____

▶ PRINT OR TYPE DOCTOR'S NAME AS SHOWN ON LICENSE   ▶ SIGNATURE OF ATTENDING DOCTOR

▶ NO. AND STREET   CITY   ZIP CODE   STATE LICENSE NUMBER   ( ) TELEPHONE NO.   DATE OF SIGNING THIS FORM

"Under Section 2116 of the California Unemployment Insurance Code, it is a violation for any individual who, with the intent to defraud, falsely certifies the medical condition of any person in order to obtain disability insurance benefits, whether for the maker or for any other person, and is punishable by imprisonment and/or a fine not exceeding twenty thousand dollars.

Figure 16–8

ASSIGNMENT **16–5** ▸ **COMPLETE TWO STATE DISABILITY INSURANCE FORMS**

Performance Objective

Task: Complete two state disability insurance forms and define patient record abbreviations.

Conditions: Use the patient's record (Figure 16–9), a Doctor's Certificate form (Figure 16–10), a Request for Additional Medical Information form (Figure 16–11), and a typewriter or computer.

Standards: Time: _____ minutes

               Accuracy: _____

               (Note: The time element and accuracy criteria may be given by your instructor.)

Directions:

1. Mr. Jake J. Burrows (Figure 16–9) has previously applied for state disability benefits. After 2 months, he is referred to another doctor for further care. Complete the form (Figure 16–10) and date it June 25. You will notice that this form is almost identical to the Doctor's Certificate and is mailed to the claimant to secure the certification of a new physician or to clarify a specific claimed period of disability. In completing this part of the assignment, look at the first three entries on the patient record only.

2. Complete the Request for Additional Medical Information form (Figure 16–11) by looking at the last entry on Mr. Burrows' record, and date the report July 15. Remember that this is not a claim for payment to the physician, and so no ledger card has been furnished for this patient.

3. Refer to Chapter 16 and Figures 16–4 and 16–6 of the *Handbook* to assist you in completing these forms.

   After the instructor has returned your work to you, either make the necessary corrections and place your work in a three-ring notebook for future reference or, if you received a high score, place it in your portfolio for reference when applying for a job.

Abbreviations pertinent to this record:

pt _____   hosp _____

c̄ _____   approx _____

C5/6 _____   retn _____

imp _____   RTO _____

adm _____   wks _____

PATIENT RECORD NO. 16-5

Burrows	Jake	J	04-26-50	M	555-478-9009
LAST NAME	FIRST NAME	MIDDLE NAME	BIRTH DATE	SEX	HOME PHONE

319 Barry Street	Woodland Hills	XY	12345
ADDRESS	CITY	STATE	ZIP CODE

555-765-9080	555-542-0979	555-478-9009	burrows@wb.net
CELL PHONE	PAGER NO.	FAX NO.	E-MAIL ADDRESS

457-XX-0801	D0453298
PATIENT'S SOC. SEC. NO.	DRIVER'S LICENSE

assembler	Convac Electronics Company
PATIENT'S OCCUPATION	NAME OF COMPANY

3440 West 7ᵗʰ Street, Woodland Hills, XY 12345	555-467-9008
ADDRESS OF EMPLOYER	PHONE

Jane B. Burrows	homemaker
SPOUSE OR PARENT	OCCUPATION

EMPLOYER	ADDRESS	PHONE

Blue Shield	Jake J. Burrows
NAME OF INSURANCE	INSURED OR SUBSCRIBER

T8471811A	53553AT
POLICY/CERTIFICATE NO.	GROUP NO.

REFERRED BY: Clarence Butler, MD, 300 Sixth Street, Woodland Hills, XY 12345   NPI# 620114352X

DATE	PROGRESS NOTES
6-02-xx	Pt. Referred by Dr. Butler. Pt states on 4-19-xx was wrestling c̄ son and jerked his neck the wrong way.
	2 days later had much pain and muscle spasm in the cervical region. X-rays show degenerated disk C5/6.
	Exam: limited range of neck motion and limited abduction both arms. Imp: Degenerated cervical disk C5/6.
	Pt unable to work as of this date. Myelogram ordered. Return for test results.
	RS/mtf *Raymond Skeleton, MD*
6-24-xx	Myelogram positive at C5/6. Scheduled for surgery the following day.
	RS/mtf *Raymond Skeleton, MD*
6-25-xx	Pt adm to College Hospital for disk excision and anterior cervical fusion at C5/6. Pt will be discharged from
	hosp on 6-29-xx. Approx date of retn to work 8-15-xx.
	RS/mtf *Raymond Skeleton, MD*
6-26 to	Pt seen daily in hospital. Discharged 6-29. RTO 2 weeks.
6-29-xx	RS/mtf *Raymond Skeleton, MD*
7-15-xx	Pt has some restriction of cervical motion. No muscle spasm. Very little cervical pain. Pt to be seen in
	2 wks. To retn to work 8-15-xx.
	RS/mtf *Raymond Skeleton, MD*

Figure 16-9

In order that any disability insurance to which you may be entitled may be paid without undue delay, please have the physician who treats or treated you during the period indicated below complete this form and return it to us at his earliest convenience.

Para que cualquier beneficio del Segurdo de Incapacidad a que Ud. pueda tener derecho a recibir sea pagado sin demoras excesivas, haga el favor de hacer que el médicio que le atiende o atiendó, durante el período indicado abajo, complete este formulario y que lo regrese a nuestra oficina cuanto antes.

Henry B. Garcia
_____
Disability Insurance Program Representative

6-2 thru 7-25-XX
_____
Period Dates - Feches del Periodo

457-XX-0801
_____
S.S.A. – No. Des S.S.

	Month	Day	Year		Month	Day	Year	

1. I attended the patient for the present medical problem from: To: At intervals of:

2. History: ,

    State the nature, severity and the bodily extent of the incapacitating disease or injury.

Findings: _____

Dianosis: _____

Type of treatment and/or medication rendered to patient: _____

3. Diagnosis confirmed by: (*Specify type of test or X-ray*)

4. Is this patient now pregnant or has she been pregnant since the date of treatment as reported above?   Yes ☐ No ☐   If "Yes", date pregnancy terminated or future EDC:

    Is the pregnancy normal?   Yes ☐ No ☐   If "No", state the abnormal and involuntary complication causing maternal disability:

5. Operation: Date performed: _____   Type of

    Date to be performed: _____   Operation:

6. Has the patient at any time during your attendance for this medical problem, been incapable of performing his/her regular work?   Yes ☐ No ☐   If "Yes", the disability commenced on:

7. APPROXIMATE date, based on your examination of patient, disability (if any) should end or has ended sufficiently to permit the patient to resume regular or customary work. Even if considerable question exists, make *SOME* "estimate." This is a requirement of the Code, and the claim will be delayed if such date is not entered. Such answers as "Indefinite" or "don't know" will not suffice.   (ENTER DATE)

8. Based on your examination of patient, is this disability the result of "occupation" either as an "industrial accident" or as an "occupational disease?" (This should include aggravation of pre-existing conditions by occupation.)   Yes ☐ No ☐

9. Have you reported this *OR A CONCURRENT DISABILITY* to any insurance carrier as a Workers' Compensation Claim? Yes ☐ No ☐   If "Yes," to whom?

10. Was or is patient confined as a registered bed patient in a hospital?   Yes ☐ No ☐

    Was patient treated in the surgical unit of a hospital or surgical unit?   Yes ☐ No ☐

    If "Yes," please provide name and address:

11. Date and hour entered as a registered bed patient and discharged pursuant to your orders:

ENTERED		STILL CONFINED	DISCHARGED	
on , 20 , at	A.M. P.M.	on , 20	on , 20 , at	A.M. P.M.

12. Would the disclosure of this information to your patient be medically or psychologically detrimental to the patient? Yes ☐ No ☐

I hereby certify that, based on my examination, the above statements truly descibe the patient's disability (if any) and the estimated duration thereof, and that I am a _____ licensed to practice by the State of _____
    (TYPE OF DOCTOR)

_____ _____
PRINT OR TYPE DOCTOR'S NAME AS SHOWN ON LICENSE   SIGNATURE OF ATTENDING DOCTOR

( )

NO. AND STREET   CITY   ZIP CODE   STATE LICENSE NUMBER   TELEPHONE NUMBER   DATE OF SIGNING THIS FORM

Certification may be made by a licensed physician and surgeon, osteopath, chiropractor, dentist, podiatrist, optometrist, designated psychologist, or an authorized medical officer of a United States Government facility. All items on this sheet must be completed.

Figure 16–10

STATE OF CALIFORNIA
EMPLOYMENT DEVELOPMENT DEPARTMENT

**REQUEST FOR ADDITIONAL
MEDICAL INFORMATION**

457-XX-0801   – Our file No,
Jake J. Burrows   – Your patient
                          – Regular or Customary Work

Raymond Skeleton, M.D.
4567 Broad Avenue
Woodland Hills, XY 12345

The original basic information and estimate of duration of your patient's disability have been carefully evaluated. At the present time, the following additional information based upon the progress and present condition of this patient is requested. This will assist the Department in determining eligibilty for further disability insurance benefits. Return of the completed form as soon as possible will be appreciated.

WM. C. SCHMIDT, M.D., MEDICAL DIRECTOR

CLAIMS EXAMINER   *DOCTOR: Please complete either part A or B, date and sign.*

PART A   IF YOUR PATIENT HAS RECOVERED SUFFICIENTLY TO BE ABLE TO RETURN TO HIS/HER REGULAR OR CUSTOMARY WORK LISTED ABOVE, PLEASE GIVE THE DATE, _____ 20 ____

PART B   THIS PART REFERS TO PATIENT WHO IS STILL DISABLED.

Are you still treating the patient? Yes ☐ No ☐   _____ 20 ____ .
                                                  DATE OF LAST TREATMENT

What are the medical circumstances which continue to make your patient disabled?
_____
_____
_____
_____

What is your present estimate of the date your patient will be able to perform his/her regular or customary work listed above?   Date _____ 20 ____ .

Further comments:
_____
_____

Would the disclosure of this information to your patient be medically or physically detrimental to the patient?   Yes ☐ No ☐

Date _____ 20 ____   _____
                                 DOCTOR'S SIGNATURE

ENCLOSED IS A STAMPED PREADDRESSED ENVELOPE FOR YOUR CONVENIENCE.

DE 2547 Rev. 17 (4-84)

Figure 16–11

ASSIGNMENT **16–6** ▸ **COMPLETE A STATE DISABILITY INSURANCE FORMS**

Performance Objective

Task: Complete a state disability insurance form and define patient record abbreviations.

Conditions: Use the patient's record (Figure 16–12), a Doctor's Certificate form (Figure 16–13), and a typewriter or computer.

Standards: Time: _____ minutes

                   Accuracy: _____

                   (Note: The time element and accuracy criteria may be given by your instructor.)

Directions:

1. Mr. Vincent P. Michael (Figure 16–12) is applying for state disability benefits. Complete the Doctor's Certificate form (Figure 16–13) and date it September 21.

   Assume that the Claim Statement of Employee has been completed satisfactorily by Mr. Michael. Remember that this is not a claim for payment to the physician, and so no ledger card has been furnished for this patient.

2. Refer to Chapter 16 and Figure 16–4 of the *Handbook* to assist you in completing this form.

   After the instructor has returned your work to you, either make the necessary corrections and place your work in a three-ring notebook for future reference or, if you received a high score, place it in your portfolio for reference when applying for a job.

Abbreviations pertinent to this record:

pt   _____   imp   _____

exam   _____   CVA   _____

L   _____   adv   _____

ESR   _____   retn   _____

mm   _____   wk   _____

hr   _____   approx _____

PATIENT RECORD NO. 16-6

Michael	Vincent	P	05-17-45	M	555-567-9001
LAST NAME	FIRST NAME	MIDDLE NAME	BIRTH DATE	SEX	HOME PHONE

1529 1/2 Thompson Boulevard	Woodland Hills	XY	12345
ADDRESS	CITY	STATE	ZIP CODE

555-398-5677	555-311-0098	555-567-9001	michael@wb.net
CELL PHONE	PAGER NO.	FAX NO.	E-MAIL ADDRESS

562-XX-8888	E0034578
PATIENT'S SOC. SEC. NO.	DRIVER'S LICENSE

assembler "A"	Burroughs Corporation
PATIENT'S OCCUPATION	NAME OF COMPANY

5411 North Lindero Canyon Road, Woodland Hills, XY 12345	555-560-9008
ADDRESS OF EMPLOYER	PHONE

Helen J. Michael	homemaker
SPOUSE OR PARENT	OCCUPATION

EMPLOYER	ADDRESS	PHONE

Blue Shield	Vincent P. Michael
NAME OF INSURANCE	INSURED OR SUBSCRIBER

T8411981A	677899AT
POLICY/CERTIFICATE NO.	GROUP NO.

REFERRED BY: Robert T. Smith (friend)

DATE	PROGRESS NOTES
9-20-xx	Pt complains of having had the flu, headache, dizziness, and of being tired. Pt unable to go to work today. Exam shows weakness of L hand. Pt exhibits light dysphasia and confusion. Chest x-ray shows cardiomegaly and slight pulmonary congestion. ESR 46 mm/hr. Imp: Post flu syndrome, transient ischemic attack, possible CVA. Prescribed medication for congestion and adv pt to take aspirin 1/day. Pt to stay off work and retn in 1 wk. Approx date of retn to work 10-16-xx.
	BC/mtf *Brady Coccidioides, MD*

Figure 16–12

DOCTOR'S CERTIFICATE
Certification may be made by a licensed medical or osteopathic physician and surgeon, chiropractor, dentist, optometrist, designated psychologist or an authorized medical officer of a United States Government facility. Certification may also be made by a licensed nurse-midwife or nurse practitioner for the purposes of disability related to normal pregnancy or childbirth. All items on this sheet must be completed legibly.

Patient File No.   Name   Social Security Number

17. I attended the patient for the present medical problem from: MONTH DAY YEAR   MONTH DAY YEAR   To   At intervals of:

18. Are you completing this form for the sole purpose of referral or recommendation to an alcoholic recovery home or drug-free residential facility? Yes   No   If yes, please enter facility name and address in item #28.

19. History: Objective Findings/Detailed Statement of Symptoms

Diagnosis:

ICD Disease Code, Primary: (REQUIRED)   ICD Disease Code, Secondary:

Type of treatment and/or medication rendered to patient:

20. Diagnosis confirmed by: **(Specify type of test or X-ray)**

21. Is this patient now pregnant or has she been pregnant since the date of treatment as reported above? Yes☐ No☐ Is the pregnancy normal? Yes☐ No☐   If "Yes," date pregnancy terminated or future EDC. If "No," state the abnormal and involuntary complication causing maternal disability.

22. Operation: Date performed or to be performed   Type of Operation: ICD Procedure Code: (REQUIRED)

23. Has the patient at any time during your attendance for this medical problem, been incapable or performing his or her regular work? Yes☐ No☐   If "Yes" the disability commenced on:

24. APPROXIMATE date, based on your examination of patient, disability (if any) should ebd or has ended sufficiently to permit the patient to resume regular or customary work. Even if considerable question exists, make SOME "estimate." This is a requirement of the Code, and the claim will be delayed if if such date is not entered. Such answers as "Indefinite" or "don't know" will not suffice.   (ENTER DATE)

25. Based on your examination of patient, is this disability the result of "occupation" either as an "industrial accident" or as an "occuaptional disease"? Yes☐ No☐ (This should include aggravation of pre-existing condiitons by occupation.)

26. Have you reported this OR A CONCURRENT DISABILITY to any insurance carrier as a Workers' Compensation claim? Yes☐ No☐ If "Yes," to whom? (Name of carrier or firm)

27. Was patient in a hospital surgical unit, surgical unit, ambulatory surgical center certified to participate in the federal Medicare program or a postsurgical recovery care unit as designated by section 1250.9 of the Health and Safety Code? Yes☐ No☐ If "Yes," please provide name and address.

28. Was or is patient in an alcoholic recovery home or drug-free residential facility? Yes☐ No☐ If "Yes," please provide name and address:

29. Would the disclosure of this information to your patient be medically or psychologically detrimental to the patient? Yes☐ No☐
Yes☐ No☐

I hereby certify that, based on my examination, the above statements truly describe the patient's disability (if any) and the estimated deration thereof, and that I am a _____ (TYPE OF DOCTOR) licensed to practice by the State of _____

▶ _____   ▶ _____
PRINT OR TYPE DOCTOR'S NAMF AS SHOWN ON LICENSE   SIGNATURE OF ATTENDING DOCTOR

▶ _____   ▶ ( ) _____
NO. AND STREET   CITY   ZIP CODE   STATE LICENSE NUMBER   TELEPHONE NUMBER   DATE OF SIGNING THIS FORM

"Under Section 2116 of the California Unemployment Insurance Code, it is a violation for any individual who, with the intent to defraud, falsely certifies the medical condition of any person in order to obtain disability insurance benefits, whether for the maker or or for any other person, and is punishable by imprisonment and/or a fine not exceeding twenty thousand dollars.

Figure 16–13

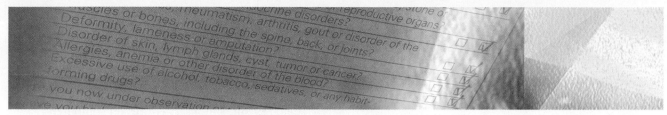

Hospital Billing

KEY TERMS

Your instructor may wish to select some specific words pertinent to this chapter for a test. For definitions of the terms, further study, and/or reference, the words, phrases, and abbreviations may be found in the glossary at the end of the Handbook. *Key terms for this chapter follow.*

admission review

ambulatory payment classifications (APCs)

appropriateness evaluation protocols (AEPs)

capitation

case rate

charge description master (CDM)

charges

clinical outliers

code sequence

comorbidity

cost outlier

cost outlier review

day outlier review

diagnosis-related groups (DRGs)

DRG validation

DRG creep

elective surgery

grouper

inpatient

International Classification of Diseases, Ninth Revision, Clinical Modification (ICD-9-CM)

looping

major diagnostic categories (MDCs)

outpatient

percentage of revenue

per diem

preadmission testing (PAT)

principal diagnosis

procedure review

quality improvement organization (QIO) program

readmission review

scrubbing

stop loss

transfer review

Uniform Bill (UB-92) paper or electronic claim form

utilization review (UR)

PERFORMANCE OBJECTIVES

The student will be able to:

■ Define and spell the key terms for this chapter, given the information from the *Handbook* glossary, within a reasonable time period and with enough accuracy to obtain a satisfactory evaluation.

■ Answer the self-study review questions after reading the chapter, with enough accuracy to obtain a satisfactory evaluation.

■ Given computer-generated UB-92 claim forms, state the reasons why claims may be either rejected or delayed or why incorrect payment is received; state these reasons within a reasonable time period

and with enough accuracy to obtain a satisfactory evaluation.

■ Analyze, edit, and insert entries on computer-generated UB-92 claim forms so that payment will be accurate, within a reasonable time period and with enough accuracy to obtain a satisfactory evaluation.

■ Answer questions about the UB-92 claim form to become familiar with the data it contains.

■ Answer questions about the UB-92 claim form to learn which hospital departments input data for different blocks on this form.

STUDY OUTLINE

Patient Service Representative
Qualifications
Primary Functions and Competencies
Principal Responsibilities

Medicolegal Confidentiality Issues
Documents
Verbal Communication
Computer Security

Admissions Procedures
Appropriateness Evaluation Protocols
Admitting Procedures for Major Insurance Programs
Preadmission Testing

Compliance Safeguards

Utilization Review
Quality Improvement Organization Program

Coding Hospital Procedures
Outpatient—Reason for Visit
Inpatient—Principal Diagnosis

Coding Inpatient Procedures
ICD-9-CM Volume 3 Procedures

Coding Outpatient Procedures
Current Procedural Terminology
Health Care Common Procedure Coding System
Modifiers

Inpatient Billing Process
Admitting Clerk
Insurance Verifier
Attending Physician, Nursing Staff, and Medical Transcriptionist
Discharge Analyst
Charge Description Master

Code Specialist
Insurance Billing Editor
Nurse Auditor

Reimbursement Process
Reimbursement Methods
Electronic Data Interchange
Hard Copy Billing
Receiving Payment

Outpatient Insurance Claims
Hospital Professional Services

Billing Problems
Duplicate Statements
Double Billing
Phantom Charges

Hospital Billing Claim Form
Uniform Bill Inpatient and Outpatient Paper or Electronic Claim Form

Diagnosis-Related Groups
History
The Diagnosis-Related Groups System
Diagnosis-Related Groups and the Physician's Office

Outpatient Classification
Ambulatory Payment Classification System

Procedure: New Patient Admission and Insurance Verification

Procedure: Coding from ICD-9-CM Volume 3

Procedure: Editing a Uniform Bill (UB-92) Paper or Electronic Claim Form

Procedure: Completing the UB-92 Paper or Electronic Claim Form

SELF-STUDY **17-1** ▶ **REVIEW QUESTIONS**

Review the objectives, key terms, glossary definitions to key terms, chapter information, and figures before completing the following review questions.

1. You are reviewing a computer-generated insurance claim before it is sent to the insurance carrier and you notice the patient's name as being that of an old friend. You quickly read the code for the diagnosis. Is this a breach of confidentiality?

   _____

2. You are coding in a medical records department when an agent from the Federal Bureau of Investigation walks in and asks for a patient's address. You ask "Why do you need Mrs. Doe's address? Do you have a signed authorization from Mrs. Doe for release of information from our facility?" The FBI agent responds "I'm trying to locate this person because of counterfeiting charges. No, I don't have a signed authorization form." Would there be any breach of confidentiality if you release the patient's

   address? Explain. _____

3. List three instances of breaching confidentiality in a hospital setting.

   a. _____

   b. _____

   c. _____

4. What is the purpose of appropriateness evaluation protocols (AEPs)?

   _____

   _____

5. If a patient under a managed care plan goes to a hospital that is under contract with the plan for admission, what is necessary for inpatient admission?

   _____

6. In what type of situation would a patient not have an insurance identification card?

   _____

7. When a patient receives diagnostic tests and hospital outpatient services before admission to the hospital and these charges are combined with inpatient services, becoming part of the diagnostic-related group payment, this regulation in hospital

   billing is known as _____.

8. The diagnosis established after study and listed for admission to the hospital for

   an illness or injury is called a/an diagnosis _____.

9. For reviewing an inpatient medical record, terminology and/or phrases to look

   for that relate to uncertain diagnoses are _____.

   _____

   _____

10. From the list of *International Classification of Diseases, 9th revision, Clinical Modification
    (ICD-9-CM)* descriptions shown, place these items in correct sequential order (1, 2, 3)
    for billing purposes. In this case, the medical procedure is a repair of other hernia of
    the anterior abdominal wall, incisional hernia repair with prosthesis, ICD-9-CM
    code 53.61

	Diagnosis	*ICD-9-CM Code*
_____	Chronic liver disease, liver damage unspecified	571.3
_____	Alcohol dependence syndrome (other and unspecified)	303.9
_____	Other hernia of abdominal cavity without mention of obstruction or gangrene (incisional hernia)	553.21

11. Mrs. Benson, a Medicare patient, is admitted by Dr. Dalton to the hospital on
    January 4 and is seen in consultation by Dr. Frank on January 5. On January 6,
    Mrs. Benson is discharged with a diagnosis of coronary atherosclerosis. State some of
    the problems regarding payment and Medicare policies that would affect this case.

    _____

    _____

    _____

12. Name five payment types under managed care contracts.

    a. _____

    b. _____

    c. _____

    d. _____

    e. _____

13. Match the words or phrases used for managed care reimbursement methods in the
    left column with the definitions in the right column. Write the correct letters in the
    blanks.

    _____ sliding scales for discounts   a. Reimbursement method that pays more for the first day
              and per diems   in the hospital than subsequent days.

    _____ discounts in the form   b. Reimbursement to the hospital on a per member per
              of sliding scale   month basis.

_____ stop loss

_____ withhold

_____ charges

_____ ambulatory payment classifications

_____ case rate

_____ diagnostic-related groups

_____ differential by service type

_____ periodic interim payments

_____ bed leasing

_____ differential by day in hospital

_____ capitation

_____ per diem

_____ percentage of revenue

c. Plan advances cash to cover expected claims to the hospital.

d. Fixed percentage paid to the hospital to cover charges.

e. Single charge for a day in the hospital regardless of actual cost.

f. Interim per diem paid for each day in the hospital; based on total volume of business generated.

g. Classification system categorizing patients who are medically related with regard to diagnosis and treatment and are statistically similar in lengths of hospital stay.

h. Hospital receives a flat per-admission payment for the particular service to which the patient is admitted.

i. An averaging after a flat rate is given to certain categories of procedures.

j. Outpatient classification based on procedures rather than on diagnoses.

k. Hospital buys insurance to protect against lost revenue and receives less of a capitation fee.

l. Method in which part of plan's payment to the hospital may be withheld and paid at the end of the year.

m. When a managed care plan leases beds from a hospital and pays per bed whether used or not.

n. A percentage reduction in charges for total bed days per year.

o. Dollar amount that a hospital bills a case for services rendered.

14. Define the term *outpatient*.

_____

_____

15. Define the term *elective surgery*.

_____

_____

16. Baby Stephens falls from a high chair, cutting his head. His mother rushes him to St. Joseph's Medical Center for emergency care. The physician examines the baby, uses two stitches to close the laceration, sends the child for skull radiographs, and then discharges him to home. Will the emergency care be billed as inpatient or outpatient services?

_____

17. The inpatient and outpatient hospital billing department uses a summary form

    for submitting an insurance claim to an insurance plan called _____

    _____

18. Why did Medicare implement the diagnosis-related groups (DRG)–based system of reimbursement?

    _____

19. Name the seven variables that affect Medicare reimbursement under the DRG system.

    a. _____

    b. _____

    c. _____

    d. _____

    e. _____

    f. _____

    g. _____

20. Define the following abbreviations.

    AEP   _____

    PAT   _____

    MDC   _____

    PPS   _____

    TEFRA   _____

    UR   _____

    IS   _____

    SI   _____

    APC   _____

21. Define cost outliers.

    _____

    _____

22. Define comorbidity.

    _____

    _____

23. You can determine whether a Uniform Bill (UB-92) claim form is for an inpatient
    or an outpatient by the following observations:

    a. When the inpatient block number 4 shows three-digit billing code/codes _____

    b. When the outpatient block number 4 shows three-digit billing code/codes _____

    c. When revenue codes and block number/numbers indicate type of service rendered _____

24. Describe the significance of Field Locators 42, 43, 44, 46, and 47 of the UB-92 claim form.

    a. FL 42   _____

    b. FL 43   _____

    c. FL 44   _____

    d. FL 46   _____

    e. FL 47   _____

To check your answers to this self-study assignment, see Appendix D.

ASSIGNMENT 17-2 ▶ LOCATE AND SEQUENCE DIAGNOSTIC CODES
FOR CONDITIONS

Performance Objective

Task: Locate the correct diagnostic code for each diagnosis listed for five
                   cases.

Conditions: Use a pen or pencil and the ICD-9-CM diagnostic code book.

Standards: Time: _____ minutes

                   Accuracy: _____

                   (Note: The time element and accuracy criteria may be given by your
                   instructor.)

Directions: These cases point out the value of proper versus improper coding with regard to correct sequence and inclusion of specific codes that indicate the variance of payment. Assign the correct ICD-9-CM code numbers. Note that the same case was assigned different DRG codes, thereby listing different principal and secondary hospital diagnoses, and that the DRG payment for each is substantially different. Also note the difference in the major diagnostic category (MDC).

CASE 1

Age: 12   Sex: Male

MDC: Four diseases and disorders of the respiratory system

DRG: Code 98: Bronchitis and asthma, age 0 to 17

Principal Diagnosis

Asthma w/o status asthmaticus_____

Secondary Diagnoses

Pneumonia, organism NOS _____

Otitis media NOS _____

DRG Payment: $2705

MDC: Four diseases and disorders of the respiratory system

DRG: Code 91: Simple pneumonia and pleurisy, age 0 to 17

Principal Diagnosis

Pneumonia, organism not otherwise

        specified (NOS) _____

Secondary Diagnoses

Asthma w/o status asthmaticus _____

Otitis media NOS _____

DRG Payment: $3246

CASE 2

Age: 77   Sex: Male

MDC: Five diseases and disorders of the circulatory system

MDC: Four diseases and disorders of the circulatory respiratory system

DRG: Code 138: Cardiac arrhythmia and conduction disorders, age >69 and/or chief complaint (CC)

Principal Diagnosis

Atrial fibrillation _____

Secondary Diagnoses

Fracture (Fx) six ribs—closed _____

Transcerebral ischemia NOS _____

Syncope and collapse _____

Fx scapula NOS—closed _____

Fall not elsewhere classifiable

(NEC) and NOS _____

    Procedures

    Contrast cerebral arteriogram _____

    Computed axial tomographic (CAT) scan of head _____

    Diagnostic (Dx) ultrasonography—heart _____

    Physical therapy NEC _____

DRG Payment: $5882

DRG: Code 83: Major chest trauma, age >69 and/or CC

Principal Diagnosis

Fx six ribs—closed _____

Secondary Diagnoses

Atrial fibrillation _____

Transcerebral ischemia NOS _____

Syncope and collapse _____

Fx scapula NOS—closed _____

Fall NEC and NOS _____

DRG Payment: $6206

Note: Because this is a hospital case, ICD-9-CM Volume 3 should be used to code the procedures. However, Volume 3 is not used in the medical office.

CASE 3

Age: 42   Sex: Male

MDC: Nineteen mental diseases and disorders

   DRG: Code 426: Depressive neuroses

Principal Diagnosis

Neurotic depression _____

Secondary Diagnoses

Acute myocardial infarction anterior wall

NEC _____

MDC: Five diseases and disorders of the circulatory system
DRG: Code 122: Circulatory disorders with ami w/o cv comp disch alive

Principal Diagnosis

Acute myocardial infarction anterior wall
   NEC _____

Secondary Diagnoses

Neurotic depression _____

Chest pain NOS _____   Chest pain NOS _____

Heart disease NOS _____   Heart disease NOS _____

Paranoid personality _____   Paranoid personality _____

Procedures

Dx ultrasound—heart _____

Other resp procedures _____

DRG Payment: $6007   *DRG Payment:* $8637

Note: Because this is a hospital case, ICD-9-CM Volume 3 should be used to code the procedures. However, as mentioned, Volume 3 is not used in the medical office.

CASE 4

Age: 65   Sex: Male

MDC: Five diseases and disorders of the circulatory system
DRG: Code 468: Unrelated OR proc

MDC: Twelve diseases and disorders of the male reproductive system
DRG: Code 336: Transurethral prostatectomy, age >69 and/or CC

Principal Diagnosis   *Principal Diagnosis*

Hypertensive heart disease NOS_____   Malig neopl prostate _____

Secondary Diagnoses   *Secondary Diagnoses*

Hematuria _____   Hematuria _____

Hyperplasia of prostate _____   Hypertensive heart disease NOS_____

Hemiplegia NOS _____   Hemiplegia NOS _____

Late eff cerebrovasc dis _____   Late eff cerebrovasc dis _____

Malig neopl prostate _____   Hyperplasia of prostate _____

Procedures

Transurethral prostatect _____

Urethral dilation _____

Cystoscopy NEC _____

Intravenous pyelogram _____

Nephrotomogram NEC _____

DRG Payment: $13,311   *DRG Payment:* $6377

Note: Because this is a hospital case, ICD-9-CM Volume 3 should be used to code the procedures. However, as mentioned, Volume 3 is not used in the medical office.

CASE 5

Age: 62   Sex: Female

MDC: Six diseases and disorders of the digestive system
DRG: Code 188: Other digestive system diagnoses, age >69 and/or CC

Principal Diagnosis

Descending colon inj—closed _____

Secondary Diagnoses

Liver injury NOS—closed _____

Open wnd knee/leg—compl _____

Firearm accident NOS _____

No procedures performed

DRG Payment: $4710

MDC: Seven diseases and disorders of the hepatobiliary system and pancreas
DRG: Code 205: Disorders of the liver exc malig, cirr, alc hepa, age >69 and/or CC

Principal Diagnosis

Liver injury NOS—closed _____

Secondary Diagnoses

Atrial fibrillation _____

Urin tract infection NOS _____

Descending colon inj—closed _____

Open wnd knee/leg—compl _____

Firearm accident NOS _____

E. coli infect NOS _____

DRG Payment: $6847

ASSIGNMENT 17-3 ▸ IDENTIFY HOSPITAL DEPARTMENTS THAT INPUT DATA FOR THE UB-92 CLAIM FORM

Performance Objective

Task: Answer questions about the hospital departments that supply data for
                   the UB-92 claim form.

Conditions: Use an ink pen.

Standards: Time: _____ minutes

                   Accuracy: _____

                   (Note: The time element and accuracy criteria may be given by your
                   instructor.)

Directions: Depending on your instructor's preference, you may complete this exercise with or without notes or other material.

You have become familiar with the information in all 86 blocks of the UB-92 claim form. This assignment will help you learn which of six hospital departments input information into the computer system to be printed out in the various blocks.

This assignment will enhance your understanding of how multiple employees in a large facility take part in helping produce a completed UB-92 claim form. It will also increase your understanding of where errors and omissions originate so that you may emend them when you start the editing and correction process. Answer the following questions.

1. Which department is responsible for inputting the charges for a blood test?

   _____

2. Which department is responsible for inputting an insurance certificate or subscriber number?

   _____

3. Which department is responsible for inputting the procedure codes?

   _____

4. Which department is responsible for inputting the patient's name and address?

   _____

5. Which department is responsible for inputting the diagnostic codes?

   _____

ASSIGNMENT **17-4** ▸ **STUDY UB-92 CLAIM FORM BLOCK DATA**

Performance Objective

Task: Answer questions about the UB-92 claim form blocks.

Conditions: Use an ink pen.

Standards: Time: _____ minutes

                      Accuracy: _____

                      (Note: The time element and accuracy criteria may be given by your
                      instructor.)

Directions: Depending on your instructor's preference, you may complete this exercise with or without notes or other material.

You have learned about a number of reimbursement methods, confidentiality issues, evaluation protocols, and the utilization review process. This information is necessary for processing an insurance claim to obtain maximum reimbursement. To the UB-92 claim form, you must become familiar with the data it contains, including codes and the location of various types of information. Answer the following questions.

1. In Block 4, state the correct billing codes for

   a. Inpatient services _____

   b. Outpatient services _____

2. What is listed in Block 7? _____

   _____

3. What insurance carriers or programs require Block 9 to be completed? _____

   _____

4. What format is required in Block 14 for the patient's date of birth? _____

   _____

5. If a patient was in the hospital for the delivery of a premature infant, what code would be used in Block 20?

   _____

6. If a patient was discharged from inpatient care at 2:15 PM, how would this be noted in Block 21?

   _____

7. What is the correct code to use in Block 22 if a patient was discharged to a home hospice situation?

   _____

8. If neither the patient nor spouse was employed, what code would be used to indicate this in Blocks 24 through 30?

_____

9. State the reason for the codes used in Blocks 32 through 35.

_____

_____

10. What revenue code must be shown on all bills as a final entry and in what block does it occur?

_____

ASSIGNMENT **17–5** ▸ **UB-92 CLAIM FORM QUESTIONS ABOUT EDITING**

Performance Objective

Task: Answer questions about editing the blocks on the UB-92 claim form.

Conditions: Use an ink pen.

Standards: Time: _____ minutes

                     Accuracy: _____

                     (Note: The time element and accuracy criteria may be given by your
                     instructor.)

Directions: You are now ready to learn more about the critical editing process for determining errors and omissions on the UB-92 claim form. This important skill may help you secure a job in the claims processing department. Refer to Figure 17–4 in the *Handbook* and, at the end of the chapter, the procedure for editing a UB-92 paper or electronic claim form, and answer the questions.

1. Where does the editing process begin on the UB-92 claim form? _____

   _____

2. What block/blocks must be filled in when insurance information on the UB-92 claim
   form is verified?

   _____

3. What block should the principal diagnostic code appear in?

   _____

4. For an inpatient claim, if Block 43 lists the hospital room, Block 44 lists the per-day
   rate, and Block 46 lists the number of hospital days, what other block is used to verify
   this claim for accuracy?

   _____

5. Besides room rate and number of inpatient days, what is another important factor in
   reviewing the services shown in Blocks 42 through 47?

   _____

   _____

6. For outpatient claims, what other item/items is/are shown besides the date, description
   of the service rendered, and fee?

   _____

7. Where can an insurance editor check when there is doubt about a service shown on a UB-92 claim form?

_____

8. Which block should show the estimated amount due from the insurance company?

_____

ASSIGNMENT 17-6 ▸ LOCATE ERRORS ON A COMPUTER-GENERATED UB-92 CLAIM FORM

Performance Objective

Task: Locate the blocks on the computer-generated insurance claim form that need completion of missing information or have data that need to be corrected before submission to the insurance company.

Conditions: Use Mary J. Torre's completed insurance claim (Figure 16–1), the checklist for editing a UB-92 claim form, and a red ink pen.

Standards: Time: _____ minutes

Accuracy: _____

(Note: The time element and accuracy criteria may be given by your instructor.)

Directions: Refer to Figure 17–4 in the *Handbook* to employ the step-by-step approach while editing the computer-generated UB-92 claim form (Figure 17–1). Use the checklist to help you when reviewing the claim form. Locate the blocks on the claim form that need completion of missing information or that have data to be corrected before submission to the insurance company. Highlight all errors you discover. Insert all corrections and missing information in red. If you cannot locate the necessary information but know it is mandatory, write "NEED" in the corresponding block.

In addition, you notice that the second line entry for pharmacy shows a total of $6,806. However, you know from reviewing the case that one injection of a drug known as TPA (revenue code 259 and fee $5,775), which dissolves clots and opens vessels when a patient has a myocardial infarction, was not broken out of the fee. Hand write this final entry. On line 2, cross out the total charge $6,806 and insert the correct pharmacy-reduced amount.

Checklist for Editing a Uniform Bill (UB-92) Claim Form: Mary J. Torre

Steps	Blocks
1	Blocks 1 _____ and 5 _____
2	Block 4: Inpatient _____ Outpatient _____
3	Blocks 12 _____, 38 _____, 58 _____
	and 59 _____
4	Block 14 _____
5	Blocks 12 _____ and 15 _____
6	Blocks 50 _____, 60 _____, 61 _____
	62 _____, 65 _____, and 66 _____
7	Blocks 67 _____, 76 _____, and 78 _____
8	Blocks 80 _____ and 81 _____
9	Blocks 82 _____ and 83 _____

10   Blocks 6 _____, 17 _____, and 32 _____

11   **Inpatient:** Blocks 42–47: 7 _____, 18 _____

          21 _____, and 46 _____

12   Block 47 _____

13   Blocks 42 _____, and 46 _____

14   **Outpatient:** Blocks 43 _____, 44 _____

          and 45 _____

15   Detailed record to be checked

16   Blocks 42 _____, 43 _____, and 47 _____

17   Block 55 _____

18   Blocks 85 _____ and 86 _____

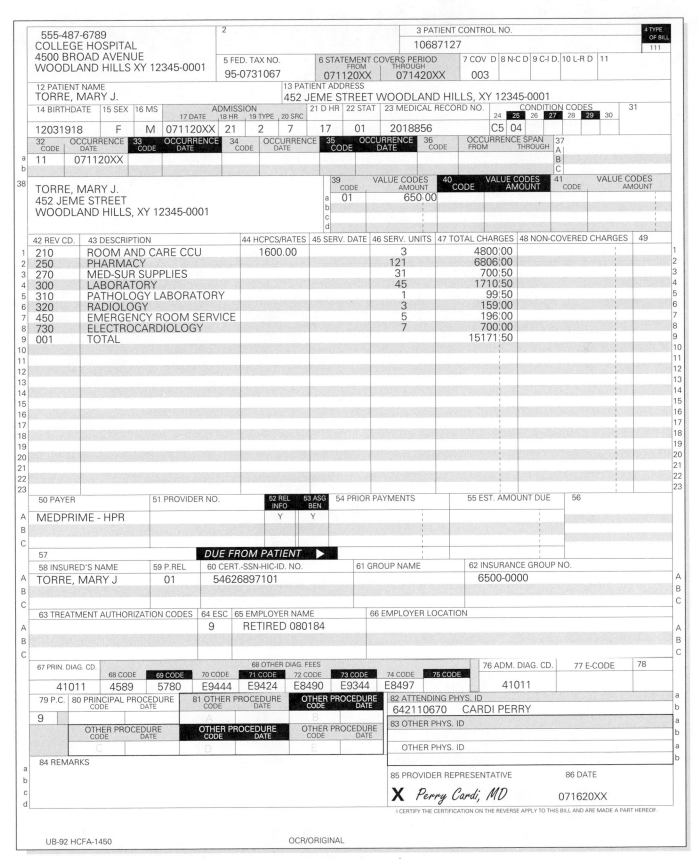

Figure 17–1

ASSIGNMENT **17-7** ▸ **LOCATE ERRORS ON A COMPUTER-GENERATED UB-92 CLAIM FORM**

Performance Objective

Task: Locate the blocks on the computer-generated insurance claim form that need completion of missing information or have data that need to be corrected before submission to the insurance company.

Conditions: Use Henry M. Cosby's completed insurance claim (Figure 16–2), the checklist for editing a UB-92 claim form, and a red ink pen.

Standards: Time: _____ minutes

Accuracy: _____

(Note: The time element and accuracy criteria may be given by your instructor.)

Directions: Refer to Figure 17–4 in the *Handbook* to employ the step-by-step approach while editing the computer-generated UB-92 claim form (Figure 17–2). Use the checklist to help you when reviewing the claim form. Locate the blocks on the claim form that need completion of missing information or that have data to be corrected before submission to the insurance company. Highlight all errors you discover. Insert all corrections and missing information in red. If you cannot locate the necessary information but know it is mandatory, write "NEED" in the corresponding block. State the reason or reasons why the claim may be rejected or delayed or why incorrect payment may be generated because of one or more errors discovered.

Checklist for Editing a Uniform Bill (UB-92) Claim Form: Henry M. Cosby

Steps	*Blocks*
1	Blocks 1 _____ and 5 _____
2	Block 4: Inpatient _____ Outpatient _____
3	Blocks 12 _____, 38 _____, 58 _____
	and 59 _____
4	Block 14 _____
5	Blocks 12 _____ and 15 _____
6	Blocks 50 _____, 60 _____, 61 _____
	62 _____, 65 _____, and 66 _____
7	Blocks 67 _____, 76 _____, and 78 _____
8	Blocks 80 _____ _____ and 81 _____
9	Blocks 82 _____ and 83 _____
10	Blocks 6 _____, 17 _____, and 32 _____

11   **Inpatient:** Blocks 42–47: 7 _____, 18 _____,

     21 _____, and 46 _____

12   Block 47 _____

13   Blocks 42 _____ and 46 _____

14   **Outpatient:** Blocks 43 _____, 44 _____,

     and 45 _____

15   Detailed record to be checked

16   Blocks 42 _____, 43 _____, and 47 _____

17   Block 55 _____

18   Blocks 85 _____ and 86 _____

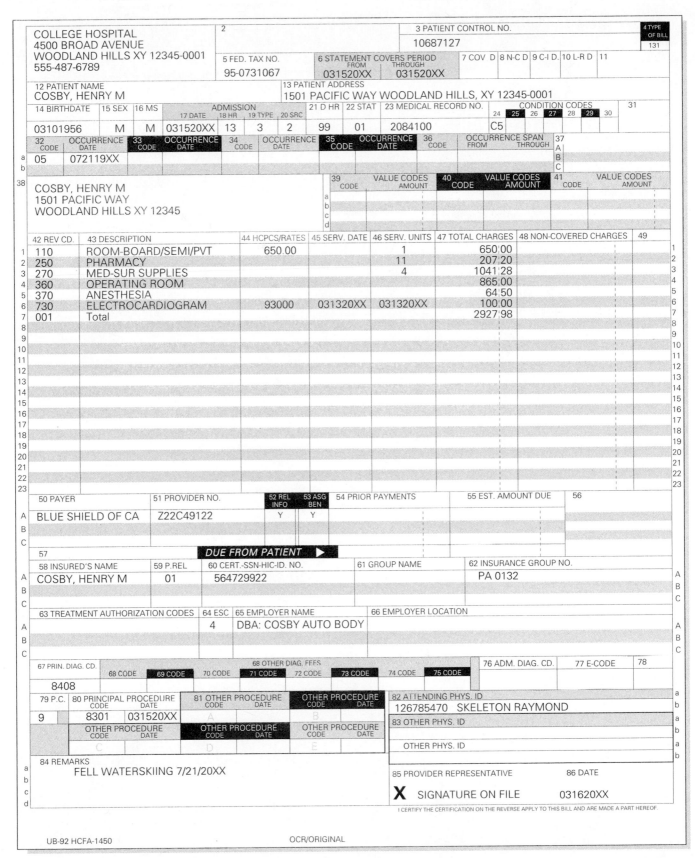

Figure 17–2

ASSIGNMENT 17–8 ▸ LOCATE ERRORS ON A COMPUTER-GENERATED
UB-92 CLAIM FORM

Performance Objective

Task: Locate the blocks on the computer-generated insurance claim form that need completion of missing information or have data that need to be corrected before submission to the insurance company.

Conditions: Use Harold M. McDonald's completed insurance claim (Figure 17–3), the checklist for editing a UB-92 claim form, and a red ink pen.

Standards: Time: _____ minutes

Accuracy: _____

(Note: The time element and accuracy criteria may be given by your instructor.)

Directions: Refer to Figure 17–4 in the *Handbook* to employ the step-by-step approach while editing the computer-generated UB-92 claim form (Figure 17–3). Use the checklist to help you when reviewing the claim form. Locate the blocks on the claim form that need completion of missing information or that have data to be corrected before submission to the insurance company. Highlight all errors you discover. Insert all corrections and missing information in red. If you cannot locate the necessary information but know it is mandatory, write "NEED" in the corresponding block.

You notice that the seventh CPT/Healthcare Common Procedure Coding System (HCPCS) code 43450 for operating room is missing. On hospital claims, the entry for operating room is usually blank and must be handwritten in, because this is the code for the surgical procedure.

Checklist for Editing a Uniform Bill (UB-92) Claim Form: Harold M. McDonald

Steps   *Blocks*

1   Blocks 1 _____ and 5 _____

2   Block 4: Inpatient _____ Outpatient _____

3   Blocks 12 _____, 38 _____, 58 _____,

and 59 _____

4   Block 14 _____

5   Blocks 12 _____ and 15 _____

6   Blocks 50 _____, 60 _____, 61 _____

62 _____, 65 _____, and 66 _____

7   Blocks 67 _____, 76 _____, and 78 _____

8   Blocks 80 _____ and 81 _____

9   Blocks 82 _____ and 83 _____

10   Blocks 6 _____, 17 _____, and 32 _____

11   **Inpatient:** Blocks 42–47: 7 _____, 18 _____,

      21 _____, and 46 _____

12   Block 47 _____

13   Blocks 42 _____ and 46 _____

14   **Outpatient:** Blocks 43 _____, 44 _____,

      and 45 _____

15   Detailed record to be checked

16   Blocks 42 _____, 43 _____, and 47 _____

17   Block 55 _____

18   Blocks 85 _____ and 86 _____

1. COLLEGE HOSPITAL 4500 BROAD AVENUE WOODLAND HILLS XY 12345-0001 555-487-6789	2		3 PATIENT CONTROL NO. 10670685	4 TYPE OF BILL 131

5 FED. TAX NO. 95-0731067 — 6 STATEMENT COVERS PERIOD FROM 070520XX THROUGH 070520XX — 7 COV D 8 N-C D 9 C-I D. 10 L-R D 11

12 PATIENT NAME: MCDONALD HAROLD M
13 PATIENT ADDRESS: 22 BEACON ROAD WOODLAND HILLS, XY 12345-0001

14. BIRTHDATE 04261929 15.SEX M 16 MS M ADMISSION 17 DATE 070520XX 18 HR 12 19 TYPE 3 20 SRC 1 21 D HR 99 22 STAT 01 23 MEDICAL RECORD NO. 2071307 CONDITION CODES 25 27 29 C5 31

38 MCDONALD HAROLD M 22 BEACON ROAD WOODLAND HILLS XY 12345-0001

42 REV CD.	43 DESCRIPTION	44 HCPCS/RATES	45 SERV. DATE	46 SERV. UNITS	47 TOTAL CHARGES	48 NON-COVERED CHARGES	49
250	PHARMACY			5	90 90		
270	MED - SUR SUPPLIES			16	2519 50		
300	DRAWING BLOOD	36415	070520XX	1	8 50		
300	13-16 BLOOD/URINE TESTS	80016	070520XX	1	28 00		
300	CREATININE CLEARANCE TEST	82575	070520XX	1	20 00		
300	CBC	85025 24	070520XX	1	16 50		
320	CONTRAST XRAY EXAM, ESOPH	74220	070520XX	1	114 00		
320	X-RAY GUIDE, GI DILATION	74360	070520XX	1	750 00		
360	OPERATING ROOM				500 00		
410	CONT OXIMETER HOURS	82805 22	070520XX	1	8 00		
001	Total				4055 40		

50 PAYER: A HEALTH PLAN REDWOOD 51 PROVIDER NO. 278654901 52 REL INFO Y 53 ASG BEN Y 54 PRIOR PAYMENTS 55 EST. AMOUNT DUE 56

57 DUE FROM PATIENT ▶

58 INSURED'S NAME: MCDONALD HAROLD M 59 P.REL 01 60 CERT.-SSN-HIC-ID. NO. 31424435401 61 GROUP NAME 62 INSURANCE GROUP NO. 1320-0000 PLAN GO

63 TREATMENT AUTHORIZATION CODES 64 ESC 9 65 EMPLOYER NAME WC PEDERSON FORD 66 EMPLOYER LOCATION

67 PRIN. DIAG. CD. 1509 68 V725

76 ADM. DIAG. CODE 77 E-CODE 78

79 P.C. 9 80 PRINCIPAL PROCEDURE 81 OTHER PROCEDURE 82 ATTENDING PHYS. ID 124589770 ANTRUM, CONCHA
83 OTHER PHYS. ID

84 REMARKS: HPR

85 PROVIDER REPRESENTATIVE: X *Concha Antrum, MD* 86 DATE 070620XX

I CERTIFY THE STATEMENTS ON THE REVERSE APPLY TO THIS BILL AND ARE MADE A PART HEREOF.

UB-92 HCFA-1450 OCR/ORIGINAL

Figure 17–3

ASSIGNMENT 17-9 ▸ LOCATE ERRORS ON A COMPUTER-GENERATED UB-92 CLAIM FORM

Performance Objective

Task: Locate the blocks on the computer-generated insurance claim form that need completion of missing information or have data that need to be corrected before submission to the insurance company.

Conditions: Use Pedro Martinez's completed insurance claim (Figure 17–4), the checklist for editing a UB-92 claim form, and a red ink pen.

Standards: Time: _____ minutes

Accuracy: _____

(Note: The time element and accuracy criteria may be given by your instructor.)

Directions: Refer to Figure 17–4 in the *Handbook* to employ the step-by-step approach while editing the computer-generated UB-92 claim form (Figure 17–4). Use the checklist to help you when reviewing the claim form. Locate the blocks on the claim form that need completion of missing information or that have data to be corrected before submission to the insurance company. Highlight all errors you discover. Insert all corrections and missing information in red. If you cannot locate the necessary information but know it is mandatory, write "NEED" in the corresponding block. Then write a list of reasons why the claim may be rejected or delayed or why incorrect payment may be generated because of errors discovered.

Checklist for Editing a Uniform Bill (UB-92) Claim Form: Pedro Martinez

Steps	Blocks
1	Blocks 1 _____ and 5 _____
2	Block 4: Inpatient _____ Outpatient _____
3	Blocks 12 _____, 38 _____, 58 _____, and 59 _____
4	Block 14 _____
5	Blocks 12 _____ and 15 _____
6	Blocks 50 _____, 60 _____, 61 _____, 62 _____, 65 _____, and 66 _____
7	Blocks 67 _____, 76 _____, and 78 _____
8	Blocks 80 _____ _____ and 81 _____
9	Blocks 82 _____ and 83 _____
10	Blocks 6 _____, 17 _____, and 32 _____

11 **Inpatient:** Blocks 42–47: 7 _____, 18 _____,

     21 _____, and 46 _____

12 Block 47 _____

13 Blocks 42 _____ and 46 _____

14 **Outpatient:** Blocks 43 _____, 44 _____,

     and 45 _____

15 Detailed record to be checked

16 Blocks 42 _____, 43 _____, and 47 _____

17 Block 55 _____

18 Blocks 85 _____ and 86 _____

COLLEGE HOSPITAL 4500 BROAD AVENUE WOODLAND HILLS XY 12345-0001 555-487-6789	2		3 PATIENT CONTROL NO. 10630911		4 TYPE OF BILL 111
	5 FED. TAX NO. 95-0731067	6 STATEMENT COVERS PERIOD FROM 06120XX THROUGH 06120XX	7 COV D 8 N-C D 9 C-I D. 10 L-R D 11 010		

12 PATIENT NAME MARTINEZ PEDRO	13 PATIENT ADDRESS 7821 SENSOR AVE WOODLAND HILLS, XY 12345-0001

14. BIRTHDATE	15.SEX	16 MS	ADMISSION 17 DATE 18 HR 19 TYPE 20 SRC	21 D HR	22 STAT	23 MEDICAL RECORD NO.	CONDITION CODES 24 25 26 27 28 29 30	31
092218	M	W	061120XX 20 1 7	19	03	3567811	C5 04	

32 CODE OCCURRENCE DATE	33 CODE OCCURRENCE DATE	34 CODE OCCURRENCE DATE	35 CODE OCCURRENCE DATE	36 CODE OCCURRENCE SPAN FROM THROUGH	37 A B C
a					
b					

38		39 CODE VALUE CODES AMOUNT		41 CODE VALUE CODES AMOUNT
MARTINEZ PEDRO 7821 SENSOR AVENUE WOODLAND HILLS XY 12345-0001		a 01 650 00 b c d		

	42 REV CD.	43 DESCRIPTION	44 HCPCS/RATES	45 SERV. DATE	46 SERV. UNITS	47 TOTAL CHARGES	48 NON-COVERED CHARGES	49	
1	110	ROOM - BOARD/SEMI/PVT	650.00		1	650 00			1
2	120	ROOM AND CARE SEMI	650.00		1	650 00			2
3	210	ROOM AND CARE CCU	1600.00		8	12800 00			3
4	250	PHARMACY			500	7133 90			4
5	270	MED - SUR SUPPLIES			149	3689 50			5
6	300	LABORATORY			97	5399 33			6
7	320	RADIOLOGY			27	1544 00			7
8	350	CT SCAN			1	622 00			8
9	410	RESPIRATORY THERAPY			240	6698 50			9
10	420	PHYSICAL THERAPY			9	470 00			10
11	450	EMERGENCY ROOM SERV			6	197 00			11
12	460	PULMONARY FUNCTION				29 00			12
13	730	ELECTROCARDIOLOGY			1	100 00			13
14	942	EDUCATION			6	82 50			14
15	001	Total				40065 73			15

	50 PAYER	51 PROVIDER NO.	52 REL INFO	53 ASG BEN	54 PRIOR PAYMENTS	55 EST. AMOUNT DUE	56
A	MEDIPRIME-HPR		Y	Y			
B							
C							

57	DUE FROM PATIENT ▶

	58 INSURED'S NAME	59 P.REL	60 CERT.-SSN-HIC-ID. NO.	61 GROUP NAME	62 INSURANCE GROUP NO.	
A	MARTINEZ PEDRO	01	55025897001		6500-0000	A
B						B
C						C

	63 TREATMENT AUTHORIZATION CODES	64 ESC	65 EMPLOYER NAME	66 EMPLOYER LOCATION	
A		5	RETIRED 1975		A
B					B
C					C

67 PRIN. DIAG. CD.	68 CODE	69 CODE	68 OTHER DIAG. FEES 70 CODE 71 CODE 72 CODE 73 CODE 74 CODE 75 CODE	76 ADM. DIAG. CODE	77 E-CODE	78
4169	51881	49121				

79 P.C.	80 PRINCIPAL PROCEDURE CODE DATE	81 OTHER PROCEDURE CODE DATE	OTHER PROCEDURE CODE DATE	82 ATTENDING PHYS. ID 642110670 COCCIDIOIDES BRADY	a b
9					
	OTHER PROCEDURE CODE DATE	OTHER PROCEDURE CODE DATE	OTHER PROCEDURE CODE DATE	83 OTHER PHYS. ID OTHER PHYS. ID	a b a b

84 REMARKS	85 PROVIDER REPRESENTATIVE 86 DATE
a b c d	X

I CERTIFY THE CERTIFICATION ON THE REVERSE APPLY TO THIS BILL AND ARE MADE A PART HEREOF.

UB-92 HCFA-1450   OCR/ORIGINAL

Figure 17–4

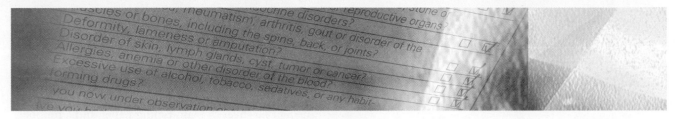

Seeking a Job and Attaining Professional Advancement

KEY TERMS

Your instructor may wish to select some specific words pertinent to this chapter for a test. For definitions of the terms, further study, and/or reference, the words, phrases, and abbreviations may be found in the glossary at the end of the Handbook. *Key terms for this chapter follow.*

alien

application form

blind mailing

business associate agreement

certification

Certified Coding Specialist (CCS)

Certified Coding Specialist-Physician (CCS-P)

Certified Medical Assistant (CMA)

Certified Medical Billing Specialist (CMBS)

Certified Professional Coder (CPC, CPC-A, CPC-H)

chronologic resume

claims assistance professional (CAP)

combination resume

continuing education

cover letter

electronic claims processor (ECP)

employment agency

functional resume

interview

mentor

National Certified Insurance and Coding Specialist (NCICS)

networking

portfolio

Professional Association of Health Care Office Managers (PAHCOM)

Registered Medical Assistant (RMA)

Registered Medical Coder (RMC)

registration

resume

self-employment

service contract

PERFORMANCE OBJECTIVES

The student will be able to:

- Define and spell the key terms for this chapter, given the information from the *Handbook* glossary, within a reasonable time period and with enough accuracy to obtain a satisfactory evaluation.
- After reading the chapter, answer the self-study review questions with enough accuracy to obtain a satisfactory evaluation.
- Research information in preparation for typing a resume, given a worksheet to complete, within a reasonable time period and with enough accuracy to obtain a satisfactory evaluation.
- Type an accurate resume in attractive format, using plain typing paper, within a reasonable time period, to obtain a satisfactory evaluation.

- Compose and type a letter of introduction to go with the resumé and place it in a typed envelope, using one sheet of plain typing paper and a number 10 envelope, within a reasonable time period, to obtain a satisfactory evaluation.
- Complete an application form for a job, given an application for position form, within a reasonable time period and with enough accuracy to obtain a satisfactory evaluation.
- Compose and type a follow-up thank-you letter and place it in a typed envelope, using one sheet of plain typing paper and a number 10 envelope, within a reasonable time period, to obtain a satisfactory evaluation.
- Access the Internet and visit Web sites to research and/or obtain data.

STUDY OUTLINE

Employment Opportunities
  Insurance Billing Specialist
  Claims Assistance Professional
Job Search
  Online Job Search
  Job Fairs
  Application
  Letter of Introduction
  Resume
  Interview
  Follow-up Letter

Self-Employment
  Setting Up an Office
  Finances to Consider
  Marketing, Advertising, Promotion, and Public
    Relations
  Documentation
  Mentor
  Networking
Procedure: Creating an Electronic Resume
Procedure: Preparing a Resume in ASCII

 SELF-STUDY **18–1 ▸ REVIEW QUESTIONS**

Review the objectives, key terms, glossary definitions of key terms, chapter information, and figures before completing the following review questions.

1. You have just completed a 1-year medical insurance billing course at a college. Name some preliminary job search contacts to make on campus.

   a. _____

   b. _____

   c. _____

   d. _____

2. Name skills that may be listed on an application form or in a resume when a person is seeking a position as an insurance billing specialist.

a. _____

b. _____

c. _____

d. _____

e. _____

f. _____

3. A question appears on a job application form about salary. Two ways in which to handle this question are

a. _____

b. _____

4. State the chief purpose of a cover letter when a resume is sent to a prospective employer.

_____

5. A resume style that emphasizes work experience dates is known as a/an _____

format; the _____ format stresses job skills.

6. When job applicants have similar skills and education, surveys have shown that hiring

by employers has been based on _____.

7. List the items to be compiled in a portfolio.

a. _____

b. _____

c. _____

d. _____

e. _____

f. _____

g. _____

h. _____

i. _____

j. _____

8. You are being interviewed for a job and the interviewer asks this question: "What is

   your religious preference?" What would you respond? _____

   _____

9. If a short period of time elapses after an interview and the applicant has received no
   word from the prospective employer, what follow-up steps may be taken?

   a. _____

   b. _____

10. If an individual creates a billing company and coding services are to be part of the
    offerings, the coding professional should have what type of professional status?

    _____

11. When an individual plans to start an insurance billing company, he or she should

    have enough funds to operate the business for a period of _____

12. Hugh Beason was the owner of XYZ Medical Reimbursement Service. A fire
    occurred, damaging some of the equipment and part of the office premises and
    requiring him to stop his work for a month so that repairs could be made. What
    type/types of insurance would be helpful for this kind of problem?

    _____

13. Under HIPAA regulations, if a physician has his insurance billing outsourced to

    a person, this individual is known as a/an _____
    because he or she uses and discloses individuals' identifiable health information.

14. When insurance billing is outsourced to a company, a document known as a _____
    should be created, signed, and notarized by both parties.

15. Gwendolyn Stevens has an insurance billing company and is attending a professional
    meeting where she has given business cards to a few attendees. Give two reasons for
    using this business marketing strategy.

    a. _____

    b. _____

16. State the difference between certification and registration.

    a. Certification: _____

    _____

    b. Registration: _____

    _____

17. Name some ways an insurance billing specialist may seek to keep knowledge current.

    a. _____

    b. _____

    c. _____

    d. _____

18. A guide who offers advice, criticism, and guidance to an inexperienced person to help

    him or her reach a goal is known as a/an _____

19. Jerry Hahn is pursuing a career as a claims assistance professional. When he markets

    his business, the target audience should be _____.

20. Jennifer Inouye has been hired as a coding specialist by a hospital and needs to keep documentation when working. This may consist of

    a. _____

    b. _____

    c. _____

21. Define the following abbreviations, which stand for validations of professionalism

    CPC   _____

    CCS   _____

    RMC   _____

    CMB   _____

    NCICS _____

22. Read each statement and indicate whether it is true (T) or false (F).

    _____   a. Enhancing knowledge and keeping up to date are responsibilities of an insurance billing specialist.

    _____   b. Professional status of an insurance billing specialist may be obtained by passing a national examination for an CMRS.

    _____   c. Professional status of a claims assistance professional may be obtained by passing a national examination as a CCS.

23. Give the names of two national organizations that certify coders.

    a. _____

    b. _____

ASSIGNMENT 18-2 ► CONSULT A RESUME WORKSHEET

Performance Objective

Task: Complete a worksheet in preparation for typing your resume.

Conditions: Use one sheet of plain typing paper and a computer or typewriter.

Standards: Time: _____ minutes

                  Accuracy: _____

                  (Note: The time element and accuracy criteria may be given by your instructor.)

Directions: Complete a worksheet in preparation for typing your resume. Some of the information requested on the worksheet should not appear on the resume but should be available if you are asked to provide it.

Checklist

1. Inserted title of personal data sheet   _____

2. Inserted heading: name, address, telephone number, and so on   _____

3. Selected one of three formats for data   _____

4. Inserted heading and data for education information   _____

5. Inserted heading and data for skill information   _____

6. Inserted heading and data for employment information   _____

7. Inserted reference information   _____

8 Printed worksheet   _____

9. Asked a classmate to review and comment on worksheet   _____

ASSIGNMENT **18-3** ▸ **TYPE A RESUME**

Performance Objective

Task: Respond to a job advertisement and type a resume by abstracting data from your worksheet developed in Assignment 18–2.

Conditions: Use one sheet of plain typing paper, a newspaper advertisement (Figure 18–1), and a computer or typewriter.

Standards: Time: _____ minutes

Accuracy: _____

(Note: The time element and accuracy criteria may be given by your instructor.)

Directions: An advertisement appeared in your local newspaper (Figure 18–1). You decide to apply for the position. Abstract data that you think are relevant from your information worksheet, and type a resume in rough draft. Ask the instructor for suggestions to improve the rough draft. Refer to Chapter 18 and Figure 18–6 in the *Handbook* to help organize your resume into an attractive format before you type the final copy.

Checklist

1. Inserted title of personal data sheet from worksheet   _____

2. Inserted heading: name, address, telephone number, and so on   _____

3. Selected one of three formats for data   _____

4. Inserted heading and data for education information   _____

5. Inserted heading and data for skill information   _____

6. Inserted heading and data for employment information   _____

7. Inserted reference information   _____

8. Proofread resume   _____

9. Printed resume   _____

MEDICAL INSURANCE CODING/REIMBURSEMENT SPECIALIST

Mid-Atlantic Clinic, a 20-physician, multi-specialty group practice in Chicago, Illinois, has a need for a coding and reimbursement specialist. Knowledge of medical terminology, CPT and ICD-9-CM coding systems, Medicare regulations, third-party insurance reimbursement and physician billing procedures required. Proficiency in the interpretation and coding of procedural and diagnostic codes is strongly preferred. Successful candidates must have excellent communication and problem-solving skills. This position offers a competitive salary and superior benefits. Please send resume to:

George B. Pason, Personnel Director
Mid-Atlantic Clinic
1230 South Main Street
Chicago, IL 60611

Figure 18–1

ASSIGNMENT 18–4 ▸ COMPLETE A COVER LETTER

Performance Objective

Task: Compose a cover letter to accompany your resume.

Conditions: Use one sheet of plain typing paper, a number 10 envelope, and a computer or typewriter.

Standards: Time: _____ minutes

                 Accuracy: _____

                 (Note: The time element and accuracy criteria may be given by your instructor.)

Directions: Compose a cover letter introducing yourself, and type a rough draft. Consult the instructor for suggestions. Type the cover letter on plain bond paper in a form that can be mailed. Refer to the sample letter in Chapter 18 and Figure 18–5 in the *Handbook* as a guide to help organize your thoughts. Type the name and address of the employer on a number 10 envelope, and insert the letter with the resume from Assignment 18–3.

Checklist

1. Assemble materials, determine the recipient's address, and decide on modified or full block letter style or format.   _____

2. Turn on the computer and select the word processing program. Open a blank document.   _____

3. Key the date line beginning at least three lines below the letterhead and make certain it is in the proper location for the chosen style.   _____

4. Double-space down and insert the inside address and make certain it is in the proper location for the chosen style. Select a style to insert an attention line, if necessary.   _____

5. Double-space and key the salutation. Use either open or mixed punctuation.   _____

6. Double-space and enter the reference line ("Re:" or "Subject:") in the location for the chosen letter style.   _____

7. Double-space and key the body (content) of the letter in single-space and make certain the paragraph style is proper for the format chosen. Double-space between paragraphs. Save the letter to the computer hard drive every 15 minutes.   _____

8. Proofread the letter on the computer screen for composition.   _____

9. Proofread the letter on the computer screen for typographical, spelling, grammatical, and mechanical errors. Use the spell-check feature of the word processing program and reference books to check for correct spelling, meaning, or usage.   _____

10. Key a complimentary close and make certain it is in the proper location for the chosen style.   _____

11. Drop down four spaces and key the sender's name and title or credentials as printed on the letterhead.   _____

12. Single- or double-space to insert copy ("CC"), or enclosure ("Enclosure" or "Enc"), or attachment notations.   _____

13. Save the file before printing a hard copy and proofread the letter once more. Make corrections, if needed.   _____

14. Print the final copy to be sent and proofread. Make a copy to be retained in the files in case it is needed for future reference.   _____

15. Save the file to a CD-ROM to be stored for future reference.   _____

16. Prepare an envelope and use the format for optical scanning recommended by the United States Postal Service.   _____

17. Clip attachments to the letter and sign.   _____

ASSIGNMENT **18-5** ▶ **COMPLETE A JOB APPLICATION FORM**

Performance Objective

Task: Complete a job application form by using data from your resume.

Conditions: Use application form (Figures 18–2, *A* and *B*), your resume, and
                            computer or typewriter.

Standards: Time: _____ minutes

                            Accuracy: _____

                            (Note: The time element and accuracy criteria may be given by your
                            instructor.)

Directions: Assume that the employer asked you to come to his or her place of business to complete an application form and make an appointment for an interview. Using your data and resume, complete an application form (Figures 18–2, *A* and *B*).

                                                                                           Checklist

1. Completed personal information on application form   _____

2. Inserted employment information   _____

3. Inserted education history on form   _____

4. Checked special skills   _____

5. Inserted employment record   _____

6. Listed reference information   _____

7. Signed and dated the form   _____

8. Proofread form   _____

APPLICATION FOR POSITION/ Medical or Dental Office
AN EQUAL OPPORTUNITY EMPLOYER

(In answering questions, use extra blank sheet if necessary)

No employee, applicant, or candidate for promotion training or other advantage shall be discriminated against (or given preference) because of race, color, religion, sex, age, physical handicap, veteran status, or national origin.
PLEASE READ CAREFULLY AND WRITE OR PRINT ANSWERS TO ALL QUESTIONS. DO NOT TYPE

Date of application

A. PERSONAL INFORMATION

Name- Last   First   Middle   Social Security No.   Area Code/Phone No. ( )

Present Address: -Street   (Apt. #)   City   State   Zip   How long at this address?

Previous Address: -Street   City   State   Zip   Person to notify in case of Emergency or Accident - Name:

From: To: Address: Telephone:

B. EMPLOYMENT INFORMATION

For what position are you applying? ☐ Full-time ☐ Part-time ☐ Either   Date available for employment?   Wage/Salary Expectations:

List hrs./days you prefer to work: List any hrs./days you are not available: (Except for times required for religious practices or observances)   Can you work overtime, if necessary? ☐ Yes ☐ No

Are you employed now?: ☐ Yes ☐ No   If so, may we inquire of your present employer?: ☐ No ☐ Yes, If yes: Name of employer: Phone number: ( )

Have you ever been bonded?: ☐ Yes ☐ No   If required for position, are you bondable? ☐ Yes ☐ No ☐ Uncertain   Have you applied for a position with this office before? ☐ No ☐ Yes, If yes, when?:

Referred by/ or where did you hear of this job?:

Can you, upon employment, submit verification of your legal right to work in the United States? ☐ Yes ☐ No Submit proof that you meet legal age requirement for employment? ☐ Yes ☐ No   Language(s) applicant speaks or writes (if use of a language other than English is relevant to the job for which applicant is applying):

C. EDUCATIONAL HISTORY

Name and address of schools attended (Include current)	Dates From	Thru	Highest grade/level completed	Diploma/degree(s) obtained/areas of study:
High school				
College				Degree/Major
Post graduate				Degree/Major
Other				Course/Diploma/License Certificate

Specific training, education, or experiences which will assist you in the job for which you have applied:

Future educational plans:

D. SPECIAL SKILLS

CHECK BELOW THE KINDS OF WORK YOU HAVE DONE:

☐ BLOOD COUNTS   ☐ DENTAL ASSISTANT   ☐ MEDICAL INSURANCE FORMS   ☐ RECEPTIONIST
☐ BOOKKEEPING   ☐ DENTAL HYGIENIST   ☐ MEDICAL TERMINOLOGY   ☐ TELEPHONES
☐ COLLECTIONS   ☐ FILING   ☐ MEDICAL TRANSCRIPTION   ☐ TYPING
☐ COMPOSING LETTERS   ☐ INJECTIONS   ☐ NURSING   ☐ STENOGRAPHY
☐ COMPUTER INPUT   ☐ INSTRUMENT STERILIZATION   ☐ PHLEBOTOMY (Draw Blood)   ☐ URINALYSIS
OFFICE EQUIPMENT USED: ☐ COMPUTER   ☐ DICTATING EQUIPMENT   ☐ POSTING   ☐ X-RAY
        ☐ WORD PROCESSOR   ☐ OTHER:

Other kinds of tasks performed or skills that may be applicable to position: Typing speed: Shorthand speed:

RM NO. 72-110 ©1976 BIBBERO SYSTEMS INC. PETALUMA, CA (MB-CO) # 2-5 (REV. 10/92)
REORDER CALL 800-BIBBERO (800) 242-2376   (PLEASE COMPLETE OTHER SIDE)

Figure 18–2, *A*

E. EMPLOYMENT RECORD

LIST MOST RECENT EMPLOYMENT FIRST   May we contact your previous Employer(s) for a reference? ☐ yes ☐ no

1) Employer

Work performed. Be specific.

Address   Street   City   State   Zip code

Phone number ( )

Type of business | Dates   Mo.   Yr.   Mo.   Yr.
                        From   To

Your position | Hourly rate/Salary
                      Starting   Final

Supervisor's name

Reason for leaving

2) Employer

Work performed. Be specific:

Address   Street   City   State   Zip code

Phone number ( )

Type of business | Dates   Mo.   Yr.   Mo.   Yr.
                        From   To

Your position | Hourly rate/Salary
                      Starting   Final

Supervisor's name

Reason for leaving

3) Employer

Work performed. Be specific:

Address   Street   City   State   Zip code

Phone number ( )

Type of business | Dates   Mo.   Yr.   Mo.   Yr.
                        From   To

Your position | Hourly rate/Salary
                      Starting   Final

Supervisor's name

Reason for leaving

F. REFERENCES: FRIENDS/ACQUAINTANCES NON-RELATED

1) _____
Name   Address   Telephone Number (☐Work ☐Home)   Occupation   Years acquainted

2) _____
Name   Address   Telephone Number (☐Work ☐Home)   Occupation   Years acquainted

Please feel free to add any information which you feel will help us consider you for employment.

READ THE FOLLOWING CAREFULLY, THEN SIGN AND DATE THE APPLICATION

I certify that all answers given by me on this application are true, correct and complete to the best of my knowledge. I acknowledge notice that the information contained in this application is subject to check. I agree that, if hired, my continued employment may be contingent upon the accuracy of that information. If employed, I further agree to comply with company/office rules and regulations.

Signature _____   Date: _____

RM NO. 72-110 ©1976 BIBBERO SYSTEMS INC. PETALUMA, CA (MB-CO) # 6-7 (REV. 4/92)   TO REORDER CALL 800-BIBBERO (800) 242-2376

Figure 18–2, *B*

ASSIGNMENT 18-6 ▸ PREPARE A FOLLOW UP THANK-YOU LETTER

Performance Objective

Task: Prepare a follow-up thank-you letter after the interview, sending it to the interviewer.

Conditions: Use one sheet of plain typing paper, a number 10 envelope, and a computer or typewriter.

Standards: Time: _____ minutes

                 Accuracy: _____

                 (Note: The time element and accuracy criteria may be given by your instructor.)

Directions: After the interview, you decide to send a follow-up thank-you letter to the person who interviewed you. Type a letter and address a number 10 envelope. Refer to Chapter 18 and Figure 18–12 in the *Handbook* to help organize your thoughts.

Checklist

1. Assemble materials, determine the recipient's address, and decide on modified or full block letter style or format.   _____

2. Turn on the computer and select the word processing program. Open a blank document.   _____

3. Key the date line beginning at least three lines below the letterhead and make certain it is in the proper location for the chosen style.   _____

4. Double-space down and insert the inside address and make certain it is in the proper location for the chosen style. Select a style to insert an attention line, if necessary.   _____

5. Double-space and key the salutation. Use either open or mixed punctuation.   _____

6. Double-space and enter the reference line ("Re:" or "Subject:") in the location for the chosen letter style.   _____

7. Double-space and key the body (content) of the letter in single-space and make certain the paragraph style is proper for the format chosen. Double-space between paragraphs. Save the letter to the computer hard drive every 15 minutes.   _____

8. Proofread the letter on the computer screen for composition.   _____

9. Proofread the letter on the computer screen for typographical, spelling, grammatical, and mechanical errors. Use the spell-check feature of the word processing program and reference books to check for correct spelling, meaning, or usage.   _____

10. Key a complimentary close and make certain it is in the proper location for the chosen style.   _____

11. Drop down four spaces and key the sender's name and title or credentials as printed on the letterhead.   _____

12. Single- or double-space to insert copy ("CC"), enclosure ("Enclosure" or "Enc"), or attachment notations.   _____

13. Save the file before printing a hard copy and proofread the letter once more. Make corrections, if needed.   _____

14. Print the final copy to be sent and proofread. Make a copy to be retained in the files in case it is needed for future reference.   _____

15. Save the file to a CD-ROM to be stored for future reference.   _____

16. Prepare an envelope and use the format for optical scanning recommended by the United States Postal Service.   _____

17. Clip attachments to the letter and sign.   _____

A S S I G N M E N T **18–7** ▸ **V I S I T   W E B   S I T E S   F O R   J O B   O P P O R T U N I T I E S**

Performance Objective

Task: Access the Internet and visit several Web sites of the World Wide Web.

Conditions: Use a computer with printer and/or a pen or pencil to make notes.

Standards: Time: _____ minutes

                      Accuracy: _____

                      (Note: The time element and accuracy criteria may be given by your
                      instructor.)

Directions: If you have access to the Internet, visit the World Wide Web and do some job searching. After obtaining the Web site data, take them to share for class discussion. Note that some sites may not be accessible if you attempt to visit them during peak hours.

1. Visit the American Association of Medical Assistants' Web site, www.aama-ntl.org, and click on "AAMA Job Source." See whether there are any new job opportunities in your state. Print a hard copy of the names, addresses, and telephone numbers of participating employers near your region while you remain online.

2. Connect to the Allied Health Opportunities for Healthcare Professionals' Web site, http://www.gvpub.com. Click on "Employment Opportunities." After you get to that screen, click on "Allied Health Opportunities," and at the next screen, click on "Medical Assistants" or "Health Information Management Professionals." Then see whether you can locate any listings for billing or coding positions. Print out some of the listings that appeal to you, and take them to class for discussion.

3. Check out an online resource, hcPro's Health Information Management Supersite, www.himinfo.com. This site has job postings for many medical job titles for people involved in health information management. Click on the Career Center under the Interactive site features to see job postings. Then click on "HIM Job Listings." Enter a job title, such as "coder" or "biller," to do a search, and see whether you can locate any job openings. Print some of these listings to share and discuss during class.

4. Visit the JustCoding Web site, www.justcoding.com, and click the link to the Coding Career Center. Then click on "Search for a Job" under the "For Employees" heading. Enter a key word, such as "coder," and see whether you can obtain any search results. Print some of these listings to share and discuss during class.

5. Access the Internet and use a search engine (Yahoo, Excite, AltaVista). Key in "Yahoo insurance billers" to search for job opportunities. See whether you can locate any jobs that are in your region or state. List three Web site addresses that you find and take them to share for class discussion.

A S S I G N M E N T **18-8** ▸ **CRITICAL THINKING**

Performance Objective

Task: Write a paragraph describing the benefits of becoming certified in this
                   field.

Conditions: Use a computer with printer and/or a pen or pencil.

Standards: Time: _____ minutes

                   Accuracy: _____

                   (Note: The time element and accuracy criteria may be given by your
                   instructor.)

Directions: Write a paragraph or two describing why you would like to become certified in this field, and incorporate a numbered list of benefits. Make sure grammar, punctuation, and spelling are correct.

Checklist

1. Composed one paragraph   _____

2. Composed a second paragraph   _____

3. Proofread the paragraphs on the computer screen for composition.   _____

4. Proofread the composition for spelling and typographical, grammatical, and
   mechanical errors. Use the spellcheck feature of the word processing program and
   reference books to check for correct spelling, meaning, and usage. Make
   corrections, if needed.   _____

5. Save the file before printing a hard copy.   _____

6. Print a copy of the composition to give to your instructor.   _____

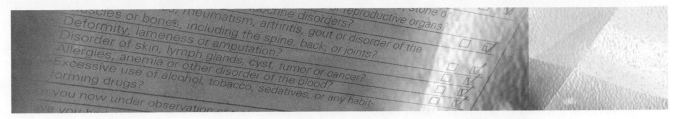

Tests

TEST 1: PROCEDURE (E/M AND MEDICINE SECTIONS) AND DIAGNOSTIC PROCEDURE CODE TEST

Directions: Using a *Current Procedural Terminology* (CPT) code book or Appendix A in this *Workbook*, insert the correct code numbers and modifiers for each service rendered. Give a brief description for each professional service rendered, although this is not needed for completing the CMS-1500 claim form. An additional optional exercise is to abstract the pertinent data from each case, use your *International Classification of Diseases, Ninth Revision, Clinical Modification* (ICD-9-CM) code book, and insert the diagnosis code.

Insert year of the CPT code book used _____

Insert year of the ICD-9-CM code book used _____

1. Dr. Input sees a new patient, Mrs. Post, in the office for acute abdominal distress. The physician spends approximately 1 hour obtaining a comprehensive history and physical examination with high-complexity decision making. Several diagnostic studies are ordered, and Mrs. Post is given an appointment to return in 1 week.

Description

_____ CPT # _____

_____ ICD # _____

2. Mr. Nakahara, an established patient, sees Dr. Practon in the office on January 11 for a reevaluation of his diabetic condition. Dr. Practon takes a detailed history and performs a detailed examination. Decision making is moderately complex.

Description

_____ CPT # _____

_____ ICD # _____

3. Dr. Cardi sees Mrs. Franklin for a follow-up office visit for her hypertension. A problem-focused history and examination of her cardiovascular system are obtained and revealed a blood pressure of 140/100. Decision making is straightforward, with medication being prescribed. The patient is advised to return in 2 weeks to have her blood pressure checked by the nurse. Mrs. Franklin returns 2 weeks later, and the nurse checks her blood pressure.

Description

_____   CPT # _____

_____   ICD # _____

_____   CPT # _____

_____   ICD # _____

4. Dr. Skeleton receives a call at 7 p.m. from Mrs. Snyder. Her husband, a patient of Dr. Skeleton's, has been very ill for 2 hours with profuse vomiting. Dr. Skeleton goes to their home to see Mr. Snyder and spends considerable time obtaining a detailed history and examination. The medical decision making is of a highly complex nature. The physician administers an injection of prochlorperazine (Compazine).

Description

_____   CPT # _____

_____   CPT # _____

_____   ICD # _____

5. Dr. Cutis sees an established patient, a registered nurse, for determination of pregnancy. A detailed history and examination are obtained, with moderate-complexity medical decision making. A Papanicolaou smear is taken, a blood sample is drawn, and the specimens are sent to an independent laboratory for a qualitative human chorionic gonadotropin (hCG) test. The patient also complains of something she has discovered under her armpit. On examination, there is a furuncle of the left axilla, which is incised and drained during this visit. The laboratory requires CPT coding on the laboratory requisition. List how these laboratory procedures would appear on the requisition sheet. The Papanicolaou smear is processed according to the Bethesda System and under physician supervision.

Professional Service Rendered by Dr. Cutis

_____   CPT # _____

_____   CPT # _____

_____   CPT # _____

_____   CPT # _____

_____   ICD # _____

_____   ICD # _____

Laboratory Service on Requisition Sheet

_____   CPT # _____

_____   CPT # _____

6. Dr. Antrum makes a house call on Betty Mason, an established patient, for a problem-focused history of acute otitis media. A problem-focused examination is performed, with straightforward medical decision making. While there, Dr. Antrum also sees Betty's younger sister, Sandra, whom she has seen previously in the office, for acute tonsillitis. A problem-focused history and examination are performed with low-complexity decision making. In addition to the examinations, Dr. Antrum gives both children injections of penicillin.

Professional Service Rendered to Betty

_____   CPT # _____

_____   CPT # _____

_____   ICD # _____

Professional Service Rendered to Sandra

_____   CPT # _____

_____   CPT # _____

_____   ICD # _____

7. Two weeks later, Dr. Antrum is called to the emergency department at College Hospital at 2 a.m. on Sunday to see Betty Mason for recurrent chronic otitis media with suppuration. A problem-focused history and examination are performed with straightforward decision making. Dr. Antrum administers a second injection of penicillin.

Description

_____   CPT # _____

_____   CPT # _____

_____   ICD # _____

8. While at the hospital, Dr. Antrum is asked to see another patient in the emergency department, who is new to her. A problem-focused history is taken. She performs a problem-focused examination and straightforward decision making for an intermediate 3.5-cm laceration of the scalp. The laceration is sutured, and the patient is advised to come to the office in 4 days for a dressing change. Four days later, the patient comes into the office for a dressing change by the nurse.

Description

_____   CPT # _____

_____   CPT # _____

_____   CPT # _____

_____   ICD # _____

9. Dr. Menter, a psychiatrist, sees the following patients in the hospital. Code each procedure.

Ms. Blake: Consultation, expanded problem-focused history and examination and straightforward decision making; referred by Dr. Practon   CPT # _____

Mrs. Clark: Group psychotherapy (50 min)   CPT # _____

Mrs. Samson: Group psychotherapy (50 min)   CPT # _____

Mr. Shoemaker: Group psychotherapy (50 min)   CPT # _____

Miss James: Individual psychotherapy (25 min)   CPT # _____

10. Dr. Input, a gastroenterologist, sees Mrs. Chan in the hospital at the request of Dr. Practon for an esophageal ulcer. In addition to the detailed history and examination and the low-complexity decision making, Dr. Input performs an esophageal intubation and washings and prepares slides for cytology. Two days later, he sees Mrs. Chan in follow-up inpatient consultation and obtains a problem-focused interval history and examination with low-complexity decision making. He performs a gastric intubation and collects washings for cytologic evaluation for a gastric ulcer.

Description

_____   CPT # _____

_____   CPT # _____

_____   ICD # _____

_____   CPT # _____

_____   CPT # _____

_____   ICD # _____

11. Mrs. Galati, a new patient, goes to Dr. Cardi because of chest pain (moderate to severe), weakness, fatigue, and dizziness. Dr. Cardi takes a comprehensive history and performs a comprehensive examination, including electrocardiography (ECG) with interpretation and report, followed by treadmill ECG. He also performs a vital capacity test and dipstick urinalysis, and draws blood for triiodothyronine (T_3) testing and for analysis by Sequential Multiple Analyzer Computer (SMAC) (16 panel tests, including complete blood cell count [CBC]), which are sent to and billed by a laboratory. Medical decision making is of high complexity.

Description

_____   CPT # _____

_____   CPT # _____

_____   CPT # _____

_____   CPT # _____

_____   CPT # _____

_____   CPT # _____

_____   ICD # _____

_____   ICD # _____

_____   ICD # _____

12. Jake Wonderhill has not had his eyes examined by Dr. Lenser for about 5 years. He is seen by Dr. Lenser, who performs the following ophthalmologic procedures in addition to a comprehensive eye examination: fluorescein angioscopy and electroretinography. Mr. Wonderhill receives a diagnosis of retinitis pigmentosa.

Description

_____   CPT # _____

_____   CPT # _____

_____   CPT # _____

_____   ICD # _____

13. Dr. Practon is making rounds at the College Hospital and answers an urgent call on 3rd Floor East. He performs resuscitation on Mr. Sanchez for cardiac arrest and orders the patient taken to the critical care unit. Chest radiographs, laboratory work, blood gas measurements, and ECG are performed. The physician is detained 2 hours in constant attendance on the patient.

Description

_____   CPT # _____

_____   CPT # _____

_____   ICD # _____

14. Mrs. Powers, a new patient, sees Dr. Skeleton for low sciatica. Dr. Skeleton takes a detailed history and performs a detailed examination of the patient's lower back and extremities. Medical decision making is of low complexity. Diathermy (30 min) is given. The next day the patient comes in for therapeutic exercises in the Hubbard tank (30 min).

Description

_____ CPT # _____

_____ CPT # _____

_____ ICD # _____

_____ CPT # _____

_____ ICD # _____

15. a. Mrs. Garcia, a new patient, is seen by Dr. Caesar for occasional vaginal spotting (detailed history/examination and low-complexity decision making). The doctor determines that the bleeding is coming from the cervix and asks her to return in 3 days for cryocauterization of the cervix. During the initial examination, Mrs. Garcia asks for an evaluation for possible infertility. Dr. Caesar advises her to wait 2 to 3 weeks and make an appointment for two infertility tests.
   b. When the patient returns in 3 days for cryocauterization, the doctor also takes a wet mount for bacteria/fungi, which is sent to and billed by a laboratory.
   c. Three weeks later, an injection procedure for hysterosalpingography and endometrial biopsy are performed.

Description

a. _____ CPT # _____

   _____ ICD # _____

b. _____ CPT # _____

   _____ CPT # _____

   _____ ICD # _____

c. _____ CPT # _____

   _____ CPT # _____

   _____ ICD # _____

Multiple Choice. After reading the boxed codes with descriptions, select the answer/answers that is/are best in each case.

59120	surgical treatment of ectopic pregnancy; tubal or ovarian, requiring salpingectomy and/or oophorectomy, abdominal or vaginal approach.
59121	tubal or ovarian, without salpingectomy and/or oophorectomy
59130	abdominal pregnancy
59135	interstitial, uterine pregnancy requiring total hysterectomy
59136	interstitial, uterine pregnancy with partial resection of uterus
59140	cervical, with evacuation

16. In regard to this section of CPT codes, which of the following statements is true about codes 59120 through 59140? *Mark all that apply.*

   a. They refer to abdominal hysterotomy.

   b. They involve laparoscopic treatment of ectopic pregnancy.

   c. They refer to treatment of ectopic pregnancy by surgery.

   d. They involve tubal ligation.

17. In regard to this section of CPT codes, for treatment of a tubal ectopic pregnancy, necessitating oophorectomy, the code to select is

   a. 59121

   b. 59120

   c. 59135

   d. 59136

   e. 59130

18. In regard to this section of CPT codes, for treatment of an ectopic pregnancy (interstitial, uterine) requiring a total hysterectomy, the code/codes to select is/are

   a. 59135

   b. 59135 and 59120

   c. 59120

   d. 59130 and 59120

   e. 59121

TEST 2: PROCEDURE CODE WITH MODIFIERS AND DIAGNOSTIC CODE TEST

Match the description given in the right column with the procedure code/modifier combination in the left column. Write the letter in the blank.

Procedure with Modifier   *Description*

1. 99245–21 _____   a. Dr. Practon assisted Dr. Caesar with a total abdominal hysterectomy and bilateral salpingo-oophorectomy.

2. 31540–57 _____   b. Dr. Skeleton interprets a thoracolumbar x-ray film that was taken at College Hospital.

3. 58150–80 _____   c. Mrs. Ulwelling saw Dr. Antrum as a new patient, and she recommended that the patient undergo a laryngoscopy, with stripping of vocal cords to be done the following day.

4. 32440–55 _____   d. Mrs. Gillenbach walked through a plate glass window and underwent a rhinoplasty, performed by Dr. Graff on February 16, 20xx. On February 26, 20xx, she came to see Dr. Graff for a consultation regarding reconstructive surgery on her right leg.

5. 72080–26 _____   e. Mr. Mercado was seen by Dr. Langerhans in the office for a complicated diabetic consultation. A comprehensive history and examination were obtained, with high-complexity medical decision making; however, the physician spent a total of 2 hours with the patient.

6. 29425–58 _____   f. Dr. Cutler performed a bilateral orchiopexy (inguinal approach) on baby Kozak.

7. 54640–99 _____   g. Dr. Skeleton applied a short leg walking cast to
   (50/51)   Mrs. Belchere's right leg 4 weeks after his initial treatment of her fractured tibia.

8. 99253–24 _____   h. Dr. Cutler went on vacation, and Dr. Coccidioides took care of Mrs. Ash during the postoperative period after her total pneumonectomy.

Directions: Using a *Current Procedural Terminology* (CPT) code book or Appendix A in this *Workbook*, insert the correct code numbers and modifiers for each service rendered. Give a brief description for each professional service rendered, although this is not needed for completing the CMS-1500 claim form.

9. Dr. Input performs a gastrojejunostomy for carcinoma in situ of the duodenum and calls in Dr. Scott to administer the anesthesia and Dr. Cutler to assist. This intraperitoneal surgery takes 2 hours, 30 minutes. The patient is otherwise normal and healthy. List the procedure and diagnostic code numbers with appropriate modifiers for each physician.

Professional Service Rendered by Dr. Input

_____ CPT # _____

_____ ICD # _____

Professional Service Rendered by Dr. Scott

_____ CPT # _____

_____ ICD # _____

Professional Service Rendered by Dr. Cutler

_____ CPT # _____

_____ ICD # _____

10. Dr. Rumsey assists Dr. Cutler with a total colectomy (intraperitoneal procedure) with ileostomy. Dr. Scott is the anesthesiologist. Surgery takes 2 hours, 55 minutes. The patient has a secondary malignant neoplasm of the colon (severe systemic disease). List the procedure code numbers with appropriate modifiers and diagnostic code numbers for each physician.

Professional Service Rendered by Dr. Rumsey

_____ CPT # _____

_____ ICD # _____

Professional Service Rendered by Dr. Scott

_____ CPT # _____

_____ ICD # _____

Professional Service Rendered by Dr. Cutler

_____ CPT # _____

_____ ICD # _____

11. Dr. Cutis removes a malignant lesion from a patient's back (1.5 cm) and does the local anesthesia herself.

Description

_____ CPT # _____

_____ ICD # _____

12. Dr. Skeleton sees Mr. Richmond, a new patient worked into the office schedule on an emergency basis after an automobile accident. Mr. Richmond has multiple lacerations of the face, arm, and chest and a fracture of the left tibia. The physician takes a comprehensive history and performs a comprehensive examination. Decision making

is moderately complex. Dr. Skeleton orders bilateral radiographs of the tibia and fibula and two views of the chest and left wrist to be taken in his office. Then he closes the following lacerations: 2.6 cm, simple, face; 2.0 cm, intermediate, face; 7.5 cm, intermediate, right arm; 4.5 cm, intermediate, chest. All radiographs are negative except that of the left tibia. Dr. Skeleton performs a manipulative reduction of the left tibial shaft and applies a cast.

Description

CPT # _____

CPT # _____

CPT # _____

CPT # _____

CPT # _____

CPT # _____

CPT # _____

CPT # _____

CPT # _____

CPT # _____

ICD # _____

ICD # _____

ICD # _____

ICD # _____

Six weeks later, Dr. Skeleton sees the same patient for an office visit and obtains radiographs (two views) of the left tibia and fibula. Treatment involves application of a cast below the patient's left knee to the toes, including a walking heel.

Description

CPT # _____

CPT # _____

CPT # _____

ICD # _____

13. Dr. Cutler performs an incisional biopsy of a patient's breast for a breast lump, which requires 40 minutes of anesthesia. Dr. Scott is the anesthesiologist. The patient is otherwise normal and healthy. List the procedure and diagnostic code numbers for each physician.

Professional Service Rendered by Dr. Cutler

_____ CPT # _____

_____ ICD # _____

Professional Service Rendered by Dr. Scott

_____ CPT # _____

_____ ICD # _____

14. Mrs. DeBeau is aware that Dr. Input will be out of town for 6 weeks; however, she decides to have him perform the recommended combined anterior-posterior colporrhaphy with enterocele repair for vaginal enterocele. Dr. Practon agrees to perform the follow-up care and assist. Dr. Scott is the anesthesiologist. The anesthesia time is 2 hours, 15 minutes. The patient is normal and healthy. List the procedure and diagnostic code numbers for each physician.

Professional Service Rendered by Dr. Input

_____ CPT # _____

_____ ICD # _____

Professional Service Rendered by Dr. Practon

_____ CPT # _____

_____ CPT # _____

_____ CPT # _____

_____ ICD # _____

Professional Service Rendered by Dr. Scott

_____ CPT # _____

_____ ICD # _____

15. Mr. Wong, a new patient, is seen in the College Hospital and undergoes a comprehensive history and physical examination (H & P) with moderately complex decision making. Dr. Coccidioides performs a bronchoscopy with biopsy. Results of the biopsy confirm the diagnosis: malignant neoplasm of upper left lobe of lung. The following day the physician performs a total pneumonectomy. Dr. Cutler assists on the total pneumonectomy (pulmonary resection), and Dr. Scott is the anesthesiologist. Surgery takes 3 hours, 45 minutes. The patient has mild systemic disease. List the procedure and diagnostic code numbers for each physician.

Professional Service Rendered by Dr. Coccidioides

_____   CPT # _____

_____   CPT # _____

_____   CPT # _____

_____   ICD # _____

Professional Service Rendered by Dr. Cutler

_____   CPT # _____

_____   ICD # _____

Professional Service Rendered by Dr. Scott

_____   CPT # _____

_____   ICD # _____

When completing the CMS-1500 claim form for Dr. Scott, in which block would you

list anesthesia minutes? _____

TEST 3: PROCEDURE (RADIOLOGY AND PATHOLOGY SECTIONS) AND DIAGNOSTIC CODE TEST

Directions: Using a CPT code book or Appendix A in this *Workbook*, insert the correct procedure code numbers and modifiers and diagnostic codes for each service rendered. Give a brief description for each professional service rendered, although this is not needed for completing the CMS-1500 claim form.

1. Mrs. Cahn sees Dr. Skeleton because of severe pain in her right shoulder. She is a new patient. Dr. Skeleton takes a detailed history and performs a detailed examination. A complete x-ray study of the right shoulder is done. Decision making is of low complexity. A diagnosis of bursitis is made, and an injection into the bursa is administered.

Description

_____   CPT # _____

_____   CPT # _____

_____   CPT # _____

_____   ICD # _____

2. John Murphy comes into the Broxton Radiologic Group, Inc., for an extended radiation therapy consultation for prostatic cancer. The radiologist takes a detailed history and does a detailed examination. Decision making is of low complexity. The physician determines a simple treatment plan involving simple simulation-aided field settings. Basic dosimetry calculations are done, and the patient returns the following day and receives radiation therapy to a single treatment area (6 to 10 MeV).

Description

_____   CPT # _____

_____   CPT # _____

_____   CPT # _____

_____   CPT # _____

_____   CPT # _____

Diagnosis: _____   ICD # _____

3. Dr. Input refers Mrs. Horner to the Nuclear Medicine department of the Broxton Radiologic Group, Inc., for a bone marrow imaging of the whole body and imaging of the liver and spleen. List the procedure code numbers after each radiologic procedure to show how the radiology group would bill. Also, list the diagnosis of malignant neoplasm of the bone marrow.

Description

Total body bone marrow, imaging   CPT # _____

Radiopharmaceuticals, diagnostic   CPT # _____

Liver and spleen imaging   CPT # _____

Radiopharmaceuticals, diagnostic   CPT # _____

Diagnosis: _____ ICD # _____

4. Dr. Input also refers Mrs. Horner to XYZ Laboratory for the following tests. List the procedure code numbers to indicate how the laboratory would bill.

Description

CBC, automated and automated differential   CPT # _____

Urinalysis, automated with microscopy   CPT # _____

Urine culture (quantitative, colony count) CPT # _____

Urine antibiotic sensitivity (microtiter)   CPT # _____

5. The general laboratory at College Hospital receives a surgical tissue specimen (ovarian biopsy) for gross and microscopic examination from a patient with Stein-Leventhal syndrome. List the procedure and diagnostic code numbers to indicate what the hospital pathology department would bill.

Description

_____ CPT # _____

Diagnosis: _____ ICD # _____

6. Dr. Langerhans refers Jerry Cramer to XYZ Laboratory for a lipid panel. He has a family history of cardiovascular disease. List the procedure and diagnostic code number or numbers to indicate how the laboratory would bill.

Description

_____ CPT # _____

Diagnosis: _____ ICD # _____

7. Dr. Caesar is an OB/GYN specialist who has her own ultrasound machine. Carmen Cardoza, age 45, is referred to Dr. Caesar for an obstetric consultation and an amniocentesis with ultrasonic guidance. The diagnosis is Rh incompatibility. The doctor performs a detailed history and physical examination, and decision making is of low complexity.

Description

_____   CPT # _____

_____   CPT # _____

_____   CPT # _____

Diagnosis: _____   ICD # _____

8. Mr. Marcos's medical record indicates that a retrograde pyelogram followed by a percutaneous nephrostolithotomy, with basket extraction of a 1-cm stone, was performed by Dr. Ulibarri for nephrolithiasis.

Description

_____   CPT # _____

_____   CPT # _____

Diagnosis: _____   ICD # _____

9. Broxton Radiologic Group, Inc., performs the following procedures on Mrs. Stephens at the request of Dr. Input. List the procedure code numbers after each radiologic procedure. On the laboratory slip, the following congenital diagnoses are listed: Diverticulum of the stomach and colon; cystic lung. Locate the corresponding diagnostic codes.

Barium enema   CPT # _____

Evaluation of upper gastrointestinal tract with small bowel   CPT # _____

Complete chest X-ray   CPT # _____

Diagnosis: _____   ICD # _____

Diagnosis: _____   ICD # _____

Diagnosis: _____   ICD # _____

10. Two weeks later, Mrs. Stephens is referred again for further radiologic studies for flank pain. List the procedure and diagnostic code numbers after each radiologic procedure.

Intravenous pyelogram (IVP) with drip infusion   CPT # _____

Oral cholecystography   CPT # _____

Diagnosis: _____   ICD # _____

TEST 4: COMPLETE A CMS-1500 CLAIM FORM

Performance Objective

Task: Complete a CMS-1500 claim form for a private case and post transactions to the patient's financial accounting record.

Conditions: Use the patient's record (Figure 1) and financial statement (Figure 2); one health insurance claim form (Figure 3); a typewriter, computer, or pen; procedural and diagnostic code books; and Appendices A and B in this *Workbook*.

Standards: Claim Productivity Management

Time: _____ minutes

Accuracy: _____

(Note: The time element and accuracy criteria may be given by your instructor.)

Directions:

1. Using OCR guidelines, complete a CMS-1500 claim form and direct it to the private carrier. Refer to Jennifer T. Lacey's patient record for information and Appendix A in this *Workbook* to locate the fees to record on the claim, and post them to the financial statement. Date the claim August 15. Dr. Caesar is accepting assignment, and the patient's signatures to release information to the insurance company and to have the payment forwarded directly to the physician are on file.

2. Use your *CPT* code book or Appendix A in this *Workbook* to determine the correct five-digit code numbers and modifiers for each professional service rendered. Use your HCPCS Level II code book or refer to Appendix B in this *Workbook* for HCPCS procedure codes and modifiers. Use your diagnostic code book to code each active diagnosis.

3. Record the proper information on the financial record and claim form, and note the date when you have billed the insurance company.

4. American Commercial Insurance Company sent a check (voucher number 5586) on November 17 in the amount of $880. The patient's responsibility is $220. Post the payment, write off (adjust) the remaining balance, and circle the amount billed to the patient.

PATIENT RECORD NO. T-5

Lacey	Jennifer	T	11-12-45	F	555-549-0098
LAST NAME	FIRST NAME	MIDDLE NAME	BIRTH DATE	SEX	HOME PHONE

451 Roberts Street	Woodland Hills	XY	12345	
ADDRESS	CITY	STATE	ZIP CODE	

555-443-9899	555-549-0098		lacey@wb.net
CELL PHONE	PAGER NO.	FAX NO.	E-MAIL ADDRESS

430-XX-7709   Y0053498
PATIENT'S SOC. SEC. NO.   DRIVER'S LICENSE

legal secretary   Higgins and Higgins Attorneys at Law
PATIENT'S OCCUPATION   NAME OF COMPANY

430 Second Avenue, Woodland Hills, XY 12345   555-540-6675
ADDRESS OF EMPLOYER   PHONE

SPOUSE OR PARENT   OCCUPATION

EMPLOYER   ADDRESS   PHONE

American Commercial Insurance Company, 5682 Bendix Blvd., Woodland Hills, XY 12345
NAME OF INSURANCE   INSURED OR SUB SCRIBER

5789022   444
POLICY/CERTIFICATE NO.   GROUP NO.

REFERRED BY: Clarence Cutler, MD

Figure 1   *Continued*

DATE	PROGRESS NOTES No. T-5
8-1-xx	New pt referred by Dr. Cutler, came into office for consultation and additional opinion.
	CC: Full feeling in stomach and low abdominal region. Difficult BM X 5 days. Sometimes
	has difficulty with urination. Irregular and painful menstruation. Ultrasonic report showed
	leiomyomata uteri and rt ovarian mass; however, visualization of mass poor and type
	cannot be identified. Pap smear Class I. No personal or family hx of CA. History of kidney
	problems in childhood. (C/HX).
	Comprehensive physical examination performed on healthy appearing white female.
	Wt: 136 lbs. BP 128/60. T 98.6 F. Palpated rt adnexal mass and
	enlarged uterus; vulva and cervix appear normal; R kidney area tender,
	UA (non-auto with micro) neg. LMP 7/16/XX.
	Tx plan: Adv hospital admit and additional tests to R/O kidney involvement and carcinoma.
	Tentatively scheduled abdominal hysterectomy with bilateral salpingo-oophorectomy.
	Pt given prep for BE (M/MDM).
	BC/llf *Bertha Caesar, MD*
8-2-xx	Adm to College Hosp (C HX/PX M/MDM). Ordered IVP and barium enema; scheduled
	surgery at 7:00 A.M. tomorrow.
	BC/llf *Bertha Caesar, MD*
8-3-xx	IVP indicated kidneys normal. No bowel involvement seen on BE. Perf abdominal
	hysterectomy with bilateral salpingo-oophorectomy.
	BC/llf *Bertha Caesar, MD*
8-4-xx	HV (EPF HX/PX M/MDM) Path report revealed interstitial leiomyomata uteri and corpus
	luteum cyst of rt ovary. Pt C/O PO pain, otherwise doing well.
	BC/llf *Bertha Caesar, MD*
8-5-xx	HV (EPF HX/PX M/MDM). Pt ambulating well, pain decreased. Dressing changed, wound
	healing well.
	BC/llf *Bertha Caesar, MD*
8-6-xx	HV (PF HX/PX SF/MDM). Pain minimal. Pt ambulating without assistance.
	Removed staples, no redness or swelling. Pln DC tomorrow.
	BC/llf *Bertha Caesar, MD*
8-7-xx	Discharge to home; pt doing well. RTO next wk.
	BC/llf *Bertha Caesar, MD*

Figure 1, cont'd

STATEMENT

Acct. No. T-5

COLLEGE CLINIC
4567 Broad Avenue
Woodland Hills, XY 12345-0001
Tel. 555-486-9002
Fax No. 555-487-8976

Jennifer T. Lacey
451 Roberts Street
Woodland Hills, XY 12345

Phone No. (H)___(555) 549-0098___(W)___(555) 540-6675___   Birthdate___11-12-45___

Insurance Co.___American Commercial Insurance Company___   Policy/Group No.___5789022 / 444___

DATE	REFERENCE	DESCRIPTION	CHARGES	CREDITS PYMNTS.	ADJ.	BALANCE
20XX			BALANCE FORWARD ⟶			
8-1-xx		Consult				
8-1-xx		UA				
8-2-xx		Admit				
8-3-xx		TAH BSO				
8-4-xx		HV				
8-5-xx		HV				
8-6-xx		HV				
8-7-xx		Discharge				

PLEASE PAY LAST AMOUNT IN BALANCE COLUMN

THIS IS A COPY OF YOUR FINANCIAL ACCOUNT AS IT APPEARS ON OUR RECORDS

Figure 2

HEALTH INSURANCE CLAIM FORM

PICA

| | | | | | | | PICA |

1. MEDICARE MEDICAID CHAMPUS CHAMPVA GROUP HEALTH PLAN FECA BLK LUNG OTHER   **1a.** INSURED'S I.D. NUMBER (FOR PROGRAM IN ITEM 1)

(Medicare #) (Medicaid #) (Sponsor's SSN) (VA File #) (SSN or ID) (SSN) (ID)

2. PATIENT'S NAME (Last Name, First Name, Middle Initial)   **3.** PATIENT'S BIRTH DATE MM DD YY SEX M F   **4.** INSURED'S NAME (Last Name, First Name, Middle Initial)

5. PATIENT'S ADDRESS (No., Street)   **6.** PATIENT RELATIONSHIP TO INSURED Self Spouse Child Other   **7.** INSURED'S ADDRESS (No., Street)

CITY   STATE   **8.** PATIENT STATUS Single Married Other   CITY   STATE

ZIP CODE TELEPHONE (Include Area Code) Employed Full-Time Student Part-Time Student   ZIP CODE TELEPHONE (INCLUDE AREA CODE)

9. OTHER INSURED'S NAME (Last Name, First Name, Middle Initial)   **10.** IS PATIENT'S CONDITION RELATED TO: **11.** INSURED'S POLICY GROUP OR FECA NUMBER

a. OTHER INSURED'S POLICY OR GROUP NUMBER   **a.** EMPLOYMENT? (CURRENT OR PREVIOUS) YES NO   **a.** INSURED'S DATE OF BIRTH MM DD YY SEX M F

b. OTHER INSURED'S DATE OF BIRTH MM DD YY SEX M F   **b.** AUTO ACCIDENT? PLACE (State) YES NO   **b.** EMPLOYER'S NAME OR SCHOOL NAME

c. EMPLOYER'S NAME OR SCHOOL NAME   **c.** OTHER ACCIDENT? YES NO   **c.** INSURANCE PLAN NAME OR PROGRAM NAME

d. INSURANCE PLAN NAME OR PROGRAM NAME   **10d.** RESERVED FOR LOCAL USE   **d.** IS THERE ANOTHER HEALTH BENEFIT PLAN? YES NO If yes, return to and complete item 9 a-d.

READ BACK OF FORM BEFORE COMPLETING & SIGNING THIS FORM.
12. PATIENT'S OR AUTHORIZED PERSON'S SIGNATURE I authorize the release of any medical or other information necessary to process this claim. I also request payment of government benefits either to myself or to the party who accepts assignment below. SIGNED DATE

13. INSURED'S OR AUTHORIZED PERSON'S SIGNATURE I authorize payment of medical benefits to the undersigned physician or supplier for services described below. SIGNED

14. DATE OF CURRENT: MM DD YY ILLNESS (First symptom) OR INJURY (Accident) OR PREGNANCY(LMP)   **15.** IF PATIENT HAS HAD SAME OR SIMILAR ILLNESS. GIVE FIRST DATE MM DD YY   **16.** DATES PATIENT UNABLE TO WORK IN CURRENT OCCUPATION MM DD YY FROM TO MM DD YY

17. NAME OF REFERRING PHYSICIAN OR OTHER SOURCE   **17a.** I.D. NUMBER OF REFERRING PHYSICIAN   **18.** HOSPITALIZATION DATES RELATED TO CURRENT SERVICES MM DD YY FROM TO MM DD YY

19. RESERVED FOR LOCAL USE   **20.** OUTSIDE LAB? $ CHARGES YES NO

21. DIAGNOSIS OR NATURE OF ILLNESS OR INJURY. (RELATE ITEMS 1,2,3 OR 4 TO ITEM 24E BY LINE) 1. 2. 3. 4.   **22.** MEDICAID RESUBMISSION CODE ORIGINAL REF. NO.   **23.** PRIOR AUTHORIZATION NUMBER

24. | A DATE(S) OF SERVICE From / To MM DD YY MM DD YY | B Place of Service | C Type of Service | D PROCEDURES, SERVICES, OR SUPPLIES (Explain Unusual Circumstances) CPT/HCPCS MODIFIER | E DIAGNOSIS CODE | F $ CHARGES | G DAYS OR UNITS | H EPSDT Family Plan | I EMG | J COB | K RESERVED FOR LOCAL USE |
|---|---|---|---|---|---|---|---|---|---|---|
| 1 | | | | | | | | | | |
| 2 | | | | | | | | | | |
| 3 | | | | | | | | | | |
| 4 | | | | | | | | | | |
| 5 | | | | | | | | | | |
| 6 | | | | | | | | | | |

25. FEDERAL TAX I.D. NUMBER SSN EIN   **26.** PATIENT'S ACCOUNT NO.   **27.** ACCEPT ASSIGNMENT? (For govt. claims, see back) YES NO   **28.** TOTAL CHARGE $ **29.** AMOUNT PAID $ **30.** BALANCE DUE $

31. SIGNATURE OF PHYSICIAN OR SUPPLIER INCLUDING DEGREES OR CREDENTIALS (I certify that the statements on the reverse apply to this bill and are made a part thereof.) SIGNED DATE   **32.** NAME AND ADDRESS OF FACILITY WHERE SERVICES WERE RENDERED (If other than home or office)   **33.** PHYSICIAN'S, SUPPLIER'S BILLING NAME, ADDRESS, ZIP CODE & PHONE # PIN# GRP#

(APPROVED BY AMA COUNCIL ON MEDICAL SERVICE 8/88) **PLEASE PRINT OR TYPE** APPROVED OMB-0938-0008 FORM CMS-1500 (12-90), FORM RRB-1500, APPROVED OMB-1215-0055 FORM OWCP-1500, APPROVED OMB-0720-0001 (CHAMPUS)

Figure 3

TEST 5: COMPLETE A CMS-1500 CLAIM FORM

Performance Objective

Task: Complete a CMS-1500 claim form for a private case and post transactions to the patient's financial accounting record.

Conditions: Use the patient's record (Figure 4) and financial statement (Figure 5); one health insurance claim form (Figure 6); a typewriter, computer, or pen; procedural and diagnostic code books; and Appendices A and B in this *Workbook*.

Standards: Claim Productivity Management

Time: _____ minutes

Accuracy: _____

(Note: The time element and accuracy criteria may be given by your instructor.)

Directions:

1. Using OCR guidelines, complete a CMS-1500 claim form and direct it to the private carrier. Refer to Hortense N. Hope's patient record for information and Appendix A in this *Workbook* to locate the fees to record on the claim, and post them to the financial statement. Date the claim July 31. Dr. Practon is accepting assignment, and the patient's signatures to release information to the insurance company and to have the payment forwarded directly to the physician are on file.

2. Use your CPT code book or Appendix A in this *Workbook* to determine the correct five-digit code numbers and modifiers for each professional service rendered. Use your Healthcare Common Procedure Coding System (HCPCS) Level II code book or refer to Appendix B in this *Workbook* for HCPCS procedure codes and modifiers. Use your diagnostic code book to code each active diagnosis.

3. Record the proper information on the financial record and claim form, and note the date you have billed the insurance company.

PATIENT RECORD NO. T-4

Hope	Hortense	N	04-12-46	F	555-666-7821
LAST NAME	FIRST NAME	MIDDLE NAME	BIRTH DATE	SEX	HOME PHONE

247 Lantern Pike	Woodland Hills	XY	12345
ADDRESS	CITY	STATE	ZIP CODE

	555-323-1687	555-666-7821		hope@wb.net
CELL PHONE	PAGER NO.	FAX NO.		E-MAIL ADDRESS

321-XX-8809	N0058921
PATIENT'S SOC. SEC. NO.	DRIVER'S LICENSE

Clerk typist	R and S Manufacturing Company
PATIENT'S OCCUPATION	NAME OF COMPANY

2271 West 74 Street, Torres, XY 12349	555-466-5890
ADDRESS OF EMPLOYER	PHONE

Harry J. Hope	carpenter
SPOUSE OR PARENT	OCCUPATION

Jesse Construction Company, 3861 South Orange Street, Torres, XY 12349	555-765-2318
EMPLOYER ADDRESS	PHONE

Ralston Insurance Company, 2611 Hanley Street, Woodland Hills, XY 12345
NAME OF INSURANCE   INSURED OR SUBSCRIBER

ATC321458809	T8471811A
POLICY/CERTIFICATE NO.	GROUP NO.

REFERRED BY: Harry J. Hope (husband)

DATE	PROGRESS NOTES
7-1-xx	New F pt comes in complaining of lt great toe pain. Incised, drained, and cleaned area around nail on lt great toe. Dx: onychia and paronychia. Started on antibiotic and adv to retn in 2 days for permanent excision of nail plate (EPF HX/PX SF/MDM). GP/llf *Gerald Practon, MD*
7-3-xx	Pt returns for nail excision. Injected procaine in lt great toe; removed entire toenail. Drs applied. PTR in 5 days for PO check. GP/llf *Gerald Practon, MD*
7-7-xx	PO check. Dressing changed, nail bed healing well. Pt to continue on AB until gone. Retn PRN (PF HX/PX SF/MDM). GP/llf *Gerald Practon, MD*

Figure 4

Acct No. T-4

STATEMENT
Financial Account
COLLEGE CLINIC
4567 Broad Avenue
Woodland Hills, XY 12345-0001
Tel. 555-486-9002
Fax No. 555-487-8976

Hortense N. Hope
247 Lantern Pike
Woodland Hills, XY 123345

Phone No. (H) 555-666-7821   (W)   555-466-5890   Birthdate 4/12/46

Primary Insurance Co.   Ralston Insurance Company   Policy/Group No. ATC321458809 / T8471811A

Secondary Insurance Co.   None   Policy/Group No.

| DATE | REFERENCE | DESCRIPTION | CHARGES | CREDITS | | BALANCE |
				PYMNTS.	ADJ.	
20xx		BALANCE FORWARD ➡				
7-1-xx		NP OV				
7-1-xx		I & D lt great toe				
7-3-xx		Excision lt great toenail				
7-7-xx		PO check				

PLEASE PAY LAST AMOUNT IN BALANCE COLUMN ⬆

THIS IS A COPY OF YOUR FINANCIAL ACCOUNT AS IT APPEARS ON OUR RECORDS

Figure 5

PLEASE
DO NOT
STAPLE
IN THIS
AREA

HEALTH INSURANCE CLAIM FORM

| | PICA | | | | | | | | PICA | | |

1. MEDICARE	MEDICAID	CHAMPUS	CHAMPVA	GROUP HEALTH PLAN	FECA BLK LUNG	OTHER	1a. INSURED'S I.D. NUMBER	(FOR PROGRAM IN ITEM 1)
(Medicare #)	(Medicaid #)	(Sponsor's SSN)	(VA File #)	(SSN or ID)	(SSN)	(ID)		

2. PATIENT'S NAME (Last Name, First Name, Middle Initial)	3. PATIENT'S BIRTH DATE MM DD YY SEX M F	4. INSURED'S NAME (Last Name, First Name, Middle Initial)

5. PATIENT'S ADDRESS (No., Street)	6. PATIENT RELATIONSHIP TO INSURED Self Spouse Child Other	7. INSURED'S ADDRESS (No., Street)

CITY	STATE	8. PATIENT STATUS Single Married Other	CITY	STATE

ZIP CODE	TELEPHONE (Include Area Code) ( )	Employed Full-Time Student Part-Time Student	ZIP CODE	TELEPHONE (INCLUDE AREA CODE) ( )

9. OTHER INSURED'S NAME (Last Name, First Name, Middle Initial)	10. IS PATIENT'S CONDITION RELATED TO:	11. INSURED'S POLICY GROUP OR FECA NUMBER

a. OTHER INSURED'S POLICY OR GROUP NUMBER	a. EMPLOYMENT? (CURRENT OR PREVIOUS) YES NO	a. INSURED'S DATE OF BIRTH MM DD YY SEX M F

b. OTHER INSURED'S DATE OF BIRTH MM DD YY SEX M F	b. AUTO ACCIDENT? PLACE (State) YES NO	b. EMPLOYER'S NAME OR SCHOOL NAME

c. EMPLOYER'S NAME OR SCHOOL NAME	c. OTHER ACCIDENT? YES NO	c. INSURANCE PLAN NAME OR PROGRAM NAME

d. INSURANCE PLAN NAME OR PROGRAM NAME	10d. RESERVED FOR LOCAL USE	d. IS THERE ANOTHER HEALTH BENEFIT PLAN? YES NO *If yes*, return to and complete item 9 a-d.

READ BACK OF FORM BEFORE COMPLETING & SIGNING THIS FORM.

12. PATIENT'S OR AUTHORIZED PERSON'S SIGNATURE I authorize the release of any medical or other information necessary to process this claim. I also request payment of government benefits either to myself or to the party who accepts assignment below.

SIGNED _____ DATE _____

13. INSURED'S OR AUTHORIZED PERSON'S SIGNATURE I authorize payment of medical benefits to the undersigned physician or supplier for services described below.

SIGNED _____

14. DATE OF CURRENT: MM DD YY ILLNESS (First symptom) OR INJURY (Accident) OR PREGNANCY(LMP)	15. IF PATIENT HAS HAD SAME OR SIMILAR ILLNESS. GIVE FIRST DATE MM DD YY	16. DATES PATIENT UNABLE TO WORK IN CURRENT OCCUPATION MM DD YY MM DD YY FROM TO

17. NAME OF REFERRING PHYSICIAN OR OTHER SOURCE	17a. I.D. NUMBER OF REFERRING PHYSICIAN	18. HOSPITALIZATION DATES RELATED TO CURRENT SERVICES MM DD YY MM DD YY FROM TO

19. RESERVED FOR LOCAL USE		20. OUTSIDE LAB? YES NO $ CHARGES

21. DIAGNOSIS OR NATURE OF ILLNESS OR INJURY. (RELATE ITEMS 1,2,3 OR 4 TO ITEM 24E BY LINE)

1. |___.___| 3. |___.___|

2. |___.___| 4. |___.___|

22. MEDICAID RESUBMISSION CODE ORIGINAL REF. NO.
23. PRIOR AUTHORIZATION NUMBER

24. A DATE(S) OF SERVICE From MM DD YY To MM DD YY	B Place of Service	C Type of Service	D PROCEDURES, SERVICES, OR SUPPLIES (Explain Unusual Circumstances) CPT/HCPCS MODIFIER	E DIAGNOSIS CODE	F $ CHARGES	G DAYS OR UNITS	H EPSDT Family Plan	I EMG	J COB	K RESERVED FOR LOCAL USE
1										
2										
3										
4										
5										
6										

25. FEDERAL TAX I.D. NUMBER SSN EIN	26. PATIENT'S ACCOUNT NO.	27. ACCEPT ASSIGNMENT? (For govt. claims, see back) YES NO	28. TOTAL CHARGE $	29. AMOUNT PAID $	30. BALANCE DUE $

31. SIGNATURE OF PHYSICIAN OR SUPPLIER INCLUDING DEGREES OR CREDENTIALS (I certify that the statements on the reverse apply to this bill and are made a part thereof.) SIGNED _____ DATE _____	32. NAME AND ADDRESS OF FACILITY WHERE SERVICES WERE RENDERED (If other than home or office)	33. PHYSICIAN'S, SUPPLIER'S BILLING NAME, ADDRESS, ZIP CODE & PHONE # PIN# GRP#

(APPROVED BY AMA COUNCIL ON MEDICAL SERVICE 8/88)   *PLEASE PRINT OR TYPE*   APPROVED OMB-0938-0008 FORM CMS-1500 (12-90),   FORM RRB-1500, APPROVED OMB-1215-0055 FORM OWCP-1500,   APPROVED OMB-0720-0001 (CHAMPUS)

Figure 6

TEST 6: COMPLETE A CLAIM FORM FOR A MEDICARE CASE

Performance Objective

Task: Complete a CMS-1500 claim form and post transactions to the patient's financial accounting record.

Conditions: Use the patient's record (Figure 7) and financial statement (Figure 8); one health insurance claim form (Figure 9); a typewriter, computer, or pen; procedural and diagnostic code books; and Appendices A and B in this *Workbook*.

Standards: Claim Productivity Management

                     Time: _____ minutes

                     Accuracy: _____

                     (Note: The time element and accuracy criteria may be given by your instructor.)

Directions:

1. Using OCR guidelines, complete a CMS-1500 claim form and direct it to the Medicare fiscal intermediary. To locate your local fiscal intermediary, go to Web site http://www.cms.hhs.gov/contacts/incardir.asp. Refer to Frances F. Foote's patient record for information and Appendix A in this *Workbook* to locate the fees to record on the claim, and post them to the financial statement. Date the claim October 31. Dr. Practon is a participating provider, and the patient's signatures to release information to the insurance company and to have the payment forwarded directly to the physician are on file.

2. Use your *CPT* code book or Appendix A in this *Workbook* to determine the correct five-digit code numbers and modifiers for each professional service rendered. Use your HCPCS Level II code book or refer to Appendix B in this *Workbook* for HCPCS procedure codes and modifiers. Use your diagnostic code book to code each active diagnosis.

3. Record the proper information on the patient's financial accounting record and claim form, and note the date when you have billed the insurance company.

PATIENT RECORD NO. T-6

Foote	Frances	F	08-10-32	F	555-678-0943
LAST NAME	FIRST NAME	MIDDLE NAME	BIRTH DATE	SEX	HOME PHONE

984 North A Street	Woodland Hills	XY	12345
ADDRESS	CITY	STATE	ZIP CODE

555-443-9908	555-320-7789	555-678-0943	foote@wb.net
CELL PHONE	PAGER NO.	FAX NO.	E-MAIL ADDRESS

578-XX-8924	B4309811
PATIENT'S SOC. SEC. NO.	DRIVER'S LICENSE

retired legal secretary	
PATIENT'S OCCUPATION	NAME OF COMPANY

ADDRESS OF EMPLOYER	PHONE

Harry L. Foote	roofer
SPOUSE OR PARENT	OCCUPATION

BDO Construction Company, 340 North 6th Street, Woodland Hills, XY 12345	555-478-9083
EMPLOYER ADDRESS	PHONE

Medicare	self
NAME OF INSURANCE	INSURED OR SUB SCRIBER

578-XX-8924A	
POLICY/CERTIFICATE NO.	GROUP NO.

REFERRED BY: G. U. Curette, MD, 4780 Main Street, Ehrlich, XY 12350 Tel: 555-430-8788   NPI #34216600XX

DATE	PROGRESS NOTES
10-11-xx	NP pt referred by Dr. Curette with a CC of foot pain centering around rt great toe and
	sometimes shooting up her leg. PF history taken. PF exam revealed severe overgrowth
	of nail into surrounding tissues. AP and lat right foot x-rays taken & interpreted which
	indicate no fractures or arthritis. Pt has had a N workup for gout by Dr. Curette.
	DX: Severe onychocryptosis both margins of rt hallux. Adv to sched. OP surgery at
	College Hospital for wedge resection of skin of nail fold to repair ingrown nail.
	No disability from work (SF/MDM).
	NP/llf *Nick Pedro, MD*
10-13-xx	Pt admitted for OP surgery at College Hospital. Complete wedge resection performed for
	repair of rt hallux ingrown nail. Pt will stay off foot over the weekend and retn next wk for
	PO re ch. Patient's occupation is sedentary and he may continue to work; no disability.
	NP/llf *Nick Pedro, MD*
10-20-xx	PO visit (PF HX/PX SF/MDM). Rt hallux healing well. RTC as necessary.
	NP/llf *Nick Pedro, MD*

Figure 7

Acct No. T-6

STATEMENT
Financial Account
COLLEGE CLINIC
4567 Broad Avenue
Woodland Hills, XY 12345-0001
Tel. 555-486-9002
Fax No. 555-487-8976

Frances F. Foote
984 North A Street
Woodland Hills, XY 12345

Phone No. (H) 555-678-0943   (W)   Birthdate   8/10/32

Primary Insurance Co.   Medicare   Policy/Group No.   578-XX-8924A

DATE	REFERENCE	DESCRIPTION	CHARGES	PYMNTS.	ADJ.	BALANCE
20xx		BALANCE FORWARD ➔				
10-11-xx		NP OV				
10-11-xx		X-rays				
10-13-xx		Wedge excision/skin of nail fold				
10-20-xx		PO				

PLEASE PAY LAST AMOUNT IN BALANCE COLUMN ⬆

THIS IS A COPY OF YOUR FINANCIAL ACCOUNT AS IT APPEARS ON OUR RECORDS

Figure 8

PLEASE
DO NOT
STAPLE
IN THIS
AREA

CARRIER

HEALTH INSURANCE CLAIM FORM

PICA

PICA

1. MEDICARE	MEDICAID	CHAMPUS	CHAMPVA	GROUP HEALTH PLAN	FECA BLK LUNG	OTHER	1a. INSURED'S I.D. NUMBER	(FOR PROGRAM IN ITEM 1)
(Medicare #)	(Medicaid #)	(Sponsor's SSN)	(VA File #)	(SSN or ID)	(SSN)	(ID)		

2. PATIENT'S NAME (Last Name, First Name, Middle Initial)

3. PATIENT'S BIRTH DATE MM DD YY   SEX   M   F

4. INSURED'S NAME (Last Name, First Name, Middle Initial)

5. PATIENT'S ADDRESS (No., Street)

6. PATIENT RELATIONSHIP TO INSURED   Self   Spouse   Child   Other

7. INSURED'S ADDRESS (No., Street)

CITY   STATE

8. PATIENT STATUS   Single   Married   Other   Employed   Full-Time Student   Part-Time Student

CITY   STATE

ZIP CODE   TELEPHONE (Include Area Code)   (   )

ZIP CODE   TELEPHONE (INCLUDE AREA CODE)   (   )

9. OTHER INSURED'S NAME (Last Name, First Name, Middle Initial)

10. IS PATIENT'S CONDITION RELATED TO:

11. INSURED'S POLICY GROUP OR FECA NUMBER

a. OTHER INSURED'S POLICY OR GROUP NUMBER

a. EMPLOYMENT? (CURRENT OR PREVIOUS)   YES   NO

a. INSURED'S DATE OF BIRTH MM DD YY   SEX   M   F

b. OTHER INSURED'S DATE OF BIRTH MM DD YY   SEX   M   F

b. AUTO ACCIDENT?   PLACE (State)   YES   NO

b. EMPLOYER'S NAME OR SCHOOL NAME

c. EMPLOYER'S NAME OR SCHOOL NAME

c. OTHER ACCIDENT?   YES   NO

c. INSURANCE PLAN NAME OR PROGRAM NAME

d. INSURANCE PLAN NAME OR PROGRAM NAME

10d. RESERVED FOR LOCAL USE

d. IS THERE ANOTHER HEALTH BENEFIT PLAN?   YES   NO   If yes, return to and complete item 9 a-d.

READ BACK OF FORM BEFORE COMPLETING & SIGNING THIS FORM.

12. PATIENT'S OR AUTHORIZED PERSON'S SIGNATURE I authorize the release of any medical or other information necessary to process this claim. I also request payment of government benefits either to myself or to the party who accepts assignment below.

SIGNED _____   DATE _____

13. INSURED'S OR AUTHORIZED PERSON'S SIGNATURE I authorize payment of medical benefits to the undersigned physician or supplier for services described below.

SIGNED _____

14. DATE OF CURRENT: MM DD YY   ILLNESS (First symptom) OR INJURY (Accident) OR PREGNANCY(LMP)

15. IF PATIENT HAS HAD SAME OR SIMILAR ILLNESS. GIVE FIRST DATE MM DD YY

16. DATES PATIENT UNABLE TO WORK IN CURRENT OCCUPATION MM DD YY FROM   TO MM DD YY

17. NAME OF REFERRING PHYSICIAN OR OTHER SOURCE

17a. I.D. NUMBER OF REFERRING PHYSICIAN

18. HOSPITALIZATION DATES RELATED TO CURRENT SERVICES MM DD YY FROM   TO MM DD YY

19. RESERVED FOR LOCAL USE

20. OUTSIDE LAB?   YES   NO $ CHARGES

21. DIAGNOSIS OR NATURE OF ILLNESS OR INJURY. (RELATE ITEMS 1,2,3 OR 4 TO ITEM 24E BY LINE)

1. |___.___   3. |___.___

2. |___.___   4. |___.___

22. MEDICAID RESUBMISSION CODE   ORIGINAL REF. NO.

23. PRIOR AUTHORIZATION NUMBER

24. A DATE(S) OF SERVICE						B Place of Service	C Type of Service	D PROCEDURES, SERVICES, OR SUPPLIES (Explain Unusual Circumstances) CPT/HCPCS MODIFIER	E DIAGNOSIS CODE	F $ CHARGES	G DAYS OR UNITS	H EPSDT Family Plan	I EMG	J COB	K RESERVED FOR LOCAL USE
From MM	DD	YY	To MM	DD	YY										
1															
2															
3															
4															
5															
6															

25. FEDERAL TAX I.D. NUMBER   SSN EIN

26. PATIENT'S ACCOUNT NO.

27. ACCEPT ASSIGNMENT? (For govt. claims, see back)   YES   NO

28. TOTAL CHARGE $

29. AMOUNT PAID $

30. BALANCE DUE $

31. SIGNATURE OF PHYSICIAN OR SUPPLIER INCLUDING DEGREES OR CREDENTIALS (I certify that the statements on the reverse apply to this bill and are made a part thereof.)

SIGNED _____   DATE _____

32. NAME AND ADDRESS OF FACILITY WHERE SERVICES WERE RENDERED (If other than home or office)

33. PHYSICIAN'S, SUPPLIER'S BILLING NAME, ADDRESS, ZIP CODE & PHONE #

PIN#   GRP#

PATIENT AND INSURED INFORMATION

PHYSICIAN OR SUPPLIER INFORMATION

(APPROVED BY AMA COUNCIL ON MEDICAL SERVICE 8/88)   **PLEASE PRINT OR TYPE**   APPROVED OMB-0938-0008 FORM CMS-1500 (12-90), FORM RRB-1500,
APPROVED OMB-1215-0055 FORM OWCP-1500,   APPROVED OMB-0720-0001 (CHAMPUS)

Figure 9

TEST 7: COMPLETE A CLAIM FORM FOR A MEDICARE/MEDIGAP CASE

Performance Objective

Task: Complete two CMS-1500 claim forms for a Medicare/Medigap case and post transactions to the patient's financial accounting record.

Conditions: Use patient's record (Figure 10) and financial statement (Figure 11); two health insurance claim forms (Figures 12 and 13); a typewriter, computer, or pen; procedural and diagnostic code books; and Appendices A and B in this *Workbook*.

Standards: Claim Productivity Management

Time: _____ minutes

Accuracy: _____

(Note: The time element and accuracy criteria may be given by your instructor.)

Directions:

1. Using OCR guidelines, complete two CMS-1500 claim forms and direct them to the Medicare fiscal intermediary. To locate your local fiscal intermediary, go to Web site http://www.cms.hhs.gov/contacts/incardir.asp. Refer to Charles B. Kamb's patient record for information and Appendix A to locate the fees to record on the claim, and post them to the financial statement. Be sure to include the Medigap information on the claim form so that it will be crossed over (sent to the Medigap insurance carrier) automatically. Date the claim June 30. Dr. Practon is a participating provider with both Medicare and the Medigap program, and the patient's signatures to release information to the insurance companies and to have the payment forwarded directly to the physician are on file.

2. Use your CPT code book or Appendix A in this *Workbook* to determine the correct five-digit code numbers and modifiers for each professional service rendered. Use your HCPCS Level II code book or refer to Appendix B in this *Workbook* for HCPCS procedure codes and modifiers. Use your diagnostic code book to code each active diagnosis.

3. Record the proper information on the patient's financial accounting record and claim form, and note the date when you have billed the insurance company.

PATIENT RECORD NO. T-7

Kamb	Charles	B	01-26-27	M	555-467-2601
LAST NAME	FIRST NAME	MIDDLE NAME	BIRTH DATE	SEX	HOME PHONE

2600 West Nautilus Street	Woodland Hills	XY	12345
ADDRESS	CITY	STATE	ZIP CODE

CELL PHONE	PAGER NO.	FAX NO.	E-MAIL ADDRESS

454-XX-9569	M3200563	
PATIENT'S SOC. SEC. NO.	DRIVER'S LICENSE	

Retired TV actor	Amer. Federation of TV & Radio Artists (AFTRA)
PATIENT'S OCCUPATION	NAME OF COMPANY

30077 Ventura Boulevard, Woodland Hills, XY 12345	555-466-3331
ADDRESS OF EMPLOYER	PHONE

Jane C. Kamb	homemaker
SPOUSE OR PARENT	OCCUPATION

EMPLOYER	ADDRESS	PHONE

Medicare (Primary)	self	National Insurance Company (Medigap)
NAME OF INSURANCE	INSURED OR SUB SCRIBER	

454-XX-9569A	Medigap Policy No. 5789002
POLICY/CERTIFICATE NO.	GROUP NO.

REFERRED BY: Mrs. O. S. Tomy (friend)   National PAYRID NAT234567

DATE	PROGRESS NOTES
6-1-xx	New pt comes into ofc to est new PCP in area; recently moved from Ohio. W obese F c/o
	nasal bleeding for two and a half months c̄ headaches and nasal congestion. Pt states she
	has had HBP for 1 yr. Taking med: Serpasil prescribed by dr in Ohio; does not know dosage.
	Took a C HX and performed a C PX which revealed post nasal hemorrhage. Coagulation
	time (Lee and White) and microhematocrit (spun) done in ofc are WNL. BP 180/100.
	Used nasal cautery and post nasal packs to control hemorrhage. Rx prophylactic antibiotic
	to guard against sinusitis NKA. Adv retn tomorrow, bring hypertensive medication.
	Pt signed authorization to request med records from dr in Ohio. D: Recurrent epistaxis
	due to nonspecific hypertension. No disability from work.
	GP/llf *Gerald Practon, MD*
6-2-xx	Pt retns and nasal hemorrhage is reevaluated (PF HX/PX SF/MDM). Postnasal packs
	removed and replaced. BP 182/98. Pt forgot medication for hypertension but states she is
	taking it 2 X d. Adv retn in 1 day, bring medication.
	GP/llf *Gerald Practon, MD*
6-3-xx	Pt retns and nasal hemorrhage is reevaluated (PF HX/PX SF/MDM). Postnasal packs
	removed. BP 178/100. Verified hypertensive medication. Pt to increase dosage to 4 X d.
	Adv retn in 5 days.
	GP/llf *Gerald Practon, MD*
6-3-xx	Pt retns and nasal hemorrhage is reevaluated (EPF HX/PX L/MDM). Prev medical records
	arrived and reviewed. BP 190/102. Pt referred to Dr. Perry Cardi (int) for future care of
	hypertension.
	GP/llf *Gerald Practon, MD*

Figure 10

Acct No. __T-7__

STATEMENT
Financial Account
COLLEGE CLINIC
4567 Broad Avenue
Woodland Hills, XY 12345-0001
Tel. 555-486-9002
Fax No. 555-487-8976

Charles B. Kamb
2600 West Nautilus Street
Woodland Hills, XY 12345

Phone No. (H) __555-467-2601__   (W) __None/retired__   Birthdate __1-26-27__

Primary Insurance Co. __Medicare__   Policy/Group No. __454-XX-9569A__

Secondary Insurance Co. __National Insurance Company (Medigap)__   Policy/Group No. __5789002__

DATE	REFERENCE	DESCRIPTION	CHARGES	CREDITS		BALANCE
				PYMNTS.	ADJ.	
20xx		BALANCE FORWARD ⟶				
6-1-xx		NP OV				
6-1-xx		Coagulation time				
6-1-xx		Microhematocrit				
6-1-xx		Post nasal pack/cautery				
6-2-xx		OV				
6-2-xx		Subsequent nasal pack				
6-3-xx		OV				
6-8-xx		OV				

PLEASE PAY LAST AMOUNT IN BALANCE COLUMN

THIS IS A COPY OF YOUR FINANCIAL ACCOUNT AS IT APPEARS ON OUR RECORDS

Figure 11

PLEASE
DO NOT
STAPLE
IN THIS
AREA

CARRIER

HEALTH INSURANCE CLAIM FORM

| | PICA | | | | | | PICA | | |

| PICA | | | | | | | | | | PICA | | |

1. MEDICARE (Medicare #) **MEDICAID** (Medicaid #) **CHAMPUS** (Sponsor's SSN) **CHAMPVA** (VA File #) **GROUP HEALTH PLAN** (SSN or ID) **FECA BLK LUNG** (SSN) **OTHER** (ID) | **1a. INSURED'S I.D. NUMBER** (FOR PROGRAM IN ITEM 1)

2. PATIENT'S NAME (Last Name, First Name, Middle Initial) | **3. PATIENT'S BIRTH DATE** MM DD YY SEX M F | **4. INSURED'S NAME** (Last Name, First Name, Middle Initial)

5. PATIENT'S ADDRESS (No., Street) | **6. PATIENT RELATIONSHIP TO INSURED** Self Spouse Child Other | **7. INSURED'S ADDRESS** (No., Street)

CITY STATE | **8. PATIENT STATUS** Single Married Other / Employed Full-Time Student Part-Time Student | CITY STATE

ZIP CODE TELEPHONE (Include Area Code) ( ) | | ZIP CODE TELEPHONE (INCLUDE AREA CODE) ( )

9. OTHER INSURED'S NAME (Last Name, First Name, Middle Initial) | **10. IS PATIENT'S CONDITION RELATED TO:** | **11. INSURED'S POLICY GROUP OR FECA NUMBER**

a. OTHER INSURED'S POLICY OR GROUP NUMBER | a. EMPLOYMENT? (CURRENT OR PREVIOUS) YES NO | a. INSURED'S DATE OF BIRTH MM DD YY SEX M F

b. OTHER INSURED'S DATE OF BIRTH MM DD YY SEX M F | b. AUTO ACCIDENT? PLACE (State) YES NO | b. EMPLOYER'S NAME OR SCHOOL NAME

c. EMPLOYER'S NAME OR SCHOOL NAME | c. OTHER ACCIDENT? YES NO | c. INSURANCE PLAN NAME OR PROGRAM NAME

d. INSURANCE PLAN NAME OR PROGRAM NAME | 10d. RESERVED FOR LOCAL USE | d. IS THERE ANOTHER HEALTH BENEFIT PLAN? YES NO If yes, return to and complete item 9 a-d.

READ BACK OF FORM BEFORE COMPLETING & SIGNING THIS FORM.
12. PATIENT'S OR AUTHORIZED PERSON'S SIGNATURE I authorize the release of any medical or other information necessary to process this claim. I also request payment of government benefits either to myself or to the party who accepts assignment below.
SIGNED _____ DATE _____ | **13. INSURED'S OR AUTHORIZED PERSON'S SIGNATURE** I authorize payment of medical benefits to the undersigned physician or supplier for services described below.
SIGNED _____

14. DATE OF CURRENT: MM DD YY ◀ ILLNESS (First symptom) OR INJURY (Accident) OR PREGNANCY(LMP) | **15. IF PATIENT HAS HAD SAME OR SIMILAR ILLNESS. GIVE FIRST DATE** MM DD YY | **16. DATES PATIENT UNABLE TO WORK IN CURRENT OCCUPATION** FROM MM DD YY TO MM DD YY

17. NAME OF REFERRING PHYSICIAN OR OTHER SOURCE | **17a. I.D. NUMBER OF REFERRING PHYSICIAN** | **18. HOSPITALIZATION DATES RELATED TO CURRENT SERVICES** FROM MM DD YY TO MM DD YY

19. RESERVED FOR LOCAL USE | | **20. OUTSIDE LAB?** YES NO $ CHARGES

21. DIAGNOSIS OR NATURE OF ILLNESS OR INJURY. (RELATE ITEMS 1,2,3 OR 4 TO ITEM 24E BY LINE)
1. _____ 3. _____
2. _____ 4. _____ | **22. MEDICAID RESUBMISSION CODE** ORIGINAL REF. NO.
23. PRIOR AUTHORIZATION NUMBER

24. A DATE(S) OF SERVICE From MM DD YY To MM DD YY	**B** Place of Service	**C** Type of Service	**D** PROCEDURES, SERVICES, OR SUPPLIES (Explain Unusual Circumstances) CPT/HCPCS MODIFIER	**E** DIAGNOSIS CODE	**F** $ CHARGES	**G** DAYS OR UNITS	**H** EPSDT Family Plan	**I** EMG	**J** COB	**K** RESERVED FOR LOCAL USE
1										
2										
3										
4										
5										
6										

25. FEDERAL TAX I.D. NUMBER SSN EIN | **26. PATIENT'S ACCOUNT NO.** | **27. ACCEPT ASSIGNMENT?** (For govt. claims, see back) YES NO | **28. TOTAL CHARGE** $ | **29. AMOUNT PAID** $ | **30. BALANCE DUE** $

31. SIGNATURE OF PHYSICIAN OR SUPPLIER INCLUDING DEGREES OR CREDENTIALS (I certify that the statements on the reverse apply to this bill and are made a part thereof.) SIGNED _____ DATE _____ | **32. NAME AND ADDRESS OF FACILITY WHERE SERVICES WERE RENDERED** (If other than home or office) | **33. PHYSICIAN'S, SUPPLIER'S BILLING NAME, ADDRESS, ZIP CODE & PHONE #** PIN# GRP#

(APPROVED BY AMA COUNCIL ON MEDICAL SERVICE 8/88) **PLEASE PRINT OR TYPE** APPROVED OMB-0938-0008 FORM CMS-1500 (12-90), FORM RRB-1500, APPROVED OMB-1215-0055 FORM OWCP-1500, APPROVED OMB-0720-0001 (CHAMPUS)

PATIENT AND INSURED INFORMATION — PHYSICIAN OR SUPPLIER INFORMATION

Figure 12

PLEASE
DO NOT
STAPLE
IN THIS
AREA

HEALTH INSURANCE CLAIM FORM

| | PICA | | | | | | | PICA | |

1. MEDICARE	MEDICAID	CHAMPUS	CHAMPVA	GROUP HEALTH PLAN	FECA BLK LUNG	OTHER	1a. INSURED'S I.D. NUMBER	(FOR PROGRAM IN ITEM 1)
(Medicare #)	(Medicaid #)	(Sponsor's SSN)	(VA File #)	(SSN or ID)	(SSN)	(ID)		

2. PATIENT'S NAME (Last Name, First Name, Middle Initial)

3. PATIENT'S BIRTH DATE   MM   DD   YY   SEX   M   F

4. INSURED'S NAME (Last Name, First Name, Middle Initial)

5. PATIENT'S ADDRESS (No., Street)

6. PATIENT RELATIONSHIP TO INSURED   Self   Spouse   Child   Other

7. INSURED'S ADDRESS (No., Street)

CITY   STATE

8. PATIENT STATUS   Single   Married   Other

CITY   STATE

ZIP CODE   TELEPHONE (Include Area Code)   (   )

Employed   Full-Time Student   Part-Time Student

ZIP CODE   TELEPHONE (INCLUDE AREA CODE)   (   )

9. OTHER INSURED'S NAME (Last Name, First Name, Middle Initial)

10. IS PATIENT'S CONDITION RELATED TO:

11. INSURED'S POLICY GROUP OR FECA NUMBER

a. OTHER INSURED'S POLICY OR GROUP NUMBER

a. EMPLOYMENT? (CURRENT OR PREVIOUS)   YES   NO

a. INSURED'S DATE OF BIRTH   MM   DD   YY   SEX   M   F

b. OTHER INSURED'S DATE OF BIRTH   MM   DD   YY   SEX   M   F

b. AUTO ACCIDENT?   PLACE (State)   YES   NO

b. EMPLOYER'S NAME OR SCHOOL NAME

c. EMPLOYER'S NAME OR SCHOOL NAME

c. OTHER ACCIDENT?   YES   NO

c. INSURANCE PLAN NAME OR PROGRAM NAME

d. INSURANCE PLAN NAME OR PROGRAM NAME

10d. RESERVED FOR LOCAL USE

d. IS THERE ANOTHER HEALTH BENEFIT PLAN?   YES   NO   *If yes,* return to and complete item 9 a-d.

READ BACK OF FORM BEFORE COMPLETING & SIGNING THIS FORM.
12. PATIENT'S OR AUTHORIZED PERSON'S SIGNATURE I authorize the release of any medical or other information necessary to process this claim. I also request payment of government benefits either to myself or to the party who accepts assignment below.

SIGNED _____   DATE _____

13. INSURED'S OR AUTHORIZED PERSON'S SIGNATURE I authorize payment of medical benefits to the undersigned physician or supplier for services described below.

SIGNED _____

14. DATE OF CURRENT: MM   DD   YY   ILLNESS (First symptom) OR INJURY (Accident) OR PREGNANCY(LMP)

15. IF PATIENT HAS HAD SAME OR SIMILAR ILLNESS. GIVE FIRST DATE   MM   DD   YY

16. DATES PATIENT UNABLE TO WORK IN CURRENT OCCUPATION   FROM   MM   DD   YY   TO   MM   DD   YY

17. NAME OF REFERRING PHYSICIAN OR OTHER SOURCE

17a. I.D. NUMBER OF REFERRING PHYSICIAN

18. HOSPITALIZATION DATES RELATED TO CURRENT SERVICES   FROM   MM   DD   YY   TO   MM   DD   YY

19. RESERVED FOR LOCAL USE

20. OUTSIDE LAB?   YES   NO $ CHARGES

21. DIAGNOSIS OR NATURE OF ILLNESS OR INJURY. (RELATE ITEMS 1,2,3 OR 4 TO ITEM 24E BY LINE)

1. |___.___| 3. |___.___|

2. |___.___| 4. |___.___|

22. MEDICAID RESUBMISSION CODE   ORIGINAL REF. NO.

23. PRIOR AUTHORIZATION NUMBER

24.	A					B	C	D		E	F	G	H	I	J	K
	DATE(S) OF SERVICE					Place of Service	Type of Service	PROCEDURES, SERVICES, OR SUPPLIES (Explain Unusual Circumstances)		DIAGNOSIS CODE	$ CHARGES	DAYS OR UNITS	EPSDT Family Plan	EMG	COB	RESERVED FOR LOCAL USE
	From			To												
	MM	DD	YY	MM	DD	YY			CPT/HCPCS	MODIFIER							
1																
2																
3																
4																
5																
6																

25. FEDERAL TAX I.D. NUMBER   SSN EIN

26. PATIENT'S ACCOUNT NO.

27. ACCEPT ASSIGNMENT? (For govt. claims, see back)   YES   NO

28. TOTAL CHARGE $

29. AMOUNT PAID $

30. BALANCE DUE $

31. SIGNATURE OF PHYSICIAN OR SUPPLIER INCLUDING DEGREES OR CREDENTIALS (I certify that the statements on the reverse apply to this bill and are made a part thereof.)

SIGNED _____   DATE _____

32. NAME AND ADDRESS OF FACILITY WHERE SERVICES WERE RENDERED (If other than home or office)

33. PHYSICIAN'S, SUPPLIER'S BILLING NAME, ADDRESS, ZIP CODE & PHONE #

PIN#   GRP#

(APPROVED BY AMA COUNCIL ON MEDICAL SERVICE 8/88)   **PLEASE PRINT OR TYPE**

APPROVED OMB-0938-0008 FORM CMS-1500 (12-90),   FORM RRB-1500,
APPROVED OMB-1215-0055 FORM OWCP-1500,   APPROVED OMB-0720-0001 (CHAMPUS)

Figure 13

TEST 8: COMPLETE A CLAIM FORM FOR A MEDICAID CASE

Performance Objective

Task: Complete a CMS-1500 claim form for a Medicaid case and post transactions to the patient's financial accounting record.

Conditions: Use the patient's record (Figure 14) and financial statement (Figure 15); one health insurance claim form (Figure 16); a typewriter, computer, or pen; procedural and diagnostic code books; and Appendices A and B in this *Workbook*.

Standards: Claim Productivity Management

Time: _____ minutes

Accuracy: _____

(Note: The time element and accuracy criteria may be given by your instructor.)

Directions:

1. Using OCR guidelines, complete a CMS-1500 claim form and direct it to the Medicaid fiscal intermediary. Obtain the address of your Medicaid fiscal agent by first going to Web site http://www.cms.hhs.gov/medicaid/allStateContacts.asp and then either sending an e-mail message to the Medicaid contact or using the toll-free number to obtain the Medicaid carrier name and address. An option might be to contact your local state medical society. Refer to Louise K. Herman's patient record for information and Appendix A to locate the fees to record on the claim, and post them to the financial statement. Date the claim May 31.

2. Use your CPT code book or Appendix A in this *Workbook* to determine the correct five-digit code numbers and modifiers for each professional service rendered. Use your HCPCS Level II code book or refer to Appendix B in this *Workbook* for HCPCS procedure codes and modifiers. Use your diagnostic code book to code each active diagnosis.

3. Record the proper information on the patient's financial accounting record and claim form and note the date when you have billed the insurance company.

4. Post the payment of $350 (voucher number 4300), received from the Medicaid fiscal intermediary 40 days after claim submission, and write off (adjust) the balance of the account.

PATIENT RECORD NO. T-8

Herman	Louise	K	11-04-50	F	555-266-9085
LAST NAME	FIRST NAME	MIDDLE NAME	BIRTH DATE	SEX	HOME PHONE

13453 Burbank Boulevard	Woodland Hills	XY	12345
ADDRESS	CITY	STATE	ZIP CODE

555-466-7003		555-266-9085	herman@wb.net
CELL PHONE	PAGER NO.	FAX NO.	E-MAIL ADDRESS

519-XX-0018	T0943995
PATIENT'S SOC. SEC. NO.	DRIVER'S LICENSE

unemployed budget analyst	
PATIENT'S OCCUPATION	NAME OF COMPANY

ADDRESS OF EMPLOYER	PHONE

Harold D. Herman	retired salesman
SPOUSE OR PARENT	OCCUPATION

EMPLOYER	ADDRESS	PHONE

Medicaid	self
NAME OF INSURANCE	INSURED OR SUBSCRIBER

0051936001X	
MEDICAID NO.	GROUP NO.

REFERRED BY: Raymond Skeleton, MD

DATE	PROGRESS NOTES
5-6-xx	NP pt referred by Dr. Skeleton. CC: Rectal bleeding. Took a comprehensive history and
	performed a comprehensive physical examination. Diagnostic anoscopy revealed
	bleeding int and ext hemorrhoids and 2 infected rectal polyps. Rx antibiotics. Retn in 2
	days for removal of hemorrhoids and polyps (M/MDM)
	RR/llf *Rex Rumsey, MD*
5-8-xx	Pt returned to office for simple internal/external hemorrhoidectomy. Rigid
	proctosigmoidoscopy also perf for removal of polyps using snare technique. Adv. sitz
	baths daily. Continue on AB until gone. Retn in 1 wk. Will be off wk today through 5/15.
	RR/llf *Rex Rumsey, MD*
5-15-xx	DNS Telephoned pt and rescheduled.
	Mary Bright, CMA
5-17-xx	PO OV (EPF HX/PX LC/MDM). Pt progressing well. No pain, discomfort or bleeding.
	Discharged from care, retn PRN.
	RR/llf *Rex Rumsey, MD*

Figure 14

Acct No. __T-8__

STATEMENT
Financial Account
COLLEGE CLINIC
4567 Broad Avenue
Woodland Hills, XY 12345-0001
Tel. 555-486-9002
Fax No. 555-487-8976

Louise K. Herman
13453 Burbank Boulevard
Woodland Hills, XY 12345

Phone No. (H) __555-266-9085__ (W) _____ Birthdate __11/4/50__

Primary Insurance Co. __Medicaid__ Policy/Group No. __0051936001X__

Secondary Insurance Co._____ Policy/Group No._____

DATE	REFERENCE	DESCRIPTION	CHARGES	CREDITS PYMNTS.	ADJ.	BALANCE
20xx		BALANCE FORWARD →				
5-6-xx		NP OV				
5-6-xx		Dx anoscopy				
5-8-xx		Int/Ext Hemorrhoidectomy				
5-8-xx		Proctosigmoidoscopy with removal of polyps				
5-17-xx		PO OV				

PLEASE PAY LAST AMOUNT IN BALANCE COLUMN

THIS IS A COPY OF YOUR FINANCIAL ACCOUNT AS IT APPEARS ON OUR RECORDS

Figure 15

PLEASE
DO NOT
STAPLE
IN THIS
AREA

CARRIER →

HEALTH INSURANCE CLAIM FORM

| | PICA | | | | | | | | PICA | |

1. MEDICARE (Medicare #)   MEDICAID (Medicaid #)   CHAMPUS (Sponsor's SSN)   CHAMPVA (VA File #)   GROUP HEALTH PLAN (SSN or ID)   FECA BLK LUNG (SSN)   OTHER (ID)   1a. INSURED'S I.D. NUMBER (FOR PROGRAM IN ITEM 1)

2. PATIENT'S NAME (Last Name, First Name, Middle Initial)

3. PATIENT'S BIRTH DATE MM DD YY   SEX M F

4. INSURED'S NAME (Last Name, First Name, Middle Initial)

5. PATIENT'S ADDRESS (No., Street)

6. PATIENT RELATIONSHIP TO INSURED   Self   Spouse   Child   Other

7. INSURED'S ADDRESS (No., Street)

CITY   STATE

8. PATIENT STATUS   Single   Married   Other   Employed   Full-Time Student   Part-Time Student

CITY   STATE

ZIP CODE   TELEPHONE (Include Area Code) ( )

ZIP CODE   TELEPHONE (INCLUDE AREA CODE) ( )

9. OTHER INSURED'S NAME (Last Name, First Name, Middle Initial)

10. IS PATIENT'S CONDITION RELATED TO:

11. INSURED'S POLICY GROUP OR FECA NUMBER

a. OTHER INSURED'S POLICY OR GROUP NUMBER

a. EMPLOYMENT? (CURRENT OR PREVIOUS) YES NO

a. INSURED'S DATE OF BIRTH MM DD YY   SEX M F

b. OTHER INSURED'S DATE OF BIRTH MM DD YY   SEX M F

b. AUTO ACCIDENT?   PLACE (State) YES NO

b. EMPLOYER'S NAME OR SCHOOL NAME

c. EMPLOYER'S NAME OR SCHOOL NAME

c. OTHER ACCIDENT? YES NO

c. INSURANCE PLAN NAME OR PROGRAM NAME

d. INSURANCE PLAN NAME OR PROGRAM NAME

10d. RESERVED FOR LOCAL USE

d. IS THERE ANOTHER HEALTH BENEFIT PLAN? YES NO *If yes*, return to and complete item 9 a-d.

READ BACK OF FORM BEFORE COMPLETING & SIGNING THIS FORM.
12. PATIENT'S OR AUTHORIZED PERSON'S SIGNATURE I authorize the release of any medical or other information necessary to process this claim. I also request payment of government benefits either to myself or to the party who accepts assignment below.

SIGNED _____ DATE _____

13. INSURED'S OR AUTHORIZED PERSON'S SIGNATURE I authorize payment of medical benefits to the undersigned physician or supplier for services described below.

SIGNED _____

PATIENT AND INSURED INFORMATION →

14. DATE OF CURRENT: MM DD YY   ◄ ILLNESS (First symptom) OR INJURY (Accident) OR PREGNANCY(LMP)

15. IF PATIENT HAS HAD SAME OR SIMILAR ILLNESS. GIVE FIRST DATE MM DD YY

16. DATES PATIENT UNABLE TO WORK IN CURRENT OCCUPATION FROM MM DD YY TO MM DD YY

17. NAME OF REFERRING PHYSICIAN OR OTHER SOURCE

17a. I.D. NUMBER OF REFERRING PHYSICIAN

18. HOSPITALIZATION DATES RELATED TO CURRENT SERVICES FROM MM DD YY TO MM DD YY

19. RESERVED FOR LOCAL USE

20. OUTSIDE LAB? $ CHARGES   YES NO

21. DIAGNOSIS OR NATURE OF ILLNESS OR INJURY. (RELATE ITEMS 1,2,3 OR 4 TO ITEM 24E BY LINE)

1. |___.___| 3. |___.___|
2. |___.___| 4. |___.___|

22. MEDICAID RESUBMISSION CODE   ORIGINAL REF. NO.

23. PRIOR AUTHORIZATION NUMBER

24. A DATE(S) OF SERVICE						B Place of Service	C Type of Service	D PROCEDURES, SERVICES, OR SUPPLIES (Explain Unusual Circumstances) CPT/HCPCS | MODIFIER	E DIAGNOSIS CODE	F $ CHARGES	G DAYS OR UNITS	H EPSDT Family Plan	I EMG	J COB	K RESERVED FOR LOCAL USE
From MM	DD	YY	To MM	DD	YY										
1															
2															
3															
4															
5															
6															

25. FEDERAL TAX I.D. NUMBER   SSN EIN

26. PATIENT'S ACCOUNT NO.

27. ACCEPT ASSIGNMENT? (For govt. claims, see back) YES NO

28. TOTAL CHARGE $

29. AMOUNT PAID $

30. BALANCE DUE $

31. SIGNATURE OF PHYSICIAN OR SUPPLIER INCLUDING DEGREES OR CREDENTIALS (I certify that the statements on the reverse apply to this bill and are made a part thereof.)

SIGNED _____ DATE _____

32. NAME AND ADDRESS OF FACILITY WHERE SERVICES WERE RENDERED (If other than home or office)

33. PHYSICIAN'S, SUPPLIER'S BILLING NAME, ADDRESS, ZIP CODE & PHONE #

PIN#   GRP#

PHYSICIAN OR SUPPLIER INFORMATION →

(APPROVED BY AMA COUNCIL ON MEDICAL SERVICE 8/88)   *PLEASE PRINT OR TYPE*   APPROVED OMB-0938-0008 FORM CMS-1500 (12-90), FORM RRB-1500, APPROVED OMB-1215-0055 FORM OWCP-1500, APPROVED OMB-0720-0001 (CHAMPUS)

Figure 16

TEST 9: COMPLETE A CLAIM FORM FOR A TRICARE CASE

Performance Objective

Task: Complete a CMS-1500 claim form for a TRICARE case and post transactions to the patient's financial accounting record.

Conditions: Use the patient's record (Figure 17) and financial statement (Figure 18); one health insurance claim form (Figure 19); a typewriter, computer, or pen; procedural and diagnostic code books; and Appendices A and B in this *Workbook*.

Standards: Claim Productivity Management

Time: _____ minutes

Accuracy: _____

(Note: The time element and accuracy criteria may be given by your instructor.)

Directions:

1. Using OCR guidelines, complete a CMS-1500 claim form and direct it to the TRICARE carrier. To locate your local fiscal intermediary, go to Web site http://www.tricare.osd.mil. Click on the area of the map you are residing in and then choose a state to access claims information for that state. Refer to Darlene M. Cash's patient record for information and Appendix A to locate the fees to record on the claim, and post them to the financial statement. Date the claim February 27. Dr. Cutler is accepting assignment, and the patient's signatures to release information to the insurance company and to have the payment forwarded directly to the physician are on file.

2. Use your CPT code book or Appendix A in this *Workbook* to determine the correct five-digit code numbers and fees for each professional service rendered. Use your HCPCS Level II code book or refer to Appendix B in this *Workbook* for HCPCS procedure codes and modifiers. Use your diagnostic code book to code each active diagnosis.

3. Record the proper information on the patient's financial accounting record and claim form, and note the date when you have billed the insurance company.

PATIENT RECORD NO. T-9

Cash	Darlene	M	3-15-70	F	555-666-8901
LAST NAME	FIRST NAME	MIDDLE NAME	BIRTH DATE	SEX	HOME PHONE

5729 Redwood Avenue   Woodland Hills   XY   12344
ADDRESS   CITY   STATE   ZIP CODE

555-290-5400   555-666-8901   cash@wb.net
CELL PHONE   PAGER NO.   FAX NO.   E-MAIL ADDRESS

298-XX-6754   J3457789
PATIENT'S SOC. SEC. NO.   DRIVER'S LICENSE

Teacher   City Unified School District
PATIENT'S OCCUPATION   NAME OF COMPANY

Century High School, 2031 West Olympic Boulevard, Dorland, XY 12345   555-678-1076
ADDRESS OF EMPLOYER   PHONE

David F. Cash   Navy Petty Officer—Grade 8 (active status)
SPOUSE OR PARENT   OCCUPATION

United States Navy   HHC, 2nd Batt, 26th Infantry, APO New York, NY, 10030
EMPLOYER   ADDRESS   PHONE

TRICARE Standard   David Cash (DOB 4-22-70)
NAME OF INSURANCE   INSURED OR SUBSCRIBER

767-XX-9080
POLICY/CERTIFICATE NO.   GROUP NO.

REFERRED BY: Hugh R. Foot, MD, 2010 Main St., Woodland Hills, XY 12345   Fed Tax ID #61 25099XX

DATE	PROGRESS NOTES
1-4-xx	New pt, referred by Dr. Foot comes in complaining of head pain which began yesterday.
	Performed an EPF history and physical exam. Lt parietal area of skull slightly tender,
	some redness of scalp. Pain localized and not consistent with HA syndromes. Rest of
	exam N. Imp: head pain, undetermined nature, possible cyst. Apply hot compresses and
	observe. Take Ibuprofen for pain prn (200 mg up to 2 q. 4 h). Retn in 1 wk, no disability
	from work (SF/MDM).
	CC/llf *Clarence Cutler, MD*
1-11-xx	Pt retns and states that the hot compresses have helped but is concerned with some
	swelling in area. On exam noticed slt elevation of skin in lt parietal area of scalp, no
	warmth over area. Slt pain on palpation. Exam otherwise neg. Imp: Subcutaneous nodule.
	Continue with same tx plan: Hot compresses daily and Ibuprofen prn. Retn in 2 to 3 wks
	if not resolved (PF HX/PX SF/MDM).
	CC/llf *Clarence Cutler, MD*
2-3-xx	Pt retns for reexamination of parietal skull. Elevation of skin still persisting. It has now
	come to a head, is warm to the touch, and consistent with an inflammatory cystic lesion.
	A decision is made to excise the benign lesion. Scalp cyst, 1.5 cm removed under
	procaine block with knife dissection; closed wound with six #000 black silk sutures.
	Adv to retn 1 wk for removal of sutures (EPF HX/PX LC/MDM).
	CC/llf *Clarence Cutler, MD*
2-10-xx	Pt presents for suture removal. Sutures removed and slight oozing occurs in midsection
	of wound. Wound dressed and pt advised to apply antibacterial cream daily. Retn in 4 to 5
	days for final check (PF HX/PX SF/MDM).
	CC/llf *Clarence Cutler, MD*
2-15-xx	Pt presents for PO check of head wound. Parietal area healed well. RTO prn
	(PF HX/PX SF/MDM).
	CC/llf *Clarence Cutler, MD*

Figure 17

Acct No. __T-9__

STATEMENT
Financial Account
COLLEGE CLINIC
4567 Broad Avenue
Woodland Hills, XY 12345-0001
Fax No. 555-487-8976

Darlene M. Cash
5729 Redwood Avenue
Woodland Hills, XY 12345

Phone No. (H) __555-666-8901__ (W) __555-678-1076__   Birthdate __3/15/70__

Primary Insurance Co. __TRICARE Standard__   Policy/Group No. __767-XX-9080__

Secondary Insurance Co.____   Policy/Group No.____

DATE	REFERENCE	DESCRIPTION	CHARGES	CREDITS PYMNTS.	ADJ.	BALANCE
20xx		BALANCE FORWARD →				
1-4-xx		NP OV				
1-11-xx		OV				
2-3-xx		OV				
2-3-xx		Excision inflammatory cystic scalp lesion				
2-10-xx		OV				
2-15-xx		OV				

PLEASE PAY LAST AMOUNT IN BALANCE COLUMN ⬆

THIS IS A COPY OF YOUR FINANCIAL ACCOUNT AS IT APPEARS ON OUR RECORDS

Figure 18

PLEASE
DO NOT
STAPLE
IN THIS
AREA

CARRIER

HEALTH INSURANCE CLAIM FORM

	PICA		PICA	

1. MEDICARE MEDICAID CHAMPUS CHAMPVA GROUP HEALTH PLAN FECA BLK LUNG OTHER

(Medicare #) (Medicaid #) (Sponsor's SSN) (VA File #) (SSN or ID) (SSN) (ID)

1a. INSURED'S I.D. NUMBER (FOR PROGRAM IN ITEM 1)

2. PATIENT'S NAME (Last Name, First Name, Middle Initial)

3. PATIENT'S BIRTH DATE MM DD YY SEX M F

4. INSURED'S NAME (Last Name, First Name, Middle Initial)

5. PATIENT'S ADDRESS (No., Street)

6. PATIENT RELATIONSHIP TO INSURED Self Spouse Child Other

7. INSURED'S ADDRESS (No., Street)

CITY STATE

8. PATIENT STATUS Single Married Other

Employed Full-Time Student Part-Time Student

CITY STATE

ZIP CODE TELEPHONE (Include Area Code) ( )

ZIP CODE TELEPHONE (INCLUDE AREA CODE) ( )

9. OTHER INSURED'S NAME (Last Name, First Name, Middle Initial)

10. IS PATIENT'S CONDITION RELATED TO:

11. INSURED'S POLICY GROUP OR FECA NUMBER

a. OTHER INSURED'S POLICY OR GROUP NUMBER

a. EMPLOYMENT? (CURRENT OR PREVIOUS) YES NO

a. INSURED'S DATE OF BIRTH MM DD YY SEX M F

b. OTHER INSURED'S DATE OF BIRTH MM DD YY SEX M F

b. AUTO ACCIDENT? PLACE (State) YES NO

b. EMPLOYER'S NAME OR SCHOOL NAME

c. EMPLOYER'S NAME OR SCHOOL NAME

c. OTHER ACCIDENT? YES NO

c. INSURANCE PLAN NAME OR PROGRAM NAME

d. INSURANCE PLAN NAME OR PROGRAM NAME

10d. RESERVED FOR LOCAL USE

d. IS THERE ANOTHER HEALTH BENEFIT PLAN? YES NO If yes, return to and complete item 9 a-d.

READ BACK OF FORM BEFORE COMPLETING & SIGNING THIS FORM.

12. PATIENT'S OR AUTHORIZED PERSON'S SIGNATURE I authorize the release of any medical or other information necessary to process this claim. I also request payment of government benefits either to myself or to the party who accepts assignment below.

SIGNED _____ DATE _____

13. INSURED'S OR AUTHORIZED PERSON'S SIGNATURE I authorize payment of medical benefits to the undersigned physician or supplier for services described below.

SIGNED _____

PATIENT AND INSURED INFORMATION

14. DATE OF CURRENT: ILLNESS (First symptom) OR INJURY (Accident) OR PREGNANCY(LMP) MM DD YY

15. IF PATIENT HAS HAD SAME OR SIMILAR ILLNESS. GIVE FIRST DATE MM DD YY

16. DATES PATIENT UNABLE TO WORK IN CURRENT OCCUPATION MM DD YY FROM TO MM DD YY

17. NAME OF REFERRING PHYSICIAN OR OTHER SOURCE

17a. I.D. NUMBER OF REFERRING PHYSICIAN

18. HOSPITALIZATION DATES RELATED TO CURRENT SERVICES MM DD YY FROM TO MM DD YY

19. RESERVED FOR LOCAL USE

20. OUTSIDE LAB? $ CHARGES YES NO

21. DIAGNOSIS OR NATURE OF ILLNESS OR INJURY. (RELATE ITEMS 1,2,3 OR 4 TO ITEM 24E BY LINE)

1. |___.___| 3. |___.___|

2. |___.___| 4. |___.___|

22. MEDICAID RESUBMISSION CODE ORIGINAL REF. NO.

23. PRIOR AUTHORIZATION NUMBER

24. A DATE(S) OF SERVICE						B Place of Service	C Type of Service	D PROCEDURES, SERVICES, OR SUPPLIES (Explain Unusual Circumstances)		E DIAGNOSIS CODE	F $ CHARGES	G DAYS OR UNITS	H EPSDT Family Plan	I EMG	J COB	K RESERVED FOR LOCAL USE
From MM	DD	YY	To MM	DD	YY			CPT/HCPCS	MODIFIER							
1																
2																
3																
4																
5																
6																

25. FEDERAL TAX I.D. NUMBER SSN EIN

26. PATIENT'S ACCOUNT NO.

27. ACCEPT ASSIGNMENT? (For govt. claims, see back) YES NO

28. TOTAL CHARGE $

29. AMOUNT PAID $

30. BALANCE DUE $

31. SIGNATURE OF PHYSICIAN OR SUPPLIER INCLUDING DEGREES OR CREDENTIALS (I certify that the statements on the reverse apply to this bill and are made a part thereof.)

SIGNED _____ DATE _____

32. NAME AND ADDRESS OF FACILITY WHERE SERVICES WERE RENDERED (If other than home or office)

33. PHYSICIAN'S, SUPPLIER'S BILLING NAME, ADDRESS, ZIP CODE & PHONE #

PIN# GRP#

PHYSICIAN OR SUPPLIER INFORMATION

(APPROVED BY AMA COUNCIL ON MEDICAL SERVICE 8/88) **PLEASE PRINT OR TYPE** APPROVED OMB-0938-0008 FORM CMS-1500 (12-90), FORM RRB-1500,
APPROVED OMB-1215-0055 FORM OWCP-1500, APPROVED OMB-0720-0001 (CHAMPUS)

Figure 19

TEST 10: COMPLETE TWO CLAIM FORMS FOR A PRIVATE PLAN

Performance Objective

Task: Complete two CMS-1500 claim forms for a private case and post transactions to the patient's financial accounting record.

Conditions: Use the patient's record (Figure 20) and financial statement (Figure 21);
two health insurance claim forms (Figures 22 and 23); a typewriter,
computer, or pen; procedural and diagnostic code books; and
Appendices A and B in this *Workbook*.

Standards: Claim Productivity Management

Time: _____ minutes

Accuracy: _____

(Note: The time element and accuracy criteria may be given by your
instructor.)

Directions:

1. Using OCR guidelines, complete two CMS-1500 claim forms and direct them to the
   private carrier. Refer to Gertrude C. Hamilton's patient record for information and
   Appendix A in this *Workbook* to locate the fees to record on the claim, and post them to
   the financial statement. Date the first claim August 15 and the second one October 15.
   Dr. Cardi is accepting assignment, and the patient's signatures to release information to
   the insurance company and to have the payment forwarded directly to the physician
   are on file.

2. Use your CPT code book or Appendix A in this *Workbook* to determine the correct
   five-digit code numbers and modifiers for each professional service rendered. Use your
   HCPCS Level II code book or refer to Appendix B in this *Workbook* for HCPCS
   procedure codes and modifiers. Use your diagnostic code books to code each active
   diagnosis.

3. Record the proper information on the financial record and claim form, and note the
   date when you have billed the insurance company.

4. Mrs. Hamilton makes a payment of $200, check number 5362, on her account on
   October 26. Post the proper entry for this transaction.

PATIENT RECORD NO. T-10

Hamilton	Gertrude	C		03-06-47	F	555-798-3321
LAST NAME	FIRST NAME	MIDDLE NAME		BIRTH DATE	SEX	HOME PHONE

5320 Phillips Street	Woodland Hills	XY	12345
ADDRESS	CITY	STATE	ZIP CODE

555-399-4990	555-312-6677	555-798-3321		hamilton@wb.net
CELL PHONE	PAGER NO.	FAX NO.		E-MAIL ADDRESS

540-XX-7677	D9043557
PATIENT'S SOC. SEC. NO.	DRIVER'S LICENSE

retired secretary	
PATIENT'S OCCUPATION	NAME OF COMPANY

ADDRESS OF EMPLOYER	PHONE

deceased	
SPOUSE OR PARENT	OCCUPATION

EMPLOYER	ADDRESS	PHONE

Colonial Health Insurance, 1011 Main Street, Woodland Hills, XY 12345	self
NAME OF INSURANCE	INSURED OR SUBSCRIBER

540XX7677	4566 (through previous employment)
POLICY/CERTIFICATE NO.	GROUP NO.

REFERRED BY: Gerald Practon, MD, 4567 Broad Avenue, Woodland Hills, XY 12345

Figure 20

DATE	PROGRESS NOTES No. T-10
7-29-xx	Dr. Practon asked me to consult on this 57-year-old pt adm to College Hosp today.
	Duplex carotid ultrasonography indicates bilateral carotid stenosis. C/HX: Suffered CVA lt
	hemisphere 1 yr prior to adm. Marked rt arm & leg weakness c̄ weakness of rt face and
	slurring of speech. C/PE revealed lt carotid bruit, II/IV, & right carotid bruit, II/IV.
	Performed hand-held Doppler vascular study on bilateral carotids which indicated
	decreased blood flow. Adv brain scan and lt carotid thromboendarterectomy; rt carotid
	thromboendarterectomy at a later date H/MDM.
	PC/llf *Perry Cardi, MD*
7-30-xx	HV (EPF HX/PX MC/MDM). Dr. Practon asked me to take over pt's care. Pt had brain scan
	done today, ECG, and lab work.
	PC/llf *Perry Cardi, MD*
7-31-xx	HV (EPF HX/PX MC/MDM). Brain scan indicates prior CVA; no new findings. ECG, normal
	sinus rhythm with occasional premature ventricular contractions. Lab work WNL.
	Discussed test results with Mrs. Hamilton.
	PC/llf *Perry Cardi, MD*
8-1-xx	HV (PF HX/PX LC/MDM). Decision made for surgery, to be scheduled tomorrow.
	PC/llf *Perry Cardi, MD*
8-2-xx	Pt taken to the operative suite. Performed lt carotid thromboendarterectomy by neck
	incision (see op report). Surgery went as planned, pt in recovery.
	PC/llf *Perry Cardi, MD*
8-3-xx	HV (PF HX/PX SF/MDM). Operative site appears normal. Pt resting comfortably.
	PC/llf *Perry Cardi, MD*
8-4-xx	DC from hosp. Pt to be seen in ofc in 1 week.
	PC/llf *Perry Cardi, MD*
8-12-xx	PO OV (D HX/PX M/MDM). Discussed outcome of surgery. Pt making satisfactory
	progress. Adv rt carotid thromboendarterectomy. Pt would like it done as soon as possible;
	next month if there is an operative time. Scheduled surgery for September 16, 20XX at
	College Hospital.
	PC/llf *Perry Cardi, MD*
9-16-xx	Adm to College Hospital. Performed a D history, D physical examination, and SF medical
	decision making. Rt. carotid thromboendarterectomy performed by neck incision.
	DX: Rt carotid stenosis.
	PC/llf *Perry Cardi, MD*
9-17-xx	HV (PF HX/PX SF/MDM). Pt stable and doing well. Operative site looks good. Plan for
	discharge tomorrow.
	PC/llf *Perry Cardi, MD*
9-18-xx	DC from hosp to home. RTC 1 wk.
	PC/llf *Perry Cardi, MD*
9-25-xx	PO visit (PF HX/PX SF/MDM). Pt making satisfactory recovery. Her neighbor will monitor
	BP daily. Retn 1 month.
	PC/llf *Perry Cardi, MD*

Figure 20, cont'd

STATEMENT
COLLEGE CLINIC
4567 Broad Avenue
Woodland Hills, XY 12345-0001
Tel. 555-486-9002
Fax No. 555-487-8976

Acct. No . T-10

Gertrude C. Hamilton
5320 Phillips Street
Woodland Hills, XY 12345

Phone No. (H)____(555) 798-3321____(W)_____   Birthdate____03-06-47____

Insurance Co____Colonial Health Insurance_____   Policy/Group No. 540Xx7677 / 4566

	REFERENCE	DESCRIPTION	CHARGES	PYMNTS.	ADJ.	BALANCE	
20xx				BALANCE FORWARD ➔			
7-29-xx		Inpatient consult					
7-30-xx		HV					
7-31-xx		HV					
8-1-xx		HV					
8-2-xx		L carotid thromboendarterectmy					
8-3-xx		HV					
8-4-xx		Discharge					
8-12-xx		PO OV					
9-16-xx		Admit					
9-16-xx		R Carotid thromboendarterectomy					
9-17-xx		HV					
9-18-xx		Discharge					
9-25-xx		PO OV					

PLEASE PAY LAST AMOUNT IN BALANCE COLUMN

THIS IS A COPY OF YOUR FINANCIAL ACCOUNT AS IT APPEARS ON OUR RECORDS

Figure 21

PLEASE
DO NOT
STAPLE
IN THIS
AREA

| | PICA | | | | | **HEALTH INSURANCE CLAIM FORM** | PICA | | |

1. MEDICARE	MEDICAID	CHAMPUS	CHAMPVA	GROUP HEALTH PLAN	FECA BLK LUNG	OTHER	1a. INSURED'S I.D. NUMBER	(FOR PROGRAM IN ITEM 1)
(Medicare #)	(Medicaid #)	(Sponsor's SSN)	(VA File #)	(SSN or ID)	(SSN)	(ID)		

2. PATIENT'S NAME (Last Name, First Name, Middle Initial)

3. PATIENT'S BIRTH DATE MM DD YY   SEX M F

4. INSURED'S NAME (Last Name, First Name, Middle Initial)

5. PATIENT'S ADDRESS (No., Street)

6. PATIENT RELATIONSHIP TO INSURED   Self Spouse Child Other

7. INSURED'S ADDRESS (No., Street)

CITY   STATE

8. PATIENT STATUS   Single Married Other

CITY   STATE

ZIP CODE   TELEPHONE (Include Area Code) (   )

Employed Full-Time Student Part-Time Student

ZIP CODE   TELEPHONE (INCLUDE AREA CODE) (   )

9. OTHER INSURED'S NAME (Last Name, First Name, Middle Initial)

10. IS PATIENT'S CONDITION RELATED TO:

11. INSURED'S POLICY GROUP OR FECA NUMBER

a. OTHER INSURED'S POLICY OR GROUP NUMBER

a. EMPLOYMENT? (CURRENT OR PREVIOUS)   YES NO

a. INSURED'S DATE OF BIRTH MM DD YY   SEX M F

b. OTHER INSURED'S DATE OF BIRTH MM DD YY   SEX M F

b. AUTO ACCIDENT?   PLACE (State)   YES NO

b. EMPLOYER'S NAME OR SCHOOL NAME

c. EMPLOYER'S NAME OR SCHOOL NAME

c. OTHER ACCIDENT?   YES NO

c. INSURANCE PLAN NAME OR PROGRAM NAME

d. INSURANCE PLAN NAME OR PROGRAM NAME

10d. RESERVED FOR LOCAL USE

d. IS THERE ANOTHER HEALTH BENEFIT PLAN?   YES NO *If yes*, return to and complete item 9 a-d.

READ BACK OF FORM BEFORE COMPLETING & SIGNING THIS FORM.
12. PATIENT'S OR AUTHORIZED PERSON'S SIGNATURE I authorize the release of any medical or other information necessary to process this claim. I also request payment of government benefits either to myself or to the party who accepts assignment below.

SIGNED _____   DATE _____

13. INSURED'S OR AUTHORIZED PERSON'S SIGNATURE I authorize payment of medical benefits to the undersigned physician or supplier for services described below.

SIGNED _____

14. DATE OF CURRENT: MM DD YY ILLNESS (First symptom) OR INJURY (Accident) OR PREGNANCY(LMP)

15. IF PATIENT HAS HAD SAME OR SIMILAR ILLNESS. GIVE FIRST DATE MM DD YY

16. DATES PATIENT UNABLE TO WORK IN CURRENT OCCUPATION FROM MM DD YY TO MM DD YY

17. NAME OF REFERRING PHYSICIAN OR OTHER SOURCE

17a. I.D. NUMBER OF REFERRING PHYSICIAN

18. HOSPITALIZATION DATES RELATED TO CURRENT SERVICES FROM MM DD YY TO MM DD YY

19. RESERVED FOR LOCAL USE

20. OUTSIDE LAB?   YES NO $ CHARGES

21. DIAGNOSIS OR NATURE OF ILLNESS OR INJURY. (RELATE ITEMS 1,2,3 OR 4 TO ITEM 24E BY LINE)

1. |___.___| 3. |___.___|

2. |___.___| 4. |___.___|

22. MEDICAID RESUBMISSION CODE   ORIGINAL REF. NO.

23. PRIOR AUTHORIZATION NUMBER

24. A DATE(S) OF SERVICE						B Place of Service	C Type of Service	D PROCEDURES, SERVICES, OR SUPPLIES (Explain Unusual Circumstances)		E DIAGNOSIS CODE	F $ CHARGES	G DAYS OR UNITS	H EPSDT Family Plan	I EMG	J COB	K RESERVED FOR LOCAL USE
From MM	DD	YY	To MM	DD	YY			CPT/HCPCS	MODIFIER							
1																
2																
3																
4																
5																
6																

25. FEDERAL TAX I.D. NUMBER   SSN EIN

26. PATIENT'S ACCOUNT NO.

27. ACCEPT ASSIGNMENT? (For govt. claims, see back)   YES NO

28. TOTAL CHARGE $

29. AMOUNT PAID $

30. BALANCE DUE $

31. SIGNATURE OF PHYSICIAN OR SUPPLIER INCLUDING DEGREES OR CREDENTIALS (I certify that the statements on the reverse apply to this bill and are made a part thereof.)

SIGNED _____   DATE _____

32. NAME AND ADDRESS OF FACILITY WHERE SERVICES WERE RENDERED (If other than home or office)

33. PHYSICIAN'S, SUPPLIER'S BILLING NAME, ADDRESS, ZIP CODE & PHONE #

PIN#   GRP#

(APPROVED BY AMA COUNCIL ON MEDICAL SERVICE 8/88)   ***PLEASE PRINT OR TYPE***   APPROVED OMB-0938-0008 FORM CMS-1500 (12-90), FORM RRB-1500, APPROVED OMB-1215-0055 FORM OWCP-1500, APPROVED OMB-0720-0001 (CHAMPUS)

Figure 22

PLEASE
DO NOT
STAPLE
IN THIS
AREA

HEALTH INSURANCE CLAIM FORM

| | PICA | | | | | | PICA | |

CARRIER

1. MEDICARE   MEDICAID   CHAMPUS   CHAMPVA   GROUP HEALTH PLAN   FECA BLK LUNG   OTHER   1a. INSURED'S I.D. NUMBER   (FOR PROGRAM IN ITEM 1)

(Medicare #)   (Medicaid #)   (Sponsor's SSN)   (VA File #)   (SSN or ID)   (SSN)   (ID)

2. PATIENT'S NAME (Last Name, First Name, Middle Initial)   3. PATIENT'S BIRTH DATE   MM   DD   YY   SEX   M   F   4. INSURED'S NAME (Last Name, First Name, Middle Initial)

5. PATIENT'S ADDRESS (No., Street)   6. PATIENT RELATIONSHIP TO INSURED   Self   Spouse   Child   Other   7. INSURED'S ADDRESS (No., Street)

CITY   STATE   8. PATIENT STATUS   Single   Married   Other   CITY   STATE

ZIP CODE   TELEPHONE (Include Area Code)   (   )   Employed   Full-Time Student   Part-Time Student   ZIP CODE   TELEPHONE (INCLUDE AREA CODE)   (   )

9. OTHER INSURED'S NAME (Last Name, First Name, Middle Initial)   10. IS PATIENT'S CONDITION RELATED TO: 11. INSURED'S POLICY GROUP OR FECA NUMBER

a. OTHER INSURED'S POLICY OR GROUP NUMBER   a. EMPLOYMENT? (CURRENT OR PREVIOUS)   YES   NO   a. INSURED'S DATE OF BIRTH   MM   DD   YY   SEX   M   F

b. OTHER INSURED'S DATE OF BIRTH   MM   DD   YY   SEX   M   F   b. AUTO ACCIDENT?   PLACE (State)   YES   NO   b. EMPLOYER'S NAME OR SCHOOL NAME

c. EMPLOYER'S NAME OR SCHOOL NAME   c. OTHER ACCIDENT?   YES   NO   c. INSURANCE PLAN NAME OR PROGRAM NAME

d. INSURANCE PLAN NAME OR PROGRAM NAME   10d. RESERVED FOR LOCAL USE   d. IS THERE ANOTHER HEALTH BENEFIT PLAN?   YES   NO   *If yes*, return to and complete item 9 a-d.

PATIENT AND INSURED INFORMATION

READ BACK OF FORM BEFORE COMPLETING & SIGNING THIS FORM.

12. PATIENT'S OR AUTHORIZED PERSON'S SIGNATURE I authorize the release of any medical or other information necessary to process this claim. I also request payment of government benefits either to myself or to the party who accepts assignment below.

SIGNED _____   DATE _____

13. INSURED'S OR AUTHORIZED PERSON'S SIGNATURE I authorize payment of medical benefits to the undersigned physician or supplier for services described below.

SIGNED _____

14. DATE OF CURRENT: MM   DD   YY   ILLNESS (First symptom) OR INJURY (Accident) OR PREGNANCY(LMP)   15. IF PATIENT HAS HAD SAME OR SIMILAR ILLNESS. GIVE FIRST DATE   MM   DD   YY   16. DATES PATIENT UNABLE TO WORK IN CURRENT OCCUPATION   MM   DD   YY   FROM   TO   MM   DD   YY

17. NAME OF REFERRING PHYSICIAN OR OTHER SOURCE   17a. I.D. NUMBER OF REFERRING PHYSICIAN   18. HOSPITALIZATION DATES RELATED TO CURRENT SERVICES   MM   DD   YY   FROM   TO   MM   DD   YY

19. RESERVED FOR LOCAL USE   20. OUTSIDE LAB?   YES   NO $ CHARGES

21. DIAGNOSIS OR NATURE OF ILLNESS OR INJURY. (RELATE ITEMS 1,2,3 OR 4 TO ITEM 24E BY LINE)

1. |___.___   3. |___.___   22. MEDICAID RESUBMISSION CODE   ORIGINAL REF. NO.

2. |___.___   4. |___.___   23. PRIOR AUTHORIZATION NUMBER

24. A DATE(S) OF SERVICE					B	C	D PROCEDURES, SERVICES, OR SUPPLIES		E	F	G	H	I	J	K
From			To		Place of Service	Type of Service	(Explain Unusual Circumstances) CPT/HCPCS	MODIFIER	DIAGNOSIS CODE	$ CHARGES	DAYS OR UNITS	EPSDT Family Plan	EMG	COB	RESERVED FOR LOCAL USE
MM	DD	YY	MM	DD	YY										
1															
2															
3															
4															
5															
6															

25. FEDERAL TAX I.D. NUMBER   SSN EIN   26. PATIENT'S ACCOUNT NO.   27. ACCEPT ASSIGNMENT? (For govt. claims, see back)   YES   NO   28. TOTAL CHARGE $ 29. AMOUNT PAID $ 30. BALANCE DUE $

31. SIGNATURE OF PHYSICIAN OR SUPPLIER INCLUDING DEGREES OR CREDENTIALS (I certify that the statements on the reverse apply to this bill and are made a part thereof.)   SIGNED   DATE   32. NAME AND ADDRESS OF FACILITY WHERE SERVICES WERE RENDERED (If other than home or office)   33. PHYSICIAN'S, SUPPLIER'S BILLING NAME, ADDRESS, ZIP CODE & PHONE #   PIN#   GRP#

PHYSICIAN OR SUPPLIER INFORMATION

(APPROVED BY AMA COUNCIL ON MEDICAL SERVICE 8/88)   *PLEASE PRINT OR TYPE*   APPROVED OMB-0938-0008 FORM CMS-1500 (12-90),   FORM RRB-1500, APPROVED OMB-1215-0055 FORM OWCP-1500,   APPROVED OMB-0720-0001 (CHAMPUS)

Figure 23

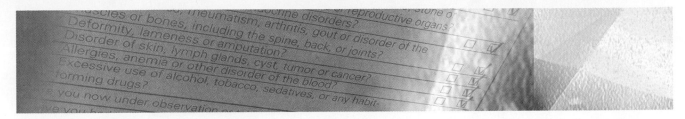

College Clinic Office Policies and Mock Fee Schedule

College Clinic

You are employed as an insurance billing specialist for an incorporated group of medical doctors, other allied health specialists, and podiatrists. These doctors are on the staff of a nearby hospital, College Hospital. Reference information to complete insurance claim forms for each assignment follows.

Office address:
  College Clinic
  4567 Broad Avenue
  Woodland Hills, XY 12345-0001
  telephone: 555-486-9002
  FAX: 555-487-8976
Group practice (employer) tax identification number:
  3664021CC
Clinic's Medicaid provider number: HSC 12345F
Medicare Durable Medical Equipment (DME) supplier
  number: 3400760001

Hospital address:
  College Hospital
  4500 Broad Avenue
  Woodland Hills, XY 12345-0001
  telephone: 555-487-6789
  FAX: 555-486-8900
Hospital provider number: 95-0731067
Hospital's Medicaid provider number: HSC43700F
Hospital's Medicare provider number: HSP43700F

College Clinic Staff

Patient records in this *Workbook* include the doctors' names, specialties, subspecialties, and physicians' identification numbers of the College Clinic staff.

Table 1. College Clinic Staff

Name	Specialty (abbreviation)	Social Security No.	State License No.	EIN No. or Federal Tax Identification No.	Medicare CMS-Assigned National Provider Identifier (NPI)*
Concha Antrum, MD	Otolaryngologist (OTO) or Ear, Nose, and Throat Specialist (ENT)	082–XX–1707	C 01602X	74–10640XX	12458977XX
Pedro Atrics, MD	Pediatrician (PD)	134–XX–7600	D 06012X	71–32061XX	37640017XX
Bertha Caesar, MD	Obstetrician and Gynecologist (OBG)	230–XX–6700	A 01817X	72–57130XX	43056757XX
Perry Cardi, MD	Internist (I) Subspecialty: Cardiovascular Disease (CD)	557–XX–9980	C 02140X	70–64217XX	67805027XX
Brady Coccidioides, MD	Internist (I) Subspecialty: Pulmonary Disease (PUD)	670–XX–0874	C 04821X	75–67321XX	64211067XX
Vera Cutis, MD	Dermatologist (D)	409–XX–8620	C 06002X	71–80561XX	70568717XX
Clarence Cutler, MD	General Surgeon (GS)	410–XX–5630	B 07600X	71–57372XX	43050047XX
Dennis Drill, DDS	Dentist	240–XX–8960	70610X	72–46503XX	74301087XX
Max Glutens, RPT	Physical Therapist (PT)	507–XX–4300	87610X	79–36500XX	65132277XX
Cosmo Graff, MD	Plastic Surgeon (PS)	452–XX–9899	C 08104X	74–60789XX	50307117XX
Malvern Grumose, MD	Pathologist (Path)	470–XX–2301	A 01602X	72–73651XX	
Gaston Input, MD	Internist (I) Subspecialty: Gastroenterologist (GE)	211–XX–6734	C 08001X	75–67210XX	32783127XX
Adam Langerhans, MD	Endocrinologist	447–XX–6720	C 06051X	60–57831XX	47680657XX
Cornell Lenser, MD	Ophthalmologist (OPH)	322–XX–8963	C 06046X	61–78941XX	54037217XX
Michael Menter, MD	Psychiatrist (P)	210–XX–5302	C 07140X	73–66577XX	67301237XX
Arthur O. Dont, DDS	Orthodontist	102–XX–4566	80530X	90–51178XX	45378247XX
Astro Parkinson, MD	Neurosurgeon (NS)	210–XX–8533	C 02600X	75–44530XX	46789377XX
Nick Pedro, DPM	Podiatrist	233–XX–4300	E 08340X	62–74109XX	54022287XX
Gerald Practon, MD	General Practitioner (GP) or Family Practitioner (FP)	123–XX–6789	C 01402X	70–34597XX	46278897XX
Walter Radon, MD	Radiologist (R)	344–XX–6540	C 05001X	95–46137XX	40037227XX
Rex Rumsey, MD	Proctologist (Proct)	337–XX–9743	C 03042X	95–32601XX	01999047XX
Sensitive E. Scott, MD	Anesthesiologist (Anes)	220–XX–5655	C 02041X	72–54203XX	99999267XX
Raymond Skeleton, MD	Orthopedist (ORS, Orthop)	432–XX–4589	C 04561X	74–65412XX	12678547XX
Gene Ulibarri, MD	Urologist (U)	990–XX–3245	C 06430X	77–86531XX	25678831XX

*Providers must begin using the NPI on May 23, 2007, except for small health plans, whose compliance date is May 23, 2008.

Abbreviations and Symbols

Abbreviations and symbols may appear on patient records, prescriptions, hospital charts, and patient ledger cards. Abbreviation styles differ, but the current trend is to omit periods in capital letter abbreviations except for doctors' academic degrees. For information on official American Hospital Association policy, refer to p. 108 in the *Handbook*. Following is a list of abbreviations and symbols used in this *Workbook* and their meanings.

Abbreviations

A	allergy
AB	antibiotics
Abdom	abdomen
abt	about
a.c.	before meals
Adj*	adjustment
adm	admit; admission; admitted
adv	advise(d)
aet	at the age of
agit	shake or stir
AgNO₃	silver nitrate
ALL	allergy
AM, a.m.	ante meridian (time—before noon)
ant	anterior
ante	before
AP	anterior-posterior; anteroposterior
approx	approximate
appt	appointment
apt	apartment
ASA	acetylsalicylic acid (aspirin)
ASAP	as soon as possible
ASCVD	arteriosclerotic cardiovascular disease
ASHD	arteriosclerotic heart disease
asst	assistant
auto	automated, automobile
AV	atrioventricular
Ba	barium (enema)
Bal/fwd*	balance forward
BE	barium enema
B/F*	balance forward; brought forward
b.i.d.	two times daily
BM	bowel movement
BMR	basal metabolic rate
BP	blood pressure
Brev	Brevital Sodium
BX, bx	biopsy
C	cervical (vertebrae); comprehensive (history/examination)
Ca, CA	cancer, carcinoma
c/a*	cash on account
CABG	coronary artery bypass graft
CAT	computed axial tomography
cau	Caucasian
CBC	complete blood count
CBS	chronic brain syndrome
cc	cubic centimeter
CC	chief complaint

chr	chronic
ck*	check
cm	centimeter
CO, c/o	complains of; care of
compl, comp	complete; comprehensive
Con, CON, Cons	consultation
Cont	continue
CPX	complete physical examination
C&R	compromise and release
Cr*	credit
C&S	culture and sensitivity
cs, CS*	cash on account
C-section	cesarean section
CT	computed or computerized tomography
CVA	cardiovascular accident; cerebrovascular accident
CXR	chest radiograph
Cysto	cystoscopy
D, d	diagnosis; detailed (history/examination); day(s)
D & C	dilatation and curettage
dc	discontinue
DC	discharge
DDS	Doctor of Dental Surgery
def*	charge deferred
Del	delivery; obstetrics and gynecology
Dg	diagnosis
dia	diameter
diag	diagnosis; diagnostic
dil	dilate (stretch, expand)
Disch	discharge
DM	diabetes mellitus
DNA	does not apply
DNS	did not show
DPM	Doctor of Podiatric Medicine
DPT	diphtheria, pertussis, and tetanus
Dr	Doctor
Dr*	debit
DRG	diagnosis-related group
Drs	dressing
DUB	dysfunctional uterine bleeding
Dx	diagnosis
E	emergency
EC*	error corrected
ECG, EKG	electrocardiogram; electrocardiograph
echo	echocardiogram; echocardiography
ED	emergency department
EDC	estimated date of confinement
EEG	electroencephalograph
EENT	eye, ear, nose, and throat
EGD	esophagogastroduodenoscopy
EKG, ECG	electrocardiogram; electrocardiograph
E/M	Evaluation and Management (*Current Procedural Terminology* code)
EMG	electromyogram
EPF	expanded problem-focused (history/examination)
epith	epithelial
ER	emergency room
Er, ER*	error corrected

---

*Bookkeeping abbreviation

ESR	erythrocyte sedimentation rate	KUB	kidneys, ureters, and bladder
est	established (patient); estimated	L	left; laboratory
Ex, exam	examination	Lab, LAB	laboratory
exc	excision	lat	lateral; pertaining to the side
Ex MO*	express money order	lbs	pound
ext	external	LC	low complexity (decision making)
24F, 28F	French (size of catheter)	LMP	last menstrual period
F	female	LS	lumbosacral
FBS	fasting blood sugar	lt	left
FH	family history	ltd	limited (office visit)
ft	foot, feet	L & W	living and well
FU	follow-up (examination)	M	medication; married
fwd*	forward	MC	moderate-complexity (decision making)
Fx	fracture	MDM	medical decision making
gb, GB	gallbladder	med	medicine
GGE	generalized glandular enlargement	mg	milligram(s)
GI	gastrointestinal	mg/dL	milligrams per deciliter
Grav, grav	gravida, a pregnant woman; used with Roman numerals (I, II, III) to indicate the number of pregnancies	MI	myocardial infarction
		micro	microscopy
		mL, ml	milliliter
GU	genitourinary	mo	month(s)
H	hospital call	MO*	money order
HA	headache	N	negative
HBP	high blood pressure	NA	not applicable
HC	hospital call or consultation; high-complexity (decision making)	NAD	no appreciable disease
		NC, N/C*	no charge
HCD	house call (day)	NEC	not elsewhere classifiable
HCN	house call (night)	neg	negative
Hct	hematocrit	NKA	no known allergies
HCVD	hypertensive cardiovascular disease	NOS	not otherwise specified
Hgb	hemoglobin	NP	new patient
hist	history	NYD	not yet diagnosed
hosp	hospital	OB, Ob-Gyn	obstetrics and gynecology
H & P	history and physical (examination)	OC	office call
hr, hrs	hour, hours	occ	occasional
h.s.	before bedtime	OD	right eye
HS	hospital surgery	ofc	office
Ht	height	OP	outpatient
HV	hospital visit	Op, op	operation
HX, hx	history	OR	operating room
HX PX	history and physical examination	orig	original
I	injection	OS	office surgery; left eye
IC	initial consultation	OV	office visit
I & D	incision and drainage	oz	ounce
I/f*	in full	PA	posterior-anterior; posteroanterior
IM	intramuscular (injection)	Pap	Papanicolaou (smear, stain, test)
imp, imp.	impression (diagnosis)	Para I	woman having borne one child
incl.	include; including	PC	present complaint
inflam	inflammation	p.c.	after meals
init	initial (office visit)	PCP	primary care physician
inj, INJ	injection	PD	permanent disability
ins, INS*	insurance	Pd, PD*	professional discount
int	internal	PE	physical examination
intermed	intermediate (office visit)	perf	performed
interpret	interpretation	PF	problem-focused (history/examination)
IUD	intrauterine device	PFT	pulmonary function test
IV	intravenous (injection)	PH	past history
IVP	intravenous pyelogram	Ph ex	physical examination
K 35	Kolman (instrument used in urology)	phys	physical
		PID	pelvic inflammatory disease

---

*Bookkeeping abbreviation

PM, p.m.	post meridian (time—after noon)	Sp gr	specific gravity
PND	postnasal drip	SQ	subcutaneous (injection)
PO, P Op	postoperative	STAT	immediately
p.o.	by mouth (per os)	strep	*Streptococcus*
post	posterior	surg	surgery
postop	postoperative	Sx	symptom(s)
PPD	purified protein derivative (such as in tuberculin test)	T	temperature
		T & A	tonsillectomy and adenoidectomy
preop	preoperative	Tb, tb	tuberculosis
prep	prepared	TD	temporary disability
PRN, p.r.n.	as necessary (pro re nata)	tech	technician
Proc	procedure	temp	temperature
Prog	prognosis	tet. tox.	tetanus toxoid
P & S	permanent and stationary	t.i.d.	three times daily
PSA	prostate-specific antigen (blood test to determine cancer in prostate gland)	TPR	temperature, pulse, and respiration
		Tr, trt	treatment
Pt, pt	patient	TURB	transurethral resection of bladder
PT	physical therapy	TURP	transurethral resection of prostate
PTR	patient to return	TX	treatment
PVC	premature ventricular contraction	u	units
PVT ck*	private check received	UA, ua	urinalysis
PX	physical examination	UCHD	usual childhood diseases
q	every	UCR	usual, customary, and reasonable (fees)
qd	one time daily, every day	UGI	upper gastrointestinal
qh	every hour	UPJ	ureteropelvic junction or joint
q.i.d.	four times daily	UR	urinalysis
QNS	insufficient quantity	URI	upper respiratory infection
qod	every other day	Urn	urinalysis
R	right; residence call; report	UTI	urinary tract infection
RBC, rbc	red blood cell (count)	W	work; white
rec	recommend	WBC, wbc	white blood cell (count); well baby care
rec'd	received	WC	workers' compensation
re ch	recheck	wk	week; work
re-exam	reexamination	wks	weeks
Reg	regular	WNL	within normal limits
ret, retn, rtn	return	Wr	Wassermann reaction (test for syphilis)
rev	review	Wt, wt	weight
RHD	rheumatic heart disease	X	-xray, x-ray(s) times (e.g., 3× means three times)
RN	registered nurse		
R/O	rule out	XR	xray, x-ray(s)
ROA*	received on account	yr(s)	year(s)
RPT	registered physical therapist		
rt	right	**Symbols**	
RTC	return to clinic		
RTO	return to office	#	pound(s)
RTW	return to work	c̄, /c	with
RX, Rx, R$_x$	prescribe; prescription; any medication or treatment ordered	s̄, /s	without
		c̄c, c̄/c	with correction (eye glasses)
S	surgery	s̄c, s̄/c	without correction (eye glasses)
SC	subcutaneous	–	negative
sched.	scheduled	ō	negative
SD	state disability	⊕	positive
SE	special examination	Ⓛ	left
SF	straightforward (decision making)	Ⓡ	right
Sig	directions on prescription	♂	male
SLR	straight leg raising	♀	female
slt	slight	–*	charge already made
Smr	smear	θ*	no balance due
SOB	shortness of breath	✓*	posted
		($0.00)*	credit

---

*Bookkeeping abbreviation

Laboratory Abbreviations

Abbreviation	*Definition*
ABG	arterial blood gas(es)
AcG	factor V (AcG or proaccelerin); a factor in coagulation that converts prothrombin to thrombin
ACTH	adrenocorticotropic hormone
AFB	acid-fast bacilli
A/C ratio	albumin-coagulin ratio
AHB	alpha-hydroxybutyric (dehydrogenase)
AHG	antihemophilic globulin; antihemolytic globulin (factor)
ALA	aminolevulinic acid
ALT	alanine aminotransferase (*see* SGPT)
AMP	adenosine monophosphate
APT test	aluminum-precipitated toxoid test
AST	aspartate aminotransferase (*see* SGOT)
ATP	adenosine triphosphate
BSP	bromsulfophthalein (Bromsulphalein; sodium sulfobromophthalein) (test)
BUN	blood urea nitrogen
CBC	complete blood count
CNS	central nervous system
CO	carbon monoxide
CPB	competitive protein binding: plasma
CPK	creatine phosphokinase
CSF	cerebrospinal fluid
D hemoglobin	hemoglobin fractionation by electrophoresis for hemoglobin D
DAP	direct agglutination pregnancy (Gravindex and DAP)
DEAE	diethylaminoethanol
DHT	dihydrotestosterone
diff	differential
DNA	deoxyribonucleic acid
DRT	test for syphilis
EACA	epsilon-aminocaproic acid (a fibrinolysin)
EMIT	enzyme-multiplied immunoassay technique (for drugs)
ENA	extractable nuclear antigen
esr, ESR	erythrocyte sedimentation (sed) rate
FDP	fibrin degradation products
FIGLU	formiminoglutamic acid
FRAT	free radical assay technique (for drugs)
FSH	follicle-stimulating hormone
FSP	fibrinogen split products
FTA	fluorescent-absorbed treponema antibodies
Gc, Gm, Inv	immunoglobulin typing
GG, gamma G, A, D, G, M	gamma-globulin (immunoglobulin fractionation by electrophoresis)
GG, gamma G E, RIA	immunization E fractionation by radioimmunoassay
GGT	gamma-glutamyl transpeptidase
GLC	gas liquid chromatography
GMP	guanosine monophosphate
GTT	glucose tolerance test
G6PD	glucose-6-phosphate dehydrogenase
HAA	hepatitis-associated agent (antigen)
HBD, HBDH	hydroxybutyrate dehydrogenase
HCT	hematocrit
hemoglobin, electrophoresis	letters of the alphabet used for different types or factors of hemoglobins (includes A_2, S, C, etc.)
Hgb	hemoglobin, qualitative
HGH	human growth hormone
HI	hemagglutination inhibition
HIA	hemagglutination inhibition antibody
HIAA	hydroxyindoleacetic acid (urine), 24-hour specimen
HIV	human immunodeficiency virus
HLA	human leukocyte antigen (tissue typing)

HPL	human placental lactogen
HTLV-III	antibody detection; confirmatory test
HVA	homovanillic acid
ICSH	interstitial cell–stimulating hormone
IFA	intrinsic factor, antibody (fluorescent screen)
IgA, IgE, IgG, IgM	immunoglobulins: quantitative by gel diffusion
INH	isonicotinic hydrazide, isoniazid
LAP	leucine aminopeptidase
LATS	long-acting thyroid-stimulating (hormone)
LDH	lactic dehydrogenase
LE Prep	lupus erythematosus cell preparation
L.E. factor	antinuclear antibody
LH	luteinizing hormone
LSD	lysergic acid diethylamide
L/S ratio	lecithin-sphingomyelin ratio
MC (*Streptococcus*)	antibody titer
MIC	minimum inhibitory concentration
NBT	nitro-blue tetrazolium (test)
OCT	ornithine carbamyl transferase
PAH	para-aminohippuric acid
PBI	protein-bound iodine
pCO_2	arterial carbon dioxide pressure (or tension)
PCP	phencyclidine piperidine
pcv	packed cell volume
pH	symbol for expression of concentration of hydrogen ions (degree of acidity)
PHA	phenylalanine
PIT	prothrombin inhibition test
PKU	phenylketonuria—a metabolic disease affecting mental development
Po_2	oxygen pressure
P & P	prothrombin-proconvertin
PSP	phenolsulfonphthalein
PT	prothrombin time
PTA	plasma thromboplastin antecedent
PTC	plasma thromboplastin component; phenylthiocarbamide
PTT	prothrombin time; partial thromboplastin time (plasma or whole blood)
RBC, rbc	red blood cells (count)
RIA	radioimmunoassay
RISA	radioiodinated human serum albumin
RIST	radioimmunosorbent test
RPR	rapid plasma reagin (test)
RT_3U	resin triiodothyronine uptake
S-D	strength-duration (curve)
SGOT	serum glutamic oxaloacetic transaminase (*see* AST)
SGPT	serum glutamic pyruvic transaminase (*see* ALT)
STS	serologic test for syphilis
T_3	triiodothyronine (uptake)
TB	tubercle bacillus, tuberculosis
TBG	thyroxine-binding globulin
T & B differentiation, lymphocytes	thymus-dependent lymphs and bursa-dependent lymphs
THC	tetrahydrocannabinol (marijuana)
TIBC	total iron-binding capacity, chemical
TLC screen	thin-layer chromatography screen
TRP	tubular reabsorption of phosphates
UA	urinalysis
VDRL	Venereal Disease Research Laboratory (agglutination test for syphilis)
VMA	vanillylmandelic acid
WBC, wbc	white blood cells (count)

Mock Fee Schedule

Refer to the mock fee schedule (Table 2) to complete the financial accounting statements (ledgers) and claim forms in this *Workbook*. The fees listed are hypothetical and are intended only for use in completing the questions. For the cases that are private, Medicaid, TRICARE, and workers' compensation, use the amounts in the column labeled Mock Fees. For Medicare cases, refer to the three columns pertaining to Medicare and use the amounts in the column labeled Limiting Charge. Follow these instructions unless your instructor wishes you to round out the amounts on the fee schedule to the next dollar.

In a real medical practice, some offices round out the amounts to the next dollar unless the physician is nonparticipating with Medicare and then by Medicare regulations the provider can only bill the exact limiting amount. Other offices may have two fee schedules. Schedule B is for Medicare participating physicians and amounts are listed in dollars and cents. Schedule A is used for other plans and the amounts are rounded to the next dollar. However, if a fee schedule is sent by the insurance plan, then the medical practice may use the dollars and cents provided.

When completing the insurance claim forms, use the latest edition of *Current Procedural Terminology* (CPT), the professional code book published by the American Medical Association, to find the correct code numbers and modifiers for the services rendered. If you do not have access to the latest edition of CPT, you may use the code numbers provided in the mock fee schedule; however, do so with the understanding that the code numbers and descriptions provided in this schedule are not comprehensive. They are based on the information found in CPT; however, students are cautioned not to use it as a substitute for CPT. Because the code numbers are subject to change, every medical office must have on hand the most recent edition of CPT.

The mock fee schedule (Tables 2 and 3) is arranged in the same sequence as the six CPT code book sections (i.e., Evaluation and Management; Anesthesia; Surgery; Radiology, Nuclear Medicine, and Diagnostic Ultrasound; Pathology and Laboratory; and Medicine), with a comprehensive list of modifiers placed at the beginning. An index at the end of the mock fee schedule can assist you in locating code numbers. Mock fees for the modifiers are not listed, because these can vary from one claim to another, depending on the circumstances.

Remember that fees can vary with the region of the United States (West, Midwest, South, East), the specialty of the practitioner, the type of community (urban, suburban, or rural), the type of practice (incorporated or unincorporated, solo, partners, or shareholders), the overhead, and a number of other factors.

TABLE 2. College Clinic Mock Fee Schedule

Modifier Code Number	Description	Mock Fee ($)
-21	*Prolonged Evaluation and Management Services:* When the face-to-face or floor/unit service(s) provided is prolonged or otherwise greater than that usually required for the highest level of evaluation and management service within a given category, it may be identified by adding modifier -21 to the evaluation and management code number. A report may also be appropriate.	Increase fee
-22	*Unusual Services:* When the service(s) provided is greater than that usually required for the listed procedure, it may be identified by adding modifier -22 to the usual procedure code number. A report may also be appropriate.	Increase fee
-23	*Unusual Anesthesia:* Occasionally a procedure that usually requires either no anesthesia or local anesthesia must be done under general anesthesia because of unusual circumstances. These circumstances may be reported by adding the modifier -23 to the procedure code number of the basic service.	Increase fee
-24	*Unrelated Evaluation and Management Service by the Same Physician During a Postoperative Period:* The physician may need to indicate that an evaluation and management service was performed during a postoperative period for a reason(s) unrelated to the original procedure. This circumstance may be reported by adding the modifier -24 to the appropriate level of E/M service.	Variable per E/M fee
-25	*Significant, Separately Identifiable Evaluation and Management Service by the Same Physician on the Same Day of a Procedure or Other Service:* The physician may need to indicate that on the day a procedure or service identified by a CPT code was performed, the patient's condition required a significant, separately identifiable E/M service above and beyond the other service provided or beyond the usual preoperative and postoperative care associated with the procedure that was performed. The E/M service may be prompted by the symptom or condition for which the procedure and/or service was provided. As such, different diagnoses are not required for reporting of the	Variable per E/M fee

---

TABLE 2. College Clinic Mock Fee Schedule—cont'd

Modifier Code Number	Description	Mock Fee ($)
	E/M services on the same date. This circumstance may be reported by adding the modifier -25 to the appropriate level of E/M service. **NOTE:** This modifier is not used to report an E/M service that resulted in a decision to perform surgery. See modifier -57.	
-26	*Professional Component:* Certain procedures are a combination of a physician component and a technical component. When the physician component is reported separately, the service may be identified by adding the modifier -26 to the usual procedure code number	Decrease fee
-27	*Multiple Outpatient Hospital E/M Encounters on the Same Date:* For hospital outpatient reporting purposes, utilization of hospital resources related to separate and distinct E/M encounters performed in multiple outpatient hospital settings on the same date may be reported by adding the modifier -27 to each appropriate level outpatient and/or emergency department E/M code(s). This modifier provides a means of reporting circumstances involving E/M services provided by physician(s) in more than one (multiple) outpatient hospital setting(s) (e.g., hospital emergency department, clinic). Do not use this modifier for physician reporting of multiple E/M services performed by the same physician on the same date. See E/M, emergency department, or preventive medicine services codes.	Variable
-32	*Mandated Services:* Services related to mandated consultation and/or related services (e.g., PRO, third party payer) may be identified by adding the modifier -32 to the basic procedure.	Use standard fee
-47	*Anesthesia by Surgeon:* Regional or general anesthesia provided by the surgeon may be reported by adding the modifier -47 to the basic service or by using the separate five-digit modifier code number 09947 (this does not include local anesthesia). **NOTE:** Modifier -47 or code number 09947 would not be used as a modifier for the anesthesia procedures 00100 through 01999.	Increase fee
-50	*Bilateral Procedure:* Unless otherwise identified in the listings, bilateral procedures that are performed at the same operative session should be identified by the appropriate five-digit code number describing the first procedure. The second (bilateral) procedure is identified either by adding modifier -50 to the procedure code number.	Paid at 50% of standard fee
-51	*Multiple Procedures:* When multiple procedures other than E/M services are performed at the same session by the same provider, the primary procedure or service may be reported as listed. The additional procedure(s) or service(s) may be identified by adding the modifier -51 to the additional procedure or service code(s). **NOTE:** This modifier should not be appended to designated "add-on" codes.	Second procedure usually paid at 50% of fee. Third procedure usually paid at 25% of fee. Fourth and subsequent procedures usually paid at 10% of fee.
-52	*Reduced Services:* Under certain circumstances a service or procedure is partially reduced or eliminated at the physician's discretion. Under these circumstances, the service provided can be identified by its usual procedure number and the addition of the modifier -52, signifying that the service is reduced. This provides a means of reporting reduced services without disturbing the identification of the basic service. Modifier code 09952 may be used as an alternative to modifier -52. **NOTE:** For hospital outpatient reporting of a previously scheduled procedure/service that is partially reduced or canceled as a result of extenuating circumstances or those that threaten the well-being of the patient before or after administration of anesthesia, see modifiers -73 and -74.	Decrease fee
-53	*Discontinued Procedure:* Under certain circumstances, the physician may elect to terminate a surgical or diagnostic procedure. Due to extenuating circumstances or those that threaten the well-being of the patient, it may be necessary to indicate that a surgical or diagnostic procedure was started but discontinued. This circumstance may be reported by adding modifier -53 to the code reported by the physician for the discontinued procedure. **NOTE:** This modifier is not used to report the elective cancellation of a procedure before the patient's anesthesia induction and/or surgical preparation in the operating suite. For outpatient hospital/ambulatory surgery center (ASC) reporting of a	Decrease fee

Continued

TABLE 2. College Clinic Mock Fee Schedule—cont'd

Modifier Code Number	Description	Mock Fee ($)
	previously scheduled procedure/service that is partially reduced or canceled as a result of extenuating circumstances or those that threaten the well-being of the patient before or after administration of anesthesia, see modifiers -73 and -74 (see modifiers approved for ASC hospital outpatient use).	
-54	*Surgical Care Only:* When one physician performs a surgical procedure and another provides preoperative and/or postoperative management, surgical services may be identified by adding the modifier -54 to the usual procedure number.	Decrease fee
-55	*Postoperative Management Only:* When one physician performs the postoperative management and another physician performs the surgical procedure, the postoperative component may be identified by adding modifier -55 to the usual procedure number.	Decrease fee
-56	*Preoperative Management Only:* When one physician performs the preoperative care and evaluation and another physician performs the surgical procedure, the preoperative component may be identified by adding the modifier -56 to the usual procedure number.	Decrease fee
-57	*Decision for Surgery:* An evaluation and management service that resulted in the initial decision to perform the surgery may be identified by adding the modifier -57 to the appropriate level of E/M service.	Use standard fee
-58	*Staged or Related Procedure or Service by the Same Physician During the Postoperative Period:* The physician may need to indicate that the performance of a procedure or service during the postoperative period was: (a) planned prospectively at the time of the original procedure (staged); (b) more extensive than the original procedure; or (c) for therapy following a diagnostic surgical procedure. This circumstance may be reported by adding the modifier -58 to the staged or related procedure. **NOTE:** This modifier is not used to report the treatment of a problem that requires a return to the operating room. See modifier -78.	Variable
-59	*Distinct Procedural Service:* Under certain circumstances, the physician may need to indicate that a procedure or service was distinct or independent from other services performed on the same day. Modifier -59 is used to identify procedures/services that are not normally reported together, but are appropriate under the circumstances. This may represent a different session or patient encounter, different procedure or surgery, different site or organ system, separate incision/excision, separate lesion, or separate injury (or area of injury in extensive injuries) not ordinarily encountered or performed on the same day by the same physician. However, when another already established modifier is appropriate it should be used rather than modifier -59. Only if no more descriptive modifier is available, and the use of modifier -59 best explains the circumstances, should modifier -59 be used.	Variable
-62	*Two Surgeons:* Under certain circumstances the skills of two surgeons (usually with different skills) may be required in the management of a specific surgical procedure. Under such circumstances the separate services may be identified by adding the modifier -62 to the procedure number used by each surgeon for reporting his or her services. **NOTE:** If a co-surgeon acts as an assistant in the performance of additional procedure(s) during the same surgical session, those services may be reported using separate procedure code(s) with the modifier -80 or modifier -81 added, as appropriate.	Use standard fee
-63	*Procedure Performed on Infants less than 4 kg:* Procedures performed on neonates and infants up to a present body weight of 4 kg may involve significantly increased complexity and physician work commonly associated with these patients. This circumstance may be reported by adding the modifier -63 to the procedure number.	
-66	*Surgical Team:* Under some circumstances, highly complex procedures (requiring the concomitant services of several physicians, often of different specialties, plus other highly skilled, specially trained personnel and various types of complex equipment) are carried out under the "surgical team" concept. Such circumstances may be identified by each participating physician with the addition of the modifier -66 to the basic procedure code number used for reporting services.	Variable
-73	*Discontinued Outpatient Hospital/Ambulatory Surgery Center (ASC) Procedure Prior to the Administration of Anesthesia:* Due to extenuating circumstances or those that threaten	Decrease fee

TABLE 2. College Clinic Mock Fee Schedule—cont'd

Modifier Code Number	Description	Mock Fee ($)
	the well-being of the patient, the physician may cancel a surgical or diagnostic procedure subsequent to the patient's surgical preparation (including sedation when provided, and being taken to the room where the procedure is to be performed), but before the administration of anesthesia (local, regional block[s] or general). Under these circumstances, the intended service that is prepared for but canceled can be reported by its usual procedure number and the addition of the modifier -73. NOTE: The elective cancellation of a service before the administration of anesthesia and/or surgical preparation of the patient should not be reported. For physician reporting of a discontinued procedure, see modifier -53.	
-74	*Discontinued Outpatient Hospital/Ambulatory Surgery Center (ASC) Procedure After Administration of Anesthesia:* Due to extenuating circumstances or those that threaten the well-being of the patient, the physician may terminate a surgical or diagnostic procedure after the administration of anesthesia (local, regional block[s] or general) or after the procedure was started (e.g., incision made, intubation started, scope inserted). Under these circumstances, the procedure started but terminated can be reported by its usual procedure number and the addition of the modifier -74. NOTE: The elective cancellation of a service before the administration of anesthesia and/or surgical preparation of the patient should not be reported. For physician reporting of a discontinued procedure, see modifier -53.	Decrease fee
-76	*Repeat Procedure by Same Physician:* The physician may need to indicate that a procedure or service was repeated subsequent to the original procedure or service. This circumstance may be reported by adding modifier -76 to the repeated service/procedure.	Decrease fee
-77	*Repeat Procedure by Another Physician:* The physician may need to indicate that a basic procedure or service performed by another physician had to be repeated. This situation may be reported by adding modifier -77 to the repeated procedure/service.	Decrease fee
-78	*Return to the Operating Room for a Related Procedure During the Postoperative Period:* The physician may need to indicate that another procedure was performed during the postoperative period of the initial procedure. When this subsequent procedure is related to the first and requires the use of the operating room, it may be reported by adding the modifier -78 to the related procedure. (For repeat procedures on the same day, see -76.)	Decrease fee
-79	*Unrelated Procedure or Service by the Same Physician During the Postoperative Period:* The physician may need to indicate that the performance of a procedure or service during the postoperative period was unrelated to the original procedure. This circumstance may be reported by using the modifier -79. (For repeat procedures on the same day, see -76.)	Use standard fee
-80	*Assistant Surgeon:* Surgical assistant services may be identified by adding the modifier -80 to the usual procedure number(s).	Billed and/or paid at approximately 20% of surgeon's fee
-81	*Minimum Assistant Surgeon:* Minimum surgical assistant services are identified by adding the modifier -81 to the usual procedure number.	Billed and/or paid at approximately 10% of surgeon's fee
-82	*Assistant Surgeon when qualified resident surgeon not available:* The unavailability of a qualified resident surgeon is a prerequisite for use of modifier -82 appended to the usual procedure code number(s).	Decrease fee
-90	*Reference (Outside) Laboratory:* When laboratory procedures are performed by a party other than the treating or reporting physician and billed by the treating physician, the procedure may be identified by adding the modifier -90 to the usual procedure number.	Fee according to contract
-91	*Repeat Clinical Diagnostic Laboratory Test:* In the course of treatment of the patient, it may be necessary to repeat the same laboratory test on the same day to obtain subsequent (multiple) test results. Under these circumstances, the laboratory test performed can be identified by its usual procedure number and the addition of modifier -91. NOTE: This modifier may not be used when tests are rerun to confirm initial results; due to testing problems with specimens or equipment; or for any other reason when a normal, one-time, reportable result is all that is required. This modifier may not be used when	Decrease fee

Continued

TABLE 2. College Clinic Mock Fee Schedule—cont'd

Modifier Code Number	Description	Mock Fee ($)
	other code(s) describe a series of test results (e.g., glucose tolerance tests, evocative/suppression testing). This modifier may only be used for laboratory test(s) performed more than once on the same day on the same patient.	
-99	*Multiple Modifiers:* Under certain circumstances two or more modifiers may be necessary to completely delineate a service. In such situations modifier -99 should be added to the basic procedure, and other applicable modifiers may be listed as part of the description of the service.	Variable

TABLE 3. Mock Fee Schedule

Code Number and Description		Mock Fees	Medicare* Participating	Nonparticipating	Limiting Charge
EVALUATION AND MANAGEMENT†					
Office					
New Patient					
99201	Level 1	33.25	30.43	28.91	33.25
99202	Level 2	51.91	47.52	45.14	51.91
99203	Level 3	70.92	64.92	61.67	70.92
99204	Level 4	106.11	97.13	92.27	106.11
99205	Level 5	132.28	121.08	115.03	132.38
Established Patient					
99211	Level 1	16.07	14.70	13.97	16.07
99212	Level 2	28.55	26.14	24.83	28.55
99213	Level 3	40.20	36.80	34.96	40.20
99214	Level 4	61.51	56.31	53.79	61.51
99215	Level 5	96.97	88.76	84.32	96.97
Hospital					
Observation Services (new or established patient)					
99217	Discharge	66.88	61.22	58.16	66.88
99218	Dhx/exam SF/LC DM	74.22	67.94	64.54	74.22
99219	Chx/exam MC DM	117.75	107.78	102.39	117.75
99220	Chx/exam HC DM	147.48	134.99	128.24	147.48
Inpatient Services (new or established patient)					
99221	30 min	73.00	66.84	63.48	73.00
99222	50 min	120.80	110.57	105.04	120.80
99223	70 min	152.98	140.03	133.03	152.98
Subsequent Hospital Care					
99231	15 min	37.74	34.55	32.82	37.74
99232	25 min	55.56	50.85	48.31	55.56
99233	35 min	76.97	70.45	66.93	76.97
99238	Discharge	65.26	59.74	56.75	65.26

*Some services and procedures may not be considered a benefit under the Medicare program and when listed on a claim form, no reimbursement may be received. However, it is important to include these codes when billing because Medicare policies may change without an individual knowing of a new benefit. For this reason, some of the services shown in this mock fee schedule do not have any amounts listed under the three Medicare columns.
†See Tables 5-1 and 5-2 in the *Handbook* for more descriptions of E/M codes 99201 through 99275.

TABLE 3. Mock Fee Schedule—cont'd

		Medicare*		
Code Number and Description	**Mock Fees**	**Participating**	**Nonparticipating**	**Limiting Charge**
Consultations				
Office (new or established patient)				
99241 Level 1	51.93	47.54	45.16	51.93
99242 Level 2	80.24	73.44	69.77	80.24
99243 Level 3	103.51	94.75	90.01	103.51
99244 Level 4	145.05	132.77	126.13	145.05
99245 Level 5	195.48	178.93	169.98	195.45
Inpatient (new or established patient)				
99251 Level 1	53.29	48.78	46.34	53.29
99252 Level 2	80.56	73.74	70.05	80.56
99253 Level 3	106.10	97.12	92.26	106.10
99254 Level 4	145.26	132.96	126.31	145.26
99255 Level 5	196.55	179.91	170.91	196.55
Follow-up Inpatient (new or established patient)				
99261 Focused	29.66	27.15	25.79	29.66
99262 Expanded	50.57	46.28	43.97	50.57
99263 Detailed	76.36	69.90	66.40	76.36
Confirmatory Second or Third Opinion (new or established patient)				
99271 Focused	45.47	41.62	39.54	45.47
99272 Expanded	67.02	61.35	58.28	67.02
99273 Detailed	95.14	87.08	82.73	95.14
99274 Comprehensive	125.15	114.56	108.83	125.15
99275 Comprehensive	172.73	158.10	150.20	172.73
Emergency Department (new/established patient)				
99281 PF hx/exam SF DM	24.32	22.26	21.15	24.32
99282 EPF hx/exam LC DM	37.02	33.88	32.19	37.02
99283 EPF hx/exam MC DM	66.23	60.62	57.59	66.23
99284 D hx/exam MC DM	100.71	92.18	87.57	100.71
99285 C hx/exam HC DM	158.86	145.41	138.14	158.86
Critical Care Services				
99291 First hour	208.91	191.22	181.66	208.91
99292 Each addl. 30 min	102.02	92.46	87.84	102.02
Neonatal Intensive Care				
99295 Initial	892.74	817.16	776.30	892.74
99296 Subsequent unstable case	418.73	383.27	364.11	418.73
Nursing Facility				
99301 30 min	64.11	58.68	55.75	64.11
99302 40 min	90.55	82.88	78.74	90.55
99303 50 min	136.76	125.18	118.92	136.76
Subsequent (new/established patient)				
99311 15 min	37.95	34.74	33.00	37.95
99312 25 min	55.11	50.44	47.92	55.11
99313 35 min	69.61	63.72	60.53	69.61
Domiciliary, Rest Home, Custodial Care				
New Patient				
99321 PF hx/exam LC DM	46.10	42.20	40.09	46.10
99322 EPF hx/exam MC DM	65.02	59.53	56.54	65.02
99323 D hx/exam HC DM	86.18	78.88	74.94	86.18

*Some services and procedures may not be considered a benefit under the Medicare program and when listed on a claim form, no reimbursement may be received. However, it is important to include these codes when billing because Medicare policies may change without an individual knowing of a new benefit. For this reason, some of the services shown in this mock fee schedule do not have any amounts listed under the three Medicare columns.

Continued

TABLE 3. Mock Fee Schedule—cont'd

Code Number and Description		Mock Fees	Medicare*		
			Participating	Nonparticipating	Limiting Charge
Established Patient					
99331	PF hx/exam LC DM	37.31	34.15	32.44	37.31
99332	EPF hx/exam MC DM	49.22	45.05	42.80	49.22
99333	D hx/exam HC DM	60.61	55.47	52.70	60.61
Home Services					
New Patient					
99341	PF hx/exam SF DM	70.32	64.37	61.15	70.32
99342	EPF hx/exam LC DM	91.85	84.07	79.87	91.85
99343	D hx/exam MC DM	120.24	110.06	104.56	120.24
Established Patient					
99347	PF hx/exam SF DM	54.83	50.19	47.68	54.83
99348	EPF hx/exam LC DM	70.06	64.13	60.92	70.06
99349	D hx/exam MC DM	88.33	80.85	76.81	88.33
Prolonged Services with Contact					
Outpatient					
99354	First hour	96.97	88.76	84.32	96.97
99355	Each addl. 30 min	96.97	88.76	84.32	96.97
Inpatient					
99356	First hour	96.42	88.25	83.84	96.42
99357	Each addl. 30 min	96.42	88.25	83.84	96.42
Prolonged Services Without Direct Contact					
99358	First hour	90.00			
99359	Each addl. 30 min	90.00			
Physician Standby Service					
99360	Each 30 min	95.00			
Case Management Services					
Team Conferences					
99361		85.00			
99362		105.00			
Telephone Calls					
99371	Simple or brief	30.00			
99372	Intermediate	40.00			
99373	Complex	60.00			
Care Plan Oversight Services					
99375	30 min or more	93.40	85.49	81.22	93.40
Preventive Medicine					
New Patient					
99381	Infant younger than 1 year	50.00			
99382	1-4 years	50.00			
99383	5-11 years	45.00			
99384	12-17 years	45.00			
99385	18-39 years	50.00			
99386	40-64 years	50.00			
99387	65 years and older	55.00			
Established Patient					
99391	Infant younger than year	35.00			
99392	1-4 years	35.00			
99393	5-11 years	30.00			
99394	12-17 years	30.00			

*Some services and procedures may not be considered a benefit under the Medicare program and when listed on a claim form, no reimbursement may be received. However, it is important to include these codes when billing because Medicare policies may change without an individual knowing of a new benefit. For this reason, some of the services shown in this mock fee schedule do not have any amounts listed under the three Medicare columns.

TABLE 3. Mock Fee Schedule—cont'd

			Medicare*		
Code Number and Description		**Mock Fees**	**Participating**	**Nonparticipating**	**Limiting Charge**
99395	18-39 years	35.00			
99396	40-64 years	35.00			
99397	65 years and older	40.00			
Counseling (new/est pt)					
Individual					
99401	15 min	35.00			
99402	30 min	50.00			
99403	45 min	65.00			
99404	60 min	80.00			
Group					
99411	30 min	30.00			
99412	60 min	50.00			
Other preventive medicine services					
99420	Health hazard appraisal	50.00			
99429	Unlisted preventive med serv	variable			
Newborn Care					
99431	Birthing room delivery	102.50	93.50	88.83	102.15
99432	Other than birthing room	110.16	100.83	95.79	110.16
99433	Subsequent hospital care	54.02	49.44	46.97	54.02
99440	Newborn resuscitation	255.98	234.30	222.59	255.98
99499	Unlisted E/M service	variable			

Anesthesiology

Anesthesiology fees are presented here for CPT codes. However, each case would require a fee for time, e.g., every 15 minutes would be worth $55. This fee is determined according to the relative value system, calculated, and added into the anesthesia (CPT) fee. Some anesthetists may list a surgical code using an anesthesia modifier on a subsequent line for carriers that do not acknowledge anesthesia codes.

99100	Anes for pt younger than 1 yr or older than 70 years	55.00			
99116	Anes complicated use total hypothermia	275.00			
99135	Anes complicated use hypotension	275.00			
99140	Anes complicated emer cond	110.00			
Physician Status Modifier Codes					
P-1	Normal healthy patient	00.00			
P-2	Patient with mild systemic disease	00.00			
P-3	Patient with severe systemic disease	55.00			
P-4	Patient with severe systemic (disease constant threat to life)	110.00			

*Some services and procedures may not be considered a benefit under the Medicare program and when listed on a claim form, no reimbursement may be received. However, it is important to include these codes when billing because Medicare policies may change without an individual knowing of a new benefit. For this reason, some of the services shown in this mock fee schedule do not have any amounts listed under the three Medicare columns.

Continued

TABLE 3. Mock Fee Schedule—cont'd

Code Number and Description		Mock Fees	Medicare*		
			Participating	Nonparticipating	Limiting Charge
P-5	Moribund pt not expected to survive for 24 hr with or without operation	165.00			
P-6	Declared brain-dead pt, organs being removed for donor	00.00			
Head					
00160	Anes for proc nose & accessory sinuses: NOS	275.00			
00172	Anes repair cleft palate	165.00			
Thorax					
00400	Anes for proc ant integumentary system of chest, incl SC tissue	165.00			
00402	Anes breast reconstruction	275.00			
00546	Anes pulmonary resection with thoracoplasty	275.00			
00600	Anes cervical spine and cord	550.00			
Lower Abdomen					
00800	Anes for proc lower ant abdominal wall	165.00			
00840	Anes intraperitoneal proc lower abdomen: NOS	330.00			
00842	Amniocentesis	220.00			
00914	Anes TURP	275.00			
00942	Anes colporrhaphy, colpotomy, colpectomy	220.00			
Upper Leg					
01210	Anes open proc hip joint; NOS	330.00			
01214	Total hip replacement	440.00			
Upper Arm and Elbow					
01740	Anes open proc humerus/ elbow; NOS	220.00			
01758	Exc cyst/tumor humerus	275.00			
Radiologic Procedures					
01922	Anes CAT scan	385.00			
Miscellaneous Procedure(s)					
01999	Unlisted anes proc	variable			
Neurology					
95812	Electroencephalogram	129.32	118.37	112.45	129.32
95819	Electroencephalogram— awake and asleep	126.81	116.07	110.27	126.81
95860	Electromyography, 1 extremity	88.83	81.31	77.24	88.83
95864	Electromyography, 4 extremities	239.99	219.67	208.69	239.99
96100	Psychological testing (per hour)	80.95	74.10	70.39	80.95

*Some services and procedures may not be considered a benefit under the Medicare program and when listed on a claim form, no reimbursement may be received. However, it is important to include these codes when billing because Medicare policies may change without an individual knowing of a new benefit. For this reason, some of the services shown in this mock fee schedule do not have any amounts listed under the three Medicare columns.

TABLE 3. Mock Fee Schedule—cont'd

Code Number and Description		Mock Fees	Medicare*		
			Participating	Nonparticipating	Limiting Charge
Physical Medicine					
97024	Diathermy	14.27	13.06	12.41	14.27
97036	Hubbard tank, each 15 min	24.77	22.67	21.54	24.77
97110	Physical therapy, initial 30 min	23.89	21.86	20.77	23.89
97140	Manual therapy (manipulation, traction), one or more regions, each 15 min	16.93	15.49	14.72	16.93
Special Services and Reports					
99000	Handling of specimen (transfer from Dr.'s office to lab)	5.00			
99025	Initial surg eval (new pt) with starred procedure	50.00			
99050	Services requested after office hours in addition to basic service	25.00			
99052	Services between 10 p.m. and 8 a.m. in addition to basic service	35.00			
99054	Services on Sundays and holidays in addition to basic service	35.00			
99056	Services normally provided in office requested by pt in location other than office	20.00			
99058	Office services provided on an emergency basis	65.00			
99070	Supplies and materials (itemize drugs and materials provided)	25.00			
99080	Special reports:				
	Insurance forms	10.00			
	Review of data to clarify pt's status	20.00			
	WC reports	50.00			
	WC extensive review report	250.00			

*Some services and procedures may not be considered a benefit under the Medicare program and when listed on a claim form, no reimbursement may be received. However, it is important to include these codes when billing because Medicare policies may change without an individual knowing of a new benefit. For this reason, some of the services shown in this mock fee schedule do not have any amounts listed under the three Medicare columns.

Continued

618   *Appendix A*   Collogo Clinic Office Policies and Mock Fee Schedule

TABLE 3. Mock Fee Schedule—cont'd

Code Number and Description		Mock Fees	Medicare*			
			Participating	Non Participating	Limiting Charge	Follow-up Days†
10060*	I & D furuncle, onychia, paronychia; single	75.92	69.49	66.02	75.92	10
11040	Debridement; skin, partial thickness	79.32	75.60	68.97	79.32	10
11044	Debridement; skin, subcu. muscle, bone	269.28	246.48	234.16	269.28	
11100	Biopsy of skin, SC tissue &/or mucous membrane; 1 lesion	65.43	59.89	56.90	65.43	10
11200*	Exc, skin tags; up to 15	55.68	50.97	45.42	55.68	10
11401	Exc, benign lesion, 0.6–1.0 cm trunk, arms, legs	95.62	87.53	8315	96.62	10
11402	1.1–2.0 cm	121.52	111.23	105.67	121.52	10
11403	2.1–3.0 cm	151.82	138.97	132.02	151.82	10
11420	Exc, benign lesion, 0.5 cm or less scalp, neck, hands, feet, genitalia	75.44	69.05	65.60	75.44	10
11422	Exc, benign lesion scalp, neck, hands, feet, or genitalia; 1.1–2.0 cm	131.35	120.23	114.22	131.35	10
11441	Exc, benign lesion face, ears, eyelids, nose, lips, or mucous membrane; 0.6–1.0 cm dia or less	119.08	109.00	103.55	119.08	10
11602	Exc, malignant lesion, trunk, arms, or legs; 1.1–2.0 cm dia	195.06	178.55	169.62	195.06	10
11719	Trimming of nondystrophic nails, any number	30.58	27.82	26.33	30.58	0
11720*	Debridement of nails, any method, 1–5	32.58	29.82	28.33	32.58	0
11721*	6 or more	32.58	29.82	28.33	32.58	0
11730*	Avulsion nail plate, partial or complete, simple repair; single	76.91	70.40	66.88	76.91	0
11750	Exc, nail or nail matrix, partial or complete	193.45	177.07	168.22	193.45	10
11765	Wedge excision of nail fold	57.95	53.04	50.39	57.95	10
12001*	Simple repair (scalp, neck, axillae, ext genitalia, trunk, or extremities incl hands & feet); 2.5 cm or less	91.17	83.45	79.28	91.17	10
12011*	Simple repair (face, ears, eyelids, nose, lips, or mucous membranes); 2.5 cm or less	101.44	92.85	88.21	101.44	10
12013*	2.6–5.0 cm	123.98	113.48	107.81	123.98	10
12032*	Repair, scalp, axillae, trunk (intermediate)	169.73	155.36	147.59	169.73	10
12034	Repair, intermediate, layer closure of wounds (scalp, axillae, trunk, or extremities) excl hands or feet; 7.6–12.5 cm	214.20	196.06	186.26	214.20	10
12051*	Repair, intermediate, layer closure of wounds (face, ears, eyelids, nose, lips, or mucous membranes); 2.5 cm	167.60	153.41	145.74	167.60	10
17000*	Cauterization, 1 lesion	52.56	48.11	45.70	52.56	10
17003	Second through 14 lesions, each	15.21	17.77	16.88	15.21	10
17100*	Destruction, any method, skin lesion (benign) any area except face—one	44.86	41.06	39.01	44.86	10
17004	Destruction (laser surgery), 15 or more lesions	52.56	48.11	45.70	52.56	10

*Codes marked with an asterisk appear in *CPT* marked as shown. See *Handbook* Chapter 5 for detailed information.
†Data for the surgical follow-up days from St. Anthony's *CPT '96 Companion: A Guide to Medicare Billing.*

TABLE 3. Mock Fee Schedule—cont'd

Code Number and Description		Mock Fees	Medicare*			
			Participating	Non Participating	Limiting Charge	Follow-up Days†
19020	Mastotomy, drainage/exploration deep abscess	237.36	217.26	206.40	237.36	90
19100*	Biopsy, breast, needle	96.17	88.03	83.63	96.17	0
19101	Biopsy, breast, incisional	281.51	257.67	244.79	281.51	10
20610*	Arthrocentesis, aspiration or injection joint (shoulder, hip, knee) or bursa	52.33	47.89	45.50	52.33	0
21330	Nasal fracture, open treatment complicated	599.46	548.71	521.27	599.46	90
24066	Biopsy, deep, soft tissue, upper arm, elbow	383.34	350.88	333.34	383.34	90
27455	Osteotomy, proximal tibia	1248.03	1142.36	1085.24	1248.03	90
27500	Treatment closed femoral shaft fracture without manipulation	554.90	507.92	482.52	554.90	90
27530	Treatment closed tibial fracture, proximal, without manipulation	344.24	315.09	299.34	344.24	90
27750	Treatment closed tibial shaft fracture without manipulation	400.94	366.99	348.64	400.94	90
27752	With manipulation	531.63	486.62	462.29	531.63	90
29280	Strapping of hand	35.13	31.36	29.79	35.13	0
29345	Appl long leg cast (thigh to toes)	123.23	112.80	107.16	123.23	0
29355	Walker or ambulatory type	133.75	122.42	116.30	133.75	0
29425	Appl short leg walking cast	102.10	93.45	88.78	102.10	0
30110	Excision, simple nasal polyp	145.21	132.92	126.27	145.21	10
30520	Septoplasty	660.88	604.93	574.68	660.88	90
30903*	Control nasal hemorrhage; unilateral	118.17	108.17	102.76	118.17	0
30905*	Control nasal hemorrhage, posterior with posterior nasal packs; initial	190.57	174.43	165.71	190.57	0
30906*	Subsequent	173.01	158.36	150.44	173.01	
31540	Laryngoscopy with excision of tumor and/or stripping of vocal cords	488.95	447.55	425.17	488.95	0
31541	With operating microscope	428.33	392.06	372.46	428.33	0
31575	Laryngoscopy, flexible fiberoptic; diagnostic	138.48	126.76	120.42	138.48	0
31625	Bronchoscopy with biopsy	312.87	286.38	272.06	312.87	0
32310	Pleurectomy	1234.79	1130.24	1073.73	1234.79	90
32440	Pneumonectomy, total	1972.10	1805.13	1714.87	1972.10	90
33020	Pericardiotomy	1289.25	1180.09	1121.09	1289.25	90
33206	Insertion of pacemaker; atrial	728.42	666.75	633.41	728.42	90
33208	AV sequential	751.57	687.89	653.50	751.57	90
35301	Thromboendarterectomy, with or without patch graft; carotid, vertebral, subclavian, by neck incision	1585.02	1450.82	1378.28	1585.02	90
36005	Intravenous injection for contrast venography	59.18	54.17	51.46	59.18	0
36248	Catheter placement (selective) arterial system, 2nd, 3rd and beyond	68.54	62.74	59.60	68.54	0
36415*	Routine venipuncture for collection of specimen(s)	10.00	—	—	—	XXX
38101	Splenectomy, partial	994.44	910.24	864.73	994.44	90
38510	Biopsy/excision deep cervical node/s	327.42	299.69	284.71	327.42	90
39520	Excision tumor, mediastinal	1436.50	1314.87	1249.13	1436.50	90
42820	T & A under age 12 years	341.63	312.71	297.07	341.63	90
42821	T & A over age 12 years	410.73	375.96	357.16	410.73	90

*Codes marked with an asterisk appear in *CPT* marked as shown. See *Handbook* Chapter 5 for detailed information.
†Data for the surgical follow-up days from St. Anthony's *CPT '96 Companion: A Guide to Medicare Billing*.

Continued

TABLE 3. Mock Fee Schedule—cont'd

Code Number and Description		Mock Fees	Medicare*			
			Participating	Non Participating	Limiting Charge	Follow-up Days†
43234	Upper GI endoscopy, simple primary exam	201.86	184.77	175.53	201.86	0
43235	Upper GI endoscopy incl esophagus, stomach, duodenum, or jejunum; complex	238.92	218.69	207.76	238.92	0
43456	Dilation esophagus	254.52	232.97	221.32	254.52	0
43820	Gastrojejunostomy	971.86	889.58	845.10	971.86	90
44150	Colectomy, total, abdominal	1757.81	108.98	1528.53	1757.81	90
44320	Colostomy or skin level cecostomy	966.25	884.44	840.22	966.25	90
44950	Appendectomy	568.36	520.24	494.23	568.36	90
45308	Proctosigmoidoscopy for removal of polyp	135.34	123.88	117.69	135.34	0
45315	Multiple polyps	185.12	169.44	160.97	185.12	0
45330	Sigmoidoscopy (rigid), diagnostic (for biopsy or collection of specimen by brushing or washing)	95.92	87.80	83.41	95.92	0
45333	Sigmoidoscopy (flexible) with removal of polyps	183.99	168.41	159.99	183.99	0
45380	Colonoscopy with biopsy	382.35	349.98	332.48	382.35	0
46255	Hemorrhoidectomy int & ext, simple	503.57	460.94	437.89	503.57	90
46258	Hemorrhoidectomy with fistulectomy	636.02	582.17	553.06	636.02	90
46600	Anoscopy; diagnostic	32.86	30.07	28.57	32.86	0
46614	With control of hemorrhage	182.10	166.68	158.35	182.10	0
46700	Anoplastic, for stricture, adult	657.39	601.73	571.64	657.39	90
47562	Cholecystectomy; laparoscopic	714.99	654.45	621.73	714.99	90
47600	Cholecystectomy; abdominal excision	937.74	858.35	815.43	937.74	90
49505	Inguinal hernia repair, age 5 or over	551.07	504.41	479.19	551.07	90
49520	Repair, inguinal hernia, any age; recurrent	671.89	615.00	584.25	671.89	90
50080	Nephrostolithotomy, percutaneous	1323.93	1211.83	1151.24	1323.93	90
50780	Ureteroneocystostomy	1561.23	1429.84	1357.59	1561.23	90
51900	Closure of vesicovaginal fistula, abdominal approach	1196.82	1095.48	1040.71	1196.82	90
52000	Cystourethroscopy	167.05	152.90	145.26	167.05	0
52601	Transurethral resection of prostate	1193.53	1092.47	1037.85	1193.53	90
53040	Drainage of deep periurethral abscess	379.48	347.35	329.98	379.48	90
53060	Drainage of Skene's gland	147.45	134.97	128.22	147.45	10
53230	Excision, female diverticulum (urethral)	859.69	786.91	747.56	859.69	90
53240	Marsupialization of urethral diverticulum, M or F	520.11	476.07	452.27	520.11	90
53270	Excision of Skene's gland(s)	184.39	168.78	160.34	184.39	10
53620*	Dilation, urethra, male	100.73	92.20	87.59	100.73	0
53660*	Dilation urethra, female	48.32	44.23	42.02	48.32	0
54150	Circumcision–newborn	111.78	102.32	97.20	111.78	10
54520	Orchiectomy, simple	523.92	479.56	455.58	523.92	90
55700	Biopsy of prostate, needle or punch	156.22	142.99	135.84	156.22	0
55801	Prostatectomy, perineal subtotal	1466.56	1342.39	1275.27	1466.56	90
57265	Colporrhaphy AP with enterocele repair	902.24	825.85	784.56	902.24	90
57452*	Colposcopy	84.18	77.05	73.20	84.18	0
57510	Cauterization of cervix, electro or thermal	115.15	105.40	100.13	115.15	10
57520	Circumferential (cone) of cervix with or without D & C, with or without Sturmdorff-type repair	387.08	354.30	336.59	387.08	90
58100*	Endometrial biopsy	71.88	65.79	62.50	71.88	0

*Codes marked with an asterisk appear in *CPT* marked as shown. See *Handbook* Chapter 5 for detailed information.
†Data for the surgical follow-up days from St. Anthony's *CPT '96 Companion: A Guide to Medicare Billing.*

TABLE 3. Mock Fee Schedule—cont'd

Code Number and Description		Mock Fees	Medicare*			
			Participating	Non Participating	Limiting Charge	Follow-up Days[†]
58120	D & C, diagnostic and/or therapeutic (nonOB)	272.83	249.73	237.24	272.83	10
58150	TAH w/without salpingo-oophorectomy	1167.72	1068.85	1015.41	1167.72	90
58200	Total hysterectomy, extended, corpus cancer, including partial vaginectomy	1707.24	1562.69	1484.56	1707.24	90
58210	With bilateral radical pelvic lymphadenectomy	2160.78	1977.83	1878.94	2160.78	90
58300*	Insertion of intrauterine device	100.00				0
58340*	Hysterosalpingography, inj proc for	73.06	66.87	63.53	73.06	0
58720	Salpingo-oophorectomy, complete or partial, unilateral or bilateral Surgical treatment of ectopic pregnancy	732.40	670.39	636.87	732.40	90
59120	Salpingectomy and/or oophorectomy	789.26	722.43	686.31	789.26	90
59121	Without salpingectomy and/or oophorectomy	638.84	584.75	555.51	638.84	90
59130	Abdominal pregnancy	699.12	639.93	607.93	699.12	90
59135	Total hysterectomy, interstitial, uterine pregnancy	1154.16	1056.44	1003.62	1154.16	90
59136	Partial uterine resection, interstitial uterine pregnancy	772.69	707.26	671.90	772.69	90
59140	Cervical, with evacuation	489.68	448.22	425.81	489.68	90
59160	D & C postpartum hemorrhage (separate proc)	293.46	268.61	255.18	293.46	10
59400	OB Care—routine, inc. antepartum/ postpartum care	1864.30	1706.45	1621.13	1864.30	N/A
59515	C-section, low cervical, incl in-hosp postpartum care (separate proc)	1469.80	1345.36	1278.09	1469.80	N/A
59510	Including antepartum and postpartum care	2102.33	1924.33	1828.11	2102.33	N/A
59812	Treatment of incompl abortion, any trimester; completed surgically	357.39	327.13	310.77	357.39	90
61314	Craniotomy infratentorial	2548.09	2332.35	2215.73	2548.09	90
62270*	Spinal puncture, lumbar; diagnostic	77.52	70.96	67.41	77.52	0
65091	Excision of eye, without implant	708.22	648.25	615.84	708.22	90
65205*	Removal of foreign body, ext eye	56.02	51.27	48.71	56.02	0
65222*	Corneal, with slit lamp	73.81	67.56	64.18	73.81	0
69420	Myringotomy	97.76	89.48	85.01	97.76	10

*Codes marked with an asterisk appear in *CPT* marked as shown. See *Handbook* Chapter 5 for detailed information.
[†]Data for the surgical follow-up days from St. Anthony's *CPT '96 Companion: A Guide to Medicare Billing.*

Continued

TABLE 3. Mock Fee Schedule—cont'd

Code Number and Description		Mock Fees	Medicare*		
			Participating	Nonparticipating	Limiting Charge
RADIOLOGY, NUCLEAR MEDICINE, AND DIAGNOSTIC ULTRASOUND					
70120	X-ray mastoids, 2 less than 3 views per side	38.96	35.66	33.88	38.96
70130	complete, min., 3 views per side	56.07	51.33	48.76	56.07
71010	X-ray chest, 1 view	31.95	29.24	27.78	31.95
71020	Chest x-ray, 2 views	40.97	37.50	35.63	40.97
71030	Chest x-ray, compl, 4 views	54.02	49.44	46.97	54.02
71060	Bronchogram, bilateral	143.75	131.58	125.00	143.75
72100	X-ray spine, LS; AP & lat views	43.23	39.57	37.59	43.23
72114	Complete, incl bending views	74.97	68.62	65.19	74.97
73100	X-ray wrist, 2 views	31.61	28.94	27.49	31.61
73500	X-ray hip, 1 view	31.56	28.88	27.44	31.56
73540	X-ray pelvis & hips, infant or child, 2 views	37.94	34.73	32.99	37.94
73590	X-ray tibia & fibula, 2 views	33.35	30.53	29.00	33.35
73620	Radiologic exam, foot; AP & lat views	31.61	28.94	27.49	31.61
73650	X-ray calcaneus, 2 views	30.71	28.11	26.70	30.71
74241	Radiologic exam, upper gastrointestinal tract, with/without delayed films with KUB	108.93	99.71	94.72	108.93
74245	Upper GI tract with small bowel	161.70	148.01	140.61	161.70
74270	Barium enema	118.47	108.44	103.02	118.47
74290	Oral cholecystography	52.59	48.14	45.73	52.59
74400	Urography (pyelography), intravenous, with or without KUB	104.78	95.90	91.11	104.78
74410	Urography, infusion	116.76	106.87	101.53	116.76
74420	Urography, retrograde	138.89	127.13	120.77	138.89
75982	Percutaneous placement of drainage catheter	359.08	328.67	312.24	359.08
76090	Mammography, unilateral	62.57	57.27	54.41	62.57
76091	Mammography, bilateral	82.83	75.82	72.03	82.83
76805	Echography, pregnant uterus, B-scan or real time; complete	154.18	141.13	134.07	154.18
76810	Echography, pregnant uterus, complete: multiple gestation, after first trimester	306.54	280.59	266.56	306.54
76946	Ultrasonic guidance for amniocentesis	91.22	83.49	79.32	91.22
77300	Radiation dosimetry	97.58	89.32	84.85	97.58
77315	Teletherapy, isodose plan, complex	213.59	195.51	185.73	213.59
78104	Bone marrow imaging, whole body	230.56	211.04	200.49	230.56
78215	Liver and spleen imaging	160.44	146.85	139.51	160.44
78800	Tumor localization, limited area	191.53	175.32	166.55	191.53

PATHOLOGY AND LABORATORY[1]

Laboratory tests done as groups or combination "profiles" performed on multichannel equipment should be billed using the appropriate code number (80048 through 80076). Following is a list of the tests. The subsequent listing illustrates how to find the correct code.

Alanine aminotransferase (ALT, SGPT)
Albumin
Aspartate aminotransferase (AST, SGOT)

Bilirubin, direct
Bilirubin, total
Calcium

Carbon dioxide content
Chloride
Cholesterol
Creatinine
Glucose (sugar)
Lactate dehydrogenase (LD)
Phosphatase, alkaline

Phosphorus (inorganic phosphate)
Potassium
Protein, total
Sodium
Urea nitrogen (BUN)
Uric acid

[1]Mock fees for laboratory tests presented in this schedule may not be representative of fees in your region due to the variety of capitation and managed care contracts, as well as discount policies made by laboratories. At the time of this edition, Medicare guidelines may or may not pay for automatic multichannel tests where a large number of tests are performed per panel. Some cases require documentation and a related diagnostic code for each test performed. Provider must have the CLIA level of licensure to bill for tests, and test results must be documented.

TABLE 3. Mock Fee Schedule—cont'd

Code Number and Description		Mock Fees	Medicare*		
			Participating	Nonparticipating	Limiting Charge
ORGAN OR DISEASE-ORIENTED PANELS					
80048	Basic metabolic panel	15.00	14.60	13.87	16.64
80050	General health panel	20.00	19.20	15.99	21.87
80051	Electrolyte panel	20.00	19.20	15.99	21.87
80053	Comprehensive metabolic panel	25.00	20.99	19.94	23.93
80055	Obstetric panel	25.00	20.99	19.94	23.93
80076	Hepatic function panel	27.00	25.00	20.88	24.98
80074	Acute hepatitis panel	27.00	25.00	20.88	24.88
80061	Lipid panel	30.00	28.60	25.97	32.16
81000	Urinalysis, non-automated, with microscopy	8.00	7.44	5.98	8.84
81001	Urinalysis, automated, with microscopy	8.00	7.44	5.98	8.84
81002	Urinalysis, non-automated without microscopy	8.00	7.44	5.98	8.84
81015	Urinalysis, microscopy only	8.00	7.44	5.98	8.84
82270	Blood, occult; feces screening 1–3	4.05	3.56	3.31	4.05
82565	Creatinine; blood	10.00	9.80	8.88	12.03
82947	Glucose; quantitative	15.00			
82951	Glucose tol test, 3 spec	40.00	41.00	36.80	45.16
82952	Each add spec beyond 3	30.00	28.60	25.97	32.16
83020	Hemoglobin, electrophoresis	25.00	20.00	19.94	23.93
83715	Lipoprotein, blood; electrophoretic separation	25.00	20.00	19.94	23.93
84478	Triglycerides, blood	20.00	19.20	15.999	21.87
84479	Triiodothyronine (T–3)	20.00	19.20	15.99	21.87
84520	Urea nitrogen, blood (BUN); quantitative	25.00	20.99	19.94	23.93
84550	Uric acid, blood chemical	20.00	19.20	15.99	21.87
84702	Gonadotropin, chorionic; quantitative	20.00	19.20	15.99	21.87
84703	Qualitative	20.00	19.20	15.99	21.87
85013	Microhematocrit (spun)	20.00	19.20	15.99	21.87
85025	Complete blood count (hemogram), platelet count, automated, differential WBC count	25.00	20.00	19.94	23.93
38220	Bone marrow, aspiration only	73.52	67.29	63.93	73.52
38221	Bone marrow aspiration (biopsy)	90.65	82.98	78.83	90.65
85345	Coagulation time; Lee & White	20.00	19.20	15.99	21.87
85032	Platelet count (manual)	20.00	19.20	15.99	21.87
86038	Antinuclear antibodies	25.00	20.00	19.94	23.93
86580	Skin test; TB, intradermal	11.34	10.38	9.86	11.34
87081	Culture, bacterial, screening for single organisms	25.00	20.00	19.94	23.93
87181	Sensitivity studies, antibiotic; per antibiotic	20.00	19.20	15.99	21.87
87184	Disk method, per plate (12 disks or less)	20.00	19.20	15.99	21.87
87210	Smear, primary source, wet mount with simple stain, for bacteria, fungi, ova, and/or parasites	35.00	48.35	45.93	55.12
88150	Papanicolaou, cytopath	35.00	48.35	45.93	55.12
88302	Surgical pathology, gross & micro exam (skin, fingers, nerve, testis)	24.14	22.09	20.99	24.14
88305	Bone marrow, interpret	77.69	71.12	67.56	77.69

*Some services and procedures may not be considered a benefit under the Medicare program and when listed on a claim form, no reimbursement may be received. However, it is important to include these codes when billing because Medicare policies may change without an individual knowing of a new benefit. For this reason, some of the services shown in this mock fee schedule do not have any amounts listed under the three Medicare columns.

Continued

TABLE 3. Mock Fee Schedule—cont'd

Code Number and Description		Mock Fees	Medicare*		
			Participating	Nonparticipating	Limiting Charge
MEDICINE PROCEDURES					
Immunization Injections					
90701	Diphtheria, tetanus, pertussis	34.00			
90703	Tetanus toxoid	28.00			
90712	Poliovirus vaccine, oral	28.00			
Therapeutic Injections					
90782	IM or SC medication	4.77	4.37	4.15	4.77
90784	IV	21.33	19.53	18.55	21.33
90788	IM antibiotic	5.22	4.78	4.54	5.22
Psychiatry					
90816	Individual psychotherapy 20–30 min	60.25	55.15	52.39	60.25
90853	Group therapy	29.22	26.75	25.41	29.22
Hemodialysis					
90935	Single phys evaluation	117.23	107.31	101.94	117.23
90937	Repeat evaluation	206.24	188.78	179.34	206.24
Gastroenterology					
91000	Esophageal incubation	69.82	63.91	60.71	69.82
91055	Gastric incubation	87.41	80.01	76.01	87.41
Ophthalmologic Services					
92004	Comprehensive eye exam	90.86	83.17	79.01	90.86
92100	Tonometry	47.31	43.31	41.14	47.31
92230	Fluorescein angioscopy	55.49	50.79	48.25	55.49
92275	Electroretinography	81.17	74.29	70.58	81.17
92531	Spontaneous nystagmus	26.00			
Audiologic Function Tests					
92557	Comprehensive audiometry	54.33	49.73	47.24	54.33
92596	Ear measurements	26.81	24.54	23.31	26.81
Cardiovascular Therapeutic Services					
93000	Electrocardiogram (ECG)	34.26	31.36	29.79	34.26
93015	Treadmill ECG	140.71	128.80	122.36	140.71
93040	Rhythm ECG, 1–3 leads	18.47	16.90	16.06	18.47
93307	Echocardiography	250.73	229.50	218.03	250.73
Pulmonary					
94010	Spirometry	38.57	35.31	33.54	38.57
94060	Spirometry before and after bronchodilator	71.67	65.60	62.32	71.67
94150	Vital capacity, total	13.82	12.65	12.02	13.82
Allergy and Clinical Immunology					
95024	Intradermal tests; immediate reaction	6.58	6.02	5.72	6.85
95028	Intradermal tests; delayed reaction	9.32	8.85	10.18	9.32
93320	Doppler echocardiography	114.60	104.90	99.65	114.60
95044	Patch tests	8.83	8.08	7.68	8.83
95115	Treatment for allergy, single inj.	17.20	15.75	14.96	17.20
95117	2 or more inj.	22.17	20.29	19.28	22.17
95165	Allergen immunotherapy, single or multiple antigens, multiple-dose vials		6.50	6.18	7.11
Neurology					
95812	Electroencephalogram, Up to 1 hr.	129.32	118.37	112.45	129.32
95819	Electroencephalogram—awake and asleep	126.81	116.07	110.27	126.81
95860	Electromyography, 1 extremity	88.83	81.31	77.24	88.83
95864	Electromyography, 4 extremities	239.99	219.67	208.69	239.99
96100	Psychological testing (per hour)	80.95	74.10	70.39	80.95

*Some services and procedures may not be considered a benefit under the Medicare program and when listed on a claim form, no reimbursement may be received. However, it is important to include these codes when billing because Medicare policies may change without an individual knowing of a new benefit. For this reason, some of the services shown in this mock fee schedule do not have any amounts listed under the three Medicare columns.

TABLE 3. Mock Fee Schedule—cont'd

Code Number and Description		Mock Fees	Medicare*		
			Participating	Nonparticipating	Limiting Charge
Physical Medicine					
97024	Diathermy	14.27	13.06	12.41	14.27
97036	Hubbard tank, each 15 min	24.77	22.67	21.54	24.77
97110	Physical therapy, initial 30 min	23.89	21.86	20.77	23.89
97140	Manual therapy (manipulation, traction), one or more regions, each 15 min.	16.93	15.49	14.72	16.93
Special Services and Reports					
99000	Handling of specimen (transfer from Dr.'s office to lab)	5.00			
99025	Initial surg eval (new pt) with starred procedure	50.00			
99050	Services requested after office hours in addition to basic service	25.00			
99052	Services between 10 p.m. and 8 a.m. in addition to basic service	35.00			
99054	Services on Sundays and holidays in addition to basic service	35.00			
99056	Services normally provided in office requested by pt in location other than office	20.00			
99058	Office services provided on an emergency basis	65.00			
99070	Supplies and materials (itemize drugs and materials provided)	25.00			
99080	Special reports:				
	Insurance forms	10.00			
	Review of data to clarify pt's status	20.00			
	WC reports	50.00			
	WC extensive review report	250.00			

*Some services and procedures may not be considered a benefit under the Medicare program and when listed on a claim form, no reimbursement may be received. However, it is important to include these codes when billing because Medicare policies may change without an individual knowing of a new benefit. For this reason, some of the services shown in this mock fee schedule do not have any amounts listed under the three Medicare columns.

INDEX

A

Abortion	59100, 59812-9852
Abscess, periurethral	53040
Allergy and clinical immunology	95004-95199
Allergy testing	95004-95199
Amniocentesis, ultrasonic guidance	76946
Anesthesia procedures	00100-01999, 99100-99140
Anoplasty	46700-46705
Anoscopy	46600-46614
Antinuclear antibodies	86038-86039
Appendix surgery	44900-44960
Arm, excision, malignant lesion	11600-11606
Arthrocentesis	20600-20610
Aspiration	
bone marrow	85095
joint or bursa	20600-20610
Audiometry	92551-92596
Avulsion, nail plate	11730-11732
Axillae	
layer closure, wounds	12031-12037
repair, simple	12001-12007

B

Barium enema	74270-74280
Biopsy	
breast	19100-19101
cervical nodes	38510-38520
cervix	57454, 57500
endometrium	58100
prostate	55700-55705
skin	11100, 11101
soft tissue (arm)	24065-24066
Blood urea nitrogen, BUN	84520-84525
Bone marrow	
aspiration	85095-85097
interpretation	88305
needle biopsy	85102
Bronchography	71040-71060
Bronchoscopy	31622-31656

C

Calcaneus, radiologic exam	73650
Care Plan Oversight Services	99375, 99376
Case management	99361, 99362
Casts and strapping	29000-29799
Catheter, drainage	75982
Cauterization benign lesion—*see* destruction	
Cauterization, cervix	57510-57513
Cesarean section	59510-59525
standby	99360
Chest, radiographs	71000-71270
Cholecystectomy	47562-47620
Cholecystography	74290, 74291
Circumcision	54150-54161
Coagulation time	85345-85348

Colectomy	44140-44160
Colonoscopy, fiberoptic	45355-45385
Colostomy, separate procedure	44320
Colporrhaphy	57240-57265, 57289
Colposcopy	57452-57460
Complete blood count	85022-85031
Conization, cervix	57520-57522
Consultation	
confirmatory	99271-99275
during surgery (pathology)	88329-88332
initial	99251-99255
inpatient follow-up	99261-99263
office	99241-99245
telephone calls	99371-99373
telephone, psychiatric patient	99371-99373
with examination and evaluation	99241-99255
Counseling	
group	99411, 99412
individual	99401-99404
Craniotomy	61314
Creatinine	82540, 82565-82570
Critical care	
initial	99291
follow-up visit	99292
neonatal	99295-99297
Culture, bacterial	87040-87088
Custodial care medical services	
established patient	99331-99333
new patient	99321-99323
Cystourethroscopy	52000-52340

D

Debridement	
nails	11720-11721
skin	11040-11044
Destruction benign lesion, any method	
face	17000-17010
other than face	17100-17105
Dentition, prolonged physician attendance	99354-99360
Dilation	
dilatation and curettage	57820, 58120, 59160, 59840, 59851
esophagus	43450-43460
urethra, female	53660-53661
urethra, male	53620-53621
Diathermy	97024
Domiciliary visits	
established patient	99331-99333
new patient	99321-99323
Dosimetry	77300, 77331

E

Ear	
excision, benign lesion, external	11440-11446
layer closure, wounds	12051-12057
simple repair, wounds	12011-12018
Echocardiography	93307
Echography, pregnant uterus	76805-76816
Electrocardiogram	93000-93042

Electroencephalogram	95819-95827
Electromyography	95858, 95860-95869
Electroretinography	92275
Emergency department services	99281-99288
Endoscopy, gastrointestinal, upper	43234-43264
Esophageal intubation	91000
Excision—see organ, region, or structure involved	
Eye	
excision	65091
removal foreign body	65205-65222
Eyelid	
excision, benign lesion	11440-11446
layer closure, wounds	12051-12057
repair, simple	12011-12018

F

Face	
excision, benign lesion	11440-11446
layer closure, wounds (intermediate)	12051-12057
simple repair, wounds	12011-12018
Feces screening; blood occult	82270
Feet—see foot	
Fluorescein angioscopy, ophthalmoscopy	92230
Foot	
excision, benign lesion, skin	11420-11426
radiologic exam	73620-73630
simple repair, wounds	12001-12007
Fracture	
femur shaft	27500-27508
nasal	21300-21339
tibia proximal, plateau	27530-27537
tibia shaft	27750-27758

G

Gastric intubation	91055
Gastrointestinal tract, radiologic examination	74210-74340
Gastrojejunostomy	43632, 43820-43825, 43860-43865
Genitalia	
excision, benign lesion	11420-11426
repair, simple	12001-12007
Glucose, quantitative	82947
Glucose tolerance test	82951, 82952
Gonadotropin, chorionic	84702, 84703

H

Handling or specimen	99000
Hands	
excision, benign lesion	11420-11426
simple repair, wounds	12001-12007
Hemodialysis	90935-90937
insertion of cannula	36800-36815
placement, venous catheter	36245-36248
Hemoglobin electrophoresis	83020
Hemorrhage, nasal	30901-30906
Hemorrhoidectomy	46221-46262
Hernia, inguinal	49495-49525
Hip, radiologic examination	73500-73540

Home visits	
established patient	99351-99353
new patient	99341-99343
Hospital visits	
discharge day	99238
first day	99221-99223
newborn, initial care	99431
prolonged service	99356, 99357
subsequent care	99231-99233
subsequent day	99433
Hubbard tank	97036, 97113
Hysterectomy	58150-58285
ectopic pregnancy	59135-59140
supracervical	58180
total	58150-58152, 58200-58240
vaginal	58260-58285
Hysterosalpingography	74740
injection procedure for	58340

I

Imaging	
bone marrow	78102-78104
liver	78201-78220
Immunotherapy	95120-95199
Incision and drainage, furuncle	10060
Incision, breast	19000-19030
Injection	
allergies, steroids	95115-95117
antibiotic	90788
arthrocentesis, small joint or bursa	20600-20610
catheter placement	36245-36248
immunization	90700-90749
intravenous	90784
IV for contrast venography	36005
medication, intravenous	90784
medication, subcutaneous or intramuscular	90782
therapeutic	90782-90784
Intrauterine device (IUD)	
insertion	58300
removal	58301

J

Joint fluid, cell count	89050, 89051

K

KUB	74400-74405, 74420

L

Laryngoscopy	31540-31575
Leg, excision, malignant lesion	11600-11606
Lip	
excision, benign lesion	11440-11446
layer closure, wounds	12051-12057
repair, superficial wound	12011-12018
Lipoprotein	83715, 83717

M

Mammography	76090, 76091
Manipulation, spine	22505, 97260
Manipulation (physical therapy)	97260, 97261
Marsupialization, urethral diverticulum	53240
Mastoids, radiologic exam	70120, 70130
Mucous membrane, cutaneous	
excision, benign lesion	11440-11446
layer closure, wounds	12051-12057
simple repair, wounds	12011-12018
Myringotomy	69420

N

Nail	
excision	11750
trim	11719
wedge excision	11765
Nasal polyp, excision	30110
Neck	
excision, benign lesion	11420-11426
simple repair, wounds	12001-12007
Neonatal critical care	99295-99297
Nephrostolithotomy	50080
Newborn care	99431-99440
Nose	
excision, benign lesion	11440-11446
layer closure	12051-12057
simple repair	12011-12018
Nursing facility care	
assessment	99301-99303
subsequent care	99311-99313
Nystagmus	
optokinetic	92534
optokinetic test	92544
positional	92532
spontaneous	92531
spontaneous test	92541

O

Obstetric care	59400-59410
Office medical service	
after hours	99050-99054
emergency care	99058
Office visit	
established patient	99211-99215
new patient	99201-99205
service at another location	99056
with surgical procedure	99025
Ophthalmologic examination	92002-92019
Orchiectomy	54520-54535
Organ- or disease-oriented laboratory panels	80049-80091
Osteotomy, tibia	27455, 27457, 27705, 27709
Outpatient visit	
established patient	99211-99215
new patient	99201-99205

P

Pacemaker, insertion	33200-33217, 71090
Papanicolaou cytopathology	88150-88155
Patch skin test	95044-95052
Pathology, surgical gross and microscopic	88302-88309
Pericardiotomy	33020
Physical medicine services	97010-97150
Platelet count	85590
Pleurectomy	32310
Pneumonectomy	32440-32450
Preventive medicine	
established patient	99391-99397
health hazard appraisal	99420
new patient	99381-99387
unlisted	99429
Proctosigmoidoscopy	45300-45321
Prolonged services	
hospital inpatient	99356-99359
office/outpatient	99354, 99355, 99358, 99359
Prostatectomy, perineal, subtotal	55801
Psychiatric evaluation of records, reports, and/or tests	90825
Psychological testing	96100
Psychotherapy	
pharmacologic management	90862
family (conjoint)	90847
group medical	90853
individual	90816
multiple-family	90849
Puncture, lumbar spine	62270, 62272

Q

Quadriceps repair	27430

R

Radiology	
dosimetry	77300, 77331
teletherapy	77305-77315, 77321
therapeutic	77261-77799
treatment delivery	77401-77417
Repair—see procedure, organ, structure, or region involved	
Reports, special	99080
Resection, prostate, transurethral	52601-54640

S

Salpingo-oophorectomy	58720
Salpingectomy and/or oophorectomy	59120-59140
excision, benign lesion	11420-11422
layer closure, wounds	12031-12037
simple repair, wounds	12001-12007
Sensitivity studies, antibiotic	87181-87192
Septum, nasal septoplasty	30520
Sigmoidoscopy	45330-45333
Skene's gland	53060-53270
Skin excision, skin tags	11200, 11201
Splenectomy	38100-38115
Smear, primary source	87205-87211

Spine, radiologic exam	72010-72120
Spirometry	94010-94070
Standby services	99360
Supplies and materials	99070, 99071

T

TB skin test	86580
Teletherapy	77305-77321
Thromboendarterectomy	35301-35381
Tibia, radiologic exam	73590
Tonometry	92100
Tonsillectomy	42820-42826
TURP	52601-52648
Treadmill exercise	93015-93018
Triglycerides	84478
Triiodothyronine	84479-84482
Trunk	
excision, malignant lesion	11600-11606
layer closure—intermediate	12031-12037
simple repair	12001-12007
Tumor localization	78800-78803

U

Ureteroneocystostomy	50780-50800
Urethral diverticulum, excision	53230-53235
Uric acid	84550-84560
Urinalysis	81000-81099
Urography	74400-74425

V

Venipuncture	36400-36425
Vesicovaginal fistula, closure	51900, 57320, 57330
Vital capacity	94010, 94150, 94160

W

Wrist, radiologic examination	73100, 73110

X

Xenograft	15400

Y

Y-plasty, bladder	51800

Z

Z-plasty	14000, 26121, 41520

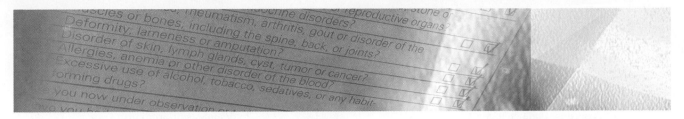

Medicare Level II HCPCS Codes

The following pages provide a partial alphanumeric list of the Centers for Medicare and Medicaid Services, referred to as Healthcare Common Procedure Coding System (HCPCS) (pronounced "hick-picks"). These Level II codes and modifiers were adopted by the Medicare program in 1984; additional codes and modifiers are added and deleted every year. This system was developed to code procedures not listed in the American Medical Association's *Current Procedural Terminology* (CPT) code book. This second level is a national standard used by all regional Medicare carriers.

Partial List of the Medicare Healthcare Common Procedure Coding System (HCPCS)

In certain circumstances, a code may need a modifier to show that the procedure has been changed by a specific situation. Remember that CPT and national modifiers apply to both CPT and HCPCS code systems. When applicable, indicate the appropriate modifier on the insurance claim form (Tables 1 and 2). Sometimes a special report may be needed to clarify the use of the modifier to the insurance company.

Table 1. Medicare HCPCS Modifiers

Modifier	Description	Modifier	Description
A1	Dressing for one wound	AK	Nonparticipating physician
A2	Dressing for two wounds	AM	Physician, team member service
A3	Dressing for three wounds	AP	No determination of refractive state
A4	Dressing for four wounds	AR	Physician scarcity area
A5	Dressing for five wounds	AS	Assistant-at-surgery service
A6	Dressing for six wound	AT	Acute treatment
A7	Dressing for seven wounds	AU	Uro, ostomy, or trach item
A8	Dressing for eight wounds	AV	Item with prosthetic/orthotic
A9	Dressing for nine or more wounds	AW	Item with a surgical dressing.
AA	Anesthesia performed by anesthetist	AX	Item with dialysis services
AD	MD supervision; more than four anesthesia procedures	BA	Item with pen services
		BO	Nutrition oral admin no tube
AE	Registered dietitian	BP	Beneficiary elected to purchase item
AF	Specialty physician	BR	Beneficiary elected to rent item
AG	Primary physician	BU	Beneficiary undecided on purch/rent
AH	Clinical psychologist	CA	Procedure payable inpatient
AJ	Clinical social worker	CB	ESRD beneficiary Part A SNF-sep pay

Continued

Table 1. Medicare HCPCS Modifiers—cont'd

Modifier	Description	Modifier	Description
CC	Procedure code change	HA	Child/adolescent program
CD	AMCC test for ESRD or MCP MD	HB	Adult program nongeriatric
CE	Med necessity AMCC test sep reimbursement	HC	Adult program geriatric
CF	AMCC test not composite rate	HD	Pregnant/parenting program
CG	Innovator drug dispensed	HE	Mental health program
E1	Upper left eyelid	HF	Substance abuse program
E2	Lower left eyelid	HG	Opioid addiction tx program
E3	Upper right eyelid	HH	Mental hlth/substance abs pr
E4	Lower right eyelid	HI	M health/m retrdtn/dev dis pro
EJ	Subsequent claim	HJ	Employee assistance program
EM	Emergency reserve supply (ESRD)	HK	spec high risk mntl hlth pop p
EP	Medicaid EPSDT program SVC	HL	Intern
ET	Emergency treatment	HM	Less than bachelor degree LV
EY	No MD order for item/service	HN	Bachelors degree level
FA	Left hand, thumb	HO	Masters degree level
FP	Service part of family planning program	HP	Doctoral level
F1	Left hand, second digit	HQ	Group setting
F2	Left hand, third digit	HR	Family/couple W client presnt
F3	Left hand, fourth digit	HS	Family/couple W/O client prs
F4	Left hand, fifth digit	HT	Child welfare agency funded
F5	Right hand, thumb	HV	Funded state addiction agency
F6	Right hand, second digit	HW	State mntl hlth agency funded
F7	Right hand, third digit	HX	County/local agency funded
F8	Right hand, fourth digit	HY	Funded by juvenile justice
F9	Right hand, fifth digit	HZ	Criminal justice agency fund
G1	URR reading of less than 60	JW	Discarded drug not administe
G2	URR reading of 60 to 64.9	K0	LWR EXT PROST FUNCTNL LVL 0
G3	URR reading of 65 to 69.9	K1	LWR EXT PROST FUNCTNL LVL 1
G4	URR reading of 70 to 74.9	K2	LWR EXT PROST FUNCTNL LVL 2
G5	URR reading of 75 or greater	K3	LWR EXT PROST FUNCTNL LVL 3
G6	ERSD patient <6 dialysis/mth	K4	LWR EXT PROST FUNCTNL LVL 4
G7	Payment limits do not apply	KA	Wheelchair add-on option/acc
G8	Monitored anesthesia care	KB	>4 modifiers on claim
G9	MAC for at risk patient	KC	Repl special pwr wc intrface
GA	Waiver of liability on file	KD	Drug/biological dme infused
GB	Claim resubmitted	KF	FDA class III device
GC	Resident/teaching phys serv	KH	DME POS INI CLM, PUR/1 MO RNT
GE	Resident primary care exception	KI	DME POS 2nd or 3rd mo rental
GF	Nonphysician serv C A hosp	KJ	DME POS PEN PMP or 4-15 mo rent
GG	Payment screen mam + diag mam	KM	RPLC facial prosth new imp
GH	Diag mammo to screening mamo	KN	RPLC facial prosth old mod
GJ	Opt out provider of ER serv	K0	Single drug unit dose form
GK	Actual item/service ordered	KP	First drug of multidrug UD
GL	Upgraded item, no charge	KQ	2nd/subsqnt drg multi DRG UD
GM	Multiple transports	KR	Rental item partial month
GN	OP speech language service	KS	Glucose monitor supply
GO	OP occupational therapy serv	KX	Documentation on file
GP	OP PT services	KZ	New cov not implement by M+C
GQ	Telehealth store and forward	LC	Left circumflex coronary artery.
GT	Interactive telecommunication	LD	Left anterior descending coronary artery.
GV	Attending phys not hospice	LL	Lease/rental (Appld to pur)
GW	Service unrelated to term CO	LR	Laboratory round trip
GY	Statutorily excluded	LS	FDA-monitored intraocular lens implant
GZ	Not reasonable and necessary	LT	Left side
H9	Court ordered	MS	6 mo maint/svc fee parts/lbr

Table 1. Medicare HCPCS Modifiers—cont'd

Modifier	Description	Modifier	Description
NR	New when rented	SW	Serv by cert diab educator
NU	New equipment	SY	Contact w/high-risk pop
PL	Progressive addition lenses	TA	Left foot, great toe
QA	FDA investigational device	TC	Technical component
QB	MD providing SVC in rural HPSA	TD	RN
QC	Single-channel monitoring	TE	LPN/LVN
QD	Recording/ storage in solid-state memory	TF	Intermediate level of care
QE	Prescribed oxygen <1 LPM	TG	Complex/high tech level care
QF	Prescribed oxygen >4 LPM & port	TH	OB tx/servcs prenatl/postpart
QG	Prescribed oxygen >4 LPM	TJ	Child/adolescent program GP
QH	Oxygen-conserving device with delivery system	TK	Extra patient or passenger
QJ	Patient in state/local custody	TL	Early intervention IFSP
QK	Med dir 2-4 concurrent anes proc	TM	Individualized ED prrm (EP)
QL	Patient died after Amb call	TN	Rural/out or service area
QM	Ambulance arrangement by hospital	TP	Med transprt unloaded vehicle
QN	Ambulance furnished by provider	TQ	Bls by volunteer amb provider
QP	Individually ordered lab test	TR	School-based IEP out of district
QQ	SOI submitted	TS	Follow-up service
QS	Monitored anesthesia care	TT	Additional patient
QT	Recording/ storage tape analog recorder	TU	Overtme payment rate
QU	MD providing service urban HPSA	TV	Holiday/weekend payment rate
QV	Item or service provided	TW	Back-up equipment
QW	CLIA waived test	Tl	Left foot, second digit
QX	CRNA service with MD med direction	T2	Left foot, third digit
QY	Medically directed CRNA	T3	Left foot, fourth digit
QZ	CRNA service: without medical direction by MD	T4	Left foot, fifth digit
Q2	HCFA/ord demo procedure/svc	T5	Right foot, great toe
Q3	Live donor surgery/services	T6	Right foot, second digit
Q4	Service exempt ordering/referring MD	T7	Right foot, third digit
Q5	Substitute MD service, recip bill arrangement	T8	Right foot, fourth digit
Q6	Locum tenens MD service	T9	Right foot, fifth digit
Q7	One Class A finding	U1	Medicaid care Level 1 state def
Q8	Two Class B findings	U2	Medicaid care Level 2 state def
Q9	One Class B and two Class C findings	U3	Medicaid care Level 3 state def
RC	Right coronary artery	U4	Medicaid care Level 4 state def
RD	Drug admin not incident-to	U5	Medicaid care Level 5 state def
RP	Replacement and repair (DMEPOS)	U6	Medicaid care Level 6 state def
RR	Rental (DME)	U7	Medicaid care Level 7 state def
RT	Right side	U8	Medicaid care Level 8 state def
SA	Nurse practitioner with physician	U9	Medicaid care Level 9 state def
SB	Nurse midwife	UA	Medicaid care Level 10 state dcf
SC	Medically necessary serv/sup	UB	Medicaid care Level 11 state def
SD	Service by home infusion RN	UC	Mcdicaid care Level 12 state def
SE	State/Fed funded program/ser	UD	Medicaid care Level 13 state def
SF	2nd opinion ordered by PRO	UE	Used durable medical equipment
SG	Ambulatory surgical center facility service	UF	Services provided, morning
SH	2nd concurrent infusion therapy	UG	Services provided afternoon
SJ	3rd concurrent infusion therapy	UH	Services provided, evening
SK	High risk population	UJ	Services provided, night
SL	State supplied vaccine	UK	Service on behalf client-collateral
SM	Second opinion	UN	Two patients served
SN	Third opinion	UP	Three patients served
SQ	Item ordered by home health	UQ	Four patients served
ST	Related to trauma or injury	UR	Five patients served
SU	Performed in phys office	US	Six or more patients served
SV	Drugs delivered not used	VP	Aphakic patient

Table 2. HCPCS Alphanumeric Index

Description	Code
A	
above-elbow endoskeletal prostheses	L6500
above-elbow prostheses	L6250
above-knee endoskeletal prostheses	L5320
acetazolamide sodium (Diamox), injection	J1120
actinomycin D, injection	J9120
adjustable arms, wheelchair	E0973
adjustable chair, dialysis	E1570
adrenaline, injection	J0170
air ambulance	A0030
air bubble detector, dialysis	E1530
air travel and nonemergency transport	A0140
alarm, pressure dialysis	E1540
alcohol	A4244
alcohol wipes	A4245
alternating pressure pad	E0180
aminophylline, injection	J0280
amitriptyline HCl (Elavil), injection	J1320
ammonia test paper	A4774
amobarbital sodium (Amytal sodium), injection	J0300
ampicillin, injection	J0290
ampicillin sodium (Omnipen-N), injection	J2430
amputee adapter, wheelchair	E0959
amputee wheelchair, detachable elevating leg rests	E1170
amputee wheelchair, detachable foot rests	E1200
amygdalin, injection	J3570
anesthetics for dialysis	A4735
ankle prostheses, Symes, metal frame	L5060
ankle prostheses, Symes, molded socket	L5050
antineoplastic drugs, not otherwise classified (NOC)	J9999
antitipping device, wheelchair	E0971
apnea monitor	E0608
appliance, pneumatic	E0655
arm rest, wheelchair	E0994
arms, adjustable, wheelchair	E0973
asparaginase (Elspar), injection	J9020
atropine sulfate, injection	J0460
aurothioglucose (Solganal), injection	J2910
axillary crutch extension	L0978
B	
back, upholstery, wheelchair	E0993
bacterial sensitivity study	P7001
bandage, elastic	A4460
bandages, gauze	A4202
bath conductivity meter, dialysis	E1550
bathroom equipment, miscellaneous	E0179
battery charger, wheelchair	E1066
BCNU (carmustine, bis-chloroethyl-nitrosourea), injection	J9050
bed accessories: boards, tables	E0315
bed pan	E0276
below-elbow endoskeletal prostheses	L6400
below-knee endoskeletal prostheses	L5300
belt, extremity	E0945

Table 2. HCPCS Alphanumeric Index—cont'd

Description	Code
belt, ostomy	A4367
belt, pelvic	E0944
bench, bathtub	E0245
benzquinamide HCl (Emete-Con), injection	J0510
benztropine, injection	J0515
bethanechol chloride, injection	J0520
bethanechol chloride (Myotonachol), injection	J0520
bethanechol chloride (Urecholine), injection	J0520
bicarbonate dialysate	A4705
bilirubin (phototherapy) light	E0202
biperiden HCl (Akineton), injection	J0190
bis-chloroethyl-nitrosourea, injection	J9050
bleomycin sulfate, injection	J9040
blood, mucoprotein	P2038
blood (split unit), specify amount	P9011
blood (whole), for transfusion, per unit	P9010
blood leak detector, dialysis	E1560
blood pressure monitor	A4670
blood pump, dialysis	E1620
blood strips	A4253
blood testing supplies	A4770
bond or cement, ostomy skin	A4364
brompheniramine maleate (Dehist), injection	J0945

C

Description	Code
calcitonin (salmon) (Calcimar), injection	J0630
calcium disodium edetate (Versenate), injection	J0600
calcium gluconate, injection	J0610
calcium glycerophosphate and calcium lactate (Calphosan), injection	J0620
calcium leucovorin, injection	J0640
calf rest, wheelchair	E0995
calibrator solution	A4256
canes	E0100
carbon filters	A4680
carmustine, injection	J9050
cast supplies	
long leg, adult (11 years +), cylinder, fiberglass	Q4034
long leg, adult (11 years +), cylinder, plaster	Q4033
long leg, adult (11 years +), fiberglass	Q4030
catheter caps, disposable (dialysis)	A4860
catheter insertion tray	A4354
catheter irrigation set	A4355
cefazolin sodium, injection	J0690
ceftriaxone sodium (Rocepin), 250-mg injection	J0696
cellular therapy	M0075
cement, ostomy	A4364
centrifuge	A4650
cephalin flocculation, blood	P2028
cephalothin sodium (Keflin), injection	J1890
cephapirin sodium, injection	J0710
cervical head harness/halter	E0942
cervical pillow	E0943
chair, adjustable, dialysis	E1570
chelation therapy, intravenous (chemical endarterectomy)	M0300
chin cup, cervical	L0150
chiropractor, manipulation of spine	A2000

Table 2. HCPCS Alphanumeric Index—cont'd

Description	Code
chloramphenicol (Chloromycetin Sodium Succinate), injection	J0720
chlordiazepoxide HCl (Librium), injection	J1990
chloroprocaine HCl (Nesacaine), injection	J2400
chloroquine HCl (Aralen HCl), injection	J0390
chlorothiazide sodium (Diuril), injection	J1205
chlorpheniramine maleate (Chlor-Trimeton), injection	J0730
chlorpromazine (Thorazine), injection	J3230
chlorprothixene (Taractan), injection	J3080
chorionic gonadotropin, injection	J0725
clamps, dialysis, venous pressure	A4918
clamps, Harvard pressure	A4920
cleansing agent, dialysis equipment	A4790
clotting time tube	A4771
codeine phosphate, injection	J0745
colchicine, injection	J0760
colistimethate sodium (Coly-Mycin M), injection	J0770
commode seat, wheelchair	E0968
compressor	E0565
compressor, pneumatic	E0650
conductive paste or gel	A4558
Congo red blood	P2029
continuous cycling peritoneal dialysis (CCPD) supply kit	A4901
contracts, repair and maintenance, ESRD	A4890
corticotropin, injection	J0800
cortisone, injection	J0810
crutches	E0110
cryoprecipitate, each unit	P9012
culture sensitivity study	P7001
cushion, one-inch, for wheelchair	E0962
Cycler, hemodialysis	E1590
Cycler dialysis machine	E1594
cyclophosphamide, injection	J9070

D

Description	Code
dactinomycin (Cosmegen) or actinomycin, injection	J9120
daunorubicin HCl, injection	J9150
decubitus care pad	E0185
deionizer, water purification system	E1615
detector, blood leak, dialysis	E1560
dexamethasone sodium phosphate, injection	J1100
dextrose/normal saline, solution	J7042
Dextrostix	A4772
dialysate concentrate additives	A4765
dialysate testing solution	A4760
dialysis, bath conductivity, meter	E1550
dialysis supplies, miscellaneous	A4913
dialyzer holder	A4919
dialyzers	A4690
diazepam (Valium), injection	J3360
diazoxide (Hyperstat), injection	J1730
dicyclomine HCl (Bentyl), injection	J0500
digoxin, injection	J1160
dihydroergotamine mesylate (D.H.E. 45), injection	J1110
dimenhydrinate (Dramamine), injection	J1240

Table 2. HCPCS Alphanumeric Index—cont'd

Description	Code
dimercaprol in peanut oil (BAL in Oil), injection	J0470
dimethyl imidazole carboxamide (DIC) (dacarbazine, DTIC-DOME), 100-mg vial	J9130
dimethyl sulfoxide, injection	J1212
dimethyl sulfoxide (DMSO) (Rimso-50), injection	J1212
diphenhydramine HCl (Benadryl), injection	J1200
disarticulation, elbow, prostheses	L6200
doxorubicin (Adriamycin), injection	J9000
drainage bag	A4358
drainage board	E0606
droperidol (Inapsine), injection	J1790
droperidol and fentanyl citrate (Innovar), injection	J1810
drugs, nonprescription	A9150
drugs, prescription, oral chemotherapy	J7150
durable medical equipment (DME) medical supplies	A4610
dyphylline (Dilor), injection	J1180

E

Description	Code
edetate sodium (ethylenediaminetetraacetic acid [EDTA], Endrate), injection	J3520
elbow protector	E0191
electrical work or plumbing, home, dialysis equipment	A4870
electrodes	A4556
elevating leg rest, wheelchair	E0990
endarterectomy, chemical	M0300
epinephrine, injection	J0170
ergonovine maleate (Ergotrate Maleate), injection	J1330
estradiol cypionate (Depo-Estradiol Cypionate), injection	J1000
estradiol valerate (Delestrogen), injection	J0970
estradiol valerate, up to 20 mg (Estraval-2X), injection	J1390
estradiol valerate, up to 10 mg (Estraval P.A.), injection	J1380
estrone, injection	J1435
ethylnorepinephrine HCl (Bronkephrine HCl), injection	J0590
etoposide, 50 mg, injection	J9181
external ambulatory infusion pump with administration equipment	E0781
extremity belt-harness	E0945

F

Description	Code
faceplate, ostomy	A4361
fentanyl citrate (Sublimaze), injection	J3010
fibrinogen unit	P9013
fistula cannulation set	A4730
flotation mattress	E0184
flotation pad gel pressure	E0185
floxuridine, 500 mg, injection	J9200
fluid barriers, dialysis	E1575
fluorouracil, injection	J9190
fluphenazine decanoate (Prolixin Decanoate), injection	J2680
foot rest, for use with commode chair	E0175
footplates, wheelchair	E0970
forearm crutches	E0110
furosemide (Lasix), injection	J1940

G

Description	Code
gamma globulin, 1 ml, injection	J1460
gauze bandages (gauze elastic)	A4202

Continued

Table 2. HCPCS Alphanumeric Index—cont'd

Description	Code
gauze, non-impregnated, sterile, 16 sq-in pad	A4200
gel, conductive	A4558
gel flotation pad	E0185
gentamicin, injection	J1580
gentamicin sulfate (Garamycin), injection	J1580
globulin, gamma, 1 ml, injection	P9014
globulin, Rh immune, 1 ml, injection	P9015
gloves, dialysis	A4927
glucose test strips	A4772
gold sodium thiosulfate, injection	J1600
Gomco drain bottle	A4912
Grade-Aid, wheelchair	E0974
gravity traction device	E0941
Gravlee Jet Washer	A4470

H

Description	Code
hair analysis	P2031
hallux-valgus dynamic splint	L3100
haloperidol (Haldol), injection	J1630
halter, cervical head	E0942
hand rims, wheelchair	E0967
harness, extremity	E0945
harness, pelvic	E0944
harness/halter, cervical head	E0942
Harvard pressure clamp, dialysis	A4920
head rest extension, wheelchair	E0966
heater for nebulizer	E1372
heel or elbow protector	E0191
heel stabilizer	L3170
helicopter ambulance	A0040
hemipelvectomy, endoskeletal prostheses	L5340
hemipelvectomy prostheses	L5280
hemodialysis, monthly capitation	E0945
hemodialysis kit	A4820
hemodialysis unit	E1590
hemostats	A4850
Hemostix	A4773
heparin	A4800
heparin infusion pump, dialysis	E1520
hexachlorophene (pHisoHex) solution	A4246
Hexcelite, cast material—see Q codes under "cast supplies" for specific casts	A4590
HN_2 (nitrogen mustard)	J9230
hot water bottle	E0220
hyaluronidase (Wydase), injection	J3470
hydralazine HCl (Apresoline), injection	J0360
hydrochlorides of opium alkaloids (Pantopon), injection	J2480
hydrocortisone, injection	J1720
hydrocortisone acetate, up to 25 mg, injection	J1700
hydrocortisone phosphate, injection	J1710
hydrocortisone sodium succinate (Solu-Cortef), injection	J1720
hydromorphone (Dilaudid), injection	J1170
hydroxyzine HCl (Vistaril), injection	J3410
hyoscyamine sulfate (Levsin), injection	J1980
hypertonic saline solution	J7130

Table 2. HCPCS Alphanumeric Index—cont'd

Description	Code
I	
ice cap or collar	E0230
imipramine HCl (Tofranil), injection	J3270
incontinence clamp	A4356
infusion pump, external ambulatory with administration equipment	E0781
infusion pump, heparin, dialysis	E1520
infusion pump, implantable	E0782
installation and/or delivery charges for ESRD equipment	E1600
insulin, injection	J1820
intercapsular thoracic endoskeletal prostheses	L6570
interferon, injection	J9213
intermittent peritoneal dialysis (IPD) supply kit	A4905
intermittent peritoneal dialysis (IPD) system, automatic	E1592
intermittent positive-pressure breathing (IPPB) machine	E0500
intraocular lenses, anterior chamber	V2630
intraocular lenses, iris supported	V2631
intraocular lenses, posterior chamber	V2632
iodine swabs/wipes	A4247
iron dextran (Imferon), injection	J1760
irrigation kits, ostomy	A4400
irrigation set, catheter	A4355
IV pole	E0776
J	
jacket, Risser	A4581
K	
kanamycin sulfate, injection	J1840
kanamycin sulfate (Kantrex), up to 75 mg, pediatric, injection	J1850
Kartop patient lift, toilet or bathroom	E0625
kit, chronic ambulatory peritoneal dialysis (CAPD) supply	A4900
kit, CCPD supply	A4901
kit, hemodialysis	A4820
L	
laetrile, amygdalin (vitamin B_{17}), injection	J3570
lancets	A4259
lead wires	A4557
leg extension, walker	E1058
leg rest, wheelchair, elevating	E0990
leukocyte-poor blood, each unit	P9016
levorphanol tartrate (Levo-Dromoran), injection	J1960
lidocaine (Xylocaine), injection	J2000
lightweight wheelchair	E1087
lincomycin, injection	J2010
liquid barrier, ostomy	A4363
liver derivative complex (Kutapressin), injection	J1910
liver injection	J2050
lubricant, ostomy	A4402
M	
manipulation, of spine, by chiropractor	A2000
mannitol, injection	J2150
measuring cylinder, dialysis	A4921
mechlorethamine, injection	J9230

Continued

Table 2. HCPCS Alphanumeric Index—cont'd

Description	Code
mechlorethamine HCl (Mustargen), injection	J9230
medical supplies used in DME	A4610
medroxyprogesterone acetate (Depo-Provera), injection	J1050
meperidine, injection	J2175
meperidine HCl and promethazine HCl (Mepergan), injection	J2180
mephentermine sulfate (Wyamine Sulfate), injection	J3450
mepivacaine HCl (Carbocaine), injection	J0670
metaraminol bitartrate (Aramine), injection	J0380
meter, bath conductivity, dialysis	E1550
methadone HCl, injection	J1230
methicillin sodium (Staphcillin), injection	J2970
methocarbamol (Robaxin), injection	J2800
methotrimeprazine (Levoprome), injection	J1970
methoxamine HCl (Vasoxyl), injection	J3390
methyldopate HCl (Aldomet Ester HCl)	J0210
methylergonovine maleate (Methergine), injection	J2210
methylprednisolone acetate (Depo-Medrol), injection	J1020
methylprednisolone sodium succinate (Solu-Medrol), injection	
up to 40 mg	J2920
up to 125 mg	J2930
metoclopramide HCl (Reglan)	J2765
metocurine iodide (Metubine Iodide), injection	J2240
microbiology tests	P7001
mini-bus, nonemergency transportation	A0120
miscellaneous dialysis supplies	A4913
mithramycin, injection	J9270
mitomycin (Mutamycin), injection	J9280
monitor, apnea	E0608
monitor, blood pressure	A4670
morphine, injection	J2270
mucoprotein, blood	P2038

N

Description	Code
nandrolone decanoate, up to 50 mg, injection	J2320
nandrolone decanoate, up to 200 mg, injection	J2322
nandrolone phenpropionate (Anabolin), injection	J0340
narrowing device, wheelchair	E0969
nasal vaccine inhalation	J3530
nebulizer, portable	E1375
nebulizer, with compressor	E0570
nebulizer heater	E1372
needle with syringe	A4206
needles	A4215
needles, dialysis	A4655
neonatal transport, ambulance, base rate	A0225
neostigmine methylsulfate (Prostigmin), injection	J2710
neuromuscular stimulator	E0745
niacin, injection	J2350
nikethamide (Coramine), injection	J3490
nitrogen mustard, injection	J9230
noncovered procedure	A9270
nonmedical supplies for dialysis (e.g., scale, scissors, stopwatch)	A4910
nonprescription drugs	A9150
nonprofit transport, nonemergency	A0120

Table 2. HCPCS Alphanumeric Index—cont'd

Description	Code
O	
occipital/mandibular support, cervical	L0160
occupational therapy	H5300
opium, injection	J2480
orphenadrine citrate (Norflex), injection	L2360
orthoses, thoracic-lumbar-sacral (scoliosis)	L1200
orthotic, knee	L1830
ostomy supplies	A4421
oxacillin sodium (Bactocill), injection	J2410
oxymorphone HCl (Numorphan), injection	J2700
oxytetracycline, injection	J2460
oxytocin (Pitocin), injection	J2590
P	
pacemaker monitor, includes audible/visible check systems	E0610
pacemaker monitor, includes digital/visible check systems	E0615
pad for water circulating heat unit	E0249
pads, flotation, electric, standard	E0192
pail or pan for use with commode chair	E0167
papaverine HCl, injection	J2440
paraffin	A4265
paraffin bath unit	E0235
paste, conductive	A4558
pelvic belt/harness/boot	E0944
penicillin G benzathine (Bicillin L-A), injection	J0560
penicillin G potassium (Pfizerpen), injection	J2540
penicillin procaine, aqueous, injection	J2510
pentazocine HCl (Talwin), injection	J3070
percussor	E0480
peritoneal straps	L0980
peroxide	A4244
perphenazine (Trilafon), injection	J3310
personal items	A9190
pessary	A4560
phenobarbital, injection	J2560
phenobarbital sodium, injection	J2515
phentolamine mesylate (Regitine), injection	J2760
phenylephrine HCl (Neo-Synephrine), injection	J2370
phenytoin sodium (Dilantin), injection	J1165
phototherapy, light	E0202
phytonadione (AquaMEPHYTON), injection, vitamin K	J3430
pillow, cervical	E0943
plasma, protein fraction, each unit	P9018
plasma, single donor, fresh frozen, each unit	P9017
platelet concentrate, each unit	P9019
platelet-rich plasma, each unit	P9020
podiatric services, noncovered	A9160
portable hemodialyzer system	E1635
portable nebulizer	E1375
postural drainage board	E0606
pralidoxime chloride (Protopam Chloride), injection	J2730
prednisolone acetate, injection	J2650
preparation kits, dialysis	A4914
prescription drug, oral	J7140
prescription drug, oral chemotherapy	J7150

Continued

Table 2. HCPCS Alphanumeric Index—cont'd

Description	Code
pressure alarm, dialysis	E1540
procainamide HCl (Pronestyl), injection	J2690
prochlorperazine (Compazine), injection	J0780
progesterone, injection	J2675
prolotherapy	M0076
promazine HCl (Sparine), injection	J2950
promethazine HCl (Phenergan), injection	J2550
propiomazine (Largon), injection	J1930
propranolol HCl (Inderal), injection	J1800
prostheses, above elbow, endoskeletal	L6500
prostheses, below elbow, endoskeletal	L6400
prostheses, hemipelvectomy	L5280
prostheses, intercapsular thoracic, endoskeletal	L6570
prostheses, knee, endoskeletal	L5300
prostheses, lower extremity, NOC	L5999
prosthetic services, NOC	L8499
protamine sulfate, injection	J2720
protector, heel or elbow	E0191

Q

Quad cane	E0105

R

rack/stand, oxygen	E1355
reciprocating peritoneal dialysis system	E1630
red blood cells, each unit	P9021
regulator, oxygen	E1353
replacement components, ESRD machines	E1640
replacement tanks, dialysis	A4880
reserpine (Sandril), injection	J2820
restraints, any type	E0710
reverse osmosis water purification, ESRD	E1610
$Rh_O(D)$ immune globulin, injection	J2790
rib belt	A4572
rims, hand (wheelchair)	E0967
Ringer's injection	J7120
rings, ostomy	A4404
Risser jacket	A4581

S

safety equipment	E0700
safety visit, wheelchair	E0980
sales tax, orthotic/prosthetic/other	L9999
scale or scissors, dialysis	A4910
seat attachment, walker	E0156
seat insert, wheelchair	E0992
secobarbital sodium (seconal sodium), injection	J2860
sensitivity study	P7001
serum clotting time tube	A4771
shunt accessories, for dialysis	A4740
sitz bath, portable	E0160
skin barrier, ostomy	A4362
skin bond or cement, ostomy	A4364
sling, patient lift	E0621

Table 2. HCPCS Alphanumeric Index—cont'd

Description	Code
slings	A4565
social worker, nonemergency transport	A0160
sodium chloride, injection	J2912
sodium succinate, injection	J1720
sorbent cartridges, ESRD	E1636
spectinomycin dihydrochloride (Trobicin), injection	J3320
sphygmomanometer with cuff and stethoscope	A4660
spinal orthosis, NOC	L1499
splint	A4570
splint, hallux-valgus, night, dynamic	L3100
stand/rack, oxygen	E1355
sterilizing agent, dialysis	A4780
streptokinase-streptodornase, injection	J2995
streptomycin, injection	J3000
streptozocin, injection	J9320
succinylcholine chloride (Anectine), injection	J0330
suction pump, portable	E0600
surgical brush, dialysis	A4910
surgical stockings, above-knee length	A4490
surgical supplies, miscellaneous	A4649
surgical trays	A4550
swabs, povidone-iodine (Betadine) or iodine	A4247
syringe	A4213
syringes, dialysis	A4655

T

Description	Code
tape, all types, all sizes	A4454
taxes, orthotic/prosthetic/other	L9999
taxi, nonemergency transportation	A0100
tent, oxygen	E0455
terbutaline sulfate, 0.5 mg, injection	J3105
terminal devices	L6700
testosterone cypionate (Depo-Testosterone), injection	J1070
testosterone cypionate and estradiol cypionate (Depo-Testadiol), injection	J1060
testosterone enanthate and estradiol valerate (Deladumone), injection	L0900
testosterone propionate, injection	J3150
testosterone suspension, injection	J3140
tetanus immune human globulin (Homo-Tet), injection	J1670
tetracycline, injection	J0120
tetracycline HCl (Achromycin), injection	J0120
theophylline and mersalyl (Salyrgan), injection	J2810
thermometer, dialysis	A4910
thiethylperazine maleate (Torecan), injection	J3280
thiotepa (triethylenethiophosphoramide), injection	J9340
thiothixene HCl (Navane IM), injection	J2330
thymol turbidity, blood	P2033
thyrotropin (TSH), exogenous, up to 10 IU, injection	J3240
tobramycin sulfate (Nebcin), injection	J3260
toilet rail	E0243
toilet seat, raised	E0244
tolazoline HCl (Priscoline), injection	J2670
tolls, nonemergency transport	A0170
tool kit, dialysis	A4910
tourniquet, dialysis	A4910
tracheotomy collar or mask	A4621

Continued

Table 2. HCPCS Alphanumeric Index—cont'd

Description	Code
traction device, gravity-assisted	E0941
traction equipment, overdoor	E0860
travel hemodialyzer system	E1635
trays, surgical	A4550
triflupromazine HCl (Vesprin), injection	J3400
trimethaphan camsylate (Arfonad)	J0400
trimethobenzamide HCl (Tigan), injection	J3250
tube-occluding forceps/clamps, dialysis	A4910
U	
ultraviolet cabinet	E0690
unclassified drugs (contraceptives)	J3490
underarm crutches, wood	E0112
unipuncture control system, dialysis	E1580
upholstery, reinforced seat, wheelchair	E0975
upholstery seat, wheelchair	E0991
urea (Ureaphil), injection	J3350
urinary drainage bag	A4357
urinary leg bag	A4358
urinary suspensory	A4359
urine control strips or tablets	A4250
urine sensitivity study	P7001
V	
vancomycin HCl (Vancocin), injection	J3370
vaporizer	E0605
vascular catheters	A4300
venous pressure clamps, dialysis	A4918
ventilator, volume	E0450
vest, safety, wheelchair	E0980
vinblastine sulfate, injection	J9360
vinblastine sulfate (Velban), injection	J9360
vitamin B_{12}, injection	J3420
vitamin K, injection	J3430
volume ventilator, stationary or portable	E0450
W	
walker, wheeled, without seat	E0141
walker attachments, platform	E0154
warfarin sodium (Coumadin), injection—unclassified	J3490
washed red blood cells, each unit	P9022
water, ambulance	A0050
water softening system, ESRD	E1625
water tanks, dialysis	A4880
wearable artificial kidney	E1632
wearable artificial kidney (WAK)	E1632
wheel attachment, walker	E0977
wheelchair, one-inch cushion for	E0962
wrist disarticulation prosthesis	L6060
Y	
youth wheelchair	E1091

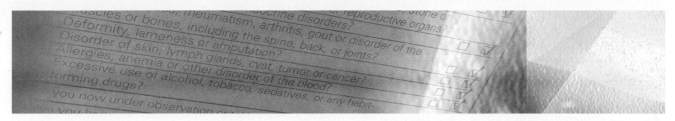

Medi-Cal

KEY TERMS

Your instructor may wish to select some words and abbreviations pertinent to the Medi-Cal program for a test. For definitions of the terms, further study, and/or reference, the words, phrases, and abbreviations may be found in the Glossary at the end of the Handbook. *Additional key terms are given in Chapter 13, "Medicaid and Other State Programs." Key terms and abbreviations for this appendix follow:*

accounts receivable (A/R) transaction

Aid to the Blind (AB)

Aid to Families with Dependent Children (AFDC)

Aid to the [permanently] Disabled (ATD)

automated eligibility verification system (AEVS)

benefits identification card (BIC)

California Children's Services (CCS)

Child Health and Disability Prevention Program (CHDP)

claim control number (CCN)

Claims and Eligibility Real-Time Software (CERTS)

Claims Inquiry Form (CIF)

Comprehensive Perinatal Services Program (CPSP)

computer media claims (CMC)

County Medical Services Program (CMSP)

Department of Health Services (DHS)

durable medical equipment (DME)

Electronic Data Systems (EDS) Corporation

electronic funds transfer (EFT)

eligibility verification confirmation (EVC)

Genetically Handicapped Persons Program (GHPP)

medically indigent (MI)

medically needy (MN)

nursing facility (NF)

Old Age Survivors, Health and Disability Insurance (OASHDI) Program

point-of-service (POS) device or network

presumptive eligibility (PE)

Provider Telecommunications Network (PTN)

Remittance Advice Details (RAD)

Resubmission Turnaround Document (RTD)

share of cost (SOC)

Treatment Authorization Request (TAR) form

Voice Drug TAR System (VDTS)

PERFORMANCE OBJECTIVES

The student will be able to:

▪ Define and spell the key terms and abbreviations for this chapter, given the information from the *Handbook* glossary, within a reasonable period of time and with enough accuracy to obtain a satisfactory evaluation.

▪ After reading the chapter, answer the self-study review questions with enough accuracy to obtain a satisfactory evaluation.

NOTE: See Chapter 13 ("Medicaid and Other State Programs"), and complete Assignments 13–2, 13–3, and 13–4, using Medi-Cal Office for Civil Rights (OCR) guidelines and block-by-block requirements found in Appendix B of the *Handbook*. Additional performance objectives will be met by completing CMS-1500 insurance claim forms for billing and posting to ledger cards.

STUDY OUTLINE

Types of Medi-Cal Plans
Managed Care Plans
Descriptions of Managed Care Plans

Medi-Cal Eligibility
Share of Cost
Identification Card
Eligibility Verification

Medi-Cal Benefits
Medi-Services

Prior Approval
Telecommunications Networks
Treatment Authorization Request

Claim Procedure
Fiscal Intermediaries
Copayment
Time Limit
Helpful Billing Tips
Medi-Cal and Other Coverage
Computer Media Claims

Uniform Bill (UB-92) Outpatient Claim Form
Instructions for Completing the UB-92
Claim Form

After Claim Submission
Remittance Advice Details
Resubmission Turnaround Document
Claims Inquiry Form

Appeal Process

Procedure: Completing a Treatment Authorization Request Form 50–1

Procedure: Instructions for Completing the CMS-1500 Claim Form for the Medi-Cal Program

Procedure: Completing the Resubmission Turnaround Document

Procedure: Completing the Claims Inquiry Form

Procedure: Completing an Appeal Form

 SELF-STUDY **C-1** ▸ **REVIEW QUESTIONS**

Review the objectives, key terms and abbreviations, chapter information, and figures in Appendix B of the *Handbook* before completing the following review questions.

1. List the Medi-Cal program managed care plan models.

a. _____

b. _____

c. _____

d. _____

e. _____

f. _____

g. _____

2. Mrs. Benson, a Medi-Cal recipient, injures her right leg in a fall. She is taken by ambulance to the emergency department of a local hospital. Must she seek treatment from a facility contracted under the Medi-Cal managed care plan, or can she be

treated wherever the ambulance takes her? _____

3. If a Medi-Cal patient receives services from outside of his or her Medi-Cal managed care plan, what must the out-of-plan physician submit with the claim form for services?

_____

_____

4. Medically indigent individuals who are unable to provide mainstream medical care for themselves and whose incomes are above the assistance level are classified under a

group called _____.

5. Name the entity that issues an identification card to each Medi-Cal recipient who is

eligible for benefits. _____

_____

6. Name the two most important verifications that are the provider's responsibilities to obtain.

a. _____

b. _____

7. List four methods used to verify eligibility.

a. _____

b. _____

c. _____

d. _____

8. Medical services to pregnant Medi-Cal recipients are available through the _____

_____ program.

9. The name of the program that offers temporary coverage for prenatal care before a

woman is officially a Medi-Cal recipient is called _____.

10. Medi-Cal recipients may receive _____ Medi-Services per calendar month.

11. An automated voice-response system for a provider to obtain before authorization for a

    Medi-Cal service is called _____.

12. Name two additional methods for obtaining prior approval for a Medi-Cal service.

    a. _____

    b. _____

13. To track a submitted Treatment Authorization Request (TAR), complete a/an _____.

14. A Medi-Cal patient seen today needs chronic hemodialysis services. You telephone for a TAR to get verbal approval. What four important items must you obtain to complete the written TAR?

    a. _____

    b. _____

    c. _____

    d. _____

15. A Medi-Cal patient comes in for an office visit, and the physician says the patient needs to undergo a cholecystectomy within the next 6 weeks to 2 months and that it needs to be scheduled when convenient (also known as elective surgery). Before scheduling surgery, what do you do?

    _____

    _____

    After you have completed this procedure, the patient is scheduled for the

    cholecystectomy. After surgery, you bill Medi-Cal, noting _____

    and _____ on the claim form. Do you need to send any

    information to the hospital? _____

16. The Medi-Cal copayment fee when a Medi-Cal patient seeks professional medical

    services from a physician is $_____.

17. The Medi-Cal copayment fee when a patient has a prescription refilled is $ _____.

18. The time limit for submission of a Medi-Cal claim to receive 100% of the maximum

    allowable is _____.

    A claim submitted within 8 months after service is rendered is reimbursed

    at _____%. A claim sent within 12 months after service is given is paid

    _____ at _____%. A claim submitted over 1 year from the month

    service is received is paid _____%.

19. State the difference in policy between the Medi-Cal global fee and the Medicare
    global package.

    _____

    _____

    _____

20. When a Medi-Cal patient has a private health insurance policy, to whom do you

    submit the initial claim? _____

21. Claims for patients who are recipients of Medicare and Medi-Cal are referred to as

    _____ claims and the claim assigned _____.

22. A Medi-Cal patient also has TRICARE. What billing procedure do you follow?
    Be exact in your steps for a dependent of an active military man.

    a. _____

    b. _____

23. Name the five categories of Medi-Cal adjudicated (resolution process) claims that
    appear on a Remittance Advice Details document.

    a. _____

    b. _____

    c. _____

    d. _____

    e. _____

24. When dollar amounts from a Remittance Advice Details document are posted to the

    patient's ledger, payments are shown as _____, and negative

    adjustments are posted as _____.

25. When the Medi-Cal fiscal intermediary makes a direct deposit into a provider's bank

    account, this is known as _____.

26. If a provider feels a claim was denied in error, he or she should submit a/an _____

    _____ for reconsideration.

27. On a Resubmission Turnaround Document, correct data are inserted into _____

    _____ of the form.

28. Dr. Practon requests an adjustment for an underpaid claim by submitting a/an _____.

29. A complaint about a Medi-Cal payment must be directed to the fiscal intermediary

    within _____ of the action that caused the complaint.

30. Define these Medi-Cal abbreviations.

    a. PE   _____   f. POS   _____

    b. RAD _____   g. CIF   _____

    c. BIC _____   h. RTD   _____

    d. TAR _____   i. SOC   _____

    e. MN   _____   j. AEVS _____

To check your answers to this self-study assignment, see Appendix D.

Claim Form Assignment

You will be completing the CMS-1500 claim form for the cases listed in Chapter 13 in this *Workbook* and directing them to your regional Medi-Cal fiscal agent. Refer to Appendix B of the *Handbook* for Medi-Cal block-by-block instructions and Figure B–7 for the Medi-Cal template. Use the claim forms and ledgers located in Chapter 13 in this *Workbook* or make copies of blank forms if the Medicaid assignments have been completed. Refer to the following assignments for specific additional information.

ASSIGNMENT **C–2** ▸ **COMPLETE A CMS-1500 CLAIM FORM
FOR A MEDI-CAL CASE**

Directions: To complete this assignment for Medi-Cal, you will need the following information in addition to that given in Chapter 13 in this *Workbook*:

1. Rose Clarkson has a share of cost (SOC) of $70.

2. Dr. James Jackson's nine-digit Medi-Cal provider number is 00G53472X.

3. Dr. Perry Cardi's nine-digit Medi-Cal provider number is 00A28695X.

4. The College Clinic's nine-digit Medi-Cal group number is ZZR1200XF.

ASSIGNMENT C-3 ▸ COMPLETE A CMS-1500 CLAIM FORM FOR A MEDI-CAL CASE

Directions: To complete this assignment for Medi-Cal, you will need the following information in addition to that given in Chapter 13 in this *Workbook*:

1. Dr. James B. Jeffers' nine-digit Medi-Cal provider number is 00C28287X.

2. Dr. Gerald Practon's nine-digit Medi-Cal provider number is 020A2365X.

3. The College Hospital's Medi-Cal facility number is HSC43700F.

4. The College Clinic's nine-digit Medi-Cal group number is ZZR1200XF.

ASSIGNMENT **C-4** ▸ **COMPLETE A CMS-1500 CLAIM FORM
FOR A MEDI-CAL CASE**

Directions: To complete this assignment for Medi-Cal, you will need the following information in addition to that given in Chapter 13 in this *Workbook*:

1. Dr. Raymond Skeleton's nine-digit Medi-Cal provider number is 000G6131X.

2. The College Hospital's Medi-Cal facility number is HSC43700F.

3. The College Clinic's nine-digit Medi-Cal group number is ZZR1200XF.

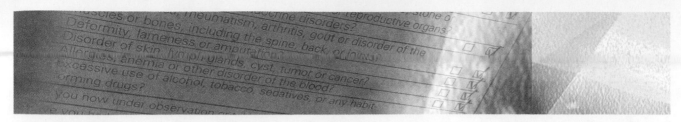

Answers to Self-Study Review Questions for Chapters

SELF-STUDY 1–1 REVIEW QUESTIONS

1. Read the job descriptions in Chapter 1 in the *Handbook*. Abilities to read handwritten and transcribed documents in the medical record, interpret information, and enter accurate code data into the computer system are technical skills required in the job of a/an **hospital coder and specialist for an acute and/or ambulatory care setting; Health Information/Medical Record Technician.**

2. Name some of the facilities where hospital billing is used.
   a. **acute care hospital**
   b. **skilled nursing facility**
   c. **long-term care facility**
   d. **rehabilitation or ambulatory surgical center**

3. Name examples of nonphysician practitioners (NPPs).
   a. **nurse practitioner**
   b. **physical therapist**
   c. **speech therapist**
   d. **licensed clinical social worker**
   e. **certified registered nurse practitioner**

4. Identify three career opportunities (job titles) available after training in diagnostic and procedural coding and insurance claims completion. Answers may vary but may consist of any three of the following:
   a. **insurance billing specialist, medical biller, reimbursement specialist, medical billing representative, senior billing representative, insurance counselor, collection manager, coding specialist**
   b. **electronic claims professional**
   c. **claims assistance professional**

5. List some of the responsibilities and duties an insurance billing specialist might perform generally as well as when acting as a collection manager. Answers may vary but should include the following comments:
   a. **Review diagnostic and procedural codes for correctness and completeness.**
   b. **Submit insurance claims promptly.**
   c. **Collect data from hospitals, laboratories, and other physicians involved in a case.**
   d. **Discuss practice's financial policies and insurance coverage and negotiate a payment plan.**
   e. **Answer routine inquiries related to account balances and insurance submission dates.**
   f. **Assist patients in budgeting.**
   g. **Follow up on delinquent accounts by tracing denied, adjusted, or unpaid claims.**

6. List the duties of a claims assistance professional.
   a. **Help patients organize, file, and negotiate health insurance claims of all types.**
   b. **Assist the consumer in obtaining maximum benefits from insurance companies.**
   c. **Tell the patient what checks to write to providers in order to eliminate overpayment.**

7. Insurance claims must be promptly submitted **within 1 to 5** business days to ensure continuous cash flow.

8. Define cash flow. **Amount of actual money available to the medical practice.**

9. Reasons for a medical practice's large accounts receivable are:
   a. **failure to verify insurance plan benefits**
   b. **failure to obtain authorization or precertification**

c. failure to collect copays or deductibles
d. inadequate claims filing

10. Skills required for an insurance billing specialist are: (Some or all of these may be mentioned by the student.)
    a. **knowledge of medical terminology**
    b. **knowledge of insurance terminology**
    c. **proficiency in completing insurance claims**
    d. **knowledge of procedural and diagnostic coding**
    e. **knowledge of anatomy and physiology, disease, and treatment (surgical, drug, and laboratory) terms**
    f. **computer skills; basic typing and/or keyboarding**
    g. **medicolegal knowledge**
    h. **knowledge of insurance carriers and Medicare policies and regulations**
    i. **basic math and use of calculator**
    j. **billing and collection techniques**
    k. **precise reading skills**
    l. **proficiency in accessing information via the Internet**
    m. **expert in legalities of collection on accounts**
    n. **use of photocopy and facsimile equipment**
    o. **knowledge of compliance issues**

11. Standards of conduct by which an insurance billing specialist determines the propriety of his or her behavior in a relationship are known as **medical ethics.**

12. Complete these statements with either the word *illegal* or *unethical.*
    a. To report incorrect information to the Aetna Casualty Company is **unethical.**
    b. To report incorrect information to a Medicare fiscal intermediary is **illegal.**
    c. It is **unethical** for two physicians to treat the same patient for the same condition.

13. When a physician is legally responsible for an employee's conduct performed during employment, this is known as **vicarious liability *(respondeat superior).***

14. A claims assistance professional neglects to submit an insurance claim to a Medicare supplemental insurance carrier within the proper time limit. What type of insurance is needed for protection against this loss for the client? **Errors and omissions insurance.**

SELF-STUDY 2–1 REVIEW QUESTIONS

1. Compliance is the process of **meeting regulations, recommendations, and expectations of federal and state agencies that pay for health care services and regulate the industry.**

2. Transactions in which health care information is accessed, processed, stored, and transferred using electronic technologies is known as **eHealth information management** and its acronym is **eHIM.**

3. Baby Nelson was born on January 20, 2005, at 7:15 AM. When using the required Health Level 7 (HL7) format for transmission, how would this appear? **200501200715**

4. A code system used for managing patient electronic health records, informatics, indexing, and billing laboratory procedures is called **Systematized**

Nomenclature of Human and Veterinary Medicine and its acronym is **SNOMED.**

5. What is the primary purpose of HIPAA Title I, Insurance Reform? **To provide continuous insurance coverage for workers and their insured dependents when they change or lose jobs.**

6. The focus on the health care practice setting and reduction of administrative costs and burdens are the goals of which part of HIPAA? **Title II, Administrative Simplification.**

7. A third-party administrator that receives insurance claims from the physician's office, performs edits, and transmits claims to insurance carriers is known as a/an **clearinghouse.**

8. Under HIPAA guidelines, a health care coverage carrier, such as Blue Cross/Blue Shield that transmits health information in electronic form in connection with a transaction is called a/an **covered entity.**

9. Dr. John Doe contracts with an outside billing company to manage claims and accounts receivable. Under HIPAA guidelines, the billing company is considered a/an **business associate** of the provider.

10. An individual designated to assist the provider by putting compliance policies and procedures in place and training office staff is known as a/an **privacy officer or privacy official** under HIPAA guidelines.

11. If you give, release, or transfer information to another entity, this is known as **disclosure.**

12. Define protected health informaton (PHI). **Data that identifies an individual and describes his or her health status, age, sex, ethnicity, or other demographic characteristics, whether or not that information is stored or transmitted electronically.**

13. Unauthorized release of a patient's health information is called **breach of confidential communication.**

14. A confidential communication related to the patient's treatment and progress that may be disclosed only with the patient's permission is known as **privileged communication.**

15. Exceptions to the right of privacy are those records involving:
    a. **industrial accidents (physician employed by insurance company)**
    b. **communicable diseases**
    c. **child abuse**
    d. **gunshot wounds**
    e. **stabbing from criminal actions**
    f. **diseases and ailments of newborns and infants**

16. At a patient's first visit under HIPAA guidelines, the document that must be given so the patient acknowledges the provider's confidentiality of their protected health information is the **Notice of Privacy Practices (NPP).**

17. Under HIPAA Privacy Regulation, state the types of information that patients do not have the right to access.
    a. **psychotherapy notes**
    b. **information compiled in anticipation of or use in legal proceedings**
    c. **information exempted from disclosure under the Clinical Laboratory Improvements Amendment (CLIA)**

18. Name the three main sections of the HIPAA Security Rule for protecting electronic health information.
   a. **administrative safeguards**
   b. **technical safeguards**
   c. **physical safeguards**
19. Indicate whether the situation is one of *fraud* or *abuse* in the following situations.
   a. Billing a claim for services not medically necessary. **abuse**
   b. Changing a figure on an insurance claim form to get increased payment. **fraud**
   c. Dismissing the copayment owed by a Medicare patient. **fraud**
   d. Neglecting to refund an overpayment to the patient. **abuse**
   e. Billing for a complex fracture when the patient suffered a simple break. **fraud**

SELF-STUDY 3–1 REVIEW QUESTIONS

1. A/an **insurance contract (policy)** is a legally enforceable agreement or contract.
2. An individual promising to pay for medical services rendered is known as a/an **guarantor.**
3. List five health insurance policy renewal provisions.
   a. **cancelable**
   b. **optionally renewable**
   c. **conditionally renewable**
   d. **guaranteed renewable**
   e. **noncancelable**
4. Insurance reimbursement or payment is also called **indemnity.**
5. Name two general health insurance policy limitations.
   a. **exclusions**
   b. **waiver or rider**
6. The act of finding out whether treatment is covered under an individual's health insurance policy is called **precertification.**
7. The steps to obtain permission for a procedure before it is done, to see whether the insurance program agrees it is medically necessary, is termed **preauthorization.**
8. Determining the maximum dollar amount the insurance company will pay for a procedure before it is done is known as **predetermination.**
9. Name three ways an individual may obtain health insurance.
   a. **Take out insurance through a group plan (contract or policy).**
   b. **Pay the premium on an individual basis.**
   c. **Enroll in a prepaid health plan.**
10. List four methods a physician's practice may use to submit insurance claims to insurance companies.
   a. **manual claims submission on the CMS-1500 claim form**
   b. **electronic claims filing from in-office computers**
   c. **contracting with an outside service bureau to prepare and submit claims electronically on behalf of the health care provider's office.**
   d. **direct data entry into the payer's system**

11. A document signed by the insured directing the insurance company to pay benefits directly to the physician is known as a/an **assignment of benefits.**
12. A patient service slip personalized to the practice of the physician and used as a communications/billing tool during routing of the patient is also known as a/an (Answers may vary but may consist of any four of the following):
   a. **encounter form**
   b. **transaction slip**
   c. **charge slip**
   d. **fee ticket**
   e. **routing form**
   f. **multipurpose billing form**
   g. **patient service slip**
   h. **superbill**
13. Electronic access to computer data may consist of the following verification or access methods.
   a. **series of numbers**
   b. **series of letters**
   c. **electronic writing (signatures or initials)**
   d. **voice**
   e. **fingerprint transmission**
   f. **computer key**
14. Guidelines for avoiding unauthorized use and preventing problems when a medical practice uses a facsimile signature stamp are:
   a. **Make only one stamp.**
   b. **Allow only long-term, trusted, bonded staff members to have access to the stamp.**
   c. **Keep the stamp in a location with a secure lock.**
   d. **Limit access to the stamp.**
15. Match the following insurance terms in the right column with their descriptions and fill in the blank with the appropriate letter.
   a. adjuster
   b. assignment
   c. carrier
   d. coordination of benefits
   e. deductible
   f. exclusions
   g. indemnity
   h. premium
   i. subscriber
   j. time limit
   k. waiting period
   d An insurance company takes into account benefits payable by another carrier in determining its own liability.
   g Benefits paid by an insurance company to an insured person.
   b Transfer of one's right to collect an amount payable under an insurance contract.
   k Time that must elapse before an indemnity is paid.
   a Acts for insurance company or insured in settlement of claims.
   h Periodic payment to keep insurance policy in force.
   e Amount insured person must pay before policy will pay.
   j Time period in which a claim must be filed.

f Certain illnesses or injuries listed in a policy that the insurance company will not cover.
c Insurance company that carries the insurance.
i One who belongs to an insurance plan.

SELF-STUDY 4–1 REVIEW QUESTIONS

1. Written or graphic information about patient care is termed a/an **health record.**
2. **Documentation** is written or dictated to record chronologic facts and observations about a patient's health.
3. Match the following terms in the right column with their descriptions and fill in the blank with the appropriate letter.
   a. Attending physician   **g** Renders a service to a patient.
   b. Consulting physician   **c** Directs selection, preparation, and administration of tests, physician medication, or treatment.
   c. Ordering physician   **a** Legally responsible for the care and treatment given to a patient.
   d. Primary care physician   **b** Gives an opinion regarding a specific problem that is requested by another doctor.
   e. Referring physician   **e** Sends the patient for tests or treatment or to another performing doctor for consultation.
   f. Teaching physician   **d** Oversees care of patients in managed care plans and refers patients to see specialists when needed
   g. Treating or performing physician   **f** Responsible for training and supervising medical students.
   h. Treating practitioner   **h** Clinical nurse specialist or physician assistant treating a patient for a medical problem
4. Performance of services or procedures consistent with the diagnosis, done with standards of good medical practice and a proper level of care given in the appropriate setting, is known as **medical necessity.**
5. If a medical practice is audited by Medicare officials and intentional miscoding is discovered, **fines and penalties** may be levied and providers may be **excluded from the program.**
6. A list of all staff members' names, job titles, signatures, and their initials is known as a/an **signature log.**
7. How should an insurance billing specialist correct an error on a patient's record? **Use legal copy pen, cross out wrong entry with a single line, write the correct entry, and date and initial entry. Never erase or use white correction paint or self-adhesive paper over errors. Or, create a typed addendum inserted below in the next available space in the patient's record.**

8. Name the five documentation components of a patient's history.
   a. **chief complaint**
   b. **history of present illness**
   c. **past history**
   d. **family history**
   e. **social history**
9. An inventory of body systems by documenting responses to questions about symptoms that a patient has experienced is called a/an **review of systems.**
10. Define the following terms in relationship to billing.
    a. New patient. **One who has not received any professional services from the physician or another physician of the same specialty who belongs to the same group practice, within the past 3 years.**
    b. Established patient. **One who has received professional services from the physician or another physician of the same specialty who belongs to the same group practice, within the past 3 years.**
11. Explain the difference between a consultation and the referral of a patient.
    a. Consultation. **Services rendered by a physician whose opinion or advice is requested by another physician or agency in the evaluation or treatment of a patient's illness or a suspected problem.**
    b. Referral. **Transfer of the total or specific care of a patient from one physician to another for known problems.**
12. Medical care for a patient who has received treatment for an illness and is referred to a second physician for treatment of the same condition is a situation called **continuity of care.**
13. If two physicians see the same patient on the same day, one for the patient's heart condition and the other for a diabetic situation, this medical care situation is called **concurrent care.**
14. When faxing a patient's medical records, a signed document **for authorizing release of information via the fax machine** must be obtained from the patient.
15. Action to take when a faxed medical document is misdirected is **telephone or fax a request to destroy the information erroneously sent.**
16. What must the former physician have from the patient before a record can be given to a new physician? **A written request from the patient or a signed authorization or release of information form.**
17. What must an insurance billing specialist do if he or she receives a request from another physician for certain records? **Obtain a written request from the patient or a signed authorization or release of information form.**
18. What must a physician have from the patient before he or she can give information to an attorney? **An authorization or release of information form signed by the patient or a subpoena.**
19. Indicate either indefinite retention or number of years for keeping records in the following situations.
    a. Computerized payroll records   **7 years**
    b. Insurance claim for Medicare patient **7 years**
    c. Medical record of a deceased patient **5 years**

d. Active patient medical records   **indefinite retention**

e. Letter to a patient about balance **1 to 5 years** due after insurance paid

20. Is it proper for an insurance billing specialist to receive a subpoena for his or her physician? **Yes, if the physician gives him or her this authority.**

21. Can a physician terminate a contract with a patient? **Yes.** If so, how? **By sending a letter of withdrawal of care, registered or certified with return signature.**

SELF-STUDY 4–2 REVIEW QUESTIONS

1. Match the following terms in the right column with the descriptions and fill in the blank with the appropriate letter.

d Pertaining to both sides   a. acute

e Decubitus ulcer   b. chronic

a Condition that runs a short but severe course   c. menopause

c Change of life   d. bilateral

f Tinnitus   e. bed sore

b Condition persisting over a long period of time in ears   f. ringing sensation in ears

2. Write in the meaning for these abbreviations and/or symbols commonly encountered in a patient's medical record.

RLQ	**right lower quadrant**
DC	**discharge**
WNL	**within normal limits**
R/O	**rule out**
URI	**upper respiratory infection**
$\bar{c}$	**with**
+	**positive**

3. When documenting incisions, the unit of measure length should be listed in **centimeters (cm).**

4. If a physician called and asked for a patient's medical record "STAT," what would he or she mean?
   a. The physician wants a statistic from a patient's record.
   b. The physician wants the record delivered on Tuesday.
   c. **The physician wants the record delivered immediately.**

5. If a physician asks you to locate the results of the last UA, what would you be searching for?
   a. **a urinalysis report**
   b. an x-ray report of the ulna
   c. uric acid test results

6. If a physician telephoned and asked for a copy of the last H&P to be faxed, what is being requested?
   a. heart and pulmonary findings
   b. H_2 antagonist test results
   c. **a history and physical examination**

7. If a hospital nurse telephoned and asked you to read the results of the patient's last CBC, what would you be searching for?
   a. carcinoma basal cell report
   b. **complete blood count**
   c. congenital blindness, complete report

8. If you were asked to make a photocopy of the patient's last CT, what would you be searching for?
   a. chemotherapy record
   b. connective tissue report
   c. **computed tomography scan**

SELF-STUDY 5–1 ICD-9-CM REVIEW QUESTIONS

1. Why is it important that diagnostic ICD-9-CM coding become routinely used in the physician's office? **Diagnostic coding should be routinely used in the physician's office to ensure accuracy of reporting a patient's diagnosis and so that the physician's future profiles reflect more realistic payments.**

2. For retrieving types of diagnoses related to pathology by an institution within an institution, the coding system is found in a book entitled *Systematized Nomenclature of Human and Veterinary Medicine (SNOMED) International.*

3. The system for coding and billing diagnoses is found in a book entitled *International Classification of Diseases, ninth revision, Clinical Modification.*

4. The abbreviation ICD-9-CM means *International Classification of Diseases, ninth revision, Clinical Modification.*

5. Volume 1, "Diseases," is a/an **tabular or numerical** listing of code numbers.

6. Volume 2, "Diseases," is a/an **alphabetic** index or listing of code numbers.

7. The coding in ICD-9-CM varies from **3** to **5** characters.

8. The abbreviation NEC appearing in the ICD-9-CM code book means **not elsewhere classifiable.**

9. To code using Volume 2, the Alphabetic Index, the main term, the **condition,** is looked up, rather than the anatomic part.

10. E codes are a supplementary classification of coding for **external causes of injury** rather than disease and of coding for **adverse reactions to medications.**

Self-Study 5–2 ICD-10-CM Review Questions

1. ICD-10 was published by the
   a. National Center for Health Statistics
   b. **World Health Organization**
   c. Centers for Disease Control and Prevention
   d. Centers for Medicare and Medicaid Services

2. ICD-10-CM is being clinically modified by the
   a. **National Center for Health Statistics**
   b. World Health Organization
   c. Centers for Disease Control and Prevention
   d. Centers for Medicare and Medicaid Services

3. ICD-10-PCS (Procedure Coding System) was developed by 3M Health Information Systems under contract with the
   a. National Center for Health Statistics
   b. World Health Organization
   c. Centers for Disease Control and Prevention
   d. **Centers for Medicare and Medicaid Services**

4. The disease codes in ICD-10-CM have a maximum of
   a. three digits
   b. four digits
   c. five digits
   d. six digits
   e. **seven digits**

5. Reason(s) the Clinical Modification was developed is/are
   a. Removal of procedural codes
   b. Removal of unique mortality codes

c. Removal of multiple codes
d. Only a and c
e. Only b
f. All of the above
6. One of the reasons for ICD-10-PCS is that
   a. ICD-9-CM was not capable of necessary expansion
   b. ICD-9-CM was not as comprehensive as it should have been
   c. ICD-9-CM included diagnostic information
   d. All of the above
7. The letters "I" and "O" are (were) used in
   a. ICD-9-CM
   b. ICD-10-CM Diseases
   c. ICD-10-PCS
   d. None of the above

SELF-STUDY 6–1 REVIEW QUESTIONS

1. The coding system used for billing professional medical services and procedures is found in a book entitled ***Current Procedural Terminology.***
2. The Medicare program uses a system of coding composed of three levels, and this is called **Healthcare Common Procedure Coding System (HCPCS).**
3. Complications or special circumstances about a medical service or procedure may be shown by using a CPT code with a/an **modifier.**
4. A relative value scale or schedule is a listing of procedure codes indicating the relative value of services performed, which is shown by **unit values.**
5. Name three methods for basing payments adopted by insurance companies and by state and federal programs.
   a. **fee schedule**
   b. **relative value schedule (RVS)**
   c. **usual, customary, and reasonable (UCR)**
6. List four situations that can occur in a medical practice when referring to charges and payments from a fee schedule.
   a. **Providers participating in the Medicare program would typically be paid by the fiscal agent an amount from a fee schedule for Medicare patients.**
   b. **Providers not participating in the Medicare program would typically be paid by the fiscal agent an amount: one based on limiting charges for each service set by the Medicare program.**
   c. **Providers that have a contractual arrangement with a managed care plan would be paid based on the fee schedule written into the negotiated contract.**
   d. **Providers rendering services to patients who have sustained industrial injuries use a separate workers' compensation fee schedule.**
7. Name the eight main sections of CPT.
   a. **Evaluation and Management**
   b. **Anesthesia**
   c. **Surgery**
   d. **Radiology, Nuclear Medicine, and Diagnostic Ultrasound**
   e. **Pathology and Laboratory**
   f. **Medicine**
   g. **Category II Codes**
   h. **Category III Codes**
8. Match the symbol in the first column with the definitions in the second column. Write the correct letters on the blanks.
   d ►◄   a. New code
   a ●   b. Modifier -51 exempt
   f ⟳   c. Add-on code
   b ⊘   d. New or revised text
   c +   e. Revised code
   e ▲   f. Service includes surgical procedure only
   g ⊙   g. Conscious sedation
9. Name five hospital departments where critical care of a patient may take place.
   a. **coronary care unit (CCU)**
   b. **intensive care unit (ICU)**
   c. **pediatric intensive care unit**
   d. **respiratory care unit (RCU)**
   e. **emergency department (ED) or emergency room (ER)**
10. A surgical package includes
    a. **surgical procedure (operation)**
    b. **local infiltration, digital block, or topical anesthesia**
    c. **subsequent to the decision for surgery, one related E/M encounter on the date immediately before or on the date of procedure (including history and physical)**
    d. **immediate postoperative care including dictating operative notes and talking with the family and other physicians**
    e. **writing orders**
    f. **evaluating the patient in the postanesthesia recovery area**
    g. **typical postoperative follow-up care (hospital visits, discharge, or follow-up office visits)**
11. Medicare global surgery policy includes
    a. **preoperative visit (1 day before or day of surgery)**
    b. **intraoperative services that are a usual and necessary part of the surgical procedure**
    c. **complications after surgery that do not necessitate additional trips to the operating room**
    d. **postoperative visits, including hospital visits, discharge, and office visit for variable postoperative period (0, 10, or 90 days)**
    e. **writing orders**
    f. **evaluating the patient in the recovery area**
    g. **normal postoperative pain management**
12. A function of computer software that performs online checking of codes on an insurance claim to detect improper code submission is called a/an **code edit.**
13. A single code that describes two or more component codes bundled together as one unit is known as a/an **comprehensive code.**
14. To group related codes together is commonly referred to as **bundled or bundling.**
15. Use of many procedural codes to identify procedures that may be described by one code is termed **unbundling, also known as "exploding" or "á la carte" medicine.**

16. A code used on a claim that does not match the code system used by the insurance carrier and is converted to the closest code rendering less payment is termed **downcoding.**

17. Intentional manipulation of procedural codes to generate increased reimbursement is called **upcoding.**

18. Give eight reasons for using modifiers on insurance claims.
    a. **A service or procedure has professional and technical components.**
    b. **A service or procedure was performed by more than one physician and/or in more than one location.**
    c. **A service or procedure has been increased or reduced.**
    d. **A service or procedure was provided more than once.**
    e. **Only part of a service was performed.**
    f. **An adjunctive service was performed.**
    g. **A bilateral procedure was performed.**
    h. **Unusual events occurred.**

19. Match the symbol in the first column with the definitions in the second column. Write the correct letters on the blanks.
    f -21   a. Unusual procedural services
    a -22   b. Multiple procedures
    e -25   c. Staged or related procedure
    h -26   d. Decision for surgery
    b -51   e. Significant, separately identifiable E/M service by the same physician on the same day of the procedure or other service
    g -52   f. Prolonged evaluation and management services
    d -57   g. Reduced services
    c -58   h. Professional component

20. What modifier is usually used in billing for an assistant surgeon? **-80**

21. Explain when to use the -99 modifier code.* **If a procedure requires more than one modifier code, a multiple two-digit code (-99) after the usual five-digit code number is typed on one line.**

SELF-STUDY 6–2 DEFINE MEDICAL ABBREVIATIONS

I & D	**incision and drainage**
IM	**intramuscular**
Pap	**Papanicolaou (smear, stain)**
ER	**emergency room**
EEG	**electroencephalograph (gram)**
DPT	**diphtheria, pertussis, tetanus**
ECG	**electrocardiogram (graph)**
IUD	**intrauterine device**
OB	**obstetrics**
D & C	**dilatation & curettage**

---

*Current Procedural Terminology codes, descriptions, and two-digit numeric modifiers only are from CPT 2005. Copyright © 2004, American Medical Association. All rights reserved.

OV	**office visit**
KUB	**kidneys, ureters, bladder**
GI	**gastrointestinal**
Hgb	**hemoglobin**
new pt	**new patient**
rt	**right**
UA	**urinalysis**
est pt	**established patient**
ASHD	**arteriosclerotic heart disease**
tet. tox.	**tetanus toxoid**
CBC	**complete blood count**
E/M	**Evaluation and Management (code)**
CPT	**Current Procedural Terminology**
Ob-Gyn	**obstetrics and gynecology**
TURP	**transurethral resection of prostate**
cm	**centimeter**
T & A	**tonsillectomy and adenoidectomy**
mL	**milliliter**
inj	**injection**
hx	**history**
NC	**no charge**

SELF-STUDY 7–1 REVIEW QUESTIONS

1. Who developed the Standard Form? **Health Insurance Association of America and American Medical Association.**

2. State the name of the insurance form approved by the American Medical Association. **Health Insurance Claim Form (CMS-1500).**

3. Does Medicare accept the CMS-1500 claim form? **Yes.**

4. What important document must you have before an insurance company can photocopy a patient's chart? **Release of information form signed by the patient.**

5. What is dual coverage? **The situation in which the patient has two insurance policies, one of which is considered primary and the other secondary.**

6. The insurance company with the first responsibility for payment of a bill for medical services is known as **the primary payer.**

7. Match the types of claims listed in the right column with their descriptions, and fill in the blanks with the appropriate letters.
    h Claim missing required information   a. clean claim
    f Phrase used when a claim is held back from payment   b. paper claim
    b Claim that is submitted and then optically scanned by the insurance carrier and converted to electronic form   c. invalid claim
    d Claim that needs manual processing because of errors or to solve a problem   d. dirty claim
    g Claim that needs clarification and answers to some questions   e. electronic claim
    e Claim that is submitted via telephone, fax, or computer modem   f. suspense claim

a Claim that is submitted the time limit and correctly completed

g. rejected claim

c Medicare claim that contains information that is complete and necessary but is illogical or incorrect

h. incomplete claim

8. If the patient brings in a private insurance form that is not group insurance, where do you send the form after completion? **To the insurance company.**

9. Match the types of number listed in the right column with their descriptions, and fill in the blanks with the appropriate letters.

c A number issued by the federal government to each individual for personal use

a. State license number

g A Medicare lifetime provider number

b. Employer identification number

f A number listed on a claim when submitting insurance claims to insurance companies under a group name

c. Social Security number

e A number issued by the Medicare program to each physician who treats and submits claims to this program

d. Provider identification number

a A number that a physician must obtain to practice in a state

e. Unique provider identification number

h A number used when billing for supplies and equipment

f. Group provider number

i A number issued to a hospital

g. National provider number

b An individual hospital physician's federal tax identification number issued by the Internal Revenue Service

h. Durable Medical Equipment number

d A number issued by the insurance carrier to every physician who renders services to patients

i. Facility provider number

10. An insurance claim is returned for the reason "diagnosis incomplete." State one or more solutions to this problem on how you would try to obtain reimbursement. **Verify and submit correct diagnostic codes by referring to an updated diagnostic code book and reviewing the patient record. Check with the physician if diagnosis code listed does not go with the procedure code shown.**

11. Indicate whether the following statements are true (T) or false (F).
    a. A photocopy of a claim form may be optically scanned. **F**
    b. Handwriting is permitted on optically scanned insurance claims. **F**
    c. Do not fold or crease an insurance form that will be optically scanned. **T**
    d. Never strike over errors when making a correction on a claim form that is to be optically scanned. **T**

12. When preparing a claim that is to be optically scanned, birth dates are keyed in with **8** digits.
13. Define this abbreviation: MG/MCD. **Medigap and Medicaid coverage.**
14. A CMS-assigned National Provider Identifier (NPI) number consists of **10** characters.

SELF-STUDY 7–6 REVIEW PATIENT RECORD ABBREVIATIONS

1. What do these abbreviations mean?
   a. PTR — **patient to return**
   b. TURP — **transurethral resection of prostate**
   c. HX — **history**
   d. IVP — **intravenous pyelogram**
   e. $\bar{c}$ — **with**
   f. Dx — **diagnosis**
   g. BP — **blood pressure**
   h. CC — **chief complaint**
   i. UA — **urinalysis**
   j. PE — **physical examination**
2. Give the abbreviation for the following terms.
   a. return — **retn, ret, rtn**
   b. cancer, carcinoma — **CA, Ca**
   c. patient — **pt, Pt**
   d. established — **est**
   e. discharged — **DC**
   f. gallbladder — **gb, GB**
   g. initial — **init (office visit)**

SELF-STUDY 8–1 REVIEW QUESTIONS

1. Exchange of data in a standardized format through computer systems is a technology known as **electronic data interchange (EDI).**
2. The act of converting computerized data into a code so that unauthorized users are unable to read it is a security system known as **encryption.**
3. Payment to the provider of service of an electronically submitted insurance claim may be received in approximately **2 weeks or less.**
4. List some benefits of using HIPAA standard transactions and code sets.
   a. **more reliable and timely processing—quicker reimbursement from payer**
   b. **improved accuracy of data**
   c. **easier and more efficient access to information**
   d. **better tacking of transactions**
   e. **reduction of data entry and manual labor**
   f. **reduction in office expenses**
5. Dr. Morgan has 10 or more full-time employees and submits insurance claims for his Medicare patients. Is his medical practice subject to the HIPAA transaction rules? **Yes.**
6. Dr. Maria Montez does not submit insurance claims electronically and has five full-time employees. Is she required to abide by HIPAA transaction rules? **No.**
7. Name the standard code sets used for the following:
   a. physician services *Current Procedural Terminology* **code set**

b. diseases and injuries *International Classification of Diseases, ninth edition, Clinical Modification, Volumes 1 and 2*

c. pharmaceuticals and biologics *National Drug Codes for Retail Pharmacy transactions*

8. Refer to Table 8–3 in the *Handbook* to complete these statements.

a. The staff at College Clinic submits professional health care claims for each of their providers and must use the industry standard electronic format called **ASC X12N 837P** to transmit them electronically.

b. The billing department at College Hospital must use the industry standard electronic format called **ASC X12N 837I** to transmit health care claims electronically.

c. The Medicare fiscal intermediary (insurance carrier) uses the industry standard electronic format called **ASC X12N 835** to transmit payment information to the College Clinic and College Hospital.

d. It has been 3 weeks since Gordon Marshall's health care claim was transmitted to the XYZ insurance company and you wish to inquire about the status of the claim. The industry standard electronic format that must be used to transmit this inquiry is called **ASC X12N 276**

e. Dr. Practon's insurance billing specialist must use the industry standard electronic format called

ASC X12N 270 to obtain information about Beatrice Garcia's health policy benefits and coverage from the insurance plan.

9. The family practice taxonomy code is **203BF10100Y**

10. A Medicare patient, Charles Gorman, signed a signature authorization form, which is on file. The patient's signature source code for data element #1351 is **B.**

11. Name the levels for data collected to construct and submit an electronic claim.

a. **High-level information**

b. **Claim-level information**

c. **Specialty claim-level information**

d. **Service line-level information**

e. **Specialty service line-level information**

f. **Other information**

12. The most important function of a practice management system is **accounts receivable.**

13. To look for and correct all errors before the health claim is transmitted to the insurance carrier, you may **print an insurance billing worksheet** or **perform a front-end edit (online error checking).**

14. Add-on software to a practice management system that can reduce the time it takes to build or review a claim before batching is known as a/an **encoder.**

15. Software that is used in a network which serves a group of users working on a related project allowing access to the same data is called a/an **grouper.**

SELF-STUDY 8–9 REVIEW PATIENT RECORD ABBREVIATIONS

Abbreviations pertinent to the record of Brad E. Diehl:

NP	new patient	exam	examination
pt	patient	LC	low complexity (decision making)
AP	anterior-posterior, anteroposterior	MDM	medical decision making
lat	lateral; pertaining to the side	cm	centimeter
neg	negative	CBC	complete blood count
BP	blood pressure	auto	automated
R/O	rule out	diff	differential
retn	return	WBC	white blood cell (count)
EPF	expanded problem-focused (history/examination)	Dx	diagnosis
hx	history	adv	advise(d)

Abbreviations pertinent to the record of Evert I. Strain:

est	established	CT	computed or computerized tomography
pt	patient	C	comprehensive (history/examination)
H & P	history and physical (examination)	hx	history
comp	comprehensive	exam	examination
PX	physical examination	MC	moderate-complexity (decision making)
BP	blood pressure	MDM	medical decision making
Lab	laboratory	hosp	hospital
SGOT	serum glutamic oxaloacetic transaminase	PF	problem focused
Dx	diagnosis	SF	straightforward
ASCVD	arteriosclerotic cardiovascular disease	neg	negative
GTT	glucose tolerance test	DC	discharged
STAT	immediately	ofc	office

SELF-STUDY 9-1 REVIEW QUESTIONS

1. Name provisions seen in health insurance policies.
   a. **The claimant is obligated to notify the insurance company of a loss within a certain time period; otherwise, the insurance company can deny benefits.**
   b. **If the insured is in disagreement with the insurer for settlement of a claim, a suit must begin within 3 years after the claim was submitted.**
   c. **An insured person cannot bring legal action against an insurance company until 60 days after a claim is submitted to the insurance company.**
   d. **The insurance company is obligated to pay benefits promptly when a claim is submitted.**
2. After an insurance claim is processed by the insurance carrier (paid, suspended, rejected, or denied), a document known as a/an **explanation of benefits** is sent to the patient and to the provider of professional medical services.
3. Name other items that indicate the patient's responsibility to pay that may appear on the document explaining the payment and check issued by the insurance carrier.
   a. **amount not covered**
   b. **copayment amount**
   c. **deductible**
   d. **coinsurance**
   e. **other insurance payment**
   f. **patient's total responsibility**
4. After receiving an explanation of benefits (EOB) document and posting insurance payment, the copy of the insurance claim form is put into a file marked **closed claims.**
5. To locate delinquent insurance claims on an insurance claim register quickly, which column should be looked at first? **Data claim paid column.** Would it appear blank or completed? **Blank.**
6. Name some of the principal procedures that should be followed in good bookkeeping and record-keeping practice when a payment has been received from an insurance company. **Pull out copies of the insurance claims that correspond with the payments and dispose of them, post payment to the patient's financial accounting record (ledger) and to the day sheet, and deposit the payment check in the bank.**
7. In good office management, a manual method used to track submitted pending or resubmitted insurance claims, a/an **tickler, suspense, or follow-up file** is used.
8. List two routine procedures to include in a manual reminder system to track pending claims.
   a. **Divide active claims by month.**
   b. **File active claims in chronologic order by date of service.**
9. In making an inquiry about a claim by telephone, efficient secretarial procedure would be to **document the date, time of the call, name of the person spoken to and his or her telephone extension, and outline or briefly note the conversation.**
10. Denied paper or electronic claims are those denied because of **benefits coverage policy issues** or **program issues.**
11. State the solution if a claim has been denied because the professional service rendered was for an injury that is being considered as compensable under workers' compensation. **Locate the insurance carrier for the industrial injury and send it a report of the case with a bill. Notify the patient's health insurance carrier monthly of the status of the case.**
12. At the time of his first office visit, Mr. Doi signed an Assignment of Benefits, and Dr. James' office submitted a claim to ABC Insurance Company. Mr. Doi received, in error, a check from the insurance company and cashed it. What steps should be taken by Dr. James' office after this error is discovered?
   a. **Call the insurance company.**
   b. **Call the patient or send a letter by certified mail.**
   c. **File a complaint with the state insurance commissioner.**
13. If an appeal of an insurance claim is not successful, the next step to proceed with is a/an **peer review.**
14. Name the five levels for appealing a Medicare claim.
   a. **Redetermination (telephone, letter, or CMS-20027 form)**
   b. **Hearing officer (HO) hearing (reconsideration)**
   c. **Administrative law judge (ALJ) hearing**
   d. **Departmental Appeal Board review**
   e. **Judicial review in U.S. District Court**
15. Medicare reconsideration by the insurance carrier is usually completed within **30** to **45** days.
16. A Medicare patient has insurance with United American (a Medigap policy), and payment has not been received from the Medigap insurer within a reasonable length of time. State the action to take in this case. **Contact the insurance company and state that if you do not receive payment, you will contact the state insurance commissioner.**
17. A TRICARE EOB is received stating that the allowable charge for Mrs. Dayton's office visit is $30. Is it possible to appeal this for additional payment? **No, in general, when the TRICARE contractor determines the allowable charge for a certain medical service, it is nonappealable.**
18. A state department or agency that helps resolve insurance conflicts and verifies that insurance contracts are carried out in good faith is known as a/an **insurance commission of the state.**
19. When an insurance company consistently pays slowly on insurance claims, it may help speed up payments if a formal written complaint is made to the **insurance commissioner.**

SELF-STUDY 10-1 REVIEW QUESTIONS

1. Third-party payers are composed of
   a. **private insurance**
   b. **government plans**
   c. **managed care contracts**
   d. **workers' compensation**
2. The unpaid balance due from patients for professional services rendered is known as a/an **accounts receivable.**
3. Write the formula for calculating the office accounts receivable (A/R) ratio. **Divide the month-end accounts**

receivable balance by the monthly average of the **medical practice charge for the prior 12-month period.**

4. What is the collection rate if a total of $40,300 was collected for the month and the total of the accounts receivable is $50,670? **80%**

5. An important document that provides identifying data for each patient and assists in billing and collection is called a/an **patient registration form or patient information sheet.**

6. A term preferable to "write-off" when used in a medical practice is **courtesy adjustment.**

7. To verify a check, ask the patient for a/an **driver's license** and **one other form of identification.**

8. The procedure of systematically arranging the accounts receivable, by age, from the date of service is called **age analysis.**

9. Are physicians' patient accounts single-entry accounts, open-book accounts, or written contract accounts? **Open-book accounts.**

10. Match the terms in the right column with the descriptions, and fill in the blank with the appropriate letter.

    d Reductions of the normal fee on the basis of a specific amount of money or a percentage of the charge   a. debtor

    g Phrase to remind a patient about a delinquent account   b. itemized statement

    h Item that permits bank customers to withdraw cash at any hour from an automated teller machine   c. fee schedule

    a Individual owing money   d. discounts

    i Claim on the property of another person as security for a debt   e. financial account record (ledger)

    e Individual record indicating charges, payments, adjustments, and balances owed for services rendered   f. creditor

    b Detailed summary of all transactions of a creditor's account   g. dun message

    f Person to whom money is owed   h. debit card

    c Listing of accepted charges or established allowances for specific medical procedures   i. lien

11. A court order attaching a debtor's property or wages to pay off a debt is known as a/an **garnishment.**

12. Match the following federal acts with their descriptions and fill in the blank with the appropriate letter.
    a. Equal Credit Opportunity Act
    b. Fair Credit Reporting Act
    c. Fair Credit Billing Act
    d. Truth in Lending Act
    e. Fair Debt Collection Practices Act

    c Law that states that a person has 60 days to complain about an error from the date that a statement is mailed.

    d Consumer protection act that applies to anyone who charges interest or agrees on payment of a bill in more than four installments, excluding a down payment.

    e Regulates collection practices of third-party debt collectors and attorneys who collect debts for others.

    a Federal law that prohibits discrimination in all areas of granting credit.

    b Regulates agencies who issue or use credit reports on consumers

13. An individual who owes on an account and moves, leaving no forwarding address, is called a/an **skip.**

14. A straight petition in bankruptcy or absolute bankruptcy is also known as a/an **Chapter 7.**

15. A wage earner's bankruptcy is sometimes referred to as a/an **Chapter 13.**

16. Translate these credit and collection abbreviations.

NSF	**not sufficient funds**	T	**telephoned**
WCO	**will call office**	SK	**skip or skipped**
PIF	**payment in full**	FN	**final notice**
NLE	**no longer employed**	UE	**unemployed**

17. State three bonding methods.
    a. **position-schedule bond**
    b. **blanket-position bond**
    c. **personal bond**

18. A system of billing accounts at spaced intervals during the month on the basis of a breakdown of accounts by alphabet, account number, insurance type, or date of service is known as **cycle billing.**

SELF-STUDY 11–1 REVIEW QUESTIONS

1. If a physician or hospital in a managed care plan is paid a fixed, per capita amount for each patient enrolled regardless of the type and number of services rendered, this is a payment system known as **capitation.**

2. When a prepaid group practice plan limits the patient's choice of personal physicians, this is termed a/an **closed panel** program.

3. In a managed care setting, a physician who controls patient access to specialists and diagnostic testing services is known as a/an **gatekeeper.**

4. Systems that allow for better negotiations for contracts with large employers are
    a. **managed care organizations (MCOs)**
    b. **physician–hospital organizations**
    c. **group practices accepting a variety of MCOs and fee for service patients**

5. The oldest type of the prepaid health plans is **health maintenance organizations (HMOs).**

6. Name three types of health maintenance organization (HMO) models.
    a. **prepaid group practice model**
    b. **staff model**
    c. **network HMO**

7. What is a foundation for medical care? **An organization of physicians sponsored by a state or local medical association concerned with the development and delivery of medical services and the cost of health care.**

8. Name two types of operations used by foundations for medical care, and explain the main feature of each.
    a. **Comprehensive type: designs and sponsors prepaid health programs or sets minimum benefits of coverage.**

h. **Claims-review type: a panel of physicians provides evaluation of the quality and efficiency of services to the numerous fiscal agents involved in its area, including the ones processing Medicare and Medicaid.**

9. A health benefit program in which enrollees may choose any physician or hospital for services but obtain a higher level of benefits if preferred providers are used is known as a/an **preferred provider organization (PPO).**

10. HMOs and preferred provider organizations (PPOs) consisting of a network of physicians and hospitals that provide an insurance company or employer with discounts on their services are referred to as a/an **point-of-service (POS) plan.**

11. An organization that reviews medical necessity and completeness of inpatient hospital care is called a/an **Quality Improvement Organization.**

12. Name at least three responsibilities and/or tasks of a quality improvement organization.
    a. **evaluates the quality and efficiency of services rendered by a practicing physician or physicians within the specialty group**
    b. **examines evidence for admission and discharge of a patient from the hospital**
    c. **settles disputes on fees**

13. To control health care costs, the process of reviewing and establishing medical necessity for services and providers' use of medical care resources is termed **utilization review.**

14. Explain the meaning of a "stop-loss" provision that might appear in a managed care contract. **If the patient's services exceed a certain cost, then the physician may ask the patient to pay.**

15. When a certain percentage of the premium fund is set aside to operate an individual practice association, this is known as a/an **withhold.**

16. Mark the following statements as true (T) or false (F).
    T a. An HMO can be sponsored and operated by a foundation.
    T b. A quality improvement organization determines the quality and operation of health care.
    F c. An employer may offer the services of an HMO clinic if he or she has five or more employees.
    F d. Medicare and Medicaid beneficiaries may not join an HMO.
    F e. Withheld managed care amounts that are not yet received from the managed care plan by the medical practice should be shown as a write-off in an accounts journal.

SELF-STUDY 12–1 REVIEW QUESTIONS

1. An individual becomes eligible for Medicare Parts A and B at age **65.**

2. Medicare Part A is **hospital** coverage and Medicare Part B is **outpatient** coverage.

3. Name an eligibility requirement that would allow aliens to receive Medicare benefits. **An applicant must have lived in the United States as a permanent resident for 5 consecutive years.**

4. Funding for the Medicare Part A program is obtained from **special contributions from employees and self-employed persons, with employers matching contributions,** and funding for the Medicare Part B program is obtained **equally from those who sign up for Medicare and from the federal government.**

5. Define a Medicare Part A hospital benefit period. **Begins the day a patient enters a hospital and ends when the patient has not been a bed patient in any hospital or nursing facility for 60 consecutive days. It also ends if a patient has been in a nursing facility but has not received skilled nursing care there for 60 consecutive days.**

6. A program designed to provide pain relief, symptom management, and supportive services to terminally ill individuals and their families is known as **hospice.**

7. Short-term inpatient medical care for terminally ill individuals to give temporary relief to the caregiver is known as **respite care.**

8. The frequency of Pap tests for Medicare patients is **once every 24 months**, and that for mammograms is **once every 12 months for women age 40 and older, plus a one-time baseline mammogram for women ages 35 to 39.**

9. Some third-party payers offer policies that fall under guidelines issued by the federal government and cover prescription costs, Medicare deductibles, and copayments; these policies are known as **Medigap or Medifill** insurance policies.

10. Name two types of HMO plans that may have Medicare Part B contracts.
    a. **HMO risk plans**
    b. **HMO cost plans**

11. The federal laws establishing standards of quality control and safety measures in clinical laboratories are known as **the Clinical Laboratory Improvement Amendment of 1988.**

12. Acceptance of assignment by a participating physician means that he or she agrees to **accept payment from Medicare (80% of the approved charges) plus payment from the patient (20% of the approved charges) after the $110 deductible has been met.**

13. Philip Lenz is seen by Dr. Doe, who schedules an operative procedure in 1 month. This type of surgery is known as **elective**, because it does not have to be performed immediately.

14. A Medicare insurance claim form showed a number, J0540, for an injection of 600,000 U of penicillin G. This number is referred to as a/an **Healthcare Common Procedure Coding System (HCPCS) Level II code number.**

15. Organizations or claims processors under contract to the federal government that handle insurance claims and payments for hospitals under Medicare Part A are known as **fiscal intermediaries,** and those that process claims for physicians and other suppliers of services under Medicare Part B are called **carriers or fiscal agents.**

16. A Centers for Medicare and Medicaid Services (CMS)–assigned provider identification number is known as a/an **PIN, UPIN, or National Provider**

Identifier (NPI). Physicians who supply durable medical equipment must have a/an **DME supplier number.**

17. If circumstances make it impossible to obtain a signature on an insurance claim from a Medicare patient, physicians may obtain a/an **lifetime beneficiary claim authorization and information release form.**

18. The time limit for sending in a Medicare insurance claim is **the end of the calendar year after the fiscal year in which services were furnished. Example: for the period Oct. 1, 2004, to Sept. 30, 2005, the claim must be sent by December 31, 2005.**

19. Mrs. Davis, a Medicare/Medicaid (Medi-Medi) patient, has a cholecystectomy. In completing the insurance claim form, the assignment portion is left blank in error. What will happen in this case? **Only Medicare processing will occur, and the payment check will go directly to the patient. Medicaid will not pay.**

20. If an individual is 65 years of age and is a Medicare beneficiary but is working and has a group insurance policy, where is the insurance claim form sent initially? **To the employer-sponsored plan.**

21. If a Medicare beneficiary is injured in an automobile accident, the physician submits the claim form to **the automobile or liability insurance company.**

SELF-STUDY 13–1 REVIEW QUESTIONS

1. Medicaid is administered by **state governments** with partial **federal funding.**
2. Medicaid is not an insurance program. It is a/an **assistance** program.
3. In all other states, the program is known as Medicaid, but in California the program is called **Medi-Cal.**
4. Because the federal government sets minimum requirements, states are free to enhance the Medicaid program. Name two ways in which Medicaid programs vary from state to state.
   a. **coverage**
   b. **benefits**
5. SCHIP means **State Children's Health Insurance Program** and MCHP **means Maternal and Child Health Program** and covers children of what age group? **Younger than 21 years.**
6. Which people might be eligible for Medicaid?
   a. **certain needy and low-income people**
   b. **older adults/elderly (65 years or older)**
   c. **the blind**
   d. **the disabled**
   e. **members of families with dependent children (one parent) financially eligible**
7. Name two broad classifications of people eligible for Medicaid assistance.
   a. **categorically needy**
   b. **medically needy**
8. When professional services are rendered, the Medicaid identification card or electronic verification must show eligibility for (circle one)
   a. day of service
   b. year of service

c. **month of service**
d. week of service

9. The name of the program for the prevention, early detection, and treatment of conditions of children receiving welfare is known as **Early and Periodic Screening, Diagnosis, and Treatment.** It is abbreviated as **EPSDT.** Optional answers: In California: **Child Health and Disability Prevention (CHDP) program.** In Ohio: **Healthcheck.**
10. Define these abbreviations.
   a. MCD — **Medicaid**
   b. SSI — **Supplemental Security Income**
   c. AFDC — **Aid to Families with Dependent Children**
   d. MI — **Medically indigent**
11. Your Medicaid patient seen today needs chronic hemodialysis services. You telephone for authorization to get verbal approval. Four important items to obtain are
   a. **date of authorization**
   b. **name of the person who provided authorization**
   c. **approximate time of day authorization was given**
   d. **verbal number given by field office**
12. The time limit for submitting a Medicaid claim varies from **2 months** to **1 year** from the date the service is rendered. In your state, the time limit is **(answer will vary, depending on state laws).**
13. The insurance claim form for submitting Medicaid claims in all states is **Health Insurance Claim Form CMS-1500.**
14. Your Medicaid patient also has TRICARE. What billing procedure do you follow? Be exact in your steps for a dependent of an active military person.
   a. **Bill TRICARE first.**
   b. **Bill Medicaid second and attach a Remittance Advice, Explanation of Benefits, or check voucher from TRICARE to the billing form.**
15. When a Medicaid patient is injured in an automobile accident and the car has liability insurance, the insurance claim is sent to the (circle one)
   a. patient
   b. **automobile insurance carrier**
   c. Medicaid fiscal agent
16. Five categories of adjudicated claims that may appear on a Medicaid Remittance Advice document are
   a. **adjustments**
   b. **approvals**
   c. **denials**
   d. **suspends**
   e. **audit/refund transactions**
17. Name three levels of Medicaid appeals.
   a. **regional fiscal intermediary or Medicaid bureau**
   b. **Department of Social Welfare or Human Services**
   c. **appellate court**

SELF-STUDY 14–1 REVIEW QUESTIONS

1. CHAMPUS, the acronym for Civilian Health and Medical Program of the Uniformed Services, is now called **TRICARE** and was organized to control escalating medical costs and to standardize benefits for active-duty families and military retirees.

2. An active duty service member is known as a/an **sponsor**; once retired, this former member is called a/an **service or military retiree**.

3. Individuals who qualify for TRICARE are known as **beneficiaries**.

4. A system for verifying an individual's TRICARE eligibility is called **Defense Enrollment Eligibility Reporting System (DEERS)**.

5. Mrs. Hancock, a TRICARE beneficiary, lives 2 miles from a Uniformed Services Medical Treatment Facility but needs to be hospitalized for mental health care services at Orlando Medical Center, a civilian hospital. What type of authorization does she require? **Inpatient nonavailability statement (INAS)**.

6. TRICARE Standard and CHAMPVA beneficiary identification cards are issued to **dependents 10 years of age and older and retirees**. Information must be obtained from **the front** and **the back** of the card and placed on the health insurance claim form.

7. Programs that allow TRICARE Standard beneficiaries to receive treatment, services, or supplies from civilian providers are called **cooperative care** and **partnership**.

8. The TRICARE Standard deductible for outpatient care is how much per patient? **$150**. Per family? **$300**.

9. What percentage does TRICARE Standard pay on outpatient services after the deductible has been met for dependents of active duty members? **80%**. For retired members or their dependents? **75%**.

10. For retired members or their dependents on TRICARE Standard, what is their responsibility for outpatient services? **$150 deductible plus 25% of TRICARE allowable**.

11. A voluntary TRICARE health maintenance organization type of option is known as **TRICARE Prime**.

12. CHAMPVA is the acronym for **Civilian Health and Medical Program of the Veterans Administration**, now known as the **Department of Veterans Affairs**.

13. Those individuals who serve in the United States Armed Forces, finish their service, and are honorably discharged are known as **veterans**.

14. CHAMPVA is not an insurance program but is considered as a/an **service benefit** program.

15. Which individuals are entitled to CHAMPVA medical benefits?
    a. **husband, wife, or unmarried child of a veteran with a total disability, permanent in nature, from a service-connected disability**
    b. **husband, wife, or unmarried child of a veteran who died because of service-connected disability or who, at the time of death, had a total disability, permanent in nature, resulting from a service-connected injury**
    c. **husband, wife, or unmarried child of an individual who died in the line of duty while on active service**

16. The public law establishing a person's right to review and contest inaccuracies in personal medical records is known as **the Privacy Act of 1974**.

17. An organization that contracts with the government to process TRICARE and CHAMPVA health insurance claims is known as a/an **fiscal intermediary**.

18. The time limit for submitting a TRICARE Standard or CHAMPVA claim for outpatient service is **within 1 year from date service is provided**; for inpatient service, it is **1 year from patient's discharge from hospital**.

SELF-STUDY 15–1 REVIEW QUESTIONS

1. Name two kinds of statutes under workers' compensation.
   a. **federal compensation laws**
   b. **state compensation laws**

2. An unexpected, unintended event that occurs at a particular time and place, causing injury to an individual not of his or her own making, is called a/an **accident**.

3. Maria Cardoza works in a plastics manufacturing company and inhales some fumes that cause bronchitis. Because this condition is associated with her employment, it is called a/an **occupational illness**. Optional answer: **industrial or workers' compensation illness**.

4. Name the federal workers' compensation acts that cover workers.
   a. **Workmen's Compensation Law of the District of Columbia**
   b. **Federal Coal Mine Health and Safety Act**
   c. **Federal Employees' Compensation Act**
   d. **Longshoremen's and Harbor Workers' Compensation Act**

5. State compensation laws that require each employer to accept its provisions and provide for specialized benefits for employees who are injured at work are called **compulsory laws**.

6. State compensation laws that may be accepted or rejected by the employer are known as **elective laws**.

7. State five methods used for funding workers' compensation.
   a. **monopolistic state or provincial fund**
   b. **qualification of employers as self-insurers**
   c. **territorial fund**
   d. **competitive state fund**
   e. **private insurance companies**

8. Who pays workers' compensation insurance premiums? **Employers**.

9. What is the time limit in your state for submitting the employer's and/or physician's report of an industrial accident? **Answers will vary; see Table 15.1 in the *Handbook***.

10. When an employee with a preexisting condition is injured at work and the injury produces a disability greater than what would have been caused by the second injury alone, the benefits are derived from a/an **subsequent or second-injury fund**.

11. Name jobs that may not be covered by workers' compensation insurance.
    a. **domestic or casual employees**
    b. **laborers**
    c. **babysitters**
    d. **charity workers**
    e. **gardeners**
    f. **newspaper vendors or distributors**

12. What are the minimum number of employees needed in your state for workers' compensation statutes to become effective? **Answers will vary; see Table 15.2 in the Handbook.**

13. What waiting period must elapse in your state before workers' compensation payments begin? **Answers will vary; see Table 15.3 in the Handbook.**

14. List five types of workers' compensation benefits.
    a. **medical treatment**
    b. **temporary disability indemnity**
    c. **permanent disability indemnity**
    d. **death benefits**
    e. **rehabilitation benefits**

15. Who can treat an industrial injury? **Licensed physician, osteopath, dentist, or chiropractor.**

16. Three types of workers' compensation claims and the differences among these are
    a. **Nondisability claim: Person is injured or ill, is treated, and goes back to work. No disability from his or her job.**
    b. **Temporary disability claim: Person is injured or ill and cannot work at his or her job and is off work for a period of time.**
    c. **Permanent disability claim: Person is injured or ill and cannot work, and the problem results in permanent injury or illness.**

17. After suffering an industrial injury, Mr. Fields is in a treatment program in which he is given real work tasks for building strength and endurance. This form of therapy is called **work hardening.**

18. Define these abbreviations.
    a. TD   **temporary disability**
    b. PD   **permanent disability**
    c. P & S   **permanent and stationary**
    d. C & R   **compromise and release**

19. Weekly temporary disability payments are based on **the employees' earnings at the time of the injury or illness.**

20. When an industrial case reaches the time for rating the disability, this is accomplished by **the state's industrial accident commission or workers' compensation board.**

21. May an injured person appeal his or her case if he or she is not satisfied with the rating? **Yes.** If so, to whom does he or she appeal? **Workers' Compensation Appeals Board or Industrial Accident Commission.**

22. When fraud or abuse is suspected in a workers' compensation case, the physician should report the situation to **the insurance carrier.**

23. Employers are required to meet health and safety standards for their employees under federal and state statutes known as the **Occupational Safety and Health Administration (OSHA) Act of 1970.**

24. A man takes his girlfriend to a roofing job and she is injured. Is she covered under workers' compensation insurance? **No.**

25. A proceeding during which an attorney questions a witness who answers under oath but not in open court is called a/an **deposition.**

26. The legal promise of a patient to satisfy a debt to the physician from proceeds received from a litigated case is termed a/an **lien.**

27. The process of carrying on a lawsuit is called **litigation.**

28. Explain third party subrogation. **A third party is responsible for the injury (person is injured by an outside party).**

29. What is the first thing an employee should do after he or she is injured on the job? **Notify his or her employer or immediate supervisor.**

30. When an individual suffers a work-related injury or illness, the employer must complete and send a form called a/an **Employer's Report of Occupational Injury or Illness** to the insurance company and workers' compensation state offices, and if the employee is sent to a physician's office for medical care, the employer must complete a form called a/an **Medical Service Order** that authorizes the physician to treat the employee,

31. If the physician believes the injured employee is capable of returning to work after having been on temporary disability, what does the physician do? **Sends in a report to the insurance company, giving the date for return to work.**

32. In a workers' compensation case, bills should be submitted **monthly** or **at the time of termination of treatment**, and a claim becomes delinquent after a time frame of **45 days.**

33. If an individual seeks medical care for a workers' compensation injury from another state, which state's regulations are followed? **The state (jurisdiction) where the claim originated and where the accident or injury occurred.**

34. When a physician treats an industrial injury, he or she must complete a/an **First Treatment Medical Report or Doctor's First Report of Occupational Injury or Illness** and send it to the following:
    a. **insurance carrier**
    b. **employer**
    c. **state workers' compensation office**
    d. **his or her files (retain a copy)**
    Is a stamped physician's signature acceptable on the form? **No; each copy must be signed in ink because it is a legal document.**

SELF-STUDY 16–1 REVIEW QUESTIONS

1. Health insurance that provides monthly or weekly income when an individual is unable to work because of a nonindustrial illness or injury is called **disability income insurance.**

2. Another insurance term for benefits is **indemnity.**

3. Some insurance contracts that pay twice the face amount of the policy if accidental death occurs may have a provision titled **double indemnity.**

4. When an individual who is insured under a disability income insurance policy cannot perform one or more of his or her regular job duties, this is known as **residual** or **partial** disability.

5. When a person insured under a disability income insurance policy cannot, for a limited time period, perform all functions of his or her regular job duties, this is known as **temporary** disability.

6. When the purchase of insurance is investigated, the word/words to look for in the insurance contract that

mean the premium cannot be increased at renewal time is/are **noncancelable clause.**

7. When an individual becomes permanently disabled and cannot pay the insurance premium, a desirable provision in an insurance contract is **waiver of premium.**

8. Provisions that limit the scope of insurance coverage are known as **exclusions.**

9. Ezra Jackson has disability income insurance under a group policy paid for by his employer. One evening he goes inline skating and suffers a complex fracture of the patella, which necessitates several months off work. Are his monthly disability benefits taxable? **Yes.** Why or why not? **Because he has not made any contribution toward the premiums.**

10. Two federal programs for individuals younger than 65 years of age who suffer from a severe disability are:
    a. **Social Security Disability Insurance (SSDI)**
    b. **Supplemental Security Income (SSI)**

11. To be eligible to apply for disability benefits under Social Security, an individual must be unable to perform any type of work for a period of **not less than 12 months.**

12. The Social Security Administration may hire a physician to evaluate an applicant's disability. A physician's role may be any one of the following:
    a. **physician treating the patient**
    b. **consultative examiner (CE)**
    c. **full- or part-time medical or psychologic consultant**

13. A Social Security Administration division that determines an individual's eligibility to be placed under the federal disability program is called **Disability Determination Services.**

14. Jamie Woods, a Navy petty officer, suffers an accident aboard the USS Denebola just before his honorable discharge. To receive veteran's benefits for this injury, the time limit in which a claim must be filed is **within 1 year from date of sustaining the injury.**

15. Name the states and the territory that have nonindustrial state disability programs.
    a. **California**
    b. **Hawaii**
    c. **New Jersey**
    d. **New York**
    e. **Puerto Rico**
    f. **Rhode Island**

16. List two states in which hospital benefits may be paid for nonoccupational illness or injury under a state's temporary disability benefit program.
    a. **Hawaii, under a prepaid health care program**
    b. **Puerto Rico, under a prepaid health care program**

17. Temporary disability insurance claims must be filed within how many days in your state? **Answers will vary. See Table 16.1 in the *Handbook*.**

18. How long can a person continue to draw temporary disability insurance benefits? **Answers will vary. See Table 16.1 in the *Handbook*.**

19. After a claim begins, when do basic state disability benefits become payable if the patient is confined to his or her home? **On the eighth day of consecutive disability or the first day of hospital confinement.**

In California, if disability extends to 22 days or beyond, benefits are paid from first day of disability. If the patient is hospitalized? **First day of hospital confinement only in Hawaii and Puerto Rico.**

20. Nick Tyson has recovered since the previous illness ended and becomes ill again with the same ailment. Is he entitled to state disability benefits? **Yes, if 15 days have elapsed.**

21. John S. Thatcher stubbed his toe as he was leaving work. Because the injury was only slightly uncomfortable, he thought no more about it. The next morning he found that his foot was too swollen to fit in his shoe, so he stayed home. When the swelling did not subside after 3 days, John went to the doctor. Radiographs showed a broken toe, which kept John home for 2 weeks. After 1 week he applied for temporary state disability benefits. Will he be paid? **Yes.** Why or why not? **Benefits become payable on the eighth day of consecutive disability. (This also may depend on whether the injury is declared a work-related or industrial injury and whether the rate of workers' compensation is less than that of state disability benefits.)**

22. Peggy Jonson has an ectopic pregnancy and is unable to work because of complications of this condition. Can she receive state temporary disability benefits? **Yes.**

23. If a woman has an abnormal condition that arises from her pregnancy (such as diabetes or varicose veins) and is unable to work because of the condition, can she receive state disability benefits? **Yes.** Four states that allow for maternity benefits in normal pregnancy are
    a. **California**
    b. **Hawaii**
    c. **New Jersey**
    d. **Rhode Island**

24. Betty T. Kraft had to stay home from her job because her 10-year-old daughter had measles. She applied for temporary state disability benefits. Will she be paid? **No.** Why or why not? **Betty herself must be ill or injured to collect benefits.**

25. Vincent P. Michael was ill with a bad cold for 1 week. Will he receive temporary state disability benefits? **No.** Why or why not? **He must be ill more than 1 week to collect state disability.**

26. Betsy C. Palm had an emergency appendectomy and was hospitalized for 3 days. Will she receive state disability benefits? **Yes.** Why or why not? **Because payment begins on the first day of hospital confinement.**

27. Frank E. Thompson is a box boy at a supermarket on Saturdays and Sundays while a full-time student at college. He broke his leg while skiing, and so he cannot work at the market, but he is able to attend classes with his leg in a cast. Can he collect state disability benefits for his part-time job? **Yes.** Why or why not? **As long as he has met the quarterly amount that is required to be put into the fund in the state, he is eligible.**

28. Jerry L. Slate is out of a job and is receiving unemployment insurance benefits. He is now suffering from severe intestinal flu. The employment office calls him to interview for a job but he is too ill to go. Can he collect temporary state disability benefits for this illness when he might have been given a job? **Yes.** Why or

why not? **Because at the time he gets the flu, he can go on state disability, inasmuch as he is not able to go for a job interview.**

29. Joan T. Corman has diabetes, which sometimes makes her so weak that she has to leave work early in the afternoon. She loses pay for each hour she cannot work. Can she collect temporary state disability benefits? **No.** Why or why not? **Because she has not been off work continuously for 7 days.**

30. While walking the picket line with other employees on strike, Gene J. Berry came down with pneumonia and was ill for 2 weeks. Can he collect temporary state disability benefits? **Yes.** Why or why not? **Because he might have become ill whether the strike was on or not.** Gene went back to work for 3 weeks and then developed a slight cold and cough, which again was diagnosed as pneumonia. The doctor told him to stay home from work. Would he be able to collect temporary disability benefits again? **Yes.** Why or why not? **Because more than 15 days had elapsed between his return to work and the recurrence of the illness.**

31. A month after he retired, Roger Reagan had a gallbladder operation. Can he receive temporary state disability benefits? **No.** Why or why not? **Because he is retired and has no state disability insurance.**

32. Jane M. Lambert fell in the backyard of her home and fractured her left ankle. She had a nonunion fracture and could not work for 28 weeks. For how long will she collect temporary state disability benefits? **Answers will vary. See Table 16.1 in the *Handbook*.**

33. Dr. Kay examines Ben Yates and completes a claim form for state disability income because of a prolonged illness. On receiving the information, the insurance adjuster notices some conflicting data. Name other documents that may be requested to justify payment of benefits.
    a. **employer's records**
    b. **employee's wage statements and/or tax forms**
    c. **medical records of attending physician**

34. Trent Walters, a permanently disabled individual, applies for federal disability benefits. To establish eligibility for benefits under this program, data allowed must be **no more than 1** year/years old.

35. A Veterans Affairs patient is seen on an emergency basis by Dr. Onion. Name the two methods or options for billing this case.
    a. **physician may bill Veterans Affairs (VA) outpatient clinic**
    b. **patient may pay physician and get reimbursed by the VA by following the instructions on the VA outpatient clinic card**

36. When a claim form is submitted for a patient applying for state disability benefits, the most important item required on the form is **the claimant's Social Security number.**

SELF-STUDY 17–1 REVIEW QUESTIONS

1. You are reviewing a computer-generated insurance claim before it is sent to the insurance carrier, and you notice the patient's name as being that of an old friend. You quickly read the code for the diagnosis. Is this a breach of confidentiality? **No. Comment: No breach of confidentiality has occurred. However, the insurance billing specialist or coding clerk must never reveal to anyone anything appearing on the insurance claim without the patient's permission.**

2. You are coding in a medical records department when an agent from the Federal Bureau of Investigation walks in and asks for a patient's address. You ask "Why do you need Mrs. Doe's address? Do you have a signed authorization from Mrs. Doe for release of information from our facility?" The FBI agent responds "I'm trying to locate this person because of counterfeiting charges. No, I don't have a signed authorization form." Would there be any breach of confidentiality if you release the patient's address? Explain. **Yes. With no signed authorization, no information may be released.**

3. List three instances of breaching confidentiality in a hospital setting. **Answers may vary and may be any three responses of the following:**
    a. **discussing patient information with coworkers or other hospital employees**
    b. **talking about patient's information with your spouse or children**
    c. **giving copies of a patient's medical reports to family members**
    d. **relaying confidential information via cellular telephone**
    e. **using samples of typed insurance claims with identifying data on the documents in your job-seeking portfolio**

4. What is the purpose of appropriateness evaluation protocols (AEP)? **These criteria are used by the review agency for admission screening. The Medicare prospective payment system (PPS) requires that all patients meet at least one severity of illness or one intensity of service to be certified for reimbursement.**

5. If a patient under a managed care plan goes to a hospital that is under contract with the plan for admission, what is necessary for inpatient admission? **Patient must be referred by a primary care physician and must obtain authorization for length of hospital stay.**

6. In what type of situation would a patient not have an insurance identification card? **Workers' compensation or industrial case.**

7. When a patient receives diagnostic tests and hospital outpatient services before admission to the hospital and these charges are combined with inpatient services, becoming part of the diagnostic-related group payment, this regulation in hospital billing is known as **the 3-day payment window or 72-hour rule.**

8. The diagnosis established after study and listed for admission to the hospital for an illness or injury is called a/an **principal** diagnosis.

9. For reviewing an inpatient medical record, terminology and/or phrases to look for that relate to uncertain diagnoses are **"rule out," "suspected," "likely," "questionable," "possible," and "still to be ruled out."**

10. From the list of *International Classification of Diseases*, ninth Revision, Clinical Modification (ICD-9-CM) descriptions shown, place these items in correct

sequential order (1, 2, 3) for billing purposes. In this case, the medical procedure is a repair of other hernia of the anterior abdominal wall, incisional hernia repair with prosthesis, ICD-9-CM code 53.61.

	Diagnosis	ICD-9-CM Code
3	Chronic liver disease, liver damage unspecified	571.3
2	Alcohol dependence syndrome (other and unspecified)	303.9
1	Other hernia of abdominal cavity without mention of obstruction or gangrene (incisional hernia)	553.21

11. Mrs. Benson, a Medicare patient, is admitted by Dr. Dalton to the hospital on January 4 and is seen in consultation by Dr. Frank on January 5. On January 6, Mrs. Benson is discharged with a diagnosis of coronary atherosclerosis. State some of the problems regarding payment and Medicare policies that would affect this case. **The diagnosis of coronary atherosclerosis is subject to review by the review agency. If a patient is admitted for consultation only, the entire payment for hospital admission, as well as any physician's fees involved, will be denied.**

12. Name five payment types under managed care contracts. **Answers will vary and may be any five of the following or a combination of some of those listed.**
    a. **ambulatory payment classifications**
    b. **bed leasing**
    c. **capitation or percentage of revenue**
    d. **case rate**
    e. **diagnosis-related groups**
    f. **differential by day in hospital**
    g. **differential by service type**
    h. **fee schedule—for example, fee maximums schedule, fee allowance schedule, workers' compensation fee schedule**
    i. **flat rate**
    j. **per diem**
    k. **periodic interim payments and cash advances**
    l. **withholds**
    m. **managed care stop loss outliers**
    n. **charges (not many of these contracts exist)**
    o. **discounts in the form of sliding scale (percentages)**
    p. **sliding scales for discounts and per diems**

13. Match the words or phrases below used for managed care reimbursement methods in the left column with the definitions in the right column.

f	sliding scales for discounts and per diems	a. Reimbursement method that pays more for the first day in the hospital than subsequent days.
n	discounts in the form of sliding scale	b. Reimbursement to the hospital on a per member per month basis.
k	reinsurance stop loss	c. Plan cash advances to cover expected claims to the hospital.
l	withhold	d. Fixed percentage paid to the hospital to cover charges.
o	charges	e. Single charge for a day in the hospital regardless of actual cost.
j	ambulatory payment classifications	f. Interim per diem paid for each day in the hospital; based on total volume of business generated.
i	case rate	g. Classification system categorizing patients who are medically related with regard to diagnosis and treatment and are statistically similar in lengths of hospital stay.
g	diagnostic-related groups	h. Hospital receives a flat per-admission payment for the particular service to which the patient is admitted.
h	differential by service type	i. An averaging after a flat rate is given to certain categories of procedures.
c	periodic interim payments	j. Outpatient classification based on procedures rather than on diagnoses.
m	bed leasing	k. Hospital buys insurance to protect against lost revenue and receives less of a capitation fee.
a	differential by day in hospital	l. Method in which part of plan's payment to the hospital may be withheld and paid at the end of the year.
b	capitation	m. When a managed care plan leases beds from a hospital and pays per bed whether used or not.
e	per diem	n. A percentage reduction in charges for total bed days per year.
d	percentage of revenue	o. Dollar amount that a hospital bills a case for services rendered.

14. Define the term *outpatient*. **An individual who receives medical service in a section or department of the hospital and goes home the same day.**

15. Define the term *elective surgery*. **A surgical procedure that may be scheduled in advance, is not an emergency, and is discretionary on the part of the physician and patient.**

16. Baby Stephens falls from a high stool, cutting his head. His mother rushes him to St. Joseph's Medical Center for emergency care. The physician examines the baby, uses two stitches to close the laceration, sends the child for skull radiographs, and then discharges him to home. Will the emergency department care be billed as inpatient or outpatient services? **Outpatient, because the patient was not admitted to stay overnight in the hospital.**

17. The inpatient and outpatient hospital billing department uses a summary form for submitting an insurance claim to an insurance plan called **Uniform Bill Claim Form (UB-92).**

18. Why did Medicare implement the diagnosis-related groups (DRG) based system of reimbursement? **To hold down rising health care costs.**

19. Name the seven variables that affect Medicare reimbursement under the DRG system.
    a. **the patient's principal diagnosis**
    b. **the patient's secondary diagnosis**
    c. **surgical procedures**
    d. **comorbidity and complications**
    e. **age and sex**
    f. **discharge status**
    g. **trim points (number of hospital days for a specific diagnosis)**

20. Define the following abbreviations.

AEP	**appropriateness evaluation protocol**
PAT	**preadmission testing**
MDC	**major diagnostic categories**
PPS	**prospective payment system**
TEFRA	**Tax Equity and Fiscal Responsibility Act of 1982**
UR	**utilization review**
IS	**intensity of service**
SI	**severity of illness**
APC	**ambulatory payment classification**

21. Define cost outliers. **Cases that cannot be assigned to an appropriate DRG because of atypical situations.**

22. Define comorbidity. **A preexisting condition that will, because of its effect on the specific principal diagnosis, require more intensive therapy or cause an increase in length of stay (LOS) by at least 1 day in approximately 75% of cases.**

23. You can determine whether a Uniform Bill (UB-92) claim form is for an inpatient or an outpatient by the following observations:
    a. When the inpatient block number 4 shows three-digit billing code/codes **111**
    b. When the outpatient block number 4 shows three-digit billing code/codes **131**
    c. When revenue codes and block number/numbers **42, 43, 44, 45, and 46** indicate type of service rendered

24. Describe the significance of field locators 42, 43, 44, 46, and 47 of the UB-92 claim form.
    a. **FL 42 is the Revenue Code that determines which per diem, case rate, flat rate, CPT code, and so on apply per contract.**
    b. **FL 43 states the descriptive category of service rendered.**
    c. **FL 44 shows room rates and HCPCS and CPT code numbers.**
    d. **FL 46 shows the number of times (units) a single procedure or service was performed.**
    e. **FL 47 is the total charges by department revenue code, total for this bill, and its purpose is to collect statistics for comparisons or to set limits for reimbursement (i.e., reimbursement maximums or stop loss).**

SELF-STUDY 18–1 REVIEW QUESTIONS

1. You have just completed a 1-year medical insurance course at a college. Name some preliminary job search contacts to make on campus.
   a. **school placement personnel**
   b. **classmates**
   c. **instructors**
   d. **school counselors**

2. Name skills that may be listed on an application form or in a resume when a person is seeking a position as an insurance billing specialist.
   a. **Procedural coding**
   b. **Diagnostic coding**
   c. **Knowledge of insurance programs**
   d. **Completing the CMS-1500 insurance claim form**
   e. **Typing or keying a specific number of words per minute**
   f. **Optional: second language, if an individual has that skill; knowledge of medical terminology; knowledge and use of computer**

3. A question appears on a job application form about salary. Two ways in which to handle this question are
   a. **write "negotiable" or "flexible" on the form**
   b. **discuss the topic during the interview**

4. State the chief purpose of a cover letter when a resume is sent to a prospective employer. **To get the employer to schedule an appointment for an interview.**

5. A resume style that emphasizes work experience dates is known as a/an **chronologic** format; the **functional** format stresses job skills or qualifications.

6. When job applicants have similar skills and education, surveys have shown that hiring by employers has been based on **physical appearance at the interview.**

7. List the items to be compiled in a portfolio.
   a. **letters of recommendation**
   b. **school diplomas or degrees**
   c. **transcripts**
   d. **certificates**
   e. **names and addresses of persons providing references**
   f. **copies of résumé**
   g. **Social Security card**
   h. **timed typing tests certified by instructor**

i. **samples of typed insurance claim forms with evidence of coding skills**
j. **other items related to education and work experience**

8. You are being interviewed for a job and the interviewer asks this question: "What is your religious preference?" What would you respond? **This is an illegal question and may be ignored, answered with "I think the question is not relevant to the requirements of this position," or you can refuse to answer and contact the Equal Employment Opportunity Commission office.**

9. If a short time period elapses after an interview and the applicant has received no word from the prospective employer, what follow-up steps may be taken?
a. **Place a telephone call.**
b. **Either write a thank-you letter immediately after the interview or send an e-mail message.**

10. If an individual creates a billing company and coding services are to be part of the offerings, the coding professional should have what type of professional status? **He or she should be certified by a reputable organization such as AAPC or AHIMA.**

11. When an individual plans to start an insurance billing company, he or she should have enough funds to operate the business for a period of **1 year or more**.

12. Hugh Beason was the owner of XYZ Medical Reimbursement Service. A fire occurred, damaging some of the equipment and part of the office premises and requiring him to stop his work for a month so that repairs could be made. What type/types of insurance would be helpful for this kind of problem? **Business interruption insurance and property insurance.**

13. Under HIPAA regulations, if a physician has his insurance billing outsourced to a person, this individual is known as a/an **business associate** because he or she uses and discloses individuals' identifiable health information.

14. When insurance billing is outsourced to a company, a document known as a **service contract** should be created, signed, and notarized by both parties.

15. Gwendolyn Stevens has an insurance billing company and is attending a professional meeting where she has given business cards to a few attendees. Give two reasons for using this business marketing strategy.
a. **advertises availability and services**
b. **helps with networking**

16. State the difference between certification and registration.
a. Certification: **A statement issued by a board or association verifying that a person meets professional standards.**
b. Registration: **Either an entry in an official registry or record that lists names of persons in an occupation who satisfy specific requirements or attain a certain level of education and pay a registration fee.**

17. Name some ways an insurance billing specialist may seek to keep knowledge current.
a. **Become a member of a professional organization.**
b. **Find a mentor for advice, criticism, wisdom, and guidance.**

c. **Network with members of a professional organization, as well as with those working in the field.**
d. **If not a member, subscribe to newsletters and journals published by professional organizations.**

18. A guide who offers advice, criticism, and guidance to someone inexperienced to help him or her reach their goal is known as a/an **mentor**.

19. Jerry Hahn is pursuing a career as a claims assistance professional. When he markets his business, the target audience should be **Medicare recipients**.

20. Jennifer Inouye has been hired as a coding specialist by a hospital and needs to keep documentation when working. This may consist of
a. **number of hours worked**
b. **quantity of work done each day**
c. **corrections applied to her work by officials in the contracting hospital**

21. Define the following abbreviations, which stand for validations of professionalism
CPC **Certified Professional Coder**
CCS **Certified Coding Specialist**
RMC **Registered Medical Coder**
CMB **Certified Medical Biller**
NCICS **National Certified Insurance and Coding Specialist**

22. Read each statement and indicate whether it is true (T) or false (F).
T a. Enhancing knowledge and keeping up to date are responsibilities of an insurance billing specialist.
T b. Professional status of an insurance billing specialist may be obtained by passing a national examination for a CMRS.
F c. Professional status of a claims assistance professional may be obtained by passing a national examination as a CCS.

23. Give the names of two national organizations that certify coders. **Answers will vary and may be any two of the following:**
a. **American Academy of Professional Coders**
b. **American Health Information Management Association**
c. **Alliance of Claims Assistance Professionals**
d. **American Association of Medical Billers**
e. **Medical Association of Billers**
f. **American Medical Billing Association**
g. **National Center for Competency Testing**
h. **National Electronic Biller's Alliance**
i. **Medical Management Institute**

SELF-STUDY C–1 REVIEW QUESTIONS

1. List the Medi-Cal program managed care plan models.
a. **MCP: County-Organized Health System (COHS)**
b. **MCP: Fee-for-Service/Managed Care (FFS/MC)**
c. **MCP: Geographic Managed Care (GMC)**
d. **MCP: Prepaid Health Plans (PHP)**
e. **MCP: Primary Care Case Management (PCCM)**
f. **MCP: Special Projects**
g. **MCP: Two-Plan Model**

2. Mrs. Benson, a Medi-Cal recipient, injures her right leg in a fall. She is taken by ambulance to the emergency department of a local hospital. Must she seek treatment from a facility contracted under the Medi-Cal managed care plan, or can she be treated wherever the ambulance takes her? **Because this case is an emergency, she can receive treatment from any facility, regardless of whether it is contracted or not.**

3. If a Medi-Cal patient receives services from outside of his or her Medi-Cal managed care plan, what must the out-of-plan physician submit with the claim form for services? **A denial letter from the Medi-Cal managed care plan.**

4. Medically indigent individuals who are unable to provide mainstream medical care for themselves and whose incomes are above the assistance level are classified under a group called **medically needy.**

5. Name the entity that issues an identification card to each Medi-Cal recipient who is eligible for benefits. **State of California, Department of Health Services**

6. Name the two most important verifications that are the provider's responsibilities to obtain.
   a. **Patient receiving care is eligible for the month when service is rendered.**
   b. **Patient is the individual to whom the Medi-Cal card was issued.**

7. List four methods used to verify eligibility.
   a. **Point of service device**
   b. **Claims and eligibility real-time software**
   c. **Computer software**
   d. **Automated eligibility verification system**

8. Medical services to pregnant Medi-Cal recipients are available through the **Comprehensive Perinatal Services** program.

9. The name of the program that offers temporary coverage for prenatal care before a woman is officially a Medi-Cal recipient is called **presumptive eligibility.**

10. Medi-Cal recipients may receive **two** Medi-Services per calendar month.

11. An automated voice-response system for a provider to obtain prior authorization for a Medi-Cal service is called **Provider Telecommunications Network.**

12. Name two additional methods for obtaining prior approval for a Medi-Cal service.
   a. **Complete a Treatment Authorization Request (TAR) Form 50-1.**
   b. **Access the Medi-Cal web site and electronically transmit an E-TAR form.**

13. To track a submitted Treatment Authorization Request (TAR), complete a/an **TAR Transmittal Form MC3020.**

14. A Medi-Cal patient seen today needs chronic hemodialysis services. You telephone for a TAR to get verbal approval. What four important items must you obtain to complete the written TAR?
   a. **date of authorization**
   b. **name of person who provided authorization**
   c. **time at which authorization was given**
   d. **log number**

15. A Medi-Cal patient came in for an office visit, and the physician said the patient needed to undergo a cholecystectomy within the next 6 weeks to 2 months and that it needed to be scheduled when convenient (also known as elective surgery). Before scheduling surgery, what do you do? **Complete a TAR form and submit it for approval.** After you have completed this procedure, the patient is scheduled for the cholecystectomy. After surgery, you bill Medi-Cal, noting **the TAR control number** and **eligibility verification** on the claim form. Do you need to send any information to the hospital? **If the hospital does not have the TAR, you may have to fax it or send a photocopy.**

16. The Medi-Cal copayment fee when a Medi-Cal patient seeks professional medical services from a physician is **$1.00.**

17. The Medi-Cal copayment fee when a patient has a prescription refilled is **$1.00.**

18. The time limit for submission of a Medi-Cal claim to receive 100% of the maximum allowable is **6 months from the end of the month of service.** A claim submitted within 8 months after service is rendered is reimbursed at **75%.** A claim sent within 12 months after service is given is paid at **50%.** A claim submitted over 1 year from the month service is received is paid **0%.**

19. State the difference in policy between the Medi-Cal global fee and the Medicare global package. **The Medi-Cal global fee includes the preoperative visit 7 days before surgery, and the Medicare global package includes preoperative visit or hospital visit 1 day before admission to the hospital.**

20. When a Medi-Cal patient has a private health insurance policy, to whom do you submit the initial claim? **The private insurance company.**

21. Claims for patients who are recipients of Medicare and Medi-Cal are referred to as **crossover** claims, and the claim **must be** assigned.

22. A Medi-Cal patient also has TRICARE. What billing procedure do you follow? Be exact in your steps for a dependent of an active military man.
   a. **Bill TRICARE first.**
   b. **Bill Medi-Cal and attach a TRICARE Summary Payment Voucher to the claim form.**

23. Name the five categories of Medi-Cal adjudicated (resolution process) claims that appear on a Remittance Advice Details document.
   a. **adjustments**
   b. **payments or approvals**
   c. **denials**
   d. **suspends**
   e. **accounts receivable transactions**

24. When dollar amounts from a Remittance Advice Details document are posted to the patient's ledger, payments are shown as **credits,** and negative adjustments are posted as **debits.**

25. When the Medi-Cal fiscal intermediary makes a direct deposit into a provider's bank account, this is known as **electronic funds transfer.**

26. If a provider feels a claim was denied in error, he or she should submit a/an **Claims Inquiry Form** for reconsideration.

27. On a Resubmission Turnaround Document, correct data are inserted into **Part B** of the form.
28. Dr. Practon requests an adjustment for an underpaid claim by submitting a/an **Claims Inquiry Form.**
29. A complaint about a Medi-Cal payment must be directed to the fiscal intermediary within **90 days** of the action that caused the complaint.
30. Define these Medi-Cal abbreviations.
    a. PE   **Presumptive eligibility**
    b. RAD   **remittance advice details**
    c. BIC   **benefits identification card**
    d. TAR   **Treatment Authorization Request**
    e. MN   **medically needy**
    f. POS   **point of service**
    g. CIF   **Claims Inquiry Form**
    h. RTD   **Resubmission Turnaround Document**
    i. SOC   **share of cost**
    j. AEVS   **Automated eligibility verification system**